P9-BBP-640

ANTI-AGING BREAKTHROUGHS

YOUR GUIDE TO LIVING YOUNGER LONGER

FROM THE EDITORS OF BOTTOM LINE

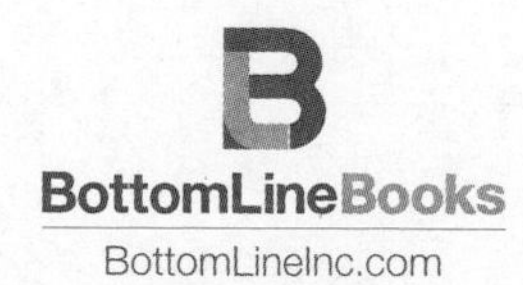

BottomLineInc.com

Anti-Aging Breakthroughs: Your Guide to Living Younger Longer

First Edition

10 9 8 7 6 5 4 3 2 1

ISBN 0-88723-821-1

Bottom Line Books® publishes the advice of expert authorities in many fields. These opinions may at times conflict as there are often different approaches to solving problems. The use of this material is no substitute for health, legal, accounting or other professional services. Consult competent professionals for answers to your specific questions.

Telephone numbers, addresses, prices, offers and websites listed in this book are accurate at the time of publication, but they are subject to frequent change.

Bottom Line Books® is a registered trademark of Bottom Line Inc.,
3 Landmark Square, Suite 201, Stamford, CT 06901

BottomLineInc.com

Bottom Line Books® is an imprint of Bottom Line Inc., publisher of print periodicals, e-letters and books. We are dedicated to bringing you the best information from the most knowledgeable sources in the world. Our goal is to help you gain greater wealth, better health, more wisdom, extra time and increased happiness.

Contents

7 • FEEL YOUNG FOREVER

8 • FOOD, NUTRITION AND DIET

9 • HEALTHY HEART

10 • LIFE HABITS FOR BETTER AGING

11 • LOOK MARVELOUS

12 • MEDICAL CARE AND PLANNING

13 • NATURAL WAYS TO LIVE LONGER

14 • SAVE YOUR SENSES

15 • STAYING SAFE

1

Anti-Aging Breakthroughs

How to Live to 100: Best Ways to Add Healthy Years to Your Life

Henry S. Lodge, MD, FACP, former internist at Columbia University Medical Center, New York City. He is author, with Chris Crowley, of *Younger Next Year* and *Younger Next Year Exercise Program*.

Will you live to 100 and beyond? Certainly genetics is a key factor, but the number of years that you actually accrue—and how healthy you are during those years—often are within your control.

Consider: The number of centenarians—people who live to the ripe old age of 100 or beyond—increased four times between 1990 and 2016. The average life expectancy in the US is now 78.7 years. In Canada and Japan, it averages at 83 years.

Improvements in health care deserve some of the credit, but personal choice is a strong predictor of how long you'll live. About 70% of "normal," age-related declines—including those caused by heart disease, diabetes and other chronic diseases—are mainly due to lifestyle factors.

But which factors are the most important? Not smoking is one. But there are four other lifestyle changes that make the biggest difference when it comes to living a healthier, longer life. They'll also improve your life right now by boosting your mood, energy and cognitive focus.

EXERCISE MORE AS YOU GET OLDER

Some exercise is better than none, but it's a myth that just a little exercise will make a difference. Walking to the mailbox or enjoying the occasional game of golf isn't enough.

Everyone should exercise hard at least five days a week. Make it six days if you're 50 or older. Tough workouts stress muscles, bones and blood vessels and cause adaptive microtrauma, small injuries that trigger the body's self-repair mechanisms.

Result: Healthier and stronger tissues.

A study that looked at 10,000 middle-aged men over a five-year period found that those who were fittest were three times less likely to die than those who were the least fit. Even more encouraging, men who were largely sedentary at the start of the study but who boosted their exercise levels reduced their mortality by half.

Suppose that you're 30 pounds overweight and a smoker, but you exercise every day. You'll still live longer than someone who is thin and doesn't smoke but does not exercise. (Obviously, you'll do even better if you give up the smokes and lose a few pounds.)

My advice: Lift weights a few days a week, and do serious aerobic exercise four days a week. You can vary your routine with other types of exercise such as yoga. Ideally, you'll exercise for about 60 minutes each time. During the aerobic workouts, keep your heart beating at approximately 60% to 65% of your maximum heart rate—and faster as you get in better shape.

I also advise patients to join a gym, even if they would rather not. Many people think that they'll get all of the exercise that they need by working out "informally"—by using a home treadmill, for example, or by going for runs or bike rides in the neighborhood. But most people don't stick with it.

In my experience, a gym membership is a good investment. Once you've written a check, you're already invested in making it work. Once you make it to the gym, you're going to exercise—and it's more fun to do it with others than alone.

Helpful: Sign up for classes or other group activities such as spin classes, aerobics sessions and Zumba that require you to be there at certain times. Or hire a personal trainer on a regular basis to give you a routine to follow.

GIVE UP WHITE FOODS

Sure, you've heard this before, but it bears repeating because it's crucial to living longer. Give up or strictly limit white potatoes, white rice, white bread and white pasta. Even though "simple" carbohydrates have only about half the calories of fat, they're more likely to cause weight gain because they act like pure sugar in the body. They cause surges in insulin that trigger inflammation and increase the risk for heart disease, diabetes and other chronic diseases.

Important: I don't recommend formal diets for weight loss. Calorie control obviously is important, but strict dieting rarely works. Most people will lose weight just by giving up junk food—and white, starchy foods are junk. Replace junk food with natural foods that haven't been processed or refined such as fruits, vegetables, whole grains, fish, etc.

Studies have shown that eating a Mediterranean-style diet (which actually is high in fat but includes the healthy foods above) is probably ideal for health as well as longevity. For more information on healthier eating, read Dr. Walter Willett's book *Eat, Drink and Be Healthy.*

LOG YOUR LIFE

Can you live longer just by writing down, every day, what you ate and how much you exercised? Surprisingly, the answer is yes.

Even though it's a bit of a hassle, keeping a daily diary of health-related details is a sign that you care. It's also a good form of accountability. You might be less likely to skip a day's exercise or chug down a supersized soft drink when you know that you'll have to confess it (if only to yourself).

The health software that now is standard issue on some smartphones makes it particularly easy to track your habits. The iPhone Health app, for example, automatically counts the number of steps you take and how far you have walked or run. You can use other features to track your weight and what you eat. I also like the apps MapMyRide (for cycling) and MapMyRun (for running).

STAY CONNECTED

People who have close friends and are engaged in their communities tend to live a lot longer than those who are loners. It makes sense because humans, like wolves, evolved as pack animals. We need people around us.

Single men, for example, have higher rates of heart disease and cancer than married men—and they tend to die years sooner. People who go home to an empty house after a heart attack are twice as likely to have a second heart attack within a few months. Those who are angry and isolated have four times the mortality rate of those who are happier.

My advice: Do whatever you can to connect with other people. Make plans with friends even when you would really rather be alone. Get involved in charities and other altruistic activities. Attend religious services. Take advantage of Meetup and other web-based social groups.

Obviously, someone who's naturally solitary will never want to become the life of the party. That's fine because what matters is the aggregate of your social connections. A few truly caring relationships can expand your life (and your life span) just as much as a wide social network.

Also, consider adopting a dog—or a cat, rabbit or bird. The emotional connections that we form with animals can rival, in terms of health benefits, those that we form with fellow humans.

One study, for example, looked at dog ownership in heart attack patients. People who didn't have a dog were six to eight times more likely to die of a second heart attack than those who did.

Not a dog lover? That's OK because any pet that you truly love and care for can offer the same benefits.

The MIT Anti-Aging Pill

Michael Fossel, MD, PhD, a leading expert on the use of telomerase for age-related diseases. He is the founder and president of Telocyte, a company that is investigating telomerase therapy for Alzheimer's disease. He is the founder of the scientific journal *Rejuvenation Research*, and the author of *The Telomerase Revolution: The Enzyme That Holds the Key to Human Aging and Will Soon Lead to Longer, Healthier Lives*. MichaelFossel.com

If there were a pill you could take to live longer, wouldn't you? Wouldn't we all?

There's a dietary supplement on the market that was developed by a famous scientist—from MIT, no less—that supposedly slows aging. It's called Basis. We decided to take a hard look at it. Is it really a fountain of youth?

Editor's note: Since this article was published, several other cell-regenerator products have been developed and are available for sale online. Most of them contain nicotinamide riboside only (see next column) at varying amounts.

THE BASICS ABOUT BASIS

You may see some wild claims about Basis (and other cell-regenerating pills) online. It's hard to filter the facts from hype! *So here's what you need to know about Basis…*

•It simulates the benefits of eating less. When animals are underfed—given an adequate diet but one with about 20% to 30% fewer calories than normal—they live longer. We humans could try to eat less, too, but it's tough to sustain when food is widely available—so anti-aging scientists have homed in on compounds called sirtuins that are stimulated during underfeeding. The theory is that sirtuins—which are proteins that protect mitochondria, tiny energy factories in each of our cells—are responsible for the longevity effect.

•It's based on science—mostly in animals. Basis, marketed by a company called Elysium Health, contains two active ingredients that have been shown in animal studies to stimulate the body's production of sirtuins…

•Nicotinamide riboside (NR)—250 mg. Your body uses NR to make a coenzyme called nicotinamide adenine dinucleotide or NAD+. We have less NAD+ in our bodies as we grow older, and it's a hot area of research for scientists who study aging. In one recent mouse study, for example, published in *Cell Metabolism*, boosting NAD+ stimulated energy metabolism, prevented weight gain and improved insulin sensitivity, eye function and bone density. (The study didn't track whether the mice lived longer, however.) NR, also being studied to protect against hearing loss, is found in tiny amounts in many foods, including edamame (young green soy beans) and broccoli.

•Pterostilbene (PT+)—50 mg. Pterostilbene is similar to resveratrol, a compound found in grapes (and wine) that has been studied for its anti-aging and disease-prevention potential, including for Alzheimer's and osteoporosis—but PT+ is more bioavailable and in some ways more powerful. In animal studies, PT+ has had biological effects that may protect against cancer, neurological disease, inflammation, cardiovascular disease and diabetes. It may lower blood pressure and body weight, although some studies suggest that it may also raise cholesterol levels. It's found in tiny amounts in grapes and berries, especially blueberries.

•Leading scientists developed it. The scientist behind Elysium Health and Basis is the well-known and well-respected biologist Leonard Guarente, PhD, who has decades of research in aging under his belt. He runs a lab that studies the biology of aging at the Massachusetts Institute of Technology.

Elysium Health's scientific board is packed with other big names in science and health, including six Nobel Prize winners.

- **It's probably safe.** As a dietary supplement, Basis isn't regulated by the US Food and Drug Administration, so it didn't need to undergo human safety studies before going on the market. But the safety research to date has been reassuring. According to anti-aging expert Michael Fossel, MD, PhD, who is not involved with Elysium Health or Basis, "I'm not aware of any safety concerns—and there may be none, but you never know."

- **It'll cost you a pretty penny.** Basis is available only online through the company's website. You can buy a single bottle—a one-month supply of the pills, which are taken twice a day—for $60. If you opt for an annual subscription, the monthly cost goes down to $40, or $480 per year.

BUT...WILL BASIS REALLY HELP YOU LIVE LONGER?

We knew you'd ask that question. We suspect you know the answer, too—no one really knows. There's no scientific evidence that Basis works in humans. Elysium Health is studying the short-term effects of the pill in people—on body weight, blood pressure, blood sugar and more—and other human trials are planned on the active ingredients (in Japan, for example), but there are no published results yet. To be fair, it's challenging to study a longevity pill in humans, especially because we live pretty long anyway, so you can't expect actual longevity results for decades. But studies can find out whether Basis reduces risk factors for chronic disease, and we'll know that in the next few years.

Dr. Fossel, for one, isn't convinced that it will actually help us live longer. Yes, we lose NAD+ as we age, he explained, but he doesn't believe that simply pouring more of it into our cells is likely to keep us on this planet longer. "Sirtuins are just part of the longevity puzzle," Dr. Fossel said. He believes a better target to get at the root causes of aging is the telomere—the protective "cap" on our chromosomes that shorten with age.

Here's why: "If I take a young cell, it's operating very nicely, but as it gets older, the pattern of gene expression changes, and that's modulated by the telomere," he said. Telomeres themselves don't cause aging, but they're the most "upstream" target that's currently within our grasp. Unfortunately, scientists still are many years away from safely and effectively being able to fiddle with telomere length and gene expression patterns in humans to extend life. "There is nothing on the market that is a miracle drug at this point," he said.

So go ahead and buy Basis if you want to—and can afford it. It's unlikely that it will hurt you, it may prime your mitochondria to work a little better, and it might reduce your risk for chronic disease. Whether it's a longevity pill is something we won't know—for ages.

If you are being treated for any health condition, let your health-care provider know that you're taking this supplement so you can be monitored for "the usual suspects," such as lipids (including cholesterol), liver function, complete blood count and blood pressure. According to Elysium, users report that they sleep better and have more energy and that their hair and nails grow faster—but that's purely anecdotal, of course. "I think it probably has about as much efficacy as a good exercise program, a reasonable diet and a safe lifestyle," concluded Dr. Fossel. It is not, of course, a substitute for those things.

Fight Aging with H2 Therapy

Sergej M. Ostojic, MD, PhD, professor of biomedical sciences at University of Novi Sad, and adjunct professor at University of Belgrade School of Medicine, both in Serbia. Dr. Ostojic has published numerous scientific papers on molecular hydrogen in many medical journals, including *Sports Medicine*, *Annals of Medicine* and *Pharmacological Research*.

Hydrogen (H2) is the most abundant element in the universe. In fact, we literally bathe in it (H2O). While tiny, scientists are discovering that the H2 molecule may have the powerful ability to help counter many of the effects of aging and related diseases with its purported antioxidant and anti-inflammatory effects. Although further research is needed to confirm the health benefits, ready-to-drink hydrogen-infused water and bath tablets are already widely available online.

WHY WE AGE

Research on the science of aging continues to evolve...

- **Free radical theory.** Free radicals are naturally occurring oxygen atoms missing an electron in their outer ring, making them unstable. Seeking stability, free radicals try to bind with other atoms and molecules. Too many free radicals can create what scientists call oxidative stress, a kind of cellular rust that ages us. Proponents of the theory claim that cellular rust is behind many of the conditions and diseases of aging, from arterial disease and arthritis to vision loss and wrinkles.

- **Telomere theory.** Telomeres are tips at the end of chromosomes that protect the genetic information within each chromosome. Throughout your life, every time a cell divides, telomeres become a little shorter. In telomere theory, the shorter the telomere, the more your body shows signs of aging. Scientific evidence links many of the ailments of aging—high blood pressure, diabetes, cancer, dementia—to shorter telomeres.

- **Mitochondrial energy theory.** Mitochondria are the energy factories in every cell. In this theory, broken-down mitochondria cause the body to work less efficiently, leading to accelerated aging and age-related diseases.

THE HOPE FOR HYDROGEN

Although hydrogen is essential to the formation of all matter, including life-giving water, it was thought to be biologically "inert," with no function in health or healing. But in 2007, Japanese scientists revolutionized the understanding of hydrogen gas. They showed in cellular and animal experiments that H2 could neutralize free radicals.

Some scientists also believe that H2 is a key signaling molecule, improving communication between brain cells and blood flow in arteries. It also activates health-protecting genes that promote the burning of fat and sugar. Plus, hydrogen may cool chronic inflammation, which fuels many diseases of aging.

In the last decade or so, there have been more than 400 cellular, animal and human studies on using H2 for health and healing, showing that hydrogen may help do many things, including...

- **Prevent muscle pain after exercise**
- **Protect skin from sun damage**
- **Protect the brain from stroke damage**
- **Improve memory and cognition in Alzheimer's disease patients**
- **Strengthen the heart in cardiovascular disease patients**
- **Lower "bad" LDL cholesterol and boost "good" HDL**
- **Balance glucose and insulin, preventing or slowing diabetes**
- **Shield the retina from damage, helping to prevent and control age-related macular degeneration and glaucoma**
- **Slow or stop the degeneration of cartilage, which can lead to osteoarthritis**

Some of the latest studies that demonstrate just how powerful molecular hydrogen can be include...

- **Heart health.** In a study of middle-aged, overweight women, published in the *Iranian Journal of Medical Sciences*, Serbian researchers found that swallowing hydrogen-producing caplets significantly reduced body fat, insulin and triglycerides—risk factors for heart disease and diabetes—during the four-week study. They theorize that H2 makes cells more sensitive to insulin, thereby improving the burning of blood fats, leading to less body fat and cardiac stress.

In a study in *Circulation Journal,* patients who inhaled hydrogen gas when they arrived at the ER after a heart attack had less long-term heart damage.

In a study in *Vascular Health and Risk Management*, a team of Japanese researchers found that people who drank hydrogen-rich water had improved arterial health within 30 minutes—with 12% greater blood flow.

- **Stroke.** In a study published in *Journal of Stroke & Cerebrovascular Disease,* Japanese scientists studied people who had a stroke, dividing them into two groups. In the 24 hours after the stroke, one group inhaled hydrogen gas for one hour twice a day and one group received a placebo treatment. Those getting the H2 had less brain injury (as shown by an MRI), less severe stroke symptoms (such as facial palsy, the inability to use limbs and problems with speech) and more and faster benefits from physical therapy, as measured by function in daily living.

• **Arthritis.** In a study published in *International Immunopharmacology* on people with painful rheumatoid arthritis, researchers found that a month of hydrogen-rich saline injections administered intravenously reduced "disease activity" by about 29%—meaning less pain, swelling and tenderness. There was no change in a placebo group.

HYDROGEN-ATE YOUR BODY

Although most studies to date involve inhaled or injected hydrogen gas (which is not yet approved by the FDA), proponents of hydrogen suggest a much simpler and more accessible method of hydrogenating—drink or bathe in it…

• **Hydrogen-infused water.** Ready-to-drink hydrogen water is available. Popular brands include HFactor and Dr. Perricone. To make hydrogen water, manufacturers add odorless and tasteless molecular hydrogen gas to water, then package it in cans or aluminum-lined pouches. (The gas can escape from glass or plastic bottles.) You need to drink the water quickly—within 30 minutes of opening it—or the hydrogen levels will dissipate.

Note: Hydrogen water is different from alkaline water, marketed under brands such as Core and Essentia. Like hydrogen water, alkaline water has been associated with antioxidant properties, but it does not contain hydrogen gas.

You also can buy tablets or powders of electrolyzed hydrogen to dissolve in water (brands include Ultra H2 and AquaH2). Or you can generate hydrogen water by mixing a powdered magnesium supplement in water and letting the water sit for a few minutes.

Another option: Putting a metallic magnesium stick in your water bottle. The most tested stick is the Dr. Hayashi Hydrogen Rich Water Stick, which uses pure magnesium and is available at Amazon.com.

Optimal dosage of hydrogen-infused water is not yet known, but proponents say that you can drink as much as you want without harm. Start with two or three eight-ounce glasses a day.

• **Hydrogen baths.** You can put a hydrogen tablet or powder, available at Amazon.com, into your bath. Bathe in hydrogen-rich water for at least 10 minutes.

Limitations: There are no known side effects of drinking hydrogen-infused water, but more study is needed to determine the possibility of long-term side effects and health benefits. Because there are no dosing guidelines yet, drink in moderation. If using magnesium to make your hydrogen water, limit daily usage to the recommended daily amount of 350 milligrams.

Living to 100—and Beyond

Michael Fossel, MD, PhD, a leading expert on the use of telomerase for age-related diseases. He is the founder and president of Telocyte, a company that is investigating telomerase therapy for Alzheimer's disease. He is the founder of the scientific journal *Rejuvenation Research*, and the author of *The Telomerase Revolution: The Enzyme That Holds the Key to Human Aging and Will Soon Lead to Longer, Healthier Lives*. MichaelFossel.com

---

The life span of the average American has increased by more than 60% in the last 100 years, and some experts believe that's just the beginning. It might be possible for people living today to extend their lives to 120 years or even more. How is this possible?

Two landmark discoveries: Genetic researchers have identified structures, known as telomeres, that appear to control how long cells live and how healthy they remain. Along with that, researchers have identified an enzyme, called *telomerase*, that maintains the integrity of these structures. These two discoveries could be the key to a much longer life.

What you need to know…

TELOMERES AND LONGEVITY

Every cell in the human body contains 46 strands of DNA. These strands (chromosomes) contain all of our genetic information—for example, the color of our hair and how tall we are as well as our propensity for certain diseases. Telomeres are structures on the ends of chromosomes that help keep these strands of gene-carrying DNA intact. Chromosomes, which are found in the nucleus of every human cell, control the cellular division and replication that are necessary for human life. As a person ages and undergoes decades of cell divisions, there's a shortening of the telomeres that help keep chromosomes intact. This process is believed to play a fundamental role in the development of genetic diseases and age-related conditions, including heart disease, cancer and Alzheimer's disease. With time, the telomeres get so short that cells can no longer survive—and, eventually, we die.

Research shows that the length of a person's telomeres is crucial. For example, people who are born with (or develop) relatively short telomeres tend to have more health problems, and die sooner, than those with longer telomeres. In a study of 780 patients with heart disease, researchers found that those with the shortest telomeres had twice the risk for heart failure and death after 4.4 years as those with the longest telomeres. Shortened telomeres have also been linked to cancer, osteoarthritis and Alzheimer's disease.

AN ANTI-AGING PLAN

When cells are damaged—due, for example, to free radicals, inflammation and excessive alcohol intake—they divide more frequently than aging healthy cells. This rapid division accelerates the rate at which telomeres shorten—and, potentially, shortens your life.

This is where telomerase, the enzyme that repairs and maintains the length of telomeres, comes into play. And the discovery of telomerase was so important scientifically that it was the basis for Carol Greider, PhD, of Johns Hopkins University School of Medicine, to be awarded the 2009 Nobel Prize in Physiology or Medicine, along with two other researchers.

Although telomerase won't keep cells alive forever, it does seem to greatly extend their lives. For example, in a laboratory study, scientists inserted a telomerase-producing gene into skin cells with short telomeres. These cells were then grafted onto the skin of mice, while untreated skin cells were grafted onto different mice.

Result: The skin grown from telomerase-containing cells looked young...skin grown from cells without telomerase was wrinkled and looked old.

Fortunately, a growing body of evidence suggests that you may be able to slow the rate at which your telomeres shorten—and, in some cases, slightly increase their length—by minimizing cell damage with certain nutrients.

While it is preferable to get one's nutrients from food sources, it is not practical for most people to get desirable levels of the following...*

- **Fish oil.** A study in *The Journal of the American Medical Association* that followed 608 heart patients for five years found that those who consumed the most fish oil had the longest telomeres. This may be the reason that people who routinely take fish oil supplements have lower rates of heart disease, arthritis and other chronic diseases.

What's behind fish oil's health-promoting effects? As an adaptogen, fish oil is a substance that helps maintain the body's normal functions. It has different effects in different parts of the body and on different cells. For example, fish oil inhibits telomerase in cancer cells (which shortens the life span of the disease-causing cells) but increases it in healthy cells (which helps them live longer).

Anti-aging dose: 1,500 mg of omega-3 twice daily with meals. Within this total, aim for 900 mg of eicosapentaenoic acid (EPA) and 600 mg of docosahexaenoic acid (DHA).

- **Acetyl-L-carnitine (ALCAR).** This supplement reduces free-radical damage to cells. It also repairs mitochondria, the structures within cells that produce energy. This is important because damaged mitochondria produce large amounts of free radicals, which accelerate cell turnover and damage to telomeres.

Every cell in the body has mitochondria, but cells that require the most energy to function, such as those in the brain, have the most—about 1,000 mitochondria per cell. ALCAR supplements

*Consult your doctor before starting this regimen. Some of these supplements may interact with blood-thinning, diabetes or other medications.

may reduce mental declines from aging and from Alzheimer's disease or chronic cerebral ischemia, a condition that reduces blood flow to the brain.

Anti-aging dose: 1,000 mg twice daily.

- **Anthocyanidins.** A type of flavonoid derived from berries, such as blueberries and bilberries, anthocyanidins have a higher antioxidant capacity than either vitamin E or vitamin C. Reducing oxidation is among the most effective ways to reduce cell damage and telomere shortening.

Anti-aging dose: 80 mg of bilberry extract twice daily.

- **N-acetylcysteine (NAC).** This amino acid is metabolized in the body into a substance that's used to manufacture the "master" antioxidant, glutathione. Glutathione improves the body's ability to remove damaged/dying cells. When this process is working well, there's a slower shortening of the telomeres.

Anti-aging dose: 600 mg twice daily.

- **Vitamin D.** It's among the most important nutrients for health and longevity. Some researchers speculate that it increases levels of telomerase—and it clearly reduces telomere shortening.

British researchers who studied more than 1,000 sets of female twins (whose average age was 49 and whose telomeres had been the same lengths at birth) found that those with higher levels of vitamin D had longer telomeres. The difference was dramatic—the telomeres in women in the higher vitamin D group showed the equivalent, in length, of five years less aging.

Anti-aging dose: 2,000 international units (IU) to 5,000 IU daily, depending on your starting blood level. A blood test for vitamin D is recommended before taking these supplements. Work with your doctor to determine the optimal vitamin D level for you.

SHOULD YOU GET TESTED?

Your doctor can order a blood test, called polymerase chain reaction (PCR), that will determine the length of your telomeres and compare it to what's normal for your age. The test can be used to track, over time, how much your telomeres are shortening.

Typical cost: About $350. Insurance will not cover the cost.

However, telomere testing is not routinely used because there's not a lot you can do with the information beyond improving your lifestyle, which you should do anyway. In the future, as more products and medications are developed that can significantly lengthen telomeres, the test could be used to determine whether the dose/medication that you're using is right for you.

CAN WE SLOW AGING?

Over-the-counter supplements known as telomerase activators are designed to help maintain and rebuild telomeres (caps at the end of each strand of DNA in our chromosomes, which help prevent deterioration of these gene-encoded structures). The supplements, available online, seem to improve some biomarkers of disease (such as cholesterol). Will this type of supplement help people live longer? There's no proof yet. Many experts on aging believe that the supplements may be somewhat helpful—although likely much less effective as they would need to be to prevent/cure age-related diseases. And they're expensive, costing several hundred dollars a month.

In the future: It may be possible to deliver an "active" telomerase gene directly to the body's cells. In theory, this could potentially prevent and even cure many—if not most—age-related diseases. While you could still die of trauma, infections, inherited genetic problems and other causes, we could essentially halt most "age-related" diseases, such as atherosclerosis, Alzheimer's, osteoarthritis, etc. You might have the health of a 30- or 40-year-old and could easily live to twice the current healthy life span.

How Your Genes Affect Your Diet and Health

Sharon Moalem, MD, PhD, a physician, scientist and inventor based in New York City. He is the author of *The DNA Restart: Unlock Your Personal Genetic Code to Eat for Your Genes, Lose Weight and Reverse Aging.*

Have you ever wondered why a cup of coffee keeps you up at night, while your spouse downs cup after cup and sleeps like a baby?

Or why a glass of wine with supper makes you tipsy, while your friends can keep sipping for hours?

You could chalk it up to random variation, but it's actually not random at all. It's largely determined by your genes. Research has shown that specific genes and gene "variants" (or mutations) can affect how your body metabolizes nutrients and other substances such as caffeine and alcohol.

For certain medical conditions, it's long been established that there is a genetic link to how specific nutrients are metabolized. For example, if you're among those of western European ancestry who have different versions of the HFE gene, it can cause you to absorb two to three times more iron than those without this genetic profile. Hereditary hemochromatosis, commonly known as iron overload disease, can be life-threatening—and is diagnosed, in part, with genetic testing.

But new research in the emerging field of nutrigenetics (the study of how individual genes affect nutrition) shows that there may be important genetic links to many more nutrients and substances than previously thought.

So far, scientists have identified hundreds of genes and gene variants that may affect how your body metabolizes different nutrients and substances.

The question is, can knowing this genetic information help people make smarter nutrition choices? Right now, the jury is still out, but some individuals find that testing helps them identify certain dietary tweaks that may improve their overall health. *Key nutrients and substances with genetic links...*

• **Folate.** Specific versions of the MTHFR gene slow the rate at which the body converts folate into a usable form of the vitamin. People who inherit this gene may be more likely to suffer a heart attack or stroke because of a folate deficiency.

Who might benefit from this test: If you have a personal or family history of heart attack, you may want to discuss this test and/or a blood test for folate deficiency with a nutritionist. If you test positive for the gene and/or a blood test identifies a folate deficiency, ask your doctor about taking a supplement with a methylated (active) form of folate.

• **Caffeine.** The body's ability to metabolize caffeine is controlled mostly by the CYP1A2 gene. People with a particular variant of this gene are "slow metabolizers"—they don't have the same ability to break down caffeine as other people. They might develop high blood pressure from drinking amounts of coffee or tea that wouldn't similarly affect a person without this gene.

Who might benefit from this test: If you have high blood pressure or become jittery when consuming caffeine, you may want to discuss this test with a nutritionist. If you test positive, you would likely benefit from reducing your intake of caffeinated beverages and foods.

• **Alcohol.** Research has found that moderate daily alcohol consumption—up to two alcoholic beverages for men...and up to one for women—can improve cardiovascular health.

But those who have the ALDH2*2 gene might want to disregard this finding. They don't have the same ability to detoxify an alcohol by-product (acetaldehyde), which increases their risk for a deadly esophageal cancer.

Who might benefit from this test: Anyone with Asian ancestry...risk factors for esophageal cancer (such as gastroesophageal reflux disease)... and those who notice their skin becoming red or flushed after drinking alcohol. If you test positive for this gene, avoid alcohol.

GETTING TESTED

A nutritionist or health-care professional (such as a doctor) can order a test kit for nutritional genetic testing online. You provide a saliva sample, and the kit is returned for analysis. The test usually costs a few hundred dollars to check for a set of genes that may have nutritional links. The professional who ordered the test will likely charge you for a follow-up consultation to discuss the results. These fees are unlikely to be covered by insurance.

SELF-TEST FOR ALCOHOL TOLERANCE

If you're interested in learning how your genes might affect the way your body metabolizes alcohol, there's a self-test I have developed based on genetic indicators found in one's earwax. It is not as accurate as genetic testing but will give you some basic information.

Moderate drinking is considered good for the heart, but some people (such as many of those who become flushed while drinking) should never drink...and everyone's alcohol tolerance is highly individualized. How much alcohol (if any) is right for you?

The earwax test: Carefully swab some of your earwax and take a look. People with flaky, dry, gray earwax probably had ancestors from eastern Asia who rarely drank. Those with the wet type of earwax (it's a yellow/brownish color and is somewhat sticky) typically had African or European ancestors who drank alcoholic beverages routinely.

My advice: If you have dry earwax, the safest approach is for you to avoid alcohol altogether—your genetic profile does not prepare you to safely metabolize alcohol. Also, people in this group are likely to have inherited the gene that predisposes them to squamous cell esophageal cancer. For this reason, it's wise to forgo alcohol since it is an important risk factor for this type of cancer. If you have wet earwax, you are unlikely to have the same difficulty metabolizing alcohol.

Can Resveratrol Replace Exercise?

Heather Hausenblas, PhD, professor of kinesiology, Jacksonville University, Florida.

Is resveratrol, a plant polyphenol found in red wine (among other places), a real-life magic potion? Recent research has shown it can slow tumor growth, improve heart health, heal inflammation-related damage and slow the ravages of aging. And now here's another study suggesting that it may be able to hold back the damage that is done when people don't exercise!

No health-conscious person would promote any pill that justifies sitting on the couch watching TV instead of living an active lifestyle—but there are times (such as when we're ill or injured or have overloaded schedules) when we just can't exercise. In that light, this research could be quite important.

SPACE-AGE FINDINGS

This is sort of an "out there" study that was inspired by space travel and involved rats—weightless ones. Even so, it's intriguing.

The study: In an effort to examine the damage that weightlessness causes for astronauts spending long periods in space, which includes loss of muscle and bone, researchers at the University of Strasbourg, France, suspended rats to approximate weightlessness. The rats were unable to move about as they usually do (though they were able to eat and drink normally). Half of these rats were dosed daily with resveratrol. After 15 days, the rats that had not received resveratrol were experiencing all the predictable problems, including loss of strength, muscle mass and bone density. They also developed insulin resistance, a precursor to diabetes. The resveratrol-taking rats, however, did not show any of these effects.

WHAT'S IN IT FOR YOU?

So resveratrol is obviously tremendously good for rodents that don't exercise...but is it reasonable to believe this is relevant to human beings when we don't exercise?

Heather Hausenblas, PhD, is a physical activity and healthy aging expert and professor of kinesiology at Jacksonville University in Florida (and scientific adviser for ResVitále, a company that makes resveratrol products). Dr. Hausenblas and her colleagues recently completed a review of the human clinical studies already done on resveratrol. She said that findings from the weightless-rats study are in line with earlier studies that show resveratrol is a powerful antioxidant that has anti-aging, anticarcinogenic and anti-inflammatory properties with few, if any, negative side effects. But as with most anti-aging supplements, more research needs to be done.

In the meantime, though, it's not surprising that resveratrol is becoming such a popular supplement. It is not easy to get from food sources—though red wine, grape juice, grapes and berries and, surprisingly, peanuts contain resveratrol, the amounts are not even close to the quantity that studies indicate would have helpful properties.

TAKE THIS LIST AND SHOP WITH IT

There now are dozens of resveratrol supplement brands on the market, but Dr. Hausenblas cautions that consumers should beware. You need to check the label carefully to be sure that the brand you choose is a high-quality product. *The label should show the following...*

- **The product doesn't contain fillers or additives, such as sugar, starch, gluten or artificial colors or flavors.** These other ingredients make it easier and cheaper for the manufacturer to produce resveratrol supplements but do not add any health value. Look for products that contain "trans" not "cis" resveratrol—trans resveratrol is the bioactive form of the resveratrol polyphenol that has been scientifically proven to enhance cellular productivity, Dr. Hausenblas said. She added that it has also been shown to increase the number of mitochondria in cells, thus boosting energy capacity.

- **The product was produced under "good manufacturing practices" (or GMP),** which are standards established by the US Food and Drug Administration to which manufacturers adhere on a voluntary basis. These standards are intended to ensure that products are consistently produced with high-quality ingredients.

Also, resveratrol is light-sensitive, so it should be protected in opaque capsules and in a bottle that shields the capsules from light.

THE DAILY DOSE

Dr. Hausenblas said that research hasn't yet pinned down what an optimal dose of resveratrol is nor who would benefit most from taking it, but she said there is enough research to indicate that a dosage of up to 500 mg a day is helpful for most people. Since the body absorbs resveratrol rapidly and its activity is fairly short-lived, she suggests splitting the daily dosage into two smaller ones that will keep some in the body most of the time. Resveratrol is safe, Dr. Hausenblas said, but she suggests starting with a low dosage so your body can adjust to it gradually—some people experience digestive upset at first. Also, pregnant women, nursing mothers and people with a medical condition should check with the doctor before taking resveratrol to be sure it is appropriate for them.

"Yo-Yo" Life Span Danger

Seung-Hwan Lee, MD, PhD, associate professor of internal medicine, College of Medicine, The Catholic University of Korea, Seoul.

When blood sugar, blood pressure, cholesterol and weight fluctuate—go up and down—by more than 5%, it can shorten a person's life span, according to a new Korean study that followed 6.7 million people for five-and-a-half years. Those who had the highest fluctuations were 41% more likely to have a stroke...and 43% more likely to have a heart attack than those whose numbers did not fluctuate by more than 5%.

Cells Are the New Cure

Max Gomez, PhD, a CBS News medical correspondent who has spent more than three decades producing health and science segments for network stations in New York City and Philadelphia. He is coauthor, with Robin Smith, MD, of *Cells Are the New Cure: The Cutting-Edge Medical Breakthroughs That Are Transforming Our Health.*

While stem cell therapies have been on the radar for decades, the recent successes in this breakthrough area of medicine are remarkable. Twenty years ago, these accomplishments would have sounded fantastic and otherworldly. But now they're a reality.

NOTEWORTHY SUCCESSES

The science is moving very quickly. It seems like every day doctors are announcing yet another advance in stem cell therapies. These successes will revolutionize the way that medicine is practiced. *Stem cells have now been used to...*

- **Build a new bladder.** It's now possible to grow a new bladder in a laboratory—stem cells are removed from the patient's injured organ and "seeded" in a bladder-shaped mold. In one patient, a made-to-order bladder continues to function more than 15 years after it was implanted.

• **Create insulin-producing cells.** Type 1 diabetes is an autoimmune disease in which the body's immune system destroys insulin-producing beta cells in the pancreas. Patients can survive only with daily injections of insulin, a treatment that's expensive and time-consuming—and not optimally effective.

There are a variety of ways to produce beta cells that can be implanted in a patient—existing beta cells can be induced to multiply using medications...non-insulin-producing cells can be manipulated to convert into beta cells...and stem cells from the patient, or more often a donor, can be induced into beta cells. The cells do not necessarily have to be injected into the pancreas, but they do need to be protected from destruction by the autoimmune system.

• **Aid in heart failure recovery.** In the largest study of this type, the University of Utah found that heart failure patients whose hearts were injected with stem cells had a 37% lower rate of death/hospitalization than those given a placebo. The stem cells, extracted from the heart patient's bone marrow, helped existing heart cells work more efficiently.

• **Repair an esophagus.** In an experimental procedure, a patient who had a damaged section of esophagus was given metal stents that were then populated with stem cells from the patient's muscle and donated skin. Four years later, the cell therapy had caused all five layers of the esophageal wall to regenerate. The patient could swallow normally, and the stents were removed.

• **Speed stroke recovery.** Even when patients survive a stroke, they often suffer from permanent neurological damage. A study conducted by researchers at Stanford University and University of Pittsburgh found that stroke patients who were injected with modified stem cells had significant improvements.

Details: Stem cells were genetically manipulated to secrete chemical factors that have been shown to support and protect damaged cells. Patients were given a one-time injection of these stem cells into an area of the brain damaged by stroke. Patients saw improvements in mobility—for example, weakened legs began to work better and some patients in wheelchairs reported the ability to walk again. It's possible that the stem cells (which began to die off a month after the treatment) secreted chemicals that improved neural circuits and reactivated impaired sections of the brain.

Outlook for the future: Right now, there are thousands of ongoing clinical trials involving stem cells.

IMPORTANT CAVEATS

Hundreds of private clinics throughout the US are getting ahead of science and offering stem cell treatments that have not been FDA-approved for conditions as varied as Parkinson's disease, spinal cord injuries and multiple sclerosis.

Some of the treatments might be helpful, but many others won't pan out...and may draw a patient away from standard treatment that could be helpful. In some cases, stem cell treatment at private clinics can be dangerous, since the source and purity of cells aren't known—for example, cells that have been multiplied in unknown labs may have been transformed into cancer cells. Also, without FDA approval, the treatments are not likely to be covered by insurance...and the cost can be enormous.

My advice: Avoid private clinics. If your doctor determines that you have a condition that might be improved with stem cell therapy, ask him/her to help you enroll in a clinical trial in your area. ClinicalTrials.gov is a good place to review ongoing stem cell clinical trials. In many cases, the sponsors of the study will pick up some or all of the costs.

How stem cell therapies work...

Most serious diseases—heart disease, diabetes, cancer and arthritis, among many others—are caused by damaged (or aging) cells in the body's tissues. The theory behind stem cell therapies is that these diseases can be cured by replacing defective cells with pristine, disease-free cells. With this groundbreaking approach, stem cells can be extracted, isolated, purified and multiplied in a lab and then implanted in the body, where they continue to divide and differentiate to regenerate healthy adult tissues. Stem cells also can act as natural healers, rather than actually replacing aging cells.

Early in your body's development, embryonic stem cells are undifferentiated. Each has the potential to eventually become any of the different types of cells that your body needs—for example, skin cells, brain cells, heart cells, etc. For medical research, embryos have either been created in the lab or obtained from in vitro fertilization clinics. But this practice is controversial—to obtain the cells, an embryo has to be destroyed.

For practical as well as moral and ethical reasons, most researchers now work with adult stem cells—stem cells that persist after birth and are found in virtually every tissue of the body. Adult stem cells have probably lost some of the potential to become any type of cell, but they can be manipulated.

Example: Adult stem cells taken from fat tissue can be coaxed to become cartilage, bone or even heart cells.

Another source of stem cells: Induced pluripotent stem cells (iPSCs). These are fully differentiated adult cells that can be transformed into embryonic-like cells via genetic manipulation in a lab.

Lithium: Not Just for Bipolar Disorder

James Greenblatt, MD, chief medical officer and vice president of medical services at Walden Behavioral Care in Waltham, Massachusetts. He is also a clinical faculty member at Tufts University School of Medicine in Boston and Geisel School of Medicine at Dartmouth College in Hanover, New Hampshire. He is author of *Nutritional Lithium: A Cinderella Story*. JamesGreenblattMD.com

Low-dose lithium may help prevent Alzheimer's...calm chronic irritability and anger...and ease depression.

Wait a second, you say to yourself—isn't lithium a serious drug for psychiatric conditions like bipolar disorder? Yes, in high doses of 150 mg to 1,800 mg. But in very low doses (say, 1 mg to 5 mg), lithium is a nutritional treatment, uniquely effective for a range of problems. *Here's what you need to know...*

ALZHEIMER'S DISEASE

It's becoming widely accepted by scientists that the neurochemical changes that lead to Alzheimer's develop over a period of decades—and that prevention is the goal.

In my medical opinion, lithium may be the most effective preventive agent. *Research is ongoing, but here are some key studies that support that statement...*

- **Low-dose lithium helps lower the risk for Alzheimer's.** A Brazilian study published in *British Journal of Psychiatry* involved 41 seniors with mild cognitive impairment, the memory loss and mental decline that often precedes Alzheimer's. Half were given low-dose lithium and half, a placebo. After one year, more of the people taking lithium had no mental decline, better memory, more focus and clearer thinking. Just 19% of those on lithium developed Alzheimer's compared with 35% in the placebo group.
- **Low-dose lithium helps treat Alzheimer's.** In another study, published in *Current Alzheimer Research*, 94 people with mild-to-moderate Alzheimer's were similarly divided into two groups. The lithium group had no cognitive decline during the 15 months of the study, while mental decline progressed by 20% in the placebo group.
- **Lithium improves sleep and eases agitation and psychosis.** In a case study report on three Alzheimer's patients with these symptoms, researchers from Columbia University Medical Center found that prescribing low-dose lithium led to dramatic changes in just two weeks—a normal sleep cycle and a marked decrease in symptoms.

How it helps: Lithium is a GSK-3 inhibitor—that means it blocks the enzyme GSK-3 to, in turn, stop the accumulation of plaques (beta-amyloid) and tangles, the changes that signal the development and advance of Alzheimer's. It improves the connections between neurons, triggers the growth of new neurons and boosts a protein that stops neurons from dying.

Lithium also protects against brain inflammation and oxidation and increases serotonin, which regulates mood and behavior.

IRRITABILITY AND ANGER

Because it improves problems with impulse control, nutritional lithium has a uniquely calming effect, demonstrated in research involving people with post-traumatic stress disorder (PTSD) and published in *Journal of Traumatic Stress*.

DEPRESSION AND SUICIDE

Lithium may be an effective way to combat the rise in suicide. Research done around the world has found that the lower the levels of lithium in the water and soil (it's a naturally occurring trace element), the higher the rate of suicide.

A study published in *Journal of Psychiatric Research* compared the suicide rate in 226 Texas counties with 3,123 lithium samples from the public water supply.

Finding: Lower suicide rates were linked to higher lithium levels in the water.

Research done in Lithuania and published in *Journal of Trace Elements in Medicine and Biology* found the same was true for men, in particular, and suggested that lithium may decrease suicide risk, which is two to four times higher among men than women.

BIPOLAR DISORDER

Pharmaceutical lithium is an effective treatment for bipolar disorder, but high doses can cause hand tremors, increased thirst, nausea, diarrhea, abdominal distress and even kidney disease. Low-dose lithium may produce positive results...without the health problems.

In fact, research published in *Experimental and Therapeutic Medicine* found that personalized dosing at lower levels than commonly prescribed can be helpful without causing the side effects of the typical prescription dose.

HOW TO USE LITHIUM

Besides drinking water, naturally occurring lithium is in vegetables, grains, eggs and milk, but you can't reliably get enough lithium from your diet to make a symptom-controlling difference.

My advice: I recommend 2.5 mg of over-the-counter lithium (see below) daily for prevention of cognitive decline or for chronic irritability...and 2.5 mg to 5 mg if you have symptoms of cognitive decline.

Also: If you have a personal or family history of bipolar disorder, substance abuse, suicide (or suicide attempts) or use prescription medication, see a physician before taking any lithium on your own.

Caution: Thyroid disorders and kidney disease can be caused by pharmaceutical lithium. If you have any health problem involving the thyroid or kidneys, talk to your doctor before using any lithium. *The right lithium...*

For low-dose nutritional lithium, look for lithium orotate or lithium citrate, available over the counter. Avoid lithium aspartate, which can cause neurons to transmit impulses at a rapid rate and trigger headaches and brain inflammation in some people.

CBD: The "No High" Marijuana Extract

Hyla Cass, MD, an integrative physician in private practice in Los Angeles. She was an assistant clinical professor of psychiatry at UCLA School of Medicine for 25 years, and is author of several books, including *Natural Highs, 8 Weeks to Vibrant Health, Supplement Your Prescription* as well as *Your Amazing Itty Bitty Guide to Cannabis* and an upcoming, more in-depth book, *The Miracle of CBD*. CassMD.com

If you follow the headlines, you know that many states have legalized the medical use of cannabis, the plant more commonly known as marijuana or hemp.

Recent development: An increasing body of scientific evidence shows comparable medical benefits from an extract of the marijuana/hemp plant that does not contain the psychoactive compound tetrahydrocannabinol (THC), which causes that signature high.

Known as cannabidiol, or CBD, it most often is taken in a formula that combines other related plant compounds (cannabinoids and terpenes) for much greater efficacy. CBD has been the focus of more than 8,000 published studies showing that it can help with a variety of common health problems.

To learn how CBD is being used, We spoke with Hyla Cass, MD, a leading integrative physician who has recommended it for many of her patients.

HOW DOES CBD WORK?

CBD's therapeutic effects are tied to the body's endocannabinoid system (ECS), a complex "communication system" that was discovered by Israeli scientist Raphael Mechoulam, PhD. The ECS is comprised of cannabinoid receptors found throughout the body to balance vital functions, including the central nervous system and the cardiovascular, hormonal and immune systems.

When there's an imbalance in the ECS, conditions such as anxiety and pain develop. CBD helps rebalance this messenger system. *Here's how CBD can help with...*

ANXIETY

Widely used antianxiety medications, such as *alprazolam* (Xanax), *lorazepam* (Ativan) and *clonazepam* (Klonopin), to mention a few, are highly addictive and commonly cause side effects, including drowsiness, dizziness, fatigue, headaches and blurred vision. CBD, on the other hand, is equally effective, much safer and rarely produces side effects (see the next column).

Scientific evidence: A review article published in *Neurotherapeutics* looked at a variety of experimental and clinical data and concluded that the evidence "strongly supports CBD as a treatment for generalized anxiety disorder, panic disorder, social anxiety disorder, obsessive-compulsive disorder and post-traumatic stress disorder."

PAIN RELIEF

Staggering numbers of people who suffer from chronic pain become addicted to opioid pain medications or, worse, die of an overdose. But CBD can often relieve chronic pain—without the risk for addiction.

Scientific evidence: In both human and animal studies, CBD is increasingly being studied for a variety of pain-relieving effects. For example, a study published in *British Journal of Pharmacology* found that CBD was "safe and effective" in the prevention and reduction of neuropathic pain due to the chemotherapy drug paclitaxel.

SEIZURES, ALZHEIMER'S, MORE

CBD can prevent seizures in patients with epilepsy. It also has been miraculous for children with Dravet's syndrome, a condition that can cause hundreds of seizures a day and has not been effectively treated with medication.

Studies are also under way to determine whether CBD can help slow the progression of Alzheimer's disease and Parkinson's disease. In addition, I often advise patients in my integrative medical practice, where I treat various conditions, to try CBD for painful health problems such as fibromyalgia, Crohn's disease, irritable bowel syndrome and migraine...to help relieve depression and improve sleep...and to help wean off prescription drugs, such as narcotics, antidepressants, antipsychotics and antianxiety drugs.

SHOULD YOU CONSIDER CBD?

Based on my clinical experience, CBD can be used effectively and safely for the conditions described earlier. Side effects are rare—generally sleepiness, diarrhea and weight gain (or weight loss).

Important: Even though CBD has a good safety profile, you should check with your doctor before trying it if you are taking medication. Certain medications, including chemotherapy agents, anti-epilepsy drugs and the blood thinner *warfarin* (Coumadin), may be affected. For a list of potential drugs that may interact with CBD, go to MedLinePlus.gov and search "cannabidiol."

HOW TO USE CBD...

Even though hemp-derived CBD oil is legal in many states, the federal Drug Enforcement Agency still classifies CBD as an illegal narcotic due to its association with the marijuana plant. To avoid any issues related to the federal regulations, which are being sorted out in the courts, CBD products often are labeled "hemp oil."

When using this type of CBD product, follow label instructions for dosing, starting low and gradually increasing the dose until you get the desired result. Response to CBD is very individualized. If you have questions, you can consult a health-care professional who has experience prescribing CBD. More and more integrative medicine practitioners are learning about and prescribing CBD in their practices. CBD is available for oral use in tincture and capsules. There also are lotions, creams and other topicals that are useful for arthritis, migraines and other painful conditions and skin ailments such as acne and psoriasis.

To ensure purity and quality: Look for a non-GMO hemp oil product that has a certificate of analysis (check the company's website), stating the amount of the various cannabinoids and terpenes, and that it does not contain chemical solvents, pesticides, mold or bacteria.

Most important, look for a reputable manufacturer, some of which are listed here: CV Sciences (CVSciences.com)...Charlotte's Web (CWHemp.com)...and Elixinol (Elixinol.com). You also can purchase the CBD that I prescribe to my patients at CassMD.com/hempoil.

2

Brain Health

Ways to Make Your Brain Act 20 Years Younger

Sandra Bond Chapman, PhD, founder and chief director of the Center for BrainHealth at The University of Texas at Dallas. She is author of *Make Your Brain Smarter: Increase Your Brain's Creativity, Energy, and Focus*, which includes all nine of the strategies used in the study.

If it seems like you've heard conflicting advice in the media about brain games and other ways to make your brain "younger," you're right. A few years ago, pricey brain-game software (and hours at the computer) were thought to accomplish this...and then, soon after, almost completely discredited. In fact, physical exercise, like Ping-Pong and dancing, have held the brain-preservation spotlight recently.

Well, our knowledge about what can really keep your brain humming keeps getting better, and now, according to a new study from the Center for BrainHealth at The University of Texas at Dallas, simple yet direct brain-training exercises—not games—should be part of any plan to keep your brain young because they can make your brain act 20 years younger. Will this be the last word on brain preservation? Of course not. But when it comes to these latest exercises, they are proved scientifically...they don't take up a lot of time...and it won't cost you anything to try them.

For the 12-week study, 58 cognitively normal people ranging in age from 56 to 75 were randomly divided into three groups—a cognitive-training group, a physical exercise group and a control group.

Members of the cognitive-training group attended weekly 60-minute sessions where they participated in cognitive exercises designed by the researchers that were intended to strengthen "innovative cognition," which is needed for adaptive and flexible thinking—the ability to react to challenging and changing life demands. They also spent two hours a week on homework assignments involving these exercises (we'll share three of them below).

Members of the exercise group did three 60-minute physical workouts per week, alternating between a treadmill and stationary bike. The control group just went on with their lives as usual.

Using MRI scanners, researchers measured how well participants' neurons were working (their "connectivity"), blood flow in the brain and the amount of glucose (energy) their brains used at the beginning, middle and end of the study. Only members of the cognitive-training group showed significant changes—a 30% increase in neuron connectivity on average, an 8% increase in blood flow, the brain's energy supply, and a 17% increase in regional white matter, the fiber bundles that connect different parts of the brain.

Translation? At the end of the study, the cognitive-training group had, on average, improved their brains' fitness so that they worked in many ways like the brains of people 20 years younger. The improved blood flow and regional connectivity were associated with an enhanced ability to think creatively and perform complex reasoning. Thus, greater brain fitness produced higher cognitive performance.

Important: Even though the physical exercise group did not show improved brain function, don't skip fitness workouts. Exercise still conveys benefits ranging from increased fitness and overall physical health to reduced inflammation—and inflammation can be harmful to the brain. So physical exercise does help your brain but in different ways.

BRAIN EXERCISES THAT WORK

Here are three of the study's cognitive exercises that you can use to improve your brain function starting right now...

- **Strategic attention.** Every day, identify two daily tasks that require fairly deep thinking, such as tracking and analyzing your budget, following a complex new recipe, writing meaningful, personal thank-you notes—or pondering the actionable takeaways from an article about the benefits of cognitive exercises.

Then carve out two 30-minute uninterrupted sessions to focus on them. Choose the time of day you usually feel sharpest. But no matter when it is, make sure that the environment is quiet—no cell phones or any other devices to distract you. And don't get up for a snack or a drink or do anything that will take you off your task during these 30-minute blocks. Why? Because it can take up to 20 minutes to get back on track after an interruption.

Benefit: Over time, you'll find that you can accomplish tasks more quickly and with greater focus.

- **Five by five.** Five times a day, intentionally do nothing for five minutes. Stop whatever you're doing—step away from your desk or laptop, for instance—and let your brain rest, empty out and reset. Just as the muscles in your body need a rest after a long run or strenuous workout, your brain needs to rest after working hard. Do not use the time to plan your vacation or the rest of your day in your head or anything of the sort. You can take a walk or sit still, but don't read, play music or listen to an audiobook. Enjoy the silence and lack of stimulation.

Sometimes it will be obvious when you need these breaks, such as when pushing yourself to keep going on a task is netting little result.

Benefit: Taking brain breaks helps you find clarity, collect your thoughts and, often, see things in a new way.

- **Innovative thinking.** Become aware of and increase the moments when your brain innovates—in other words, create more "aha" moments. You say that it's not possible to purposely create innovative thoughts? Oh, yes, it is! The trick is to get yourself out of your familiar ruts—try a new experience, take on a new challenge, seek ways to improve an existing relationship or an ongoing logistical challenge. Brain "aha" moments usually come when you have brain downtime, when you are in the shower, driving without the radio on or in nature with no earbuds. The more you embrace the brain's capacity to improve even routine activities, tasks and conversations, the greater will be your innovative brainpower.

Start by trying to have at least one innovative thought each day, and work your way up from there as you get better at it. But don't just think these thoughts. As soon as you realize that you see a better way to do or say something, write it down and put some aspect of it into practice. Keep an innovation diary, and challenge yourself to see how many times you innovate each day or week. The strongest brain changes come with the implementation of innovative ideas—just thinking them is not enough.

Benefit: By challenging yourself to do and act on innovative thinking, you put your brain in unknown territory and activate the neurotransmitter norepinephrine, the brain's wonder drug that speeds learning and makes it longer lasting. Additionally, innovative problem-solving helps reduce your fear of failure and fear of the unknown—the awe of a new experience actually recharges the brain.

Carving out blocks of time and keeping a tally of your brain breaks and innovation attempts can seem daunting at first. It's OK to start slowly and gradually add to the time you spend on cognitive exercises. Once you start seeing the benefits in your daily life, you'll want to make more time for these exercises, and they will become a habit.

And that's key: For cognitive exercises to work, you need to do them regularly.

The One-Week Plan to a Better Brain

Dean Sherzai, MD, PhD, and **Ayesha Sherzai, MD,** neurologists and codirectors of the Brain Health and Alzheimer's Prevention Program at Loma Linda University in California. They are authors of the newest book from Bottom Line Inc., *The Alzheimer's Solution* (BottomLineStore.com), and creators of a free brain-health app at www.BrainXQ.com. TeamSherzai.com

---

With researchers clamoring to unlock the mystery of what causes memory loss and related cognitive difficulties, it's easy to assume that some elusive discovery will banish these brain problems forever.

The truth is, the key to a better brain—sharper mental focus, improved memory, clearer thinking, balanced emotions, and a lower risk for dementia and stroke—is largely within our control now.

Based on the body of research we have analyzed, nine out of 10 cases of Alzheimer's disease could be prevented by changes in lifestyle—what you do day by day...day after day—to improve the health of brain cells (neurons) and build more connections between them.

After 15 years of treating thousands of patients with Alzheimer's disease and its frequent precursor known as mild cognitive impairment (MCI), we've devised a simple one-week plan that will help you form habits to protect and enhance your brain in the weeks, months and years to come. *Better-brain lifestyle strategies to adopt...*

***Day #1:* Don't rely on supplements to protect your brain.** There are only two supplements we think are worth taking for brain health—an omega-3 supplement with at least 250 mg daily of docosahexaenoic acid (DHA), the most important omega-3 fatty acid for brain health...and 500 micrograms (mcg) daily of vitamin B-12, which is linked to reduced risk for Alzheimer's.*

Our recommendation: Opt for an algae-derived omega-3 supplement over fish oil—it is highly absorbable and toxin- and pollutant-free.

***Day #2:* Add a "superstar" food to your diet.** A whole-food, plant-based diet reduces brain-damaging inflammation and oxidation...protects the small arteries of the brain that are damaged by saturated fats and cholesterol...supplies the brain with the nutrients and phytochemicals it needs for optimal functioning...and minimizes or eliminates refined carbohydrates and other processed foods—all of which weaken neurons and their connections.

Among plant foods, mushrooms are a surprising superstar. In fact, a study published in *Phytotherapy Research* found that older people with MCI had improved cognitive function after 16 weeks of taking dried mushroom powder. Plus, mushrooms deliver umami—the pleasant, savory taste found mainly in cooked meat, making them a great meat substitute.

Our recommendation: Include mushrooms in your meals at least two to three times a week—button mushrooms, portobello, cremini, porcini, maitake, shiitake, you name it.

A Mediterranean diet or MIND diet, which focuses on leafy greens, nuts, berries, beans, whole grains, and fish and poultry, is advised.

***Day #3:* Choose the right fats.** More than 60% of the brain is comprised of fat, and the brain constantly uses those fats in the process of rebuilding neurons and their support structures. But for optimal brain health, you need to consume the right kind of fats—not saturated fat, for example, but plant-based fats, such as the mono- and polyunsaturated fats found in nuts, seeds, avocados and olives.

Omega-3 fatty acids—found in nuts, seeds, marine algae and fish—are especially critical for brain health.

*Before taking any supplement, check with your doctor if you have a medical condition or take medication.

Note: We don't recommend fish because it often has high levels of mercury and other toxic chemicals that are bad for the brain. If you must eat fish, stick with small, low-mercury fish such as sardines and anchovies.

Our recommendation: As part of a plant-based diet, get plenty of good fats and limit bad fats. *To do this...*

- **Minimize or eliminate sweets...**processed junk food...sugary cereals...baked packaged goods...chips and other salty snacks...processed white bread products...meats, processed meats and poultry...and canned soups.

- **Maximize fresh and frozen vegetables** and fruits...beans and lentils...100% whole grains... seeds and nuts...brain-healthy oils, such as olive and avocado...low-calorie, plant-based sweeteners, such as date sugar and stevia...nondairy plant milks...and spices (turmeric is particularly brain protective at a dose of one teaspoon daily—consult your doctor before adding turmeric to your daily diet if you have a chronic condition, such as a gallbladder problem...or take medication, such as a diabetes drug).

Day #4: **Protect sleep.** During sleep, we "consolidate" memory—turning daily experience into long-term memories. Sleep also detoxifies the brain when "janitor" brain cells (microglia) are activated to remove toxins that accumulate during the day.

Our recommendation: Aim for seven to eight hours of sleep a night.

Avoid foods that are particularly disruptive to sleep, such as sugary foods, high-fat foods, and chocolate and other caffeine-containing foods. Stop eating at least three hours before going to sleep at night...and stop drinking fluids at least two hours before.

Day #5: **Increase your "klotho" with exercise.** Klotho is a little-known but important anti-aging hormone linked in animal studies to protection against cognitive decline. Studies show that klotho levels increase after only 20 minutes of intense aerobic exercise. "Intense" means that you'll have difficulty finishing a sentence.

Our recommendation: Aim for 25 to 30 minutes of intense aerobic exercise, four to five days a week, such as brisk walking, biking or working out on a treadmill, an elliptical, a stair-climber or other type of cardio machine.**

Day #6: **Get rid of clutter**—and clean out your brain. Stress exhausts the brain. And a surprising source of stress is a cluttered environment—when our homes or offices become disorderly, we experience more stress and anxiety. A clean, orderly space encourages sustained quiet and self-reflection, both of which positively impact cognition.

Our recommendation: As part of a stress-reducing plan, keep your home and office clean and uncluttered.

Day #7: **Put on your dancing shoes.** Brain-protective cognitive reserve develops from any challenging mental activity, such as learning to play a musical instrument or mastering a new language. But one of the best and most enjoyable ways to build cognitive reserve is dancing. When you dance, it activates various parts of the brain such as your motor cortex...your parietal lobe...your frontal lobe...and your occipital lobe. Plus, dancing is a social activity—and research shows social interaction also builds cognitive reserve.

Our recommendation: Find a dance studio and take dance classes—and then go out dancing. Or buy a DVD and learn to dance at home. Ballroom, jazz, folk—the possibilities are endless!

**Speak to your primary care physician before starting this (or any new) exercise program.

Consume the "Big 3" for Brain Health

Dean Sherzai, MD, PhD, and **Ayesha Sherzai, MD,** neurologists and codirectors of the Brain Health and Alzheimer's Prevention Program at Loma Linda University in California. They are authors of the newest book from Bottom Line Inc., *The Alzheimer's Solution* (BottomLineStore.com), and creators of a free brain-health app at www.BrainXQ.com. TeamSherzai.com

The Mediterranean diet, which includes fish, fruit, beans, vegetables, whole grains and monounsaturated fat (such as olive oil), has been widely promoted for brain health. But which specific foods are most likely to help keep you mentally sharp? *There's strong evidence for...*

• **Fruit and vegetable juices, such as pomegranate, blueberry and grape.** A nine-year study of 1,836 participants found that those who drank fruit or vegetable juices at least three times a week were 76% less likely to develop Alzheimer's than those who had them less than once a week.

Possible reason: Juices have a high concentration of anti-inflammatory antioxidants—and this may help interrupt some of the brain changes (such as beta-amyloid deposits) that occur in Alzheimer's patients. A daily serving of a juiced mixture of fresh vegetables and low-sugar fruits, such as berries, lime or cantaloupe, is a good source of antioxidants and nutrients. Fruits high in sugar, such as bananas and mangoes, should be avoided, since recent research has linked higher sugar levels with cognitive decline and dementia.

• **Fatty fish.** Researchers recently announced that people with high blood levels of omega-3 fatty acids had increased volume in the hippocampus, a part of the brain that's affected in those with cognitive decline. Other research has shown that there's less Alzheimer's in parts of the world where people eat the most fish.

One problem is that people often eat the wrong kind of fish. It must be omega-3–rich, fatty fish.

Best choices: Salmon, herring, mackerel, sardines or tuna, eaten at least twice a week. If you don't like fish, you can take a daily supplement. Lovaza is the only fish oil supplement approved by the FDA. Because it's available by prescription, it may be covered by your insurance. Alternatively, you can take an over-the-counter fish oil supplement (check with your doctor first—fish oil can raise risk for bleeding). Flaxseed, chia seeds and walnuts contain a plant-based omega-3.

• **Vegetables—and more vegetables.** With all the focus on brain-healthy fruits such as blueberries, vegetables are often forgotten. That's a mistake. In a study of more than 3,700 people, those who consumed the most vegetables (a median of 4.1 daily servings) had 38% less cognitive decline than those who ate the least. Good choices for those four or more daily servings are kale, spinach, brussels sprouts, broccoli and red bell peppers.

Daily Greens Keep Your Brain Young

Martha Clare Morris, ScD, is director, nutrition and nutritional epidemiology, at Rush University Medical Center, Chicago, and lead author of a study of 960 adults, published in *Neurology*.

Daily greens keep the brain 11 years younger. Older adults who ate the most leafy greens such as spinach and kale—a little more than one serving a day—had "younger" brain function (such as memory) than people who ate fewer or no greens. One serving is one-half cup of cooked or one cup of uncooked greens. Add olive oil to better absorb brain-healthy nutrients.

Memory Trouble?—The Solution Could Be Simple: Vitamin B-12

Sally M. Pacholok, RN, BSN, an emergency nurse, Trauma Nursing Core Course provider and a member of the Emergency Nurses Association who has worked in health care for 32 years. She started the public education website B12Awareness.org. Based in Detroit, she is author, with Jeffrey J. Stuart, DO, of *Could It Be B12? An Epidemic of Misdiagnoses*.

No one's surprised when Grandpa Joe gets more and more forgetful. We just assume that getting older is accompanied by memory loss, as well as other problems such as a tendency to fall or a failing heart.

What's often overlooked: The possibility of a critical vitamin deficiency. Many of the so-called age-related diseases actually are caused by a deficiency of vitamin B-12.

Studies have shown that B-12 deficiency occurs in 15% to 25% of people 65 and older—in the US, that's at least 6 million seniors. The Centers for Disease Control and Prevention has reported that one in every 31 adults age 51 and older is deficient in B-12.

Troubling: Few doctors routinely test for B-12 even when patients have signs and symptoms that are clearly consistent with a deficiency. And even when doctors suspect a B-12 deficiency, they often rely on a complete blood cell count (CBC) versus specific B-12 testing. This is problematic because untreated B-12 deficiency can cause permanent brain and/or nervous system injury.

WHAT HAPPENS

A deficiency of B-12 causes demyelination, or damage to our nerves and brain. Nerves have an insulating coating known as the myelin sheath, and B-12 deficiency damages this sheath—in a manner somewhat similar to the fraying of an electrical wire—making it harder for nerve cells to carry messages. This causes balance and gait disorders, which frequently cause falls and fall-related trauma (such as hip fractures). B-12 deficiency also causes brain atrophy (shrinkage) and a resulting decline in memory and cognitive functioning. I estimate that at least 20% of patients with a diagnosis of dementia or Alzheimer's disease actually are suffering from a B-12 deficiency.

B-12 also is crucial to the function of osteoblasts (bone-forming cells). Thus, people with B-12 deficiency are at greater risk for osteoporosis and non-fall–related fractures.

In addition, researchers have discovered that B-12 is just as important as another B vitamin, folate, for lowering our level of homocysteine, a toxic amino acid that can cause blood clots, heart attacks and strokes when elevated.

MISSED DIAGNOSES

Most physicians get little training in nutrition. And it's easy for doctors to mistake a B-12 deficiency for other disorders that share the same signs and symptoms. In addition to dementia and Alzheimer's, it is common for B-12 deficiency to be misdiagnosed as depression, mental illness, vertigo, chronic fatigue syndrome, multiple sclerosis, fibromyalgia and diabetic neuropathy.

When diagnosing a B-12 deficiency, most doctors look for macrocytic anemia, a condition in which red blood cells are abnormally large and hemoglobin counts are low. But you don't have to have macrocytic anemia to be B-12 deficient. Sometimes blood test results may appear normal even when there is a B-12 deficiency. For example, when people take supplements that contain folic acid, the folic acid can "mask" such a deficiency.

WHO'S AT RISK?

A B-12 deficiency can occur at any age, but older adults are at greater risk.

Reasons: You need adequate amounts of hydrochloric acid in the stomach to break down and absorb B-12. Nearly one-third of those age 50 and older don't produce enough stomach acid.

Also, a stomach protein called intrinsic factor is needed for B-12 absorption. The body's production of intrinsic factor may decline with age—or stop altogether in people with an autoimmune disease called pernicious anemia.

Also at risk: Vegetarians or vegans who eat little or no animal foods...heavy drinkers...people with eating disorders...patients who have had stomach surgery (including gastric bypass for weight loss)...those with intestinal diseases, such as Crohn's and celiac disease...patients who take the diabetic drug *metformin* (Glucophage)...and certain women who are breast-feeding.

TESTS AND TREATMENTS

Your B-12 level should be tested annually, just as you have your cholesterol and glucose screened annually.

Best tests: The serum B-12 test measures the amount of B-12 in the blood. It costs less than $100 and is covered by insurance. Another useful test for a B-12 deficiency is the urinary methylmalonic acid test (uMMA).

There still is controversy about what level of serum (blood) B-12 is needed. A serum B-12 of less than 200 picograms per milliliter (pg/mL) is considered a deficiency. However, it has been well-documented in medical literature that symptomatic patients with serum B-12 between 200 pg/mL and 400 pg/mL actually are B-12 deficient. A level of at least 450 pg/mL is the minimum required. For brain and nerve health a serum B-12 level of at least 1,000 pg/mL needs to be maintained. It is very difficult to get enough B-12 from your diet. *If you test low...*

- **Start with injections.** B-12 injections assure proper absorption. Unlike oral forms of B-12, the injections bypass the stomach and small intestine, where malabsorption and transport problems occur.

B-12–deficient patients should be given a series of injections—1,000 micrograms (mcg) every day for seven days—followed by weekly injections for two months. Maintenance therapy typically is an injection every two weeks.

Injections actually are the cheapest treatment, once the patient or family member is taught by a health-care provider to self-administer them properly. A 30-milliliter multidose vial of a form of vitamin B-12 called hydroxocobalamin costs an average of $36 and typically is enough to treat a patient for one year. Microfine needles make the injections almost painless.

Ask your doctor about B-12 lozenges. After an initial series of injections, some people can switch to B-12 lozenges. A typical dose is 2,000 mcg daily of methylcobalamin, another form of B-12. That sounds like a lot, especially because the recommended daily allowance (RDA) for B-12 is 2.4 mcg daily (2.6 mcg and 2.8 mcg during pregnancy and lactation, respectively)—but only about 1% of oral B-12 is absorbed.

- **Beware of acid-suppressing drugs.** Millions of Americans depend on medications such as *omeprazole* (Prilosec) and *ranitidine* (Zantac) to reduce stomach acid. These drugs are prescribed for patients who have ulcers, heartburn or GERD. People who take them long-term have a high risk of developing a B-12 deficiency.

My advice: If you are on acid-suppressing medications long-term, your B-12 level must be monitored and your doctor should place you on high-dose B-12 lozenges or injections.

Stay Sharp As You Age—Surprising Causes of Memory Loss

Pamela W. Smith, MD, MPH, MS, a diplomat of the Board of the American Academy of Anti-Aging Physicians...founder and director of The Fellowship in Metabolic, Anti-Aging and Functional Medicine, Boca Raton, Florida...and codirector of the master's program in medical sciences with a concentration in metabolic and nutritional medicine, University of South Florida College of Medicine, Tampa. She is author of *What You Must Know About Memory Loss & How to Stop It.*

It is no secret that age and memory are intertwined. But age itself is not the sole reason that we forget things. Memory loss often can be traced to specific factors, including hormonal changes, inflammation and exposure to mercury and other toxins.

Common causes of memory loss—and what you can do to control them...

LOW TESTOSTERONE

After a man reaches age 30, his testosterone goes into free fall. Levels drop by about 1% a year. At least 30% of men in their 70s are hypogonadal, with very low testosterone.

Low testosterone increases the death of brain cells. It also has been linked to an increase in amyloid-B, proteins that are associated with Alzheimer's disease and other forms of dementia.

What to do: If a saliva test shows low testosterone, your doctor may recommend creams, injections or other forms of testosterone replacement. Men who supplement with testosterone have been shown to have improvements in verbal memory (the recall of verbal information) and spatial memory (the part of the memory responsible for recording information about one's environment and spatial orientation).

Important: Women need testosterone, too, and should get tested. Testosterone replacement in women with low levels can help preserve memory.

LOW ESTROGEN

Women often refer to the "brain fog" that occurs during menopause. It's a real phenomenon that is caused in part by declining levels of estrogen. Every brain cell is affected by estrogen, which conducts chemical signals through the hippocampus and other areas of the brain.

Low-dose estrogen replacement can improve brain circulation and reduce the risk for Alzheimer's disease by up to 54%.

Men also depend on estrogen for brain function, although they require smaller amounts than women.

What to do: Both men and women should ask their doctors for a saliva-estrogen test. It measures "free" levels of the three different forms of estrogen (estrone, estradiol and estriol). Free estrogen is the form that is active and available for immediate use in the body.

If your estrogen is low, your doctor may prescribe supplemental hormones. I advise patients to use bioidentical hormones that are made from natural substances. They may be more effective—and cause fewer side effects—than synthetic forms of estrogen.

LOW THYROID

People with low levels of thyroid hormone (hypothyroidism) often experience memory loss. Unfortunately, doctors don't routinely test for it. They mistakenly attribute the symptoms—such as memory loss, fatigue, increased sensitivity to cold, apathy or weight gain—to other conditions, including depression.

What to do: Get a thyroid test if you have any of the above symptoms. A diet high in B vitamins (from meats, whole grains and fortified cereals) and vitamin A (from brightly colored produce) can help improve thyroid function. An adequate intake of iodine (iodized salt is a source) also is important.

If your level of thyroid hormones is too low, your doctor probably will prescribe a thyroid replacement, such as *levothyroxine* (Synthroid) or Armour Thyroid.

IMPAIRED CIRCULATION

If you have high cholesterol or other cardiovascular risk factors—you smoke, have high blood pressure, are sedentary, overweight, etc.—you probably have at least some atherosclerosis, fatty plaques in the arteries that reduce the flow of blood and oxygen to the brain.

What to do: In addition to the obvious—more exercise, weight loss, not smoking—I strongly advise patients to eat a Mediterranean-style diet. This features lots of fruits, vegetables and grains along with healthy amounts of olive oil and fish. A recent study found that people who closely followed this diet were 28% less likely to develop mild cognitive impairment and 48% less likely to get Alzheimer's disease.

Also helpful: Eating more soluble fiber (such as that found in oatmeal, beans, fruit and nuts) or taking a fiber supplement has been shown in both men and women to decrease hardening of the arteries and improve circulation.

EXPOSURE TO MERCURY

Americans are exposed to mercury all the time. It is present in soil, the water supply and some foods, including many fish. It also is used in many dental fillings. Over time, the mercury from fillings and other sources can cause inflammation and oxidative stress in the brain, both of which can damage the neurotransmitters that are essential for memory and other brain functions.

What to do: You can get tested for mercury and other heavy metals, but the tests will be positive only after long-term exposure. I advise patients to reduce their exposure long before it will show up on any test.

If you have dental fillings made of amalgam (an alloy of mercury and other metals), consider replacing them with fillings made from plastics or other materials. The work should be done by an environmental dentist who specializes in the safe removal of mercury.

Also important: Avoid eating shark, swordfish, king mackerel, marlin, orange roughy, ahi tuna and tilefish, which tend to accumulate mercury. Limit canned albacore tuna to three servings or less per month and canned light tuna to six servings or less per month.

Best: Cold-water salmon.

A Sniff Test for Alzheimer's Disease

Study titled "Odor Identification Screening Improves Diagnostic Classification in Incipient Alzheimer's Disease" by David R. Roalf, PhD, research assistant professor, department of behavioral neuroscience and psychiatry, University of Pennsylvania, Philadelphia, and colleagues, published in *Journal of Alzheimer's Disease*.

A simple sniff test can help in the early diagnosis of Alzheimer's disease. Combined with standard cognitive tests, it enhances the ability to identify the disease before there are any other symptoms. That means better care.

Background: Brain degeneration can begin as early as 10 years before a definitive diagnosis. Many people develop mild cognitive impairment (MCI) first—a condition marked by problems with memory and thinking that are not serious enough to affect daily functioning. Many people with MCI don't know they have it—and while having MCI increases your risk of developing Alzheimer's, it's not a sure thing. Better tests are needed to identify people with MCI in the first place...and to figure out which ones are at highest risk for Alzheimer's.

Smell might be key. A sharp decline in the sense of smell is one of the earliest warning signs—areas in the brain that process odors are often the first to be affected by the disease. Smell affects taste, too—one reason why many Alzheimer's patients often complain that food doesn't taste as good as it once did. So researchers decided to test a commercially available "sniff" test to see if it could improve early diagnosis.

Study: Researchers at University of Pennsylvania studied 262 people with Alzheimer's disease, 198 with mild cognitive impairment and 292 healthy older adults. On average, subjects were in their early-to-mid-70s. Some with MCI were further classified based on the severity of their condition, since people with more severe memory loss and other symptoms are more likely to progress to Alzheimer's.

Each participant had been painstakingly diagnosed by an experienced clinician using a battery of tests including neuroimaging and advanced cognitive testing. Then researchers used the "Sniffin' Sticks Odor Identification Test," which asks participants to identify 16 common odors and takes about eight minutes. Everyone also took a standard cognitive test called the Montreal Cognitive Assessment (MoCA). It's a one-page, 30-point test that measures such skills as short-term memory recall. A health professional can give it in about 10 minutes.

Findings: The healthy older adults did best on the smell test, followed by those with MCI, followed by those with Alzheimer's. Within the MCI group, the test also sniffed out those most at risk—patients on the milder side did better identifying odors than those who were more impaired.

Surprising finding: The sniff test was pretty good on its own but it really made a difference when combined with MoCA, the standard cognitive test. By itself, MoCA correctly identified 77% of those with mild cognitive impairment and 93% of those with Alzheimer's. Add the sniff test, and the accuracy rate went up to 92% of those with MCI and 98% of those with Alzheimer's.

Bottom line: This finding may change the landscape of Alzheimer's screening, making it easier to identify people at highest risk of developing the disease quickly and relatively inexpensively.

Here's why that matters: Knowing you're at high risk means you can get targeted medical care if symptoms develop, work with your doctor to stop taking medications that can increase dementia risk, improve lifestyle factors linked to improved cognition, make plans for future care and finances—and perhaps sign up for new clinical trials in the future. That's why an annual "cognitive checkup" is now covered by insurance.

Should you try the sniff test yourself? You could buy it—it's commercially available and easy to self-administer—but it's pricey ($325 for a 12-odor version), and best given along with cognitive testing, as this study showed. If your doctor orders it, it's at least possible that insurance might pick up all or part of the tab.

Do see your doctor if you find that your sense of smell or taste seems to be declining. Rest assured—a loss of smell or taste can be caused by many things other than incipient dementia, including medical problems such as a thyroid condition, certain drugs such as nasal steroid sprays, even a zinc deficiency. Best to find out.

Does Cholesterol Cause Dementia?

Alina Solomon, MD, PhD, department of neurology, University of Kuopio, Kuopio, Finland.

Rachel Whitmer, PhD, research scientist, division of research, Kaiser Permanente Northern California, Oakland, California.

It's beginning to seem that there's no end to the possible number of pathways leading to dementia—the latest, according to new research, is elevated cholesterol earlier in life. It's not only bad for your heart but also for your brain. So, what does this mean for those of us who didn't take steps to bring down—or didn't even know about—our high cholesterol when we were younger?

HOW HIGH IS TOO HIGH?

At Kaiser Permanente of Northern California, Rachel Whitmer, PhD, and her colleagues analyzed the records of 9,844 patients who completed health evaluations as part of a preventive screening program in the 1960s and 1970s, when they were 40 to 45 years old. Decades later (when the participants were 61 to 88 years old), 596 of them had been diagnosed with dementia—either Alzheimer's disease or vascular dementia, the second most common type of dementia.

Dr. Whitmer looked back at all participants' cholesterol levels—and found that those who had had high total cholesterol (240 mg/dL or higher) when screened in their 40s now had a 57% higher risk for Alzheimer's and a 26% higher risk for vascular dementia. Participants whose cholesterol had been borderline-high (200 mg/dL to 239 mg/dL) when screened now had a 23% higher risk for Alzheimer's and a 50% higher risk for vascular dementia than those with cholesterol under 200 mg/dL.

The study had some limitations, including a lack of information about whether participants had cholesterol-lowering therapy and no differentiation among types of cholesterol, which we now know is an important health factor. Additional research also is needed to answer some key questions, including why high cholesterol raises dementia risk. Findings were published in *Dementia & Geriatric Cognitive Disorders*.

FOR A LONG, HAPPY, HEALTHY LIFE...

It's fair to say that these results do suggest that you have a higher risk of dementia if you have even moderately high cholesterol earlier in life. Study coauthor Alina Solomon, MD, PhD, of the department of neurology at the University of Kuopio in Finland, says that this doesn't mean that people with elevated cholesterol should automatically begin taking statin drugs—as we've pointed out before, they have potentially serious side effects. Consult with your doctor, suggests Dr. Solomon, and if appropriate look first at making lifestyle changes, which will definitely have a positive effect on your cholesterol and your brain. Though you may not be able to control such risk factors as age and genetics, you can help prevent age-related diseases by eating well, exercising, maintaining a healthy weight and controlling stress. Not only are these measures key to living a good, long life but also, it seems, to being able to enjoy it.

Lung Disease Linked to Dementia Risk

Pamela L. Lutsey, PhD, MPH, associate professor, Division of Epidemiology & Community Health, University of Minnesota, Minneapolis.

Compared to those with healthy lungs, people with obstructive lung disease, such as chronic obstructive pulmonary disease (COPD) and asthma, had a 33% higher risk of developing dementia, according to a 23-year study of 14,000 men and women.

Theory: The low blood oxygen levels resulting from these conditions lead to inflammation, stress and damage to the brain's blood vessels.

Curcumin Fights Dementia

Bill Gottlieb, CHC, is a natural health coach in Middletown, California, certified by the American Association of Drugless Practitioners. He is author of 16 health books that have sold three million copies including *Speed Healing*. His Bottom Line videos can be found at BottomLineInc.com/author/bill-gottlieb. BillGottliebHealth.com

Specially formulated supplements of curcumin—the active ingredient in the spice turmeric—improve memory and focus in people who don't have dementia. They also may reduce the risk of developing Alzheimer's disease.

Scientific evidence: Researchers at UCLA Longevity Center recruited 40 healthy middle-aged and elderly people. For 18 months, 21 of them took a curcumin supplement twice daily, while 19 took a placebo. At the beginning and again at the end of the study, their short-term verbal and visual memory abilities—such as recalling memorized words and images—were tested. And their brains were scanned for toxic amyloid plaques and tau tangles, two signs of Alzheimer's.

Key findings: After 18 months, participants taking curcumin had significantly improved results on the memory tests. (*Bonus:* They also had improved mood.) Participants taking the placebo had little or no improvement in memory. What's more, the follow-up brain scans showed that the curcumin group, compared with the placebo group, had lower levels of amyloid and tau deposits.

THE RIGHT KIND OF CURCUMIN SUPPLEMENT

While curcumin in its natural state—in the spice turmeric and in many supplements—is poorly absorbed by the body, there are five formulations that research has shown are well-absorbed. The UCLA researchers used one of them, Theracurmin, at a dose of 90 mg twice daily. (A one-month supply costs about $53.) The other four are Meriva, Curcumin C3 Complex, BCM-95 and CurcuWIN. All are available online.

More research is needed before we know whether curcumin supplements actually prevent Alzheimer's disease. Curcumin supplements have a strong safety record, but they can cause stomach upset in some people. And they act as blood thinners, so doctors generally say that curcumin should not be taken by people using blood-thinning drugs. To determine whether curcumin is safe for you—and what a proper dose might be—it's best to work with a doctor who has studied this supplement.

If you take curcumin, though, you may find that you experience more benefits. It's a powerful anti-inflammatory and antioxidant that has been found to help relieve arthritis pain, ease muscle soreness after exercise and relieve allergy symptoms.

Gum Disease and Brain Health

Plos One.

Oral bacteria can travel to the brain and might trigger Alzheimer's disease. A laboratory study found that animals exposed to periodontal-disease bacteria had higher amounts of amyloid beta, the same plaque that occurs with Alzheimer's.

For a Healthier Brain, Go Dancing!

Marc E. Agronin, MD, a geriatric psychiatrist at Miami Jewish Health in Florida, MarcAgronin.com. He is author of *The End of Old Age: Living a Longer, More Purposeful Life*.

The study "Dancing or Fitness Sport? The Effects of Two Training Programs on Hippocampal Plasticity and Balance Abilities in Healthy Seniors" was published on June 15, 2017, in *Frontiers in Human Neuroscience*.

If you'd rather crank up the music and boogie down than spend a single minute in a gym, we have some good news—dancing may improve brain health more than regular aerobic workouts.

Exercise has long been recognized as a smart way to help prevent age-related cognitive declines—including mental impairments that are caused (or worsened) by Alzheimer's disease and other forms of dementia. Questions have remained, however, regarding the type of exercise that works best.

Do we have a winner? Dancing may offer special benefits, according to a report published in *Frontiers in Human Neuroscience*. In this study, researchers looked at two groups of adults with an average age of 68. Some of the people in the study slogged through traditional endurance workouts, such as cycling or Nordic walking. Others danced.

After 18 months of weekly exercise, people in both groups showed increases in the volume of the hippocampus, the part of the brain that plays a key role in memory and learning—and the same brain region that's often affected by dementia. But the dancers had an edge. They showed more improvement in balance than those in the workout group.

Why is dancing such an effective way to help your brain stay sharp?

Part of the benefit from dancing comes from the mental workout—memorizing arm movements, step patterns, rhythms, etc., explains Kathrin Rehfeld, MD, of the German Center for Neurodegenerative Diseases and the lead author of the study.

In the study, dance routines were changed every two weeks—for example, mambo, cha-cha and jazz square—which challenged the dancer's balance system and required mental effort to learn the choreographies.

Bottom Line's takeaway: "Dance provides the ultimate cross-fit for your brain," says Marc E. Agronin, MD, a geriatric psychiatrist at Miami Jewish Health in Florida and the author *The End of Old Age: Living a Longer, More Purposeful Life*. The aerobic conditioning and endurance promote optimal blood flow to the brain and the release of neural growth factors. "There's also musical inspiration combined with coordinated movements that enhance memory, balance, dexterity and visuospatial abilities," he continues.

Another advantage: Dancing, for many people, is more fun than a sweaty gym workout...and it's one more tool for challenging your body as well as your mind. Plus, there's less risk for injury than there is with many other physical activities.

If you'd like to start dancing, Dr. Agronin suggests Zumba Gold, a modified, lower-intensity version of traditional Zumba classes. Typically offered in classes, it provides a highly stimulating and fun way to exercise with multiple forms of upbeat music and dance. You may even be able to find an instructor who will provide one-on-one instruction. And don't forget ballroom dancing. It's another great way to boost memory, coordination and socialization with partners, says Dr. Agronin.

So what are you waiting for? It's time to kick up your heels!

Beware of "Skinny Fat"—a New Dementia Risk

James E. Galvin, MD, MPH, associate dean for clinical research and professor of integrated medical science, Schmidt College of Medicine, Florida Atlantic University, Boca Raton.

In a study of more than 350 people, average age 69, participants who were "skinny fat" (an age-related combination of loss of muscle mass, known as sarcopenia, and high body fat) performed worse on tests of executive function and cognition, including memory, mental flexibility and self-control, than those who were sarcopenic or obese alone.

If you are "skinny fat": Talk to your doctor about your risk for dementia.

You Can't Beat Beets!

Christopher Bell, PhD, department of health and exercise science, Colorado State University, Fort Collins.

When obese people drank 17 ounces of beet juice before consuming a large amount of sugar, their insulin sensitivity and blood sugar improved.

Probable reason: Nitrate-rich beet juice helps the body make nitric oxide, which is typically low in obese people but improves blood flow and helps the body metabolize sugar faster. The amount of beet juice used in the study may be unpalatable to many people, but other research has shown that just five ounces of beetroot juice concentrate before eating may provide some benefit to obese people with elevated blood sugar levels.

Caution: If you've been advised to avoid nitrate-rich foods (if you have kidney stones, for example), skip the beets.

How a Harvard Brain Specialist Keeps Her Own Brain Healthy

Marie Pasinski, MD, a memory specialist and neurologist who is on the faculty of Harvard Medical School and a staff neurologist at Massachusetts General Hospital, both in Boston. She is author, with Liz Neporent, of *Chicken Soup for the Soul: Boost Your Brain Power!*.

Scientists used to believe that memory and other mental abilities inevitably declined with age. Not anymore. We now know that the brain has the ability to form new neurons and create new neural pathways throughout life. This means that your ability to remember and learn actually can get better as you age.

It doesn't take hard work—or complicated mental "workouts"—to improve mental agility. *Here's what Marie Pasinski, MD, a memory specialist at Harvard Medical School, does to keep her own brain healthy...*

HANG OUT WITH FRIENDS

Close relationships are good for the brain. We have found that people who have supportive friends (or spouses) and rich social networks have better cognitive function and lower rates of dementia than those who spend more time alone.

When I take a break during my workday to go for a walk, I like to find someone to go with me. Exercising with friends is ideal because you can catch up on one another's lives while you get in shape.

It's not entirely clear why friendships are so important. One reason is purely mental—the brain is stimulated when you share ideas with other people. Mental stimulation increases the number of neurons and the connections among neurons. Social engagement lowers levels of stress hormones, which appear to be toxic to the neurons in the hippocampus—the brain's memory center. It also appears to lower blood pressure and reduce the risk for stroke.

Spend as much time as you can with people you care about—getting together with one close friend can be just as beneficial as hanging out with a group. Meeting new people is beneficial because it adds an extra jolt of stimulation. You can broaden your social network by volunteering or joining community groups.

DON'T LIVE ON AUTOPILOT

Routine is seductive. People like going to the same restaurants or taking the same route to work. The problem with routine is that it literally creates mental ruts—the brain uses only preexisting pathways and neural connections to complete familiar tasks. It stops growing and improving.

By embracing new experiences, you stimulate your brain to create neurons and forge additional neural pathways. This happens every time you extend your scope of experience and think in new ways. The more you challenge your brain—even when the "challenge" is as simple as looking at unfamiliar scenery—the more its functions improve.

For me, writing is a new experience. I can't spell to save my life. My worst course in college was English 101. When a friend suggested that I write a book about memory, I immediately dismissed the idea. Then, a few weeks later, I learned that Harvard was offering a course on publishing. I decided to take it. Now I've completed two books.

For me, shifting attention from medicine to writing was a radical change. But any change, even a small one, can help boost memory and thinking. If you take a new route to work, you will see different buildings. You will have to think about where you're going. This alone is enough to stimulate the brain's circuitry.

WORK BOTH SIDES OF THE BRAIN

A lot of my patients love to do crossword or other puzzles. They enjoy the challenge, and they've heard that mental activities improve memory. They're right—but only up to a point.

The improvements that you get from mental challenges quickly level off as you gain expertise.

Better: In addition to taking on new challenges, do things that work the underused side of your brain. If you're an accountant who crunches numbers all day, you're drawing heavily on the logical left side of the brain. Take up a hobby that works the right side, the imaginative side, such as painting or making pottery.

For me, playing the piano is a creative and welcome distraction from my work in medicine. I tried to learn to play when I was young, but my teacher was awful! I took it up again later in life. This time, I got to choose my own teacher, who has since become a close friend.

HAVE FUN

People who enjoy what they're doing get a mental boost. "Forcing" yourself to do things that aren't fun won't be anywhere near as good for your brain as activities that you genuinely enjoy. Also, enjoyment triggers the release of dopamine, a neurotransmitter that enhances learning and retention of new material.

I often ask patients to describe some of the things that they would like to do but have never done. Some would like to learn a new language. Others want to take up a new hobby, such as bird-watching or playing a sport. Ideally, whatever you choose will be both unfamiliar and fun.

I've tried all sorts of things in recent years, from joining Facebook and taking improv classes to competing in triathlons and gardening.

MOVE!

I do something physical every day. I enjoy biking, running, swimming, tennis and skiing. I also take jazz-dance classes.

Exercise triggers the release of brain-derived neurotrophic factor, a growth factor that promotes the formation of new synapses in the brain—the connections among brain cells that are critical for memory and other cognitive functions.

Exercise also increases the size of the brain. In one study, nonexercisers were given MRI scans to measure their brain volume. Then they were instructed to walk for 60 minutes, three days a week. After six months, they were given another MRI. The scans showed that they had an increase in the size of the prefrontal cortex, the part of the brain that is involved in reasoning, problem-solving and other "executive" functions.

Exercise also increases the size of the hippocampus, the area of the brain that is closely involved with memory. It improves circulation and helps prevent hypertension and other conditions that increase the risk for dementia.

Even if you don't enjoy "formal" exercise, you can get similar benefits just by moving more. I spend a lot of time at my computer, but I take a break every hour or so just to move around.

EAT BRAIN FOOD

A Mediterranean-style diet, with relatively little red meat and lots of fish, vegetables and whole grains, is the best diet for brain health. People who follow this diet have less atherosclerosis, hypertension and diabetes, conditions that cause inflammation and other brain changes that impair thinking and memory. *Fish and olive oil, two staples of the Mediterranean diet, are particularly good for the brain...*

- **Fish and omega-3s.** About two-thirds of the brain consists of fat. When you eat salmon, sardines or other cold-water fish, the omega-3s from the fish are incorporated into brain tissue. A study published in *American Journal of Clinical Nutrition*, which looked at more than 2,000 men and women ages 70 to 74, found that those who ate, on average, one-third of an ounce or more of fish daily did better on cognitive tests than those who ate less.

I try to eat fish at least a few days a week. If you're not fond of fish, you can get some of the same benefits from eggs or milk that is fortified with omega-3s. Other less potent sources of omega-3s include walnuts, pumpkin seeds and soybeans. You also can take fish-oil supplements. The usual dose is 1,000 milligrams (mg) to 2,000 mg daily. Because the supplements can have a blood-thinning effect and/or interact with some medications, check with your doctor before taking them.

• **Olive oil.** It's a healthy fat that reduces inflammation, improves cholesterol and helps reduce the risk for stroke. I use it for cooking almost every day. People who use olive oil regularly tend to have lower rates of dementia and better cognitive function.

Don't Let Your Brain Shrink

Daniel G. Amen, MD, a brain-imaging specialist and assistant clinical professor of psychiatry and human behavior at the University of California, Irvine, School of Medicine. He is the founder, CEO and medical director of The Amen Clinics and the author of several books, including *Use Your Brain to Change Your Age: Secrets to Look, Feel, and Think Younger Every Day*. AmenClinics.com

When scientists talk about memory and learning, the hippocampus, a small, seahorse-shaped structure located deep inside the brain, gets most of the credit for these vital cognitive functions.

What you don't hear much about: The prefrontal cortex (PFC), a much larger part of the brain located just behind and slightly beneath the forehead. Known as the "executive" part of the brain because it controls judgment, insights and impulse control, the PFC is just as important when it comes to staying sharp mentally, learning new information and controlling processes involved in memory.

Unfortunately, millions of Americans don't follow simple lifestyle habits that promote optimal functioning of the PFC.

Result: Lapses in judgment (such as making risky maneuvers when driving)...disorganized thinking (including an inability to prioritize tasks)...shorter attention spans (resulting in difficulty with reading and other activities that require focus)...and impairments in learning and memory.

IMPROVE YOUR BRAIN—LIVE LONGER

The PFC needs good "fuel" to thrive. That's why people with healthful habits tend to have a larger PFC than those who don't take good care of themselves. As a result, they're more likely to live longer (because their judgment about risks is better), and they're less likely to develop Alzheimer's disease.

Important findings: A 2007 study of Catholic nuns and priests found that those who had the most self-discipline were 89% less likely to develop Alzheimer's disease. Self-discipline is one of the traits that is enhanced when you have a robust PFC.

POWER UP YOUR "WIRING"

People with healthful habits have less damage to myelin, the fatty coating on brain cells, than people who are less conscientious about their health. Brain cells that are sheathed in myelin work 10 to 100 times faster than unmyelinated cells. People with healthful habits also tend to have better blood circulation in the brain, which improves thinking as well as memory. *To protect your PFC—and other key parts of the brain...*

• **Rethink your alcohol intake.** Millions of Americans drink a glass or two of red wine a day because it's good for the heart. But the cardio-protective properties of alcohol—it raises HDL "good" cholesterol and reduces clots, thus reducing the risk for a heart attack—may be offset by the damage it can do to the brain. Alcohol decreases the size and functioning of the PFC. What's more, even moderate drinking (two drinks daily for men and one for women) can impair brain circulation.

My advice: If your doctor agrees that you can forgo the cardiovascular benefits of drinking wine, limit your intake to no more than two or three alcoholic beverages per week.

• **"Water" your brain.** The brain is 80% water. People who don't drink enough water or who drink a lot of dehydrating liquids, such as alcohol or caffeinated coffee or tea, often have impairments in cognition and judgment, which can occur when the PFC is damaged.

My advice: Drink plenty of water—eight glasses (64 ounces) of water every day is typically sufficient. If you like, add a splash of lemon or lime juice for flavor.

• **Slow down on the omega-6s.** Most Americans get far too many inflammation-promoting omega-6 essential fatty acids in their diets—primarily from cooking oils (such as corn and vegetable), fatty red meats and processed foods—that are harmful to the brain. That's why a plant-based, anti-inflammatory diet is among the most effective ways to reduce damage to the PFC and other areas of the brain.

My advice: Eat lots of greens—including salads—along with vegetables, fruit, whole grains and legumes. Approximately three servings of lean protein daily will help balance blood sugar and keep you feeling sharp. Also, eat at least three servings weekly of cold-water fish such as salmon, mackerel and sardines. The omega-3s in these fish have potent anti-inflammatory effects. Fish oil supplements (1 g to 3 g daily) are also helpful. Check with your doctor first if you use a blood thinner.

Aim to change your diet so that your intake of omega-6 fatty acids is no more than three times higher than your intake of omega-3s.

Good rule of thumb: A plant-based diet that's high in fish provides the ideal 3:1 (or lower) ratio of omega-6s to omega-3s.

• **Try green tea and rhodiola.** Distractibility, disorganization and poor impulse control are commonly associated with children who may be suffering from attention-deficit/hyperactivity disorder (ADHD), but many adults (who may or may not have ADHD) also struggle with such symptoms.

Often linked to low activity in the PFC, these symptoms can be reversed, in part, with green tea and rhodiola, a plant-based supplement frequently used as an energy booster. In one study, researchers at my clinic did brain scans before and after giving patients green tea and rhodiola. Two months later, scans showed a significant increase in circulation in the PFC.

How it helps: Green tea appears to benefit the PFC by increasing the availability of dopamine, a brain chemical that controls the brain's reward and pleasure centers. It also helps regulate emotional responses, such as the motivation to take positive actions. Rhodiola is an "adaptogen," a substance that normalizes the body's functions by boosting blood flow to the brain and raising dopamine and serotonin levels.

My advice: Take 200 mg of rhodiola and drink two to three cups of green tea daily (avoid drinking it in the evening since the tea's caffeine can interfere with sleep...or drink decaffeinated green tea).

• **Keep your BMI in check.** People who are overweight—with a body mass index (BMI) of 25 or higher—have less circulation in the PFC than those of normal weights. Excess body weight is associated with atherosclerosis, diabetes and other conditions that impede circulation throughout the body.

Danger: A high BMI can cause the brain to shrink. Research has shown that people who are obese typically have about 8% less brain tissue than normal-weight adults.

My advice: At least once a year, check your BMI by using an online calculator. Go to NHLBI.NIH.gov and search "BMI Calculator." A BMI of 18.5 to 24.9 is considered normal. If your BMI is 25 or higher, you need to lose weight.

• **Don't ignore sleep problems.** An estimated 18 million Americans have sleep apnea, a condition in which breathing intermittently stops during sleep. Unfortunately, the condition is undiagnosed in most of these people.

Why does this matter? Scans on patients with sleep apnea show brain changes that resemble early Alzheimer's disease. Poor sleep decreases blood flow to the PFC and other parts of the brain. Snoring, daytime fatigue and morning headaches are common symptoms of sleep apnea. Your doctor may recommend tests in a sleep laboratory.

My advice: If you're overweight, sleep apnea can often be reduced or even eliminated with weight loss. Many patients also benefit from continuous positive airway pressure (CPAP) units, which help keep the airways open during sleep.

Also important: Avoid sleepless nights. Patients with chronic insomnia have a higher risk for cognitive declines than people who sleep well. To prevent insomnia, follow the tried-and-true strategies—relax in a warm bath before bed...reduce arousal by not watching TV or using a computer in the hour before bedtime...and go to bed and wake up at the same times every day.

Also helpful: Melatonin. The standard dose of this sleep hormone supplement is 1 mg to 6 mg taken a half hour before bed. Start with the lower dose and increase it over a period of weeks, if necessary.

Check with your doctor first if you take an antidepressant, blood pressure medication, blood thinner, steroid or nonsteroidal anti-inflammatory drug—melatonin may interact with these medications.

Why Vegetarians Have It All Wrong

Terry Wahls, MD, an internist and a clinical professor of medicine at the University of Iowa Carver College of Medicine in Iowa City. She is the author of *The Wahls Protocol: A Radical New Way to Treat All Chronic Autoimmune Conditions Using Paleo Principles* and founder of The Wahls Foundation, which educates the public and health-care practitioners on the benefits of integrative treatment for multiple sclerosis and other chronic diseases.

A diet rich in fruits and vegetables and whole grains, but with little or no meat, has long been touted as the best way to lower your risk for heart disease, prevent weight gain and reduce risk for certain cancers.

But as a medical doctor with progressive multiple sclerosis (MS), I believe that meat (grass-fed beef...organic chicken, pork and lamb...and wild game and fish) has played a critical role in my recovery—and that meat can help protect against other autoimmune diseases, Parkinson's disease, Alzheimer's disease and early cognitive impairment.

HOW MEAT BENEFITS THE BRAIN

- **Meat provides vitamin B-12.** A diet without meat raises your risk for vitamin B-12 deficiency. If your body doesn't get enough B-12, you can develop neurological symptoms such as problems with balance and coordination, difficulties with decision-making and cognitive decline. Vitamin B-12 is found naturally only in animal foods such as clams, liver, salmon and beef. A synthetic form is often added to cereals and nutritional yeast, but I recommend avoiding gluten because many people are sensitive to it. Alternatively, you could take a B-12 supplement, but I prefer natural food sources, which supply additional vitamins and nutrients.

- **Meat is the best source of complete proteins.** Protein is essential to make, repair and maintain the structure of all the cells in our bodies, including cells in the brain. The amino acids found in protein help the brain produce crucial neurotransmitters that regulate mood and maintain and repair brain cells. If you don't have enough protein to do this, brain function deteriorates.

Meat contains all of the essential amino acids your body needs to manufacture protein. To get a complete protein from a nonmeat source, you would have to combine a grain and a legume, for example.

- **Certain meats provide omega-3 fatty acids.** Cell membranes throughout the body, including in the brain, rely on essential fatty acids to stay healthy. The brain is especially dependent on the omega-3 fatty acids *docosahexaenoic acid* (DHA) and *eicosapentaenoic acid* (EPA) that are found in fish such as sardines, herring and anchovies (the fish I prefer to eat because small fish have less risk for heavy metal and plastic contamination) as well as organic chicken and grass-fed beef. These omega-3s help preserve the integrity of cell membranes in the brain and stave off neurological problems like mood disorders and cognitive decline.

While you can get alpha linolenic acid (ALA), another omega-3, from plant sources, your body can convert only small amounts of ALA into DHA and EPA. DHA and EPA supplements are available, but numerous studies have shown that foods high in omega-3s are more beneficial to brain health than supplements.

THE BEST MEAT FOR YOUR BRAIN

Most grass-fed beef, organic chicken and wild game and fish are beneficial for brain health, but organ meats (particularly heart, liver and tongue) provide the most nutrition. Organ meats are chock-full of vitamins A and B and essential nutrients such as creatine, carnitine and coenzyme Q10 (CoQ10). There are a variety of ways to add organ meats to your meals and make them more palatable. *To get the most nutrition from meat...*

- **Start with heart.** Beef and bison heart taste a lot like steak, especially if you serve them up with mushrooms. Just don't overcook organ meat, or it will be dry and tough. Cooking it to medium rare also helps the meat retain vitamins.

• **Disguise liver.** If you don't like the taste of liver, purée small raw pieces of it in a blender with water to make a slurry. Add this mixture to soups, stews or chili, and let the food simmer a few minutes.

• **Try sausage or liver pâté.** Your local butcher can make a sausage out of ground liver and some other ground meat, such as pork or chicken. Start with a ratio of one part liver to six parts ground meat, and work up to a ratio of one to three. If you don't like the taste of liver, ask the butcher to add spices to conceal it.

• **Make a bone broth.** Put the carcass of a chicken or beef or pork knuckle bones into a pot. Add one tablespoon of vinegar per one quart of water, and toss in one whole onion and carrot and a few cloves of garlic. Let the broth simmer for at least six hours, then strain out the bone, vegetables and foam. Use the broth as a stock for soup or drink it.

• **Consider an organ meat supplement.** If you just can't stomach the idea of eating organ meat, consider taking a supplement.

Good choice: Organ Delight from Dr. Ron's Ultra-Pure (DrRons.com).

THE WAHLS PROTOCOL

Keep in mind that I'm not advocating a meat-only diet. In fact, the Wahls Protocol diet (the eating plan I developed to combat my own MS) starts by recommending six to nine cups a day (depending on your size and gender) of vegetables, fruits and berries (get twice as many veggies as fruits and berries).

In particular, I prefer green, leafy vegetables...sulfur-rich vegetables in the cabbage and onion families...deeply colored vegetables such as yams, beets, peppers and tomatoes...and brightly colored berries such as raspberries, strawberries and cranberries.

For meat, I recommend six to 12 ounces a day (depending on your size and gender) for disease treatment and prevention.

My regimen also incorporates a CoQ10 supplement, a spirulina or chlorella algae supplement and green tea—which is high in quercetin, an antioxidant with anti-inflammatory properties.

Add 5 Years of Brainpower

Yian Gu, PhD, assistant professor, neuropsychology, Columbia University College of Physicians & Surgeons, New York City.

Eating the right five foods can postpone brain aging by five years.

New study: Adults age 65 and older who frequently ate at least five foods from the Mediterranean diet (such as fish, vegetables, fruit, whole grains, legumes and olive oil) and consumed moderate amounts of wine and low amounts of dairy, meat and poultry were found to have larger brain volumes than those who didn't eat this way. The difference in brain volume was comparable to about five fewer years of brain aging.

Theory: The Mediterranean diet may help slow the loss of brain cells during aging.

The Vitamin That Sharpens Memory

Daniel G. Amen, MD, a brain-imaging specialist and assistant clinical professor of psychiatry and human behavior at the University of California, Irvine, School of Medicine. He is the founder, CEO and medical director of The Amen Clinics and the author of several books, including *Use Your Brain to Change Your Age: Secrets to Look, Feel, and Think Younger Every Day*. AmenClinics.com

Can supplements help you find your car keys? Some just might. Research shows that taking the right supplements, in combination with a healthy lifestyle, can preserve and improve brain function.

Renowned brain specialist Daniel G. Amen, MD, knows this firsthand. During his studies of single-photon emission computerized tomography (SPECT) imaging, he decided to have some scans done of his own brain. What he found was that years of unhealthy habits—drinking diet soda, eating fast food, not exercising—had caught up with him. He started a healthy brain program, which included brain-building supplements. Now his brain is healthier than it was 20 years earlier.

Here, the best supplements for your brain.

Caution: Most people can safely take all of them daily, but always check with your health-care provider first, particularly if you have any health problems such as high blood pressure or if you are on any medications, including blood thinners.

MEMORY VITAMIN

Americans don't get enough sun, and because of this, about two-thirds of adults don't meet their vitamin D needs through sunshine exposure.

You probably know that vitamin D is essential for bone strength as well as for preventing some cancers, including breast cancer.

What's new: Vitamin D appears to help the immune system remove beta-amyloid, an abnormal protein, from the brain. This is important because beta-amyloid causes the "tangles" that are associated with Alzheimer's disease.

Brain cells use vitamin D for learning, memory and other cognitive functions. It also is an antioxidant that protects neurons from cell-damaging inflammation. A Tufts University study found that elderly adults with optimal levels of vitamin D performed better on cognitive tests and had better brain-processing speeds than those with lower levels.

Recommended: 2,000 international units (IU) of vitamin D daily is a typical dose, but I advise patients to get their blood levels of vitamin D tested before taking supplements. Everyone synthesizes and absorbs vitamin D differently.

FISH OIL

There's compelling evidence that the omega-3 fatty acids in fish-oil supplements can improve your mood as well as your memory and other cognitive functions. I take fish oil every day, and I advise everyone to do so.

A large portion of the brain consists of *docosahexaenoic acid* (DHA), one of the main omega-3s in fish oil. The brain uses DHA to form cell membranes. People who consume fish oil, either by taking supplements or eating fish, have better brain functions, including a faster transmission of nerve signals and improved cerebral blood flow.

When Danish researchers compared the diets of more than 5,000 older adults, they found that those who ate the most fish were less likely to get dementia and more likely to maintain robust memories.

Important: The American diet is high in omega-6 fatty acids—found in processed foods, red meats, cooking oils, etc. Even if you eat a lot of fish, you still will need supplements to achieve the recommended ratio of one part omega-3s to every three parts omega-6s.

Recommended: 1 to 2 grams daily. Look for a supplement that provides roughly equal amounts of DHA and *eicosapentaenoic acid* (EPA).

MULTIVITAMIN

Most Americans don't eat the recommended five daily servings of fruits and vegetables. A multivitamin, particularly one that includes B vitamins, is good insurance and can help your brain. In a 2010 study, researchers tested the mental performance of 215 participants. The participants then were given either a daily multivitamin or a placebo. When they were retested a month later, those in the vitamin group showed better mental performance than they had in the beginning. There wasn't a change in the control group.

B vitamins nourish the myelin layer that covers brain cells. Studies have shown that adults who don't get enough of these nutrients, particularly vitamins B-6, B-12 and folic acid, tend to have the greatest declines in memory and other cognitive functions.

Recommended: Look for a product with all seven of the major B vitamins.

VINPOCETINE

This vasodilator comes from the periwinkle plant. Unlike many supplements, it's able to cross the blood-brain barrier and improve brain circulation. Studies show that it significantly increases the oxygenation of brain tissue and improves memory, particularly when used in combination with other brain-boosting supplements.

Recommended: 5 milligrams (mg) to 10 mg daily.

GINKGO

When I examine blood flow and activity patterns with SPECT, the "prettiest" brains often are found in people who take ginkgo. This popular herb is among the best-studied supplements. It dilates blood vessels and reduces the "stickiness" of platelets, cell-like structures in blood that increase the risk for clots. Ginkgo contains flavonoids as well as terpenoids, potent antioxidants that prevent damage to brain cells.

There's strong evidence that ginkgo improves memory. It is also thought to help reduce the risk for vascular dementias and, possibly, Alzheimer's disease.

Recommended: 60 mg to 120 mg, twice daily.

ST. JOHN'S WORT

Anxiety, stress and depression cause serious impairments in mental functions. Chronic stress, for example, increases levels of hormones that can damage the hippocampus (the part of the brain involved in memory). People who are depressed tend to sleep poorly and don't take care of themselves. These and other factors can interfere with clear thinking.

The herb St. John's wort is one of the best treatments for depression. It also is used for treating anxiety and stress. It improves mental focus and helps stop your mind from "spinning."

A review of 29 studies involving 5,489 patients, published by *The Cochrane Collaboration* (an organization that analyzes medical research), concluded that St. John's wort was just as effective as prescription antidepressants, while causing fewer side effects.

Recommended: If you feel depressed or anxious, take 900 mg of St. John's wort daily, divided into two doses.

Caution: St. John's wort rarely causes side effects, but it can interact with other medications. Talk to your doctor.

It's Teatime for Your Brain!

Feng Lei, PhD, assistant professor, Yong Loo Lin School of Medicine, National University of Singapore.

A single cup of black, green or oolong tea daily was linked to a 50% reduction in the risk of developing dementia, according to a study involving 957 people over age 55. Why? These teas are made from the Camellia sinensis plant and are full of catechins and theaflavins—both of which have anti-inflammatory and antioxidant properties that appear to protect against vascular damage and neurodegeneration. While tea bags are OK, the tea should be freshly brewed.

Even Moderate Drinking Is Bad for the Brain

Anya Topiwala, MD, PhD, is clinical lecturer in old age psychiatry in the department of psychiatry at University of Oxford, UK.

Even moderate drinking is bad for the brain, reports Anya Topiwala, MD, PhD. Over a 30-year period, people who drank as few as four pints of strong beer or five large glasses of wine a week had hippocampal atrophy, a type of brain damage often found in people with Alzheimer's disease. Light drinkers—up to three small glasses of wine or two pints of beer a week—showed no decrease in brain function.

Make Your Brain Younger

Clinton Wright, MD, scientific director, Evelyn F. McKnight Brain Institute, University of Miami.

Older adults who did regular moderate-to-intense exercise like running or swimming laps had the memory and other cognitive skills of someone a decade younger than those who were sedentary or did light exercise such as gardening, a new study of 900 older adults found.

Possible reason: Exercise boosts blood flow to the brain and enhances brain cell connections. It also lowers risk for high blood pressure, elevated cholesterol and diabetes—all of which can impair cognitive function.

To Protect Your Brain: Hold Off on Retirement

Analysis of the records of more than 400,000 retired workers in France by researchers at National Institute of Health and Medical Research, Paris, presented at the 2013 Alzheimer's Association International Conference.

Delaying retirement may protect your brain. For each additional year that a person worked before retiring, dementia risk dropped by 3% in a recent analysis. That means someone who retired at age 60 had a 15% greater chance of developing dementia, on average, than someone who retired at 65.

Theory: The mental stimulation and social connections at work may keep the brain healthy.

Why Your Neurons Hate High Blood Sugar (And How to Protect Them)

Robert Krikorian, PhD, director of the Cognitive Disorders Center and associate professor of clinical psychiatry at the University of Cincinnati College of Medicine.

Richard Anderson, PhD, a researcher at the USDA's Beltsville Human Nutrition Center in Maryland.

Sugar isn't sweet to your brain. That's the conclusion of several new studies, which show that people with chronically high levels of blood sugar (glucose) and insulin (the glucose-controlling hormone that shoots up when blood sugar levels are high) are more likely to have memory problems and other types of cognitive decline.

- **"Greater cognitive decline."** Dutch researchers measured memory and other mental abilities at the beginning and end of a five-year study of 2,613 people who were 43 to 70 years old. People with type 2 diabetes—a disease of chronically high blood sugar and insulin—had a rate of cognitive decline that was 2.6 times higher than people who didn't have diabetes. Among those 60 and older, the five-year decline was 3.6 times greater among those with diabetes. "Middle-aged individuals with type 2 diabetes showed a greater decline in cognitive function than middle-aged individuals without diabetes," concluded the researchers in *Diabetes Care.*

- **From mild cognitive impairment to dementia—via diabetes.** Mild cognitive impairment (MCI) is the stage of memory loss and mental decline before dementia. A study by British researchers found that people with MCI and diabetes are three times more likely to develop dementia than people with MCI who don't have diabetes.

- **Higher glucose and insulin, more Alzheimer's.** In a 15-year study, Japanese researchers performed autopsies on people who had been tested for glucose and insulin levels during their lifetime. Those with the highest levels of glucose were 71% more likely to have the brain plaques that are the hallmark of Alzheimer's disease. Those with the highest levels of insulin were 203% more likely to have the plaques. "Adequate control of diabetes might contribute to a strategy for the prevention of Alzheimer's disease," concluded the researchers in *Neurology.*

Surprising new risk factor: "High brain levels of insulin are neurodegenerative," says Robert Krikorian, PhD, director of the Cognitive Disorders Center and associate professor of clinical psychiatry at the University of Cincinnati College of Medicine. "Excess insulin produces higher levels of brain-harming inflammation and higher levels of beta-amyloid, the neuron-destroying plaques that are a feature of Alzheimer's."

But a new study by Dr. Krikorian and his colleagues shows that chromium—a glucose-balancing, insulin-controlling nutritional supplement—may help stop cognitive decline.

CHROMIUM FOR YOUR CRANIUM

Dr. Krikorian studied 26 people with MCI, dividing them into two groups. One group took a daily supplement of 1,000 mcg of chromium, which dozens of studies show can balance blood levels of glucose and regulate the body's production and use of insulin. The other group took a placebo.

Results: After three months, those taking the chromium had an improved ability to remember and learn. There was little change in the placebo group.

These findings suggest that supplementation with chromium can enhance cognition and brain function in older adults at risk for neurodegeneration, concluded Dr. Krikorian and his colleagues in the journal *Nutritional Neuroscience*.

How it works: Chromium controls blood sugar by improving the functioning of insulin receptors, the structures on cells that allow insulin to move glucose out of the bloodstream. (If your insulin receptors don't work, you have insulin resistance.) *Specifically, chromium...*

- **Helps cells make more insulin receptors**
- **Boosts an enzyme that helps those receptors work**
- **Blocks an enzyme that turns those receptors off.**

"If chromium were a drug for diabetes, everyone would have touted it as a wonder drug," says Richard Anderson, PhD, a researcher at the Beltsville Human Nutrition Center and author of more than 70 studies on chromium.

MCI AND INSULIN RESISTANCE

Dr. Krikorian thinks that just about everyone with MCI has blood sugar and insulin problems—and therefore needs more chromium.

"We've enrolled more than 150 people with mild cognitive impairment in studies I've conducted," he says. "Their average waist circumference is 40 inches—a very reliable indicator of insulin resistance.

"We've also found that the average fasting glucose level of people with MCI is 98 milligrams per deciliter (mg/dL), just a couple of points below the standard measurement for borderline diabetes." (Levels above 83 mg/dL harm the brain, he adds.)

Recommendation: Dr. Krikorian routinely recommends that all his patients with MCI take a daily dose of 400 mcg (micrograms) of chromium picolinate, the best-absorbed form of the supplement. The chromium picolinate supplement used in the study was Chromax, from Nutrition 21.

"I think everyone with MCI—and even people who don't have MCI—should be supplementing their diet with chromium. That's because everyone eats some sugary, starchy junk food, which routinely raises glucose and insulin levels."

Video Games Are Good for Your Brain

Gregory West, PhD, associate professor of psychology, Université de Montréal, Canada, and coauthor of a study published in *PLOS One*.

Video games may help protect the brain. Older adults who played Super Mario 64, a 3-D logic-and-puzzle game, for 30 minutes a day, five days a week, for six months, had increased volume of gray matter in the brain's hippocampus and cerebellum regions—and their short-term memory improved. The effects were not seen in people who took piano lessons for six months or in a control group that did neither activity. Gray matter normally atrophies as people age. Learning new things may help slow the atrophy—but the reason for the specific effectiveness of the video game in this study remains unknown.

3

Cancer Breakthroughs and Care

6 Ways to Beat Back Cancer

Lorenzo Cohen, PhD, the Richard E. Haynes Distinguished Professor in Clinical Cancer Prevention and director of the Integrative Medicine Program at The University of Texas MD Anderson Cancer Center in Houston.

From time to time, we all hear about cancer patients who defy the odds and live longer than anyone predicted—or even, in some cases, have a complete remission. Why does this happen? No one knows for sure. Researchers are trying to understand this puzzle. *Here's what we've learned so far...*

SPONTANEOUS REMISSIONS

Some cancers simply disappear. We know, for example, that about 5% of patients with advanced kidney cancer will have spontaneous remissions. This doesn't mean that they're cured—the cancer could return at some point. But for some reason, these patients do much better than others.

Genetic factors surely play a role. Researchers have identified a number of "response mutations" in various types of tumors that somehow make them more likely to respond positively to treatments such as chemotherapy or radiation.

IMPROVE YOUR ODDS

Research is ongoing, but there's evidence suggesting that the six steps below are important in getting the best possible outcome—and can help prevent cancer from developing in the first place...

- **Take control and manage stress.** "Negative" emotions, such as anxiety and depression, are a normal response to a life-changing illness. Yet there's good evidence (both from human and animal studies) that chronic stress can make your body more susceptible to cancer growth—and that reducing stress may make a difference.

Important research: A study published in the journal *Biological Psychiatry* found that breast cancer patients who participated in a 10-week stress-management program had an increase in cancer-controlling gene expression (such as type 1 interferon response genes) for improved immune function and a decrease in genes that control inflammatory molecules that promote cancer growth. An analysis of the 11-year survival data found that the women in the stress-management group lived significantly longer than those in the control group.

My advice: Engage in a stress-management activity every day (for example, meditation, yoga, relaxation techniques, etc.)...strive to bring that state of calm with you throughout the day...and get counseling if you need it.

- **Get a good night's sleep.** Poor sleep and disruptions in the body's biological clock (as occurs with shift work, for example) have been linked to the development of certain malignancies, including breast and prostate cancer. Now research is suggesting that sleep may play a role in cancer survival.

My advice: The sweet spot seems to be about seven hours of sleep a night. Some people need a bit more, but you don't want to get much less. Research has shown that the risk of dying from all causes—not just cancer—is higher in those who get less than six hours of sleep a night.

• **Watch your weight.** People with a higher body mass index (BMI) have greater concentrations of inflammatory molecules...more insulin resistance...and more estrogen and cancer-related growth factors.

And the effects can be significant. Obese patients are not only more likely to be diagnosed with cancer but also to have a cancer recurrence. They tend to have more complications from surgery, chemotherapy or other treatments as well.

My advice: People with a BMI of 27 or higher should make a serious effort to lose weight. They'll get a double benefit because the two main weight-loss strategies—a healthier diet and more exercise—will also improve cancer recovery and survival.

Important: Consult your doctor about the ideal time to lose weight during your treatment—it may not be appropriate at all stages of cancer care.

• **Get more exercise.** It is well known that regular exercise can help prevent many types of cancer. But can it also help cancer patients live longer? The jury is still out.

Thus far, observational studies—those that look at large populations of people—do suggest that it might make a difference. Exercise is believed to decrease circulating levels of cancer-promoting inflammatory markers and increase aspects of immune function that can help to control cancer growth.

My advice: Exercise at least 30 minutes a day at least five or six days a week. Any amount of activity helps—even 10-minute bouts every few hours count. Also avoid sitting for hours at a time.

• **Reduce exposure to toxins.** Cancer-causing chemicals are all around us. Hormone disrupters, such as bisphenol A (BPA) and parabens, are in some plastic bottles and cosmetics and can alter hormonal functioning and increase cancer risk. Carcinogens, such as formaldehyde and benzene, can be in wallpaper, paint, wood floor finishes and other household products.

My advice: Avoid personal-care products that contain parabens, phthalates, triclosan and synthetic fragrance. Use glass and stainless steel containers instead of plastic. Ventilate your home when painting or refinishing floors.

THE HEALTHY PLATE FORMULA

To help fight cancer, it's important to make wise food choices throughout the day.

Here's how: Fill half your plate with vegetables (organic, if possible) at every meal, including breakfast. The other half should contain protein, fruits (preferably organic) and whole grains. Try replacing meat with sardines, salmon and other cold-water fish (loaded with omega-3 fatty acids) and beans at least four times a week for a healthy source of animal and plant proteins. Add spices and herbs, which are filled with healthy phytochemicals. It's also smart to eat fewer "white" foods, including white bread, white rice, etc. These and other high-glycemic foods are quickly converted to glucose, which increases levels of insulin and insulin-like growth factor (a cancer promoter).

Helpful: Meet with a dietitian to help guide you in healthy eating. To find a registered dietitian near you, consult the Academy of Nutrition and Dietetics, EatRight.org.

Breakthrough Cancer Drug

Ulrik Lassen, MD, PhD, head, department of oncology, Rigshospitalet, Copenhagen.

Breakthrough cancer drug gets accelerated FDA approval. *Larotrectinib* (Vitrakvi) is the first primary tumor-agnostic therapy—it attacks malignancies that have specific genetic characteristics regardless of where the cancer is in the body. In three separate studies, 122 patients with 24 cancer types, including breast, pancreatic, lung and thyroid (with an NTRK gene fusion) that had not spread to other parts of the body but could not be safely surgically removed, had an overall response rate—meaning tumors shrank either partially or completely—of more than 80%.

Breakthrough Cancer Therapy: Blood Cancers Have a Response Rate Up to 80%

Caron A. Jacobson, MD, medical oncologist and assistant professor of medicine at Dana-Farber Cancer Institute and Harvard Medical School, both in Boston. She is the medical director of the Immune Effector Cell Therapy Program at Dana-Farber, which houses its CAR T-cell program. Dr. Jacobson, who specializes in lymphoma treatment and is affiliated with Brigham and Women's Hospital in Boston, is the principal investigator of CAR T-cell trials in lymphoma there and at Dana-Farber.

When it comes to the development of cancer treatments, the decades-long arc of progress is slow and incremental. Then something truly significant happens to change the course of the disease. What's happening now appears to be one of those moments.

Latest development: A type of blood-cancer treatment that has already shown remarkable success in clinical trials is beginning to receive FDA approvals. Two of these treatments, for example, have recently been approved (see next page).

With the new treatment, known as CAR T-cell therapy, blood is drawn from a patient to isolate his/her T-cells, the powerhouses of the body's immune system. The T-cells are genetically altered and reprogrammed to recognize and kill tumor cells and then infused back into the patient.

The treatment has been called a "living drug" because it's hoped that the enhanced T-cells will continue to multiply and remain active in the body, possibly providing lifelong protection against the cancer.

A GAME CHANGER

Researchers at universities and pharmaceutical companies have now developed CAR T-cell therapy for leukemia, multiple myeloma and lymphoma—blood cancers that account for about 10% of all cancer cases diagnosed in the US each year.

The hope is that similar treatments eventually will be used for tumors affecting the breast, lung, prostate and other parts of the body.

Important: The treatment of "solid" tumors with this type of gene therapy still presents formidable obstacles that will have to be overcome.

CAR T-cell therapies have mainly been studied in patients with lymphoma or other blood cancers that didn't respond well to standard treatments or that later recurred.

Example: Lymphoma patients are typically given several types and/or protocols of standard chemotherapy without a sure result. These patients are thought to be good candidates for CAR T-cell therapy—and the early results are promising. Studies show that up to 80% of such patients respond to CAR T- cell therapy, and about 30% to 40% of patients were still in remission after six months. In earlier studies, some patients have remained in remission for more than five years.

Important caveat: So far, hundreds of patients have been treated with CAR T-cell therapy. We're seeing remarkable response rates, with many patients achieving a "complete" response—meaning that no cancer is detectable in the body with current methods. But the treatments are too new—and patients haven't been followed for a long enough time—to say for sure that the treatments promise a cure.

HOW IT WORKS

Except for cases for which FDA-approved CAR T-cell therapy now is available (see next page), adult patients who are eligible for this treatment receive it by participating in a clinical trial. They report to a laboratory or clinic, where they undergo a four-to-six-hour process to collect blood cells, which are then sent to a company that reengineers the patient's T-cells, giving them the ability to recognize a protein (for example, CD19) on the surface of blood-cancer cells. The engineering process takes two to four weeks.

The patients are given several days of routine chemotherapy. After that, the engineered T-cells are given back to the patient via infusion. This treatment, which takes about 15 minutes, usually is administered just once, though some studies allow a second infusion if there is a partial response or relapse. The cell infusion and period of observation thereafter are typically done on an inpatient basis.

The reengineered cells circulate throughout the body and quickly begin to multiply and attack the tumor cells. Even though it's hoped that the reengineered cells will stay active in the body indefinitely, it's too early to know if this will happen. The cells might last for six months, 12 months...or forever.

NOT RISK-FREE

With the treatment beginning to get FDA approval, it is expected to be very expensive—possibly costing hundreds of thousands of dollars. At this point, it's unclear the extent to which insurance will cover the cost.

For now, the CAR T-cell treatments are somewhat risky. The genetically altered T-cells, when activated by cancer cells, can trigger a condition known as cytokine release syndrome. Many patients experience intense flulike symptoms, including a high fever, aches and fatigue. About 10% to 15% will get sick enough that they require ICU-level care, but these side effects can be treated with steroids and other drugs. Mild-to-severe confusion may develop in up to 30% of patients. While this too is reversible, there have been cases of fatal brain swelling.

The cardiac stress and respiratory distress due to the "inflammatory cascade" that is triggered by the treatment also can be life-threatening. The risks will undoubtedly decline as doctors gain more experience with the therapy.

HOW TO ACCESS THIS THERAPY...

Latest development: Based on the results of trials of CAR T-cells in children and young adults with acute lymphoblastic leukemia, in August 2017, the FDA approved a CD19-targeted CAR T-cell therapy called *tisagenlecleucel* (Kymriah). In October 2017, a second CAR T-cell therapy, *axicabtagene* (Yescarta), was approved for patients with large B-cell lymphomas who have not responded to other treatments.

For patients with lymphoma, leukemia or multiple myeloma for whom an FDA-approved CAR T-cell therapy is not available, a clinical trial may be an option. If your doctor believes that you're a candidate for CAR T-cell therapy, discuss whether it makes sense for you to participate in an ongoing study. Your oncologist can advise you about clinical trials in your area. If accepted into the trial, the CAR T-cell therapy is covered but supportive care is billed to insurance.

Breakthroughs in Lung Cancer

Timothy Burns, MD, PhD, assistant professor of medicine in the department of medicine, Division of Hematology/Oncology, at UPMC Hillman Cancer Center in Pittsburgh, where his laboratory focuses on discovering targeted therapies for lung cancer.

Lung cancer kills more Americans—both smokers and nonsmokers—than colon, breast and prostate cancers combined. But the good news is, treatment options are now extending the lives of many people affected by this formidable disease.

Latest development: Recently announced treatment breakthroughs provide new hope for people with non-small cell lung cancer (NSCLC)—the type of malignancy responsible for 85% of all lung cancers.

THE NEW HEAVY HITTERS

- **Immunotherapy.** Some of the newest treatments for NSCLC are immune checkpoint inhibitors—drugs that energize the immune system to kill cancer cells by blocking one of two cancer-promoting proteins, PD-1 and PD-L1. These drugs include *pembrolizumab* (Keytruda), the immunotherapy treatment credited with saving the life of former President Jimmy Carter when melanoma spread to his brain...*nivolumab* (Opdivo)...*atezolizumab* (Tecentriq)...and *durvalumab* (Imfinzi).

Typically, these drugs are used only as second-line therapies for patients with advanced disease who haven't responded to other types of treatments, such as chemotherapy. But several studies presented at the 2018 annual meeting of the American Association for Cancer Research show that immunotherapy can work as a first-line therapy for people with advanced NSCLC, improving survival.

New scientific findings: A combination of the immunotherapy drug pembrolizumab and chemotherapy worked better than chemo alone as a first-line treatment for patients with metastatic NSCLC—69% were still alive after one year in the combo group, with only 49% alive in the chemo-only group, according to a one-year study published in *The New England Journal of Medicine.*

In a similar one-year study, patients with stage IV lung cancer were given either chemotherapy or two immunotherapy drugs—nivolumab and *ipilimumab* (Yervoy), which blocks CTLA-4, a protein similar to PD-1. Those treated with immunotherapy were 42% less likely to have their disease progress than those who received other treatment.

Meanwhile, research focusing on the use of immunotherapy without chemotherapy as a first-line treatment—reported at a recent meeting of the American Society of Clinical Oncology—also delivered positive results. The stage IV NSCLC patients getting pembrolizumab lived four to eight months longer than those getting chemo. Only 18% of the immunotherapy patients suffered severe side effects, such as inflammation of the lung, liver or colon, versus 41% of those in the chemo group.

Takeaway: With the impressive results of these studies, first-line treatment with an immunotherapy drug with or without chemotherapy is now the standard-of-care for most cases of advanced NSCLC. If a test of your tumor tissue shows that you have a high PD-L1 activity—and one-third of patients with NSCLC do—then single-agent immunotherapy might be the best first treatment for you with or without chemotherapy. Patients whose tumor does not express high levels of this marker still benefit from the combination of immunotherapy with chemotherapy in the majority of cases. Talk to your oncologist.

- **Gene-modulating drugs.** This type of therapy uses drugs to turn off one of several genetic mutations (oncogenes) that can drive lung cancer. As estimated 10% to 20% of NSCLC patients have the epidermal growth factor receptor (EGFR) mutation, which is treated with drugs such as *erlotinib* (Tarceva), *afatinib* (Gilotrif), *gefitinib* (Iressa) and *osimertinib* (Tagrisso). An estimated 5% have the anaplastic lymphoma kinase (ALK) mutation, which is treated with drugs such as *crizotinib* (Xalkori), *ceritinib* (Zykadia), *alectinib* (Alecensa) and *brigatinib* (Alunbrig).

These oral drugs are so powerful that they can, in rare cases, extend life by five years or more. However, the newer and more effective of these drugs—such as alectinib for ALK—has been used as a second-line therapy. Now this treatment paradigm is changing.

New scientific findings: In a study published in 2018, more than 500 NSCLC patients with an EGFR mutation got either osimertinib as a first-line treatment or the previous standard therapy (erlotinib or gefitinib). After 12 months, those taking osimertinib had a 54% lower risk for disease progression or death. In April 2018, the FDA approved osimertinib for first-line treatment of metastatic NSCLC.

In a study of more than 300 metastatic NSCLC patients with the ALK mutation, the disease progressed or death occurred in 41% of those receiving alectinib (a newer more effective drug) compared with 68% receiving crizotinib, an older drug, after about a year and a half. The alectinib group also had fewer side effects. Patients receiving alectinib had control of their tumors for almost three years, on average.

Takeaway: If you are diagnosed with NSCLC, get tested to find out if you have a genetic mutation driving the disease. If you do, talk to your oncologist about the best gene-targeting drug for you—patients with these mutations often do not benefit from immunotherapy.

The liquid biopsy option...

The gold standard for biopsies in NSCLC is a tissue biopsy—removing a portion of the tumor and testing it—to identify the specific type of cancer and genetic mutations that inform treatment decisions.

Problem: In many cases, a tissue biopsy isn't possible—for example, the position of the tumor in the lung or other organ may make it too difficult to biopsy, or the patient may have emphysema.

Solution: A liquid (blood-based) biopsy can be used when a tissue biopsy is not an option. The FDA approved liquid biopsy for lung cancer in 2016. A recent study published in *JAMA Oncology* suggests that combining liquid biopsies with tumor biopsies can improve the chance of finding a targetable mutation. Ask your oncologist if this is right for you. FoundationOne and Guardant360 are the two most widely used liquid biopsies.

9 Ways to Prevent Breast Cancer—Before and After Menopause

Anne McTiernan, MD, PhD, research professor at Fred Hutchinson Cancer Research Center in Seattle, Washington, and author of *Starved: A Nutrition Doctor's Journey from Empty to Full.*

What are the most effective things women can do to avoid getting breast cancer? A team of researchers at the World Cancer Research Fund asked that question. Here's what they found.

Background: Every year, 315,000 American women are newly diagnosed with breast cancer. Although new treatments have improved survival, breast cancer remains the second-leading cause of cancer deaths in American women. Many known risk factors are hard to change—such as getting your first period before age 12...not ever having children or having your first child after age 30... hitting menopause after age 55...a family history of breast cancer...being exposed to high levels of radiation. But many lifestyle factors do make a difference—some, a big difference.

Study: The World Cancer Research Fund International and the American Institute for Cancer Research gathered an international panel of experts to review 119 scientific studies involving 12 million women about the ways diet, weight and physical activity affect a woman's risk of developing breast cancer. They then determined which of those factors protected women the most from getting the disease—both before and after menopause. (Since men account for only 1% of breast cancer cases, the panel limited its recommendations to women.)

Convincing evidence found that...

- **Physical activity and breastfeeding decrease the risk for breast cancer.**
- **Drinking alcohol increases the risk.**
- **Eating certain kinds of vegetables and fruits reduces risk.**

Surprisingly, women who were overweight or obese between the ages of 18 and 30 were less likely to develop breast cancer, either before or after menopause, compared with women who were of normal weight between the ages of 18 and 30. The reasons aren't well understood. But while being overweight or obese throughout adulthood was still associated with less risk for premenopausal breast cancer, a pattern of adult weight gain—defined in different studies as after age 35 or age 50—was strongly associated with increased postmenopausal breast cancer risk.

Bottom line: These evidence-backed lifestyle habits can help prevent breast cancer...

BEFORE MENOPAUSE

- **If you have children, breastfeed if you are able to.** The longer you nurse and the more children you nurse, the more you reduce breast cancer risk thanks to the resulting hormonal changes that reduce estrogen exposure throughout your life.
- **Watch out for weight gain in your 30s, 40s and 50s.** Being overweight before age 30 is protective against breast cancer. But take steps to prevent the weight gain that tends to creep up after age 30.

AFTER MENOPAUSE

• **Redouble efforts to manage your weight.** Once through menopause, obesity increases breast cancer risk by a whopping 40%, according to some studies. Women who get and eliminate breast cancer have a higher chance of their cancer returning and a higher chance of dying of the disease if they are obese.

• **Whittle your waistline.** It's not just how much you weigh, but where weight lodges on your body. Extra fat around your middle can lead to inflammation, increased levels of estrogen (produced by the fat) and higher insulin levels—all of which can set the stage for breast cells to mutate and turn cancerous. It's tough to avoid turning apple-shaped after menopause. Try to keep your waist measurement less than 32 inches by eating healthy foods and staying active.

AT EVERY AGE

These lifestyle factors can help prevent breast cancer throughout life—and it's never too late to start them…

• **Curb your drinking.** Even one drink a day increases breast cancer risk by 5% if you're premenopausal —and by 9% if you're postmenopausal. Each additional daily drink increases risk, on average, by the same percentages. So if you like to have a glass of wine with a meal, do not pour more than five ounces—that is one drink.

• **Step up your activity level.** Any type of exercise reduces breast cancer risk. Aim for about 30 minutes at least five days a week. While moderately-intense activity such as brisk walking counts, exercising vigorously—running versus walking, kickboxing versus yoga—is particularly protective.

Higher-intensity workouts not only help you get rid of harmful belly fat but also boost the immune system so your body is better able to kill mutating cells before they form a tumor. (Exercise also can improve outcomes for people who have cancer, research finds.)

• **Get your calcium.** Diets rich in calcium protect against breast cancer both before and after menopause.

One reason: Calcium helps regulate cell growth, especially in breast tissue.

• **Load up on nonstarchy veggies.** There is evidence that eating nonstarchy vegetables—such as broccoli, leafy greens, summer squash, asparagus, tomatoes—is especially helpful in reducing the risk of estrogen-negative breast cancer, which tends to grow at a faster rate than hormone-positive cancers. Aim for at least one cup a day. (Starchy veggies such as potatoes don't count.)

• **Eat your carotenoids.** When choosing fruits and vegetables, go for color. Animal and test-tube studies have shown that carotenoids—fat-soluble pigments that give produce its coloring—have protective properties. Choose red, orange and yellow fruits and vegetables such as berries, beets, peppers and carrots.

How much can these healthy lifestyle habits help reduce breast cancer risk? By about one-third, the researchers estimate. That would be about 100,000 US women every year.

An Inside Look at BRCA-Related Cancer

Pamela N. Munster, MD, professor of medicine at University of California, San Francisco, where she is leader of the Helen Diller Family Comprehensive Cancer Center and coleader of the Center for BRCA Research. She is author of *Twisting Fate: My Journey with BRCA—from Breast Cancer Doctor to Patient and Back.*

In 2012, Pamela N. Munster, MD, was discussing a new breast cancer medication with a colleague when her phone vibrated. The voice on the other end told the BRCA expert that multiple "irregularities" had been detected on her own breast scan.

At age 48, Dr. Munster was diagnosed with an early form of breast cancer…subsequent genetic testing revealed she was BRCA2 positive, meaning that she was far more likely to develop breast cancer and ovarian cancer than the general population. She went from doctor to patient, undergoing treatment and recovery, to then see her father get diagnosed with a BRCA-related pancreatic cancer.

Here, she shares the details of her experience, along with important facts about the BRCA genetic mutation that could save your life or the life of someone you love.

The 411 on BRCA: Everybody has two copies of the BRCA1 and BRCA2 genes. Their everyday role is to produce special tumor-suppressing proteins that help to repair any DNA damage that occurs constantly as part of a normal process in all cells.

Problems can arise when either of these two genes is abnormal. A faulty BRCA gene can allow DNA damage to go unrepaired and give cancer more opportunities to develop. For reasons that are not yet completely clear, BRCA genes are particularly important in certain tissues causing specific cancers.

A woman with a BRCA mutation has a 60% to 80% lifetime risk of developing breast cancer, compared with 12% for the average woman. Her lifetime ovarian cancer risk is also higher—about 40% to 50% for those with a BRCA1 mutation and approximately 20% to 30% for those with a BRCA2 mutation, compared with less than 2% for the average woman.

An underrecognized problem: Men can carry BRCA mutations, too, driving their lifetime breast cancer risk up to 5% to 10% versus 0.1% for the average man. They are also seven times more likely to develop prostate cancer, often a very aggressive form and at an earlier age than usual.

A study presented at the 2017 Annual Scientific Meeting of the American Urological Association found that men with BRCA mutations are also at greater risk of developing multiple other types of cancer. Particularly, BRCA2 mutations are linked to skin, pancreatic, digestive tract and colorectal cancers. Women with BRCA2 mutations also are at increased risk for these cancers.

Criteria for getting tested: Many people think, "My mother didn't have breast cancer, so I don't have to worry." But anyone with a BRCA1 or BRCA2 mutation, male or female, can pass it on to their daughters and sons, who will each have a 50% chance of inheriting the mutation, and the cancer doesn't necessarily need to be in an immediate relative for you to have a mutation. *Consider BRCA mutation testing if you...*

- **Have a relative,** on either side, who was diagnosed with breast cancer before age 50, had cancer in both breasts or was a male with breast cancer.
- **Have both breast and ovarian cancers in your family,** on either side, especially multiple people with breast cancer, or if you're of Ashkenazi Jewish descent.
- **Have any relative with pancreatic cancer** or male relatives with prostate cancer at a younger age.
- **Are adopted or have few close relatives** and therefore an unknown or limited family medical history.

It's never too late for testing. Once I tested positive, I knew it had to be from my dad or my mom. So I encouraged my then-78-year-old father to get tested. His own mother survived breast cancer in her 60s, so my mutation was likely passed down through him. He tested positive for the BRCA2 mutation.

One year later, he began complaining of unexplained abdominal pain. This vague symptom might be waved off in most patients, but knowing his BRCA status and increased cancer risk, I urged him to get a full workup. An MRI revealed pancreatic cancer, with a large tumor that was deemed inoperable. But because he received a chemo targeted to BRCA tumors, despite his age, his tumor shrunk by half, rendering it operable. He just surpassed his five-year survival mark.

Given the high lifetime risk for breast cancer in BRCA mutation carriers, prophylactic mastectomy or very close monitoring is suggested. When it comes to ovarian cancer, most women with a BRCA mutation will opt to have their ovaries removed once they have completed childbearing. If you're past menopause and have already gone through the changes that come from the loss of estrogen, the effects of the surgery may be more tolerable. Hormone replacement therapy may ease the transition for those undergoing the surgery in their 30s or 40s.

Be cautious with at-home tests. Last year, the FDA approved 23andMe's direct-to-consumer BRCA test. While advances have been made in this field, there can be perils. You may not want to find out potentially life-altering news for yourself and your family via mail without the counseling and support of a health-care provider who can put the relevance of your mutation into perspective or refer you to a clinic for screening and prophylactic surgeries if you indeed carry a mutation.

Also, many tests only screen for certain mutations—23andMe screens for three mutations in the BRCA1 and BRCA2 genes out of more than 1,000. These three variants are almost exclusively found in the Ashkenazi Jewish population. So if you are of another ethnicity, your results will likely come back negative even if you are, in fact, BRCA positive. I'm of Swiss-French ancestry, and my own 23andMe results showed no BRCA mutations.

Bottom line: Consult a specialist for a full screening if you want testing. Find one via the National Society of Genetic Counselors at NSGC.org/page/find-a-genetic-counselor. Insurance covers testing if you meet certain criteria such as a family history of breast cancer.

Plant-Based Diet Increases Breast Cancer Survival

Susan E. McCann, PhD, RD, associate member, Division of Cancer Prevention and Population Sciences, Roswell Park Cancer Institute, Buffalo, New York.

We already know that plant-rich diets are rich in health benefits, but it's always a pleasure to see research supporting the evidence as to when and why it matters, since it serves to reinforce the fact that enhancing wellness can measurably improve our health, even in the face of disease. A recent study demonstrated that lignans, a class of chemicals in such foods as seeds, whole grains, fruits and vegetables, may contribute to survival in women with breast cancer. Researchers from Roswell Park Cancer Institute in Buffalo, New York, asked 1,122 women who had been diagnosed with breast cancer between 1996 and 2001 to answer a questionnaire concerning their intake of more than 100 foods. The results showed that postmenopausal patients who ate a high-lignan diet were about 70% less likely to die from the cancer. Curiously, lignan intake didn't make a difference in survival among premenopausal women.

WHY DID SOME WOMEN LIVE LONGER?

Susan E. McCann, PhD, RD, in the Division of Cancer Prevention and Population Sciences, was the lead study author. She acknowledged there are several possible alternate explanations for the difference in survival between pre- and postmenopausal women—for instance, in younger women, breast cancer often is especially aggressive. Also, the fact that there were fewer of these younger, pre-menopausal women in the study may have affected the statistical significance of the results. Then again, she says, the younger women reported eating fewer lignans—and perhaps this is what made the difference in survival odds. Previous studies have shown lignans inhibit tumor growth by preventing fresh blood vessels from forming in them and interfering with growth factors that help fuel them.

But might a high-lignan intake help prevent cancer from developing in the first place? Interestingly, several small studies have shown this may help protect premenopausal women against breast cancer, but Dr. McCann says that the findings overall are inconsistent. For example, she did a study that showed lignans seemed to help protect women with genetic susceptibility to breast cancer, which some other studies replicated... and others did not. Dr. McCann is now conducting new research to investigate further what properties of lignans contribute to their cancer-fighting effectiveness.

PLAN TO BE A PLANT-EATER

A wide variety of foods contain lignans. Flax seeds are rich in them, but lignans are present as well in wheat, oats, barley and rye, fruit (especially berries), legumes, seeds (pumpkin and sesame, for example), a wide variety of vegetables, tea and even coffee, which after all starts out as a bean. Dr. McCann says that researchers are currently investigating more about the question of lignan intake and cancer, but in the meantime, you can pick from any number of reasons to eat lots of lignans—in addition to possible cancer protection, doing so will make it easier to maintain a normal weight, keep diabetes under control and help protect against a host of other chronic diseases.

Better Ovarian Cancer Detection

Edward J. Pavlik, PhD, director, Ovarian Screening Research Program, University of Kentucky, Lexington.

Among 37,000 healthy women (average age 57) who took part in studies to investigate the effectiveness of transvaginal ultrasound screening, 72 ovarian cancers were detected. Of these, 70% were early stage, and 88% of these women had a five-year survival rate, compared with about 50% of unscreened women who were diagnosed with ovarian cancer.

Theory: Ultrasound detects changes in size and structure of the ovary. Women at risk for ovarian cancer (due to family history, for example) should discuss transvaginal screening with their doctors.

PSA Screening Support

Ruth B. Etzioni, PhD, is an epidemiologist at Fred Hutchinson Cancer Research Center, Seattle.

New research offers support for PSA screening. Two major PSA studies show that prostate-cancer screening may reduce the chance of dying from that cancer by 25% to 30%. But the chance of being overdiagnosed is about five times the chance of having one's life saved—this can lead to unneeded, potentially harmful treatments. Men should be screened if they are willing to consider not being treated—a low-risk prostate cancer may be better left alone.

Moderate Exercise Boosts Cancer Treatment

Study led by researchers at Kansas State University, Manhattan, published in *Journal of the National Cancer Institute*.

Regular activities that use 30% to 60% of a patient's aerobic capacity—not less and not more—can make radiation treatment for cancer more effective by enhancing oxygen delivery and blood flow to the tumors. Examples of this type of exercise are a brisk walk or a slow jog. Too much exercise may have a negative impact by shutting down blood flow to the tumor region or harming the immune system. Each patient should talk to his/her doctor for specific recommendations.

For Prostate Cancer, Continuous Treatment Beats Intermittent Therapy

Maha Hussain, MD, FACP, professor and associate director for clinical research, University of Michigan Comprehensive Cancer Center, Ann Arbor. Her study was published in *The New England Journal of Medicine*.

For men with advanced prostate cancer, androgen deprivation therapy helps control the disease for a period of time—but this treatment also causes troublesome side effects. To limit the side effects, many men opt for intermittent rather than continuous therapy.

But: What do these patients gain in terms of quality of life...and what do they lose in terms of how long they live?

A new study provides answers that could dramatically alter doctors' treatment recommendations and patients' decisions about how to fight their prostate cancer. *Here's why...*

ON AGAIN, OFF AGAIN?

Background: Male hormones (androgens) fuel the growth of most types of prostate cancer. The point of androgen deprivation therapy is to coax advanced prostate cancer into shrinking by using drugs that either block androgens from being used by the body or that stop the production of androgens altogether. The side effects include hot flashes, decreased libido, thinning bones and increased risk for cardiovascular problems. Men who are wary of or unable to tolerate these side effects often choose to take the drugs only when their cancer shows signs of increased activity...and to halt the therapy when cancer activity wanes.

Researchers wanted to gauge the pros and cons of this intermittent approach as compared with the standard continuous therapy. The study included 1,535 men with newly diagnosed, advanced prostate cancer that had spread outside of the prostate gland. Prior to treatment, the men had their baseline prostate-specific antigen (PSA) levels measured. PSA is a protein produced by the prostate gland, with higher levels generally correlating to higher prostate cancer risk and/or increased prostate cancer activity.

All the participants underwent seven months of androgen deprivation therapy. Then, those whose PSA had declined to a score of four or less were randomly assigned to one of two groups (this point was called the "time of randomization"). Half of the men were placed in the continuous-therapy group, so their treatment continued nonstop. The other half were assigned to the intermittent-therapy group, so their treatment was halted at the time of randomization—but whenever a patient's PSA rose back up to his baseline level or to 20 (whichever was lower), that patient resumed his androgen deprivation therapy. For members of the intermittent group, this on-again, off-again treatment continued based on individual PSA scores.

The patients were followed for up to 10 years. Men in the intermittent group ended up receiving treatment about 47% of the time during the study period. Also, at various times during the study, all the men answered questions about their quality of life in five areas—erectile function, libido, vitality, physical functioning and mental health.

REVEALING RESULTS

Over the course of the study, 928 of the original 1,535 participants died, most from their prostate cancer. Among those in the continuous-therapy group, 58% died...while among those in the intermittent group, 63% died. The group that received continuous therapy had a median survival period of 5.8 years from the time of the randomization, while the group that received intermittent therapy had a median survival period of 5.1 years. That difference in survival time is not huge—but it's certainly something that patients would want to be aware of.

And what about those tough-to-tolerate side effects of androgen deprivation therapy? Men in the intermittent group did experience modest, temporary improvements in some aspects of quality of life when they put the therapy on pause after that initial seven-month course of treatment. For instance, three months later, they reported fewer erectile problems and better mental health. However, by nine months and again 15 months later, the quality-of-life improvements they reported were so minor that the researchers deemed them "not statistically significant." Meanwhile, the rates of serious physical side effects (such as cardiovascular events) were similar in both groups—30.4% of the intermittent group and 32.7% of the continuous group.

What this means: The totality of the data from this study and another smaller clinical trial indicate that intermittent therapy is not as promising as once thought. For men with advanced prostate cancer, the benefits in terms of reduced side effects from intermittent androgen deprivation therapy are modest, given the potential for improved longevity with continuous treatment. Patients will want to discuss the pros and cons of each therapy schedule with their doctors in light of this new information—and some may find the drugs' side effects easier to tolerate over time once they consider the likely advantages in terms of time gained.

New Prostate Cancer Test

Alison L. Allan, PhD, associate professor of oncology, Schulich School of Medicine and Dentistry, Western University, London, Ontario, Canada.

A new blood test, which reveals whether a patient's circulating tumor cells contain the protein AR-V7, determines the most effective treatment for patients with advanced prostate cancer. Participants who tested positive for AR-V7 survived twice as long when they were treated with a specific chemotherapy than with hormone-targeting therapy, the two standard treatments. Those who tested negative for the protein lived seven months longer when they took the hormone-targeting drugs, compared with chemotherapy.

4 Dangerous Myths About Testicular Cancer

Ajay Nangia, MD, professor of urology at University of Kansas Medical Center, with a practice at the University of Kansas Hospital, both in Kansas City. He is a leading male infertility specialist

Women learn early about breast cancer. It's got ribbons and races. But men tend to know almost nothing about testicular cancer...and some of what they think they know is actually wrong—which could be putting their health and even their lives in danger. *Here's the truth regarding four common myths about this male cancer...*

***MYTH #1*: Testicular cancer is mostly a problem for older men.**

Truth: Not even in the ballpark. Even though prostate cancer rates rise with age, especially after age 60, the majority of the approximately 8,850 cases of testicular cancer diagnosed each year in the US are found in men ages 15 to 40. It's the most common cancer to strike young men. It does occur in older men, though—about 7% of new cases are in men over age 55.

***MYTH #2:* Testicular cancer is less "serious" than other types of cancers.**

Truth: Testicular cancer does have a relatively high cure rate—even if the cancer has spread. The five-year survival rate is 95%. When caught early and localized to the testicles, it's 99%. If it has spread to nearby tissue and/or lymph nodes, the survival rate is 96%. Even if the cancer has spread to other parts of the body, the five-year survival rate is 73%.

But these reassuring statistics mask the bigger truth that this is indeed a serious cancer. For starters, testicular cancer can't be easily diagnosed via a biopsy—the removal of a tiny piece of a potentially cancerous tissue for testing—because it could cause the cancer to spread.

Note: Biopsies do not cause most other types of cancer to spread.

So if symptoms (see the next page) or a physical exam lead to a suspicion of testicular cancer, and serum tumor marker blood tests and testicular ultrasound also point to cancer, an accurate diagnosis often involves removing the entire affected testicle—a procedure called radical inguinal orchiectomy.

That's traumatic enough...leaving men self-conscious about their altered appearance. Then there's chemotherapy or radiation, and sometimes a second surgery to remove nearby lymph nodes.

What's more, both the cancer itself and treatment (especially chemotherapy) can lead to infertility—even in the 97% of cases in which only one testicle is removed. As a result, men who may wish to father children in the future are advised to bank sperm before treatment—or if they haven't, to wait for a year or two after chemo before attempting impregnation to reduce the likelihood of having DNA-damaged sperm.

Finally, sexual performance may be affected. Treatment often leads to low testosterone levels, which can increase the risk for high cholesterol and high blood pressure—and erectile dysfunction.

***MYTH #3:* Injuring your testicles ups your chances of getting testicular cancer.**

Truth: There's no evidence that a swift kick or some other assault you-know-where impacts your testicular cancer risk. Nor will certain sexual practices, having a vasectomy or infection with human papillomavirus (HPV) increase your risk.

What are the risk factors? There's a strong genetic link, so family history matters. Being born with an undescended testicle also is a risk factor.

Sophisticated new genetic tests can help identify, for example, the risk that a man born with undescended testicles actually has of developing the cancer. Unfortunately, there are no preventive steps a man can take.

***MYTH #4:* Testicular self-exams are a waste of time and effort.**

Truth: This is where there's some disagreement. The US Preventive Services Task Force (USPSTF), an independent panel of national experts that makes recommendations about health-screening practices, has concluded from a review of studies that the benefit of self-exams is small. But I, along with many other doctors in the field, disagree. The USPSTF's rationale is that there's no evidence that self-examination is effective at reducing mortality. Even without screening, if testicular cancer is discovered, "current treatment options provide very favorable health outcomes." But I see men who are dealing with the aftermath of testicular cancer, chemotherapy and/or surgery, and who are infertile and regret not having frozen their sperm. Plus, what harm is there in doing something that's free and can be handled, so to speak, in the shower?

HOW TO DO A TESTICULAR SELF-EXAM

Testicular self-exams are easy and painless. The hardest part is remembering to do it once a month. *Here are some guidelines from the Testicular Cancer Society...*

1. Do the exam during or right after a warm shower or bath, when the scrotum is most relaxed and easy to examine by hand.

2. Use both hands to examine each testicle. Place your index and middle fingers on the underside and your thumbs on top. Firmly yet gently roll the testicle between your thumbs and fingers to check for surface or texture irregularities (see next column).

3. Find the epididymis, a rope-like structure on the back of the testicle. Become familiar with how it feels so you won't mistake it for a lump.

4. If you do the exam outside the shower, stand in front of a mirror and check for any visible swelling of the skin on your scrotum. It's not essential but provides an additional check.

5. If you notice irregularities or changes in your testicles, make an appointment to see your doctor as soon as possible.

TESTICULAR CANCER SYMPTOMS

Testicular cancer is often diagnosed when a man notices something unusual and goes to his doctor. *If you have any of these signs, it's best to get checked out...*

- **A painless lump or swelling,** usually hard, on the surface of either testicle.
- **A dull ache in the lower abdomen or in the groin**—especially if it lasts for more than an hour. It could be something else such as an infection or a physical twisting, but it's worth checking out, even going to the ER. Most guys wait too long—hours, days or even months!
- **A sudden buildup of fluid in the scrotum,** forming a soft or hard swelling.
- **Pain or discomfort in a testicle or in the scrotum.**

Eat Omega-3s

Theodore M. Brasky, PhD, is a cancer epidemiologist in the Public Health Sciences Division of the Fred Hutchinson Cancer Research Center, Seattle, and leader of a study published in *American Journal of Epidemiology*.

Men should not change their diets despite recent findings that omega-3 fatty acids increase risk for aggressive prostate cancer...and trans-fatty acids reduce risk, says Theodore M. Brasky, PhD. These findings are contrary to what researchers would have expected, because omega-3 fatty acids typically are good for the heart...and trans-fatty acids are linked to inflammation and heart disease.

Reality: Men's risk of dying from heart disease is so much greater than their risk of dying from aggressive prostate cancer that a diet high in omega-3s and low in trans-fatty acids still is best for most men.

Deadly Melanoma: Best Prevention, Detection and Treatment Breakthroughs

Albert Lefkovits, MD, an associate clinical professor of dermatology at Mount Sinai School of Medicine and codirector of the Mount Sinai Dermatological Cosmetic Surgery Program, both in New York City. He is a member of the Medical Advisory Council of The Skin Cancer Foundation and a past-president of the Dermatology Society of Greater New York.

Melanoma is the most dangerous form of skin cancer. It's particularly frightening because it's more likely than other cancers to spread (metastasize) to other parts of the body. More than 76,000 Americans are diagnosed with melanoma each year, and between 8,000 and 9,000 will die from it.

Good news: New technology increases the chances that a melanoma will be detected early—and when it is, you have a 95% to 97% chance of surviving. The prognosis is worse after the disease has spread, but two new drugs can significantly increase survival times—and medications that may be even more effective already are in the pipeline.

WHO'S AT RISK?

A study published in *Journal of Investigative Dermatology* found that melanoma rates increased by 3.1% annually between 1992 and 2004—and the incidence continues to rise.

The increase is due to several reasons. The US population is aging, and older adults are more likely to get melanoma (though it is a leading cause of cancer death in young adults). Public-awareness campaigns have increased the rate of cancer screenings (though officials would like the screening rates to be even higher), and more screenings mean an increase in melanoma diagnoses.

If you are a fair-skinned Caucasian, your lifetime risk of getting melanoma is about one in 50. The risk is lower among African Americans, Hispanics and Asians, but they're more likely to die from it because they often develop cancers on "hidden" areas (such as the soles of the feet), where skin changes aren't readily apparent.

Important: Don't be complacent just because you avoid the sun or use sunscreen. Many cancers appear in areas that aren't exposed to the sun, such as between the toes or around the anus.

STATE-OF-THE-ART SCREENING

Melanomas grow slowly. Patients who get an annual skin checkup are more likely to get an early diagnosis than those who see a doctor only when a mole or skin change is clearly abnormal.

Doctors used to depend on their eyes (and sometimes a magnifying glass) to examine suspicious areas. But eyes-only examinations can identify melanomas only about 60% of the time.

Better: An exam called epiluminescence microscopy. The doctor takes photographs of large areas of skin. Then he/she uses a device that magnifies suspicious areas in the photos. The accuracy of detecting melanomas with this technique is about 90%.

The technology also allows doctors to look for particular changes, such as certain colors or a streaked or globular appearance, that indicate whether a skin change is malignant or benign. This can reduce unnecessary biopsies.

Few private-practice physicians can afford the equipment that's used for these exams. You might want to get your checkups at a medical center or dermatology practice that specializes in early melanoma detection. If this isn't possible, ask your doctor if he/she uses a handheld dermatoscope. It's a less expensive device that's still superior to the unaided eye.

NEW TREATMENTS

In the last two years, the FDA has approved two medications for patients with late-stage melanoma. These drugs don't cure the disease but can help patients live longer.

- ***Ipilimumab* (Yervoy)** is a biologic medication, a type of synthetic antibody that blocks a cellular "switch" that turns off the body's ability to fight cancer. A study of 676 patients with late-stage melanoma found that those who took the drug survived, on average, for 10 months after starting treatment, compared with 6.4 months for those in a control group.
- ***Vemurafenib* (Zelboraf)** may double the survival time of patients with advanced melanoma. It

works by targeting a mutation in the BRAF V600E gene, which is present in about 50% of melanoma patients. Researchers who conducted a study published in *The New England Journal of Medicine* found that more than half of patients who took the medication had at least a 30% reduction in tumor size. In about one-third of patients, the medication slowed or stopped the progression of the cancer.

- **Combination treatment.** Each of these medications attacks tumors in different ways. They can be used in tandem for better results. For example, a patient might start by taking the first drug, then, when it stops working, he/she can switch to the second drug. This approach can potentially extend survival by up to a year.

Both drugs can have serious side effects. For now, they're recommended only for a select group of patients.

SELF-PROTECTION

Take steps to protect yourself...

- **Check your skin monthly.** It's been estimated that deaths from melanoma could be reduced by 60% if everyone would do a monthly skin exam to look for suspicious changes. Look for asymmetric moles in which one part is distinctly different from the other part...moles with an irregular border... color variations...a diameter greater than 6 millimeters (mm), about one-quarter inch...or changes in appearance over time.

- **Get a yearly checkup with a dermatologist.** It's nearly impossible to self-inspect all of the areas on your body where melanoma can appear. I advise patients to see a dermatologist every year for full-body mapping. The doctor will make a note (or photograph) of every suspicious area and track the areas over time.

Important: New moles rarely appear in people over the age of 40. A mole that appears in patients 40 years and older is assumed to be cancer until tests show otherwise.

- **Use a lot of sunscreen.** Even though melanoma isn't caused only by sun exposure, don't get careless. Apply a sunscreen with an SPF of at least 30 whenever you go outdoors. Use a lot of sunscreen—it takes about two ounces of sunscreen (about the amount in a shot glass) to protect against skin cancer. Reapply it about every two hours or immediately after getting out of the water.

- **Don't use tanning salons.** Researchers who published a study in *Journal of the National Cancer Institute* found that people who got their tans at tanning salons—that use tanning lamps and tanning beds that emit UV radiation—at least once a month were 55% more likely to develop a malignant melanoma than those who didn't artificially tan.

Get an Extra Edge Against Cancer

Mark A. Stengler, NMD, a naturopathic physician and founder of The Stengler Center for Integrative Medicine in Encinitas, California (MarkStengler.com). He has served on a medical advisory committee for the Yale University Complementary Medicine Outcomes Research Project and is author of *Outside the Box Cancer Therapies: Alternative Therapies That Treat and Prevent Cancer* and coauthor of *Prescription for Natural Cures and Prescription for Drug Alternatives* (both from Bottom Line Books, BottomLineStore.com).

More than one-third of American adults reach for vitamins, herbs or other natural medicines when they have colds or other routine (and hopefully mild) health problems. Similar remedies can help when you have cancer.

To learn more about the best and safest ways to use natural therapies—also known as complementary and alternative medicine (CAM)—to fight cancer and its complications, we spoke with Mark A. Stengler, NMD, a naturopathic physician who treats cancer patients.

HOW CAM CAN WORK

Research has shown that many so-called "alternative" treatments can enhance the effects of conventional cancer care such as surgery, radiation or chemotherapy...reduce treatment side effects...and possibly improve survival.

This type of integrative care doesn't replace conventional cancer treatments. Rather, with the guidance of a doctor, complementary therapies are added to a patient's treatment plan.

Important: To ensure that the therapies described below would be appropriate for you, consult the Society for Integrative Oncology (IntegrativeOnc.org) to find an integrative oncologist near you...or check with The American Association of Naturopathic Physicians (Naturopathic.org) to locate a naturopathic doctor who also treats cancer patients.

Also: Be sure to ask the doctor you choose to be in touch with your oncologist. *Here's how CAM can help with problems that plague most cancer patients...*

• **Get relief from "chemo brain."** It's estimated that three-quarters of cancer patients will experience some degree of mental cloudiness. Known as "chemo brain," it can include mood swings, memory loss and mental fatigue. It eventually improves, but some patients will feel like they're in a mental fog years after their treatments have ended.

What helps: The omega-3 fatty acids in fish oil supplements—a typical daily dose is 1,000 mg total of *eicosapentaenoic acid* (EPA) and *docosahexaenoic acid* (DHA) combined—help regulate acetylcholine, a neurotransmitter that increases nerve growth factor and improves memory as well as energy levels.

The omega-3s also increase the effectiveness of 5-fluorouracil and other chemotherapy drugs, according to a study published in *Clinical Nutrition Research*. In research published in *Cancer*, lung cancer patients who took fish oil along with chemotherapy had a greater one-year survival rate than those who didn't take the supplements.

Note: Fish oil may cause stomach upset in some patients, along with bleeding in those who are taking anticoagulant medications such as *warfarin* (Coumadin), *apixaban* (Eliquis) and *rivaroxaban* (Xarelto).

• **Boost energy levels.** Ginseng is one of the more effective supplements for cancer patients. A number of studies have shown that it reduces treatment-related side effects, including weakness and fatigue. A double-blind study in *Journal of the National Cancer Institute* found that patients who took ginseng had less fatigue than those given placebos.

My advice: The American form of ginseng (*Panax quinquefolius*) is more effective than the Asian form.

Typical dose: 1,300 mg to 2,000 mg daily. It rarely causes side effects, although it may lower blood sugar in those with diabetes.

Also helpful: Glutathione, a "super antioxidant" that can be combined with chemotherapy to reduce toxin-related fatigue and other side effects. It's usually given in an IV solution. Side effects are unlikely, but it may interfere with some chemotherapy drugs. Be sure to consult an integrative oncologist to see whether you will/won't benefit from glutathione.

• **Improve immune response.** Turkey tail is one of the best-studied medicinal mushrooms. Available in capsule form, the supplement has chemical compounds (beta-glucans) that stimulate many aspects of the immune response, including antibody activity—important for inducing the death of cancer cells.

Impressive research: A study published in *Cancer Immunology and Immunotherapy* found that post-surgical remissions in colorectal cancer patients were twice as common in those who were given turkey tail.

Typical dose: 3,000 mg daily. Side effects are unlikely.

A NUTRITIONAL BOOST

Conventional oncologists receive little training in nutrition, but it's a critical issue for cancer patients. One study found that 91% of cancer patients had nutritional impairments, and 9% were seriously malnourished. Research shows that malnutrition contributes directly or indirectly to a significant number of cancer deaths due to poor appetite and the disease process of advanced cancer.

Loss of appetite is a major cause of malnutrition and muscle loss (cachexia). I advise patients who are losing weight to address these problems by getting more calories.

With every meal, include high-fat foods such as olive oil, coconut oil, avocado, nuts and seeds. A 10-year study, published in *Archives of Internal Medicine*, looked at more than 380,000 adults and found that a Mediterranean-style diet, which is high in olive oil and other healthy fats, reduced cancer deaths in men by 17% and 12% in women.

Also helpful: Protein shakes. They can provide the extra protein that's critical for cancer patients. Up to 80% of those with advanced cancer experience muscle loss. Protein shakes can help reverse it.

Best option: Ready-made whey protein or pea protein shakes—both are nutritious, have 5 g of sugar or less per serving and are readily available in health-food stores.

My advice: Get 1 g to 1.2 g of protein per kilogram (2.2 pounds) of body weight daily. This means that someone who weighs 150 pounds will need about 68 g to 82 g of protein daily. You can get that much from two or three servings of a typical whey protein beverage, which comes ready-mixed or in powdered form.

Caution: If you have moderate or severe kidney disease, check with your doctor for advice on your protein intake.

The Sugar–Cancer Link

Patrick Quillin, PhD, RD, CNS, a clinical nutritionist who served for 10 years as director of nutrition for Cancer Treatment Centers of America, CancerCenter.com. Currently CEO of American Eagle Nutrition in Carlsbad, California, he is the author of numerous books, including *Beating Cancer with Nutrition* and also edited the textbook *Adjuvant Nutrition in Cancer Treatment*.

With all the negative publicity that high-fructose corn syrup (HFCS) has been getting, an increasing number of food and beverage manufacturers are beginning to replace the processed sweetener with old-fashioned white sugar in products ranging from tomato sauce and soft drinks to salad dressing and bread.

But is sugar really more healthful than HFCS? The truth is, it can be harmful as well.

That's because every time a person eats a gooey donut packed with sugar or downs some other refined carbohydrate, such as a fluffy roll packed with bleached white flour, it can wreak havoc with his/her blood sugar (glucose) levels. We all know that elevated glucose levels can result in diabetes, but that's not the only risk.

Latest development: There is growing scientific evidence that consistently high levels of blood sugar may be linked to an increased risk for, and faster progression of, some cancers.

What you need to know: Reducing one's intake of any type of processed sugar and refined carbohydrates could reduce cancer risk and enhance cancer treatments in those battling the disease, according to many experts. Interestingly, the nutrients in fresh and frozen fruit, which are high in natural sugar, have been linked to reduced cancer risk.

KEY RESEARCH FINDINGS

Important studies have linked high blood glucose levels with...

- **Liver, gallbladder and other cancers.** In a study that appeared in the journal *PLoS Medicine*, Swedish investigators tracked blood glucose and rates of cancer and cancer deaths among more than 500,000 men and women for 10 years.

The researchers found that men with the highest blood glucose levels had a significantly higher risk of developing and dying of such cancers as those of the liver, gallbladder and respiratory tract than those with the lowest glucose levels. Women with the highest glucose levels had an increased risk of developing cancers of the pancreas and bladder and dying of cancers of the pancreas, uterus, cervix and stomach. In general, cancer risk increased right along with blood glucose readings for both men and women.

These risks were independent of body weight—an important point, since doctors have traditionally attributed any potential link between cancer and high intakes of dietary sugar and other refined carbohydrates to obesity, a known risk factor for various cancers.

- **Pancreatic cancer.** In a study published in *Cancer Epidemiology, Biomarkers & Prevention* in 2010, researchers followed more than 60,000 men and women in Singapore for 14 years and found that those who consumed two or more sugared sodas per week had almost twice the risk of developing pancreatic cancer as those who didn't.

The mechanisms linking high sugar intake to increased cancer risk are still being studied. But the likeliest reason is that it leads to higher circulating levels of insulin, as well as a related hormone, known as insulin-like growth factor, both of which scientists think may promote the growth of some cancers, including malignancies of the pancreas and colon.

Elevated blood glucose also suppresses the immune system. Perhaps even more important, cancer cells are believed to feed directly on blood glucose, which means that elevated blood glucose ensures a ready supply of "fuel" for cancer growth.

CANCER-FIGHTING ACTION PLAN

Even though the scientific evidence linking cancer to sugar consumption is not yet definitive, I believe that it's prudent for everyone to take steps to regulate blood glucose levels to reduce cancer risk. It's also wise for cancer patients to follow these steps, as an adjunct to their cancer treatment, to help the disease from progressing. *My advice...*

- **Adopt a low-glycemic-index diet.** Glycemic index (GI) indicates how quickly your digestive tract converts a given food into blood glucose. High-GI foods cause blood glucose (and the insulin production that results) to spike sharply, while lower-GI foods produce a more gradual rise. *What to do...*

  - Reduce your intake of refined simple carbohydrates, most of which have a high GI. Simple carbohydrates include sugared soda, candy and any other foods containing sugars, such as sucrose, fructose, corn syrup, dextrose and maltose...foods containing refined flour, which includes any type of flour not listed as "whole grain," such as white rice and white bread...processed snack foods...and high-GI vegetables, such as white and red potatoes, corn and turnips.

    Important: Do not limit the amount of colorful fruits and vegetables you eat—the fiber in these foods will improve the GI, and their phytochemicals help prevent cancer.

  - Eat more low-GI foods, which are typically high in protein and complex carbohydrates that produce a mild, gradual rise in blood glucose levels.

Good choices include: Legumes...nuts and seeds...low-fat proteins, such as fish, chicken and lean beef (some fatty fish, such as salmon, have fatty acids that may help guard against cancer)...cheese...nonsweetened yogurt...eggs...low-GI vegetables, such as artichokes, asparagus, bell peppers, broccoli, Brussels sprouts, cabbage, cauliflower and onions...and low-GI fruits, such as cherries, grapefruit, plums, apricots and oranges. To check the GI of various foods, consult the Glycemic Index and GI Database website at GlycemicIndex.com.

My advice: If you have cancer and receive intravenous nutrition at any point during your treatment, ask your doctor about receiving a low-glucose solution (40% glucose) to help control your glucose levels and replacing the calories with protein (amino acids) and fats (lipids). The typical IV solution is 75% glucose.

- **Take nutritional supplements.** If you have cancer or are concerned about your cancer risk, ask your doctor about taking magnesium and chromium supplements to help stabilize your blood glucose levels. Also discuss the dosages he considers most beneficial for you.

Important: If you have a chronic medical condition or take any prescription medication, be sure to consult your doctor before taking these or any supplements.

- **Get serious about exercise.** Regular exercise lowers blood glucose (because your muscles burn more glucose during activity) and makes your body more responsive to the blood sugar–regulating properties of insulin. Exercising (ideally, strength training plus a cardio routine, such as brisk walking) for 30 minutes three times a week will have maximum benefit, but any amount of exercise is better than none.

ON THE HORIZON

There's also growing interest among scientists as to whether drugs that affect blood glucose mechanisms can be used to treat cancer. *For example...*

Important finding I: A small study in Japan, which was published in *Cancer Prevention Research*, found that when people with precancerous colorectal cells received a low dose of the diabetes drug *metformin* (Glucophage)—which works, in part, by reducing circulating insulin levels—for one month, these cells were significantly reduced, compared with those in a control group.

More extensive trials of metformin's effects on lung, prostate and breast cancers are now being coordinated by the National Cancer Institute.

Important finding II: In a study published in *The Journal of Biological Chemistry* in 2010, researchers reported that by tweaking the structure of the experimental diabetes drug *ciglitazone*, they produced a compound that killed prostate and breast cancer cells in the lab by preventing glucose from entering the cancer cells and by suppressing their ability to metabolize glucose. More research on the drug is under way.

Remember: If you're getting too much sugar in your diet, diabetes may not be the only potential threat to your health.

Take an Aspirin After Chemo...Live Longer

Study titled "Aspirin in the Treatment of Cancer: Reductions in Metastatic Spread and in Mortality: A Systematic Review and Meta-Analyses of Published Studies" by researchers at Cardiff University, Hywel Dda University Health Board, University of Cambridge, all in the UK, published in *PLOS One*.

Aspirin, already known to reduce risk of getting cancer, may soon become part of the regimen for patients who already have cancer. Researchers at University of Cardiff conducted a meta-analysis of 47 studies—two randomized trials and 42 observational studies—of people with cancers of the breast, bowel and prostate, some of whom took low-dose aspirin in addition to their regular cancer treatment.

Results: For those who had aspirin therapy added at some point to their cancer treatments, their cancers were less likely to spread and, over the five-year period studied, they were 20% less likely to die.

Aspirin has been around for more than 100 years and is one of the most researched medicines in the world. It's easily available, cheap and relatively safe. But it's not risk-free. For one thing, taking aspirin regularly increases the chance for internal bleeding, although the researchers did report that no serious or life-threatening bleeding was reported in the studies that they analyzed.

For someone who is being treated for cancer, the best advice is to discuss with your doctor whether it makes sense to add low-dose aspirin to your treatment plan. Given the strength of the potential benefit, it's an essential conversation.

The Right Team to Treat Your Cancer

Richard A. Ehlers II, MD, associate professor, department of breast surgical oncology and associate vice president in the Division of Houston Area Locations at The University of Texas MD Anderson Cancer Center. He is also adjunct assistant professor in the department of surgery at The University of Texas Medical Branch at Galveston.

If you or a loved one is being treated for cancer, you may not be aware of so-called "tumor boards." But if you're getting care at a major academic or cancer-specific medical center, these regular face-to-face gatherings of cancer specialists—oncologists, radiologists, surgeons, pathologists, psychologists and others—play a key role in assessing individual cases. This may involve reviewing the pathology report...tracking disease progression...and discussing the treatment options for different types of cancer.

What gets reviewed: If your case comes before a tumor board, the doctors likely will address a variety of issues. Is surgery an option or will radiation and/or chemotherapy be more appropriate? If surgery can be done, should it or chemotherapy be used first, followed by other treatments? Is this patient battling mental health issues...or getting the runaround from insurance to get coverage for certain drugs?

HOW TUMOR BOARDS HELP

Cancer care is rarely a straightforward process. From the time you are diagnosed until your treatments end, your care will depend on the opinions of a surprising number of specialists—and good communication among those experts can strongly affect how well you do.

Important recent finding: Among nearly 5,000 patients with colorectal and lung cancers, those whose doctors participated in weekly tumor boards lived longer, according to a study presented at a symposium of the American Society of Clinical Oncology.

To ensure that the medical center where you're being treated relies on a tumor board's guidance, you should seek out a cancer center designated by the National Cancer Institute or accredited by the Commission on Cancer.

Large cancer centers usually have separate tumor boards for different types of cancer. At smaller programs, a single board will review all or most cancer cases.

Tumor boards provide important oversight because what seems like a perfect treatment plan can fall short in real-world circumstances. For example, chemotherapy might be the recommended treatment for a specific cancer, but a tumor-board oncologist might argue that a particular patient isn't healthy enough to withstand the treatment. A psychologist or social worker at a meeting might point out that the patient will need transportation to and from the chemotherapy clinic.

WHO GETS REVIEWED?

At MD Anderson Cancer Center and other large cancer centers, virtually all cases are discussed at a tumor board, although doctors give most of their attention to rare/complicated cases. There's no separate charge to patients for the review.

My advice: If you're not sure that your case has been discussed at your treatment center's tumor board, ask your doctor whether it has been (or will be). Your doctor should not be offended by this question—especially if he/she will be presenting the case. If your case hasn't been reviewed, ask why not. You have the right to request a tumor board review, but it might not be available at a smaller medical center.

Most tumor boards meet weekly or twice a month and are comprised of a dozen or more specialists, including surgeons, medical oncologists, radiation oncologists and pathologists. Depending on the cancer, other doctors—gynecologists, urologists, etc.—may participate. Meetings often include a nutritionist, nurses, mental health experts and a social worker.

THE BENEFITS

Your case might go before a tumor board prior to treatment...after a preliminary treatment plan has been initiated...or during treatment when there is an important change in clinical circumstances.

Important finding: When the records of more than 200 pancreatic cancer patients collected from various institutions without tumor boards were later evaluated by a panel at Johns Hopkins University School of Medicine that included medical and radiation oncologists, surgical oncologists, pathologists and other experts, treatment changes were recommended in nearly 25% of these cases.

Research also shows that patients tend to have better outcomes in terms of treatment responsiveness, recovery times and survival, among other factors, when their cases are discussed at a tumor board.

Also: Patients whose cases are reviewed are more likely to be guided to a clinical trial—one that their primary oncologist might not be aware of. Many cancer patients are eligible for these trials, which provide excellent care...yet only about 3% of patients ever participate. The more patients there are enrolled, the more quickly important clinical questions can be answered.

The National Cancer Institute website lists thousands of clinical trials that are looking for participants—to compare drug treatments, study new surgical techniques or radiation treatments, etc. Most tumor boards have a "checklist," which includes the question of whether there is a trial for which the patient might be eligible.

THE PERSONAL TOUCH

The services provided by tumor boards go beyond the nuts and bolts of treatment. For example, many cancer patients lose weight during chemotherapy or radiation treatments. If poor nutrition is threatening your recovery—or even your ability to continue treatments, a nutritionist might recommend nutritional counseling, or even help you find a free meal service in your area.

Many cancer patients suffer from mental health issues—depression, bipolar disorder, etc. The best cancer plan won't help if you're unable (or unwilling) to continue treatments. A tumor board will attempt to address—or correct—all the issues that can affect how well or poorly you respond to treatments.

Patients don't typically attend tumor boards. Many different cases are reviewed at any one meeting. The presence of a patient would affect the confidentiality of others' personal health information.

"I'm Scared My Cancer Will Come Back"

Kathleen Ashton, PhD, a health psychologist at Cleveland Clinic who works with breast cancer patients and patients at risk for breast cancer, and a faculty member of Lerner College of Medicine, both in Cleveland.

You made it through cancer treatment. You should be feeling free and happy, but you can't stop feeling like there's a sword hanging over your head. For many, if not most, survivors, fear of cancer coming back is a persistent concern. It can affect quality of life for many years after treatment, and for some, the fear becomes severe and disabling.

The risk of recurrence varies widely between types of cancer. For each type of cancer, the stage, cell type, treatment and genetic makeup of the patient also affect risk of recurrence. For some common cancers like colon, breast and prostate cancers, the overall risk is about 20% to 30%, but for others, such as bladder cancer and lymphoma, it can be twice as high, so it's normal for patients to have worries.

But for some, normal worries build into significant fear and anxiety...into a condition that even has its own name, FOCR—fear of cancer recurrence. Some people are at higher risk for FOCR than others, such as those whose cancer has a high recurrence rate, such as ovarian, lung and brain cancers. Another risk factor is having a history of anxiety or depression before cancer.

HOW TO RECOGNIZE FOCR

People with FOCR are unable to escape worry and anxiety. Similar to people with PTSD, they may avoid anything that reminds them of cancer, including skipping follow-up appointments and cancer surveillance testing—the very things that could help protect them. *Other clues to watch for include...*

- **Sleep problems**
- **Racing thoughts**
- **Constant tension or anxiety**
- **Irritability**
- **Loss of interest in the future**
- **Feeling that life is out of control**

Obviously, FOCR will affect your quality of life. If you have symptoms, let your doctor know so it can be diagnosed and, most important, treated.

TAKE ACTION TO MANAGE FOCR

Step one to manage FOCR is a cancer survivorship plan, which should be set up with your cancer team soon after treatment. This is a must for any cancer survivor, so if you've been putting it off or have one but aren't following through, it's time for a reboot. *A survivorship plan includes...*

- **An honest discussion about the realistic risk for recurrence**
- **The type of surveillance testing you will follow**
- **Signs and symptoms of recurrence to look for**
- **A plan for what happens if recurrence occurs**
- **Lifestyle strategies to reduce the risk of recurrence**

If you've been afraid to verbalize any of these issues (maybe you feel talking about them makes recurrence loom even more), you might be surprised to learn that, for many survivors, having a plan actually reduces unreasonable fears of recurrence.

Feeling that life is out of your control is one of the hardest things cancer survivors live with. Taking back some control with lifestyle changes that reduce your risk of recurrence can be empowering. *For many cancer survivors, these include...*

- **Losing weight if you are overweight or maintaining a healthy weight**
- **Eating a healthy diet**—and, in particular, eating lots of vegetables and avoiding sugar and refined carbohydrates
- **Getting daily exercise**
- **Getting enough sleep**
- **Avoiding alcohol**
- **Not smoking**

Self-help strategies can also help. You might practice a formal stress reduction method such as meditation or guided relaxation or join a cancer recovery support group.

It can be difficult to cope with FOCR alone. Treatment from a mental health provider can help you conquer fears of recurrence. *Effective treatments include...*

- **Cognitive behavioral therapy,** a form of psychotherapy that helps you recognize unhealthy or unreasonable thoughts and behaviors and replace them with healthy coping strategies and an action plan.
- **Mindfulness and exposure therapies,** psychotherapies that teach you to be present with your thoughts. You may learn to face your fears without judgment and reduce the power of fearful thoughts over time.

Talking about cancer recurrence and planning for a healthy survivorship will control FOCR for most people, allowing for an active recovery and a full life.

Smog Linked to Several Cancers

Thuan Quoc Thach, PhD, scientific officer, School of Public Health, The University of Hong Kong.

Long-term exposure to microscopic airborne particulates of dust, dirt, soot, smog or smoke raised risk of dying not only from lung cancer but also malignancies of the liver, pancreas, breast and other organs by 22% or more, according to a new 10-year study of nearly 67,000 adults age 65 and older. Risk increased with greater concentration of particulates in the air.

Possible reason: Particulates can impair DNA repair, weaken immunity and trigger inflammation.

4

Dodge Deadly Diseases

Simple Ways to Cut Your Disease Risk by 80%

David L. Katz, MD, MPH, internist and preventive medicine specialist. He is cofounder and director of the Yale Prevention Research Center and clinical instructor at the Yale School of Medicine, both in New Haven. He is author, with Stacey Colino, of *Disease-Proof: The Remarkable Truth About What Makes Us Well.*

If you were to boil down all of our medical wisdom to just a few words, you would already know them—exercise, eat well, don't smoke and maintain a healthy weight. But a shocking number of people are not following through. Only 9% of adults meet all of the criteria for a healthy lifestyle—that's right, only 9%!

The study, which looked at more than 23,000 participants between the ages of 35 and 65, found that those who improved any one of the factors above were 50% less likely to develop a chronic disease. Those who did all four at the start of the study had a nearly 80% reduced risk for any chronic disease.

So why aren't we doing what we should? Because it seems too hard! *Here are little ways to get started...*

• **Stand up.** A report in *BMJ Open* suggests that you could gain an extra two years of life just by standing up. Researchers found that people who reduced their daily sitting to less than three hours tended to live longer than those who spent more of their days in a chair.

My advice: Remind yourself to move. At least once an hour, stand up for a few minutes. A fast walk through the halls will get the blood moving.

Better: Do high knee raises, jumping jacks or other calisthenics.

When I'm on a long car trip, I do isometric exercises by flexing my arms against the steering wheel. At home, stand up and flex your calves while talking on the phone or watching TV.

• **Eat popcorn.** Even if your diet is mainly healthy, you still will gain weight if you don't keep an eye on portion sizes. This is particularly important for those who eat processed foods, which typically pack a lot of calories into surprisingly small servings.

My advice: Eat foods with a high satiety index. Even small servings of these foods will fill you up, so you consume fewer calories. Popcorn is a good example. It contains a lot of air, which takes up space in the stomach. (But avoid chemical-laden packaged microwave popcorn.)

Other high-satiety foods include those with a lot of water (such as soup or fruits)...protein (beans, lean meats, nuts, etc.)...and low-glycemic foods (such as sweet potatoes or whole grains), which are absorbed slowly into the bloodstream.

•Go caveman. Our Stone Age ancestors probably got about half of their calories from meat. This wasn't a problem because the meats they ate were much leaner than today's steaks and hamburgers. You don't have to avoid meat to be healthy. You do have to limit saturated fat.

The mass-produced beef, pork and poultry that most of us eat come from confined animals. They're fattened with grains and manufactured foods, an unnatural diet that makes meat tender but also increases saturated fat.

My advice: Eat meats only from animals that were given a more or less natural diet. Game meats, such as venison and antelope, are leaner than traditional beef and pork—and rich in omega-3 fatty acids.

If you don't care for the "wild" taste of game, look for beef or pork that is grass-fed and buy free-range poultry.

•Get the right fiber. The Centers for Disease Control and Prevention has reported that the prevalence of diabetes has increased by 45% in the last 20 years, with the greatest increase occurring in people 65 years old and older.

Self-defense: Studies have shown that soluble fiber—the type found in beans, lentils, berries, vegetables and whole grains, particularly oats—slows the rate at which sugar enters the bloodstream. If you eat oatmeal for breakfast, you will have a lower blood sugar response to whatever you eat for lunch.

My advice: In addition to adding more fiber to your diet—the optimal amount is 35 grams or more a day—include foods with a high percentage of soluble fiber. For example, add a whole grain, an apple or avocado, raw spinach or cooked broccoli, or a bean dish to every meal.

•Think movement, not exercise. Even people who exercise often approach it as a formal, and not particularly fun, activity. This mind-set might explain why lack of physical activity now accounts for nearly 10% of premature deaths in the world each year.

In my experience, most people want to exercise, but they haven't found a natural way to integrate it into their lives. You might not realize that the accumulation of 20 to 30 minutes of daily physical activity provides up to 85% of the cardiovascular benefits of hard exercise.

My advice: Think about what you already do—and do those things more often. Dancing is good exercise. So is a stroll through a park. An hour spent gardening counts. So does moving furniture...a bike ride...and a yoga class.

How to Survive Sepsis

Steven Q. Simpson, MD, professor of medicine at University of Kansas, Kansas City, and chief medical officer of the Sepsis Alliance, Sepsis.org. He was among the authors of the *2016 International Guidelines for Management of Sepsis and Septic Shock.*

When it comes to medical emergencies, we all know that heart attack, stroke and asthma attacks are among the most serious. But there's a medical emergency that most people don't know about even though it kills 270,000 people in the US each year. That's one death every two minutes...and more deaths than those caused by prostate cancer, breast cancer and AIDS combined.

This runaway killer is known as sepsis. It is a life-threatening condition that occurs when the body goes into overdrive to fight an infection, such as pneumonia, the flu or even a urinary tract infection.

Sepsis causes a deadly cascade of events when the chemicals that the immune system releases into the blood to fight infection trigger inflammation throughout the body that leads to tissue damage, organ failure and death. If not recognized and treated promptly, sepsis can worsen—and kill—within a matter of days...or even hours.

Latest development: New efforts are under way to help people identify sepsis more quickly and get the right treatment promptly so they can survive this devastating illness.

What you need to know to protect yourself and your family...

THE DANGER SIGNS

While anyone who is battling a bacterial, viral or fungal infection can develop sepsis, the old and very young are at particular risk. So are people with chronic diseases such as diabetes, cancer, chronic obstructive pulmonary disease (COPD) and kidney disease.

Sepsis is commonly misdiagnosed because its symptoms—including fast breathing (greater than 20 breaths per minute—the normal rate is 12 to 20)...a racing pulse (above 90 beats per minute)... the chills...pale, clammy skin...and extreme fatigue—can be mistaken for any number of health problems such as heart attack, stroke, pulmonary embolism, exacerbations of chronic lung disease or heart failure.

Misdiagnosis also can occur because there is no definitive test for sepsis—it is diagnosed based on a checklist of signs and symptoms.

To help people identify the red flags of sepsis, the Sepsis Alliance has created the TIME acronym...

Temperature: It can be either above normal (such as 100.4°F or higher) or below normal (such as 96.8°F or lower). Severe chills or burning fever are common.

Infection: It may be obvious, such as the flu or an abscess, or there could be less obvious signs and symptoms, including intense pain in some part of one's body, profound weakness or loss of appetite for both food and water.

Mental decline: People with sepsis are often confused or disoriented. They may be very sleepy and hard to rouse.

Extremely ill: Sufferers often experience intense, sharp pain in the chest, belly or elsewhere. They may be short of breath. Many survivors recall, "I felt like I was going to die."

If you think you may have sepsis, seek immediate medical attention. If your doctor isn't available, call 911 or get to an emergency room.

Important: Whether you're seeing your own physician or an ER doctor, make sure he/she knows your concerns.

Ask straight out: "Could this be sepsis?" Don't be shy about pushing for tests for impaired organ function such as creatinine for kidney function, lactate (lactic acid) level, platelet count, bilirubin and liver enzyme studies.

Keep in mind that the diagnosis of sepsis is missed completely about half of the time—and a delay in treatment can be fatal. Untreated sepsis can rapidly turn into shock, in which blood pressure plummets and tissues are starved for oxygen and nutrients. For every hour that treatment is delayed, the likelihood of septic shock increases.

NEWEST TREATMENT OPTIONS

The latest sepsis practice guidelines, jointly issued by American and European critical care medicine societies, more strongly emphasize the urgency of sepsis diagnosis and treatment.

Under these guidelines, a main goal is to eradicate infection with antibiotics that cover a wide variety of bacteria. Equally important is raising blood pressure to restore delivery of oxygen and nutrients to the organs and normalize their ability to function. This means intravenous fluids and, if needed, vasopressor drugs, such as norepinephrine, that stimulate the heart and tighten blood vessels to improve function.

Drugs to reduce immune system activity, once a mainstay of treatment, are no longer standard, reflecting a better understanding of the complex biology involved. Instead, researchers are exploring the use of anti-inflammatory drugs early in the condition's course and immune-stimulating drugs later.

Another change involves medical centers' adoption of highly organized procedures to bring optimal treatment to their patients in the shortest time.

For example, in New York State, which mandates this approach, patients who were diagnosed and treated for sepsis after three hours (and up to 12 hours) of an exam were 14% more likely to die in the hospital than those treated within three hours, according to a 2017 study published in *The New England Journal of Medicine*.

To be alert for possible sepsis: If you have a loved one in the ICU, ask the doctors every day if there are signs of infection, especially if the person is on a mechanical ventilator.

LINGERING AILMENTS

Scientists are discovering increasing evidence that the effects of sepsis can linger. Up to half of survivors suffer "post-sepsis syndrome" (PSS). Physical aspects of PSS reflect damage to vital organs and other tissues. There can be impaired breathing and liver and kidney function, which are often irreversible. Gangrene due to tissue death caused by infecting organisms can necessitate amputation. Fatigue and muscle and joint pain are sometimes disabling.

Recent discovery: The long-term mental impact has only recently been recognized. This may include insomnia, hallucinations, panic attacks, poor concentration, impaired memory and even post-traumatic stress disorder (PTSD).

While the reasons for such mental effects are not yet known, it's believed that sepsis may disrupt the protective blood-brain barrier, leaving the brain vulnerable to damaging inflammation.

Medications used in the ICU—especially sedative agents, including benzodiazepines such as *midazolam*—also may have negative effects on mental functioning, sometimes lasting for years.

Much remains to be learned about PSS, but it seems likely that quick action early in the course of sepsis could cut the risk.

AVOIDING SEPSIS

The key to preventing sepsis is to prevent infection. *To do this...*

- **Get recommended vaccinations, including yearly flu shots and vaccination against pneumonia.**

Also: Sepsis can occur with shingles if the skin becomes infected with bacteria. This is an additional reason to consider getting the shingles vaccine.

- **Practice good hygiene.** Wash your hands frequently and thoroughly (for at least 20 seconds).
- **Clean any cut, scrape or burn quickly and apply antiseptic or antimicrobial cream.** If a wound shows signs of a worsening infection—redness, swelling, red streaks radiating up the arm or leg—seek immediate medical attention.

Note: Sepsis is not generally contagious, but some infections that cause sepsis are, such as plague or meningococcal meningitis.

The Tango Fix for Parkinson's Disease

Gammon M. Earhart, PhD, assistant professor of physical therapy, anatomy and neurobiology and neurology, Washington University School of Medicine, St. Louis, and coauthor of a study reported in *Scientific American.*

The tango can help Parkinson's patients in a variety of areas.

Recent study: People with Parkinson's disease who took tango lessons improved their mobility compared with study subjects who attended traditional exercise classes instead. The dancers also had better balance and were at lower risk for falling.

If You Have Diabetes, Do This to Live Up to 14 Years Longer

Darren McGuire, MD, MHSc, international researcher, cardiologist, distinguished teaching professor of medicine at University of Texas Southwestern Medical Center in Dallas, deputy editor of *Circulation* and one of the authors of "Risk Factors, Mortality, and Cardiovascular Outcomes in Patients with Type 2 Diabetes" published in the *New England Journal of Medicine*.

People with type 2 diabetes almost always die from heart disease or stroke, and usually about 10 years before people without diabetes. But if you have diabetes, that doesn't have to be your fate...if you're willing to follow a very specific five-point strategy.

This plan, developed from a study of more than 250,000 people with diabetes, is a game-changer because it can put a full, healthy life back within reach, adding 12 to 14 years to the average life span of someone with type 2 diabetes. The plan takes aim at the five leading risk factors for heart disease and stroke in people with diabetes—high blood pressure, high LDL cholesterol, little physical activity, insulin resistance and smoking. If you already don't smoke and/or already get lots of exercise, good for you—you've already handled part of the plan. But you can't get away with stopping there. The cumulative effect of the five points is what reduces heart and stroke risks enough to get you back to "even."

Do the following, and your chances for a heart attack or stroke will be the same as for someone without diabetes...

• **Take a statin.** These drugs are affordable, widely available, easy to remember to take once a day and have the best evidence of any type of drug that they will quickly reduce your body's cholesterol levels.

Note: Statins aren't without side effects, and not everyone tolerates them well, but there are many different statins available to try if you do get side effects.

• **Take metformin.** This drug enhances the effects of insulin so that it can better control blood sugar. It has a long, positive track record of effectiveness and safety and is typically the first drug prescribed to patients newly diagnosed with diabetes.

Important: If metformin doesn't do enough to control blood sugar or if, independent of your blood sugar, you develop coronary artery disease or have a stroke, you might want to talk to your doctor about SGLT2 inhibitors and/or GLP-1 receptor agonists, the latest generation of diabetes drugs that reduce the risks for heart disease, stroke and cardiovascular death.

• **Keep your blood pressure in a healthy range.** Check yours at least once a week with a home monitor, sitting upright with feet uncrossed and flat on the floor with your arm resting comfortably on an armrest or table. If your pressure is higher than 130/80, take steps to reduce it, which may require medication.

Note: It's important to point out that obesity often sets the stage for many heart and stroke risk factors because it triggers an escalation of high blood pressure as well as increasing risk for high cholesterol and insulin resistance. A loss of just five to 10 pounds can make a difference in all these health checkpoints.

• **Get into a regular exercise program.** Exercise has been found to normalize the structure of blood vessels, improving circulation and reducing stress on the heart. The effect is immediate and can last for up to 24 hours. Exercise also helps you reduce cholesterol, keep blood sugar in line and knock off any extra weight. Studies have shown the best effects from a combination of aerobic exercise and strength training, but it does not have to be high intensity or exhausting—a brisk walk for 30 minutes most days of the week serves this purpose for most.

• **Stop smoking.** If you still smoke, this could be the hardest of the five steps. If you've tried and failed to quit in the past, don't throw up your hands—try a different approach. Maybe what was lacking in the past was a support system of successful quitters to lean on...or maybe nicotine replacement therapy would do the trick for you. You can get help with both those approaches and others—including the ability to create your own customized "quit plan"—through the federally sponsored website Smokefree.gov. There's advice for coping with triggers, nicotine withdrawal and blue moods, and support is provided through online chats, smartphone apps, texting programs and social media. There's even targeted advice specifically for men, women, vets, teens and seniors.

Thin People Get Diabetes Too...and It's More Deadly

Mercedes Carnethon, PhD, associate professor of preventive medicine and epidemiology at Northwestern University Feinberg School of Medicine in Chicago, where she specializes in population studies of diabetes, obesity, cardiovascular disease and fitness.

Nearly 20% of people with this disease are not overweight...

It's widely known that type 2 diabetes tends to strike people who are overweight. In fact, about 85% of people with diabetes are carrying extra pounds. But what about those who aren't overweight?

A popular misconception: It's commonly believed—even by many doctors—that lean and normal-weight people don't have to worry about diabetes. The truth is, you can develop diabetes regardless of your weight.

An unexpected risk: For those who have this "hidden" form of diabetes, recent research is now showing that they are at even greater risk of dying than those who are overweight and have the disease.

What you need to know about diabetes—no matter what you weigh...

THE EXTRA DANGER NO ONE EXPECTED

No one knows exactly why some people who are not overweight develop diabetes. There's some speculation that certain people are genetically primed for their insulin to not function properly, leading to diabetes despite their weight.

Still, because diabetes is so closely linked to being overweight, even researchers were surprised by the results of a recent analysis of 2,600 people with type 2 diabetes who were tracked for up to 15 years.

Startling new finding: Among these people with diabetes, those who were of normal weight at the time of diagnosis were twice as likely to die of non–heart-related causes, primarily cancer, during the study period as those who were overweight or obese.* The normal-weight people were also more likely to die of cardiovascular disease, but there weren't enough heart-related events to make that finding statistically significant.

Possible reasons for the higher death rates among normal-weight people with diabetes...

- **The so-called obesity paradox.**

Even though overweight and obese people have a higher risk of developing diabetes, kidney disease and heart disease, they tend to weather these illnesses somewhat better, for unknown reasons, than lean or normal-weight people.

*Normal weight is defined as a body mass index (BMI) of 18.5 to 24.9...overweight is 25 to 29.9...and obese, 30 or above. To calculate your BMI, go to NHLBI.NIH.gov and search for "BMI Calculator."

Visceral fat, a type of fat that accumulates around the internal organs, isn't always apparent. Unlike the fat you can grab, which is largely inert, visceral fat causes metabolic disturbances that increase the risk for diabetes, heart disease and other conditions. You can have high levels of visceral fat even if you're otherwise lean. Visceral fat can truly be measured only by imaging techniques such as a CT scan (but the test is not commonly done for this reason). However, a simple waist measurement can help indicate whether you have visceral fat (see next page).

- **Lack of good medical advice.**

In normal-weight people who are screened and diagnosed with diabetes, their doctors might be less aggressive about pursuing treatments or giving lifestyle advice than they would be if treating someone who is visibly overweight.

HOW TO PROTECT YOURSELF

It's estimated that about 25% of the roughly 29 million Americans with diabetes haven't been diagnosed. *Whether you're heavy or lean...*

- **Get tested at least once every three years starting at age 45**—regardless of your weight. That's the advice of the American Diabetes Association (ADA). You may need even earlier testing and/or more frequent tests if you have risk factors, such as a family history of diabetes and/or a sedentary lifestyle. Talk to your doctor.

Remember: If your weight is normal, your doctor may have a lower clinical suspicion of diabetes—a fancy way of saying he/she wouldn't even wonder if you have the condition. As a result, the doctor might think it's OK to skip the test or simply forget to recommend it. Ask for diabetes testing—even if your doctor doesn't mention it.

The HbA1c blood test is recommended by the ADA because it shows your average blood glucose levels over the previous two to three months. Many people prefer the A1c test because it doesn't require fasting. Both types of tests are usually covered by insurance.

- **Pull out the tape measure.**

Even if you aren't particularly heavy, a large waist circumference could indicate high levels of visceral fat. "Abdominal obesity" is defined as a waist circumference of more than 35 inches in women and more than 40 inches in men. Even if you are under these limits, any increase in your waist size could be a warning sign. Take steps such as diet and exercise to keep it from increasing.

To get an accurate measurement: Wrap a tape measure around your waist at the level of your navel. Make sure that the tape is straight and you're not pulling it too tight. And don't hold in your stomach!

- **Watch the sugar and calories.**

The Harvard Nurses' Health Study found that women who drank just one daily soft drink (or fruit punch) had more than an 80% increased risk of developing diabetes.

Research has consistently linked sweetened beverages with diabetes. But it's not clear whether the culprits are the sweeteners (such as high-fructose corn syrup) or just the extra calories, which lead to weight gain. Either way, it's smart no matter what you weigh to eliminate soda and other supersweet beverages from your diet—or if you don't want to give them up, have no more than one soft drink a week.

- **Get the right type of exercise.**

People who want to lose weight often take up aerobic workouts, such as swimming or biking, which burn a lot of calories. But if you don't need to lose weight, strength training might be a better choice. When you add muscle, you significantly improve insulin sensitivity and enhance the body's ability to remove glucose from the blood.

Walking may not sound very sexy, but it's one of the best exercises going because it has both aerobic and muscle-building effects. In fact, walking briskly (at a pace that causes sweating and mild shortness of breath) for half an hour daily reduces the risk for diabetes by nearly one-third. That's pretty impressive!

Don't Let Your Feet Kill You

David G. Armstrong, DPM, MD, PhD, a podiatric surgeon and professor of surgery at Keck School of Medicine of University of Southern California in Los Angeles. Dr. Armstrong is coeditor of the *American Diabetes Association's Clinical Care of the Diabetic Foot*. He is also founder and cochair of the International Diabetic Foot Conference (DFCon.com).

Feet are easy to ignore...unless they hurt. That's one big reason many people with diabetes are at risk for losing their feet—their disease has robbed them, to a large extent, of what doctors call "the gift of pain."

Here's what happens: Diabetes damages nerves, which can lead to a loss of feeling. This means that an ill-fitting shoe or an ingrown toenail can start a silent cascade of injury, leading to a foot ulcer (open sore or wound) and infection.

Many people with diabetes also have poor blood flow, and that can allow an infection to fester—raising the risk that an unnoticed cut or blister could lead to the loss of toes, a foot or even an entire lower leg. Such amputations happen nearly 75,000 times each year in the US.

Even worse danger: Once a person with diabetes has a foot ulcer, his/her chance of dying in the next 10 years doubles. If the foot ulcer leads to amputation, the five-year risk for death is 70%.

But those tragic complications don't have to happen to you. *Here are five simple steps to help prevent foot ulcers and limb loss...*

STEP #1: **Watch your blood sugar—and more.** If you maintain good control of your blood sugar, your heart and kidneys will thank you—and so will your feet. Of course, you need to take your medications, watch your diet, and if your feet are still healthy, use them to stay active—walking is good preventive medicine for your whole body.

Warning: If you already have nerve damage in your feet, talk to your primary care doctor or foot doctor (podiatrist) about the right dose of walking for you. There may be times when you have to stay off your feet to save them.

STEP #2: **Be smart about your shoes and socks.** You need to wear both—whether you're inside or outside your house. (If you've lost sensation in your feet, don't walk around the house barefoot! At least wear house slippers.)

In choosing your socks, start with a clean, lightly padded pair with no irritating seams. Choose well-fitted, supportive shoes with plenty of room for your toes (no pointy-toed shoes!)—and get in the habit of checking inside for foreign objects before slipping them on. Even though high heels aren't recommended, women with diabetes may want to wear moderate heels (no more than two inches) for special occasions.

Buying tip: It's widely known that you should shop for shoes late in the day, when your feet may have swelled a bit, but this is vital for people with diabetes so that they don't buy shoes that are too tight. And stay away from cheap plastic and vinyl shoes—they may be less expensive, but they don't breathe enough, which causes your feet to perspire, increasing the chance for a blister to develop.

If diabetes has already caused changes, such as neuropathy and especially a previous blister or wound on your feet, talk with a podiatrist about the best shoes and inserts for you. These supportive shoes can be pricey (more than $100), but insurers often cover at least one pair per year—though you may want more so that you can allow your shoes to air out for a day between wearings.

Also: See your podiatrist at least once a year to make sure your feet are healthy and you're wearing the right shoes.

STEP #3: **Knock your socks off! You need to do this every day to get a good look at your feet.** Carefully examine the tops, the soles, the heels—and between your toes, where moisture and friction can lead to trouble. Use a mirror (or ask a family member to help if needed).

Goal: Get to know your feet so well that you will notice changes from day to day. Any new redness could signal trouble. Look for swelling, calluses, sores, blisters or ingrown toenails, and let your primary care physician or podiatrist know about these warning signs.

Important: There's one other time to strip off your shoes and socks—each and every time that you see your primary care doctor (not just your podiatrist). Take off your socks as soon as you reach the exam table. That way, both of you will remember to look at and talk about your feet.

STEP #4: **Watch out for hot spots.** If areas of your skin heat up, that can be a sign of inflammation. If you detect that heat early enough, you may be able to head off an ulcer.

Helpful: Consider doing your foot check in the morning before you've been walking on your feet all day. But if that doesn't work for your schedule, just be sure you do your foot check regularly.

Do not be surprised if your doctor asks you to take the temperature of your feet in several spots each day—looking for areas of one foot that are a few degrees warmer than the same areas of the other foot. This can be done with an inexpensive thermometer that can be purchased online, such as Advocate's Non-Contact Infrared Thermometer or Equinox Digital Non-Contact Infrared Thermometer.

Also: If you and your podiatrist are game, you can try out newer heat-sensing socks. These can be paired with your smartphone or other devices to send alerts to you. One such product, Siren's Diabetic Socks, is expected to hit the market soon. You can preorder these socks at Siren.care or 888-459-5470.

STEP #5: **Pamper those puppies.** Dry skin is more easily damaged, so after washing your feet in warm (not hot) water, apply a rich moisturizing cream. Keep toenails trimmed, straight across—and if that becomes difficult for you, ask your health-care providers for nail-trimming help. Make sure to ask your podiatrist before going to a nail salon. *Also, avoid these missteps...*

- **Do not put moisturizer between your toes—** excess moisture there can promote infection. Use talcum powder or cornstarch in those areas.
- **Do not warm your feet with hot-water bottles or heating pads—**you might not feel when it's too hot. Wear warm socks instead.
- **Do not use acids or chemical corn removers,** which could damage the skin and lead to foot ulcers. See a podiatrist for help.
- **Do not attempt "bathroom surgery" on corns, calluses or ingrown toenails.** Consult a podiatrist.

• **Do not smoke.** Quitting is one of the best things you can do to improve blood flow—to your feet and everywhere else. Do not give up trying if you have not quit yet.

Metformin: New Benefits (and Risks) for This Old Diabetes Drug

Kevin M. Pantalone, DO, Endocrine Certification in Neck Ultrasound (ECNU), FACE, is a staff endocrinologist at Cleveland Clinic and serves as the director of clinical research for Cleveland Clinic's department of endocrinology, diabetes and metabolism. Dr. Pantalone's clinical focus is on the glycemic management of type 2 diabetes, and his research interests are related to the adverse effects of diabetes therapies.

If type 2 diabetes is part of your life—whether you have the condition or are at risk of developing it—you've probably heard of a drug called metformin. Perhaps your doctor has told you about it, has recently started you on it or has been prescribing it to you for years to keep your blood sugar under control.

It's no newbie. Metformin has been available by prescription in the US for more than 20 years and in Europe for more than 40 years. US doctors write nearly 60 million prescriptions a year. It's recommended as the go-to-first prescription for people with diabetes by the American Diabetes Association, the American Association of Clinical Endocrinologists and the American College of Physicians.

Yet, in many ways, metformin remains a mystery. We know broadly but still not exactly, how it works. Even more surprising, new health benefits—and side effects—keep popping up. In fact, we've only recently learned that metformin might protect the heart, fight cancer and even boost longevity. On the other hand, it can, rarely, lead to a potentially fatal side effect, and it can even make a common diabetes complication worse.

It's time to take a closer look at metformin.

MEDIEVAL FLOWER REMEDY, MODERN DRUG

In medieval times, herbalists prescribed *Galega officinalis*—the bloom of the French lilac, also known as goat's rue and Italian fitch—for patients with what we now recognize as diabetes. In the 1950s, medical researchers identified a compound in the lilac, metformin, that appeared to reliably and safely reduce high blood sugar. Metformin became widely available in Europe in the 1970s and was approved by the US Food and Drug Administration in 1995 to treat type 2 diabetes. Some combination prescriptions include metformin with other prescription medications.

HOW IT WORKS

We now know what medieval herbalists didn't—metformin increases the sensitivity of muscle and fat tissue to the hormone insulin. That makes it easier for your body to drive blood glucose (aka blood sugar) into the body's cells where it can be metabolized into energy. It also cuts the amount of sugar that the liver pushes out into the bloodstream. The exact mechanisms aren't known, but the result is lower blood sugar.

WHY IT'S THE BEST FIRST DRUG FOR DIABETES

There are three great things about metformin that set it apart from other diabetes medications. It is very inexpensive. It won't cause your blood sugar to plummet, as some diabetes drugs do. That's a complication that can range from merely bothersome to so dangerous that it lands you in the hospital. Metformin doesn't have that risk.

And it doesn't cause weight gain as many other diabetes drugs do—and may even help some people lose a few pounds. One explanation for this is that the drug enhances the effect of the appetite-suppressing hormone leptin. The weight story is important because many diabetes patients stop taking medications that make them gain weight. Metformin doesn't present that problem.

CANCER PREVENTION...AND LONGEVITY?

It's amazing that this French lilac has been a diabetes remedy for centuries, and metformin has been a drug for more than 50 years, yet every few years there's a new study highlighting a potential new benefit—or entirely new use. *Promising findings...*

• **Cardiovascular protection.** Some observational studies have reported that people with type 2 diabetes who take the drug are less prone to heart disease than those who don't.

• **Cancer treatment.** Metformin's potential to prevent, treat or enhance other treatments for certain cancers has recently emerged. These are based on small, preliminary studies, however. The drug's ability to reduce both blood sugar and insulin levels may play a part in its possible anticancer properties.

• **Longevity.** The latest area of research is the potential for metformin to improve longevity by slowing physiological aging and increasing life span. These studies are based on preliminary observations using animal models (roundworms). Much more research in animals—and eventually, humans—will be needed to determine if metformin can have a similar effect in humans...with or without diabetes.

SIDE EFFECTS, OLD AND NEW

The most common complaint with metformin is that it can cause gastrointestinal issues such as abdominal discomfort and diarrhea. Although this may sound minor, it keeps some people from being able to take the drug. An extended-release metformin is available, and in some patients, this version may be better tolerated. *Other side effects include...*

• **A very rare but potentially fatal reaction.** It has been known for many years that if a patient's kidney function is poor when they are taking metformin, there is an increased risk for lactic acidosis, a condition in which too much lactic acid builds up in the blood. This metformin side effect occurs in fewer than 10 out of every 100,000 patients—0.005%—but it's fatal half the time it occurs. That's why your doctor should test you regularly for kidney function if you're taking metformin. Metformin does not cause kidney damage—it is just not safe to take if a patient already has a significant impairment in his or her kidney function.

• **B-12 deficiency.** A recently discovered side effect of metformin, particularly after long-term use, is a deficiency of vitamin B-12. People who are B-12 deficient for a long time may develop cognitive problems and even dementia. Ironically, a B-12 deficiency can also contribute to neuropathy—a burning sensation or lack of sensation in the legs and feet. This common diabetes symptom is usually the effect of high blood sugar causing nerve damage, but B-12 deficiency can cause leg neuropathy or make it worse. It can also cause a form of anemia. If you have type 2 diabetes, have been taking metformin for a long time—and especially if you are experiencing neuropathy or cognitive issues—ask your doctor to check your B-12 level. The fix can be as simple as a B-12 pill or a monthly B-12 injection.

Generally, metformin is a safe medication. Under the care of a physician, it is safe to take this drug for decades so long as a patient's kidney function remains good and B-12 levels are checked in the appropriate clinical situations, such as in cases of longstanding use, anemia, neuropathy or cognitive issues.

IS METFORMIN RIGHT FOR YOU?

Now that you've got the scoop on this drug—its past, present and future potential—how can you tell if it's right for you? *The following are general guidelines, which may inform you as you tailor your individual treatment plan with your doctor...*

• **If you have type 2 diabetes.** You may be able to control your blood sugar with lifestyle changes alone, including a healthy diet, weight loss and exercise. However, it is generally recommended that patients start metformin along with lifestyle changes at the time of type 2 diabetes diagnosis. It's an important discussion to have with your doctor.

• **If you are at risk for developing type 2 diabetes.** People at risk include not only those with prediabetes but also women who developed diabetes during pregnancy (gestational diabetes), because they have a greatly increased risk of developing type 2 diabetes over their lifetimes. It is best to try lifestyle modifications before considering metformin. If that isn't working for you, ask your doctor about metformin.

•If you are a woman with polycystic ovary syndrome (PCOS). This condition increases the risk of developing type 2 diabetes and often leads to infertility. It is marked by high insulin levels, which contribute to a hormonal imbalance. In patients with PCOS, metformin, which tends to reduce insulin resistance, is sometimes prescribed in an attempt to restore ovulation and to improve fertility. If pregnancy is confirmed, metformin is usually continued for at least the first trimester. Always talk with your doctor about your treatment options.

There are, however, practical concerns to be aware of if you don't have diabetes but are taking metformin. Insurers tend to assume that anyone on metformin may have diabetes...even if you're taking it to prevent diabetes. That could affect medical and life insurance coverage. If you are not diabetic but need to take metformin, you may need your doctor to write a letter to your insurer confirming that you do not have diabetes. While there may be many medical reasons to take metformin beyond just type 2 diabetes, a thorough discussion about the role of metformin therapy, and the risks versus benefits, should take place before a patient starts any medication, including metformin.

Drug-Free Way to Remission

Gerald Bernstein, MD, FACP, is director of the diabetes management program at The Gerald J. Friedman Diabetes Institute in New York City.

Losing 15% of your weight starts diabetes remission.

Recent finding: The pancreas's insulin-producing beta cells began functioning normally again when people lost 15% of their weight (about 30 pounds for a 200-pound person), reversing their type 2 diabetes. It's not yet known how long this benefit will last.

Diabetes Risk for Women

Mark Woodward, PhD, director, epidemiology and biostatistics division, The George Institute for International Health, University of Sydney, Camperdown, Australia, and leader of a study of 450,000 people, presented at the Second International Conference on Women, Heart Disease, and Stroke.

The risk of dying from heart disease associated with diabetes is 50% greater for women than for men. Women with diabetes also have a nearly threefold greater risk for fatal heart disease than women without diabetes.

Self-defense: Talk with your doctor about ways to treat blood pressure and cholesterol as well as diabetes.

New Dangers to Your Kidneys

Orlando Gutiérrez, MD, an associate professor of medicine in the division of nephrology and assistant professor of epidemiology at The University of Alabama at Birmingham School of Medicine.

Your kidneys are two of your body's best friends. Besides filtering and cleaning your blood, they also regulate fluids, acidity and key minerals...produce hormones that control blood pressure...and manufacture a form of vitamin D that strengthens bones.

But modern life can really clobber your kidneys—high blood pressure, elevated blood sugar and obesity all can damage these vital organs and are major risk factors for chronic kidney disease (CKD).

THE BEST DEFENSE

Controlling the big risk factors mentioned above are the best ways to prevent or control CKD. But recent studies have revealed several new risk factors that might threaten your kidneys. *These include...*

PROTON PUMP INHIBITORS

Americans spend about $11 billion yearly on acid-reducing, heartburn-easing proton pump inhibitors (PPIs), such as *esomeprazole* (Nexium) and *omeprazole* (Prilosec).

New finding: Researchers at Johns Hopkins University studied more than 10,000 people with normal kidney function. After 15 years, those using PPIs were 20% to 50% more likely to develop CKD.

Possible explanation: PPIs may cause interstitial nephritis—inflammation and scarring in the kidneys.

What to do: The researchers found that people who took an H2 blocker—such as *ranitidine* (Zantac) or *famotidine* (Pepcid)—instead of a PPI for heartburn did not have a higher risk for CKD.

Note: Many of my patients find that TUMS and lifestyle changes, such as avoiding spicy and fatty foods and eating more slowly, can greatly reduce heartburn.

HIGH-ACID DIET

Just as our oceans are becoming more acidic and threatening marine life, scientists are finding that an acidic diet threatens our kidneys.

New finding: When researchers analyzed 14 years of health data for nearly 1,500 people with CKD, they found that those who ate a high-acid, junk food–laden diet that included red meat, processed foods, sweets and few fruits and vegetables were three times more likely to develop kidney failure.

What to do: Adopt a more alkaline diet. In a recent study, researchers from Columbia University Medical Center followed 900 people for nearly seven years and found that those who routinely ate a Mediterranean-type diet—rich in alkaline foods such as vegetables, fruits, beans and heart-healthy fats like olive oil—were 50% less likely to develop CKD than those who didn't eat these foods.

TOO MUCH PHOSPHORUS

The mineral phosphorus is a must—for cellular health, energy and digestion, a steady heartbeat and strong bones and teeth. But too much phosphorus damages the kidneys and the circulatory system.

New findings: In a study I conducted with fellow kidney specialists involving nearly 10,000 people, we found that an excess of phosphorus in the diet was linked to more than double the risk of dying from any cause and three times the risk of dying from heart disease. In another study, higher levels of dietary phosphorus sped up the decline from CKD to end-stage renal disease.

Red meat and dairy products are rich in phosphorus, but about 40% of the phosphorus in our daily diets is from phosphorus-containing additives used to extend shelf life and improve flavor and texture. Those additives are just about everywhere—including in many flavored waters, iced teas, nondairy creamers and bottled coffee beverages.

What to do: Whenever possible, choose a natural food over a processed food—eat fresh green beans, for example, rather than canned...and homemade bread rather than highly processed bread.

Also helpful: If you must eat a processed food, check the label for the word phosphate or phosphoric acid, which indicates the presence of phosphorus—and try to pick a product without the additive.

SITTING TOO MUCH

It's not just lack of regular exercise that contributes to chronic health problems such as heart disease—it's also excessive sitting. And sitting takes a toll on your kidneys, too.

New finding: In a study of nearly 6,000 people, every 80-minute period of sitting during the day increased the likelihood of CKD by 20%, according to research from the University of Utah School of Medicine. That was true whether or not the person exercised regularly or had diabetes, high blood pressure or obesity.

What to do: When the same team of researchers looked at people with CKD, they found that standing up and/or walking around for just two minutes an hour lowered the risk for death by 41%. Research also shows that regular exercise is good for your kidneys.

My advice: Walk at least 30 minutes, three times a week (in addition to getting up every hour you sit)...or check with your doctor for advice on the best type of exercise for you.

MORE FROM DR. GUTIÉRREZ

Should You Be Tested for Kidney Disease?

More than 25 million Americans have chronic kidney disease (CKD)—but only 6% know it!

Beware: The symptoms of kidney disease (such as swollen legs, feet and/or ankles...frequent urination...fatigue...and/or dry, itchy skin) are not likely to be noticed until you reach end-stage renal disease because the body is very good at adapting to loss of kidney function until most of the function is gone.

Blood test for measuring kidney function: Estimated Glomerular Filtration Rate (eGFR). A filtration rate of less than 60 mL/min for more than three months means that you have CKD. Most insurance companies pay for the cost of the test if the patient has a risk factor for kidney disease—such as high blood pressure...type 2 diabetes...obesity...age (65 or older)...or a family history of the disease (a parent or sibling who has CKD). If you have a risk factor for CKD, get the test every year. Otherwise, there's usually no need for testing, but be sure to consult your doctor for advice.

Strong Muscles Fight Kidney Disease

K. Kalantar-Zadeh, et al., "Mid-Arm Muscle Circumference and Quality of Life and Survival in Maintenance Hemodialysis Patients," *Clinical Journal of the American Society of Nephrology* (2010).

Strong muscles help kidney disease patients live longer. Kidney disease patients on dialysis live longer—and are happier—if they have robust muscles. Measuring lean muscle mass in the arm, researchers found that patients with the highest amount of lean muscle mass were 37% less likely to die during the five-year study period than those with the least amounts. Techniques such as weight training to build lean muscle mass can help kidney disease patients.

Liver Disease Is Rampant

Rich Snyder, DO, nephrologist, osteopathic physician and clinical professor at Philadelphia College of Osteopathic Medicine. He is author of *What You Must Know About Liver Disease: A Practical Guide to Using Conventional and Complementary Treatments.*

Alarming fact—about 30 million Americans have some form of liver disease. That's one-tenth of the population. Yet it's normal for people to go undiagnosed for years or even decades.

Unless liver disease is detected and treated early, it can cause severe inflammation that can lead to scarring (cirrhosis), organ failure and/or cancer—and it even may require a transplant. It is a leading cause of death in the US.

Important: I advise patients who have risk factors for liver disease to get their livers checked—the inexpensive group of blood tests can be done during routine checkups. Risk factors include obesity, metabolic syndrome (see next page), hepatitis and a history of alcohol or drug abuse.

If you have liver disease, medications may be required, but herbs and supplements can help reduce inflammation, improve liver function and slow ongoing damage. Always speak with your doctor before taking any natural supplements.

I usually advise patients to start with just one remedy at a time. After six to eight weeks, we reassess to see if there's improvement and if an additional supplement is required. Any of the herbs below can be started first, but milk thistle and turmeric are among the more common options.

MILK THISTLE

Milk thistle has been used for thousands of years for liver health. It's among the most studied herbs for treating hepatitis and other liver diseases.

Milk thistle (a member of the plant family that includes daisies and sunflowers) contains a flavonoid called silymarin. It's an antioxidant that reduces inflammation, blocks the movement of toxins into liver cells and increases the output of enzymes that prevent toxin-related damage.

Research suggests that milk thistle can improve liver function and improve survival in patients with chronic hepatitis and/or cirrhosis. One study found that it reduced the viral load (the amount of viral particles in the blood) in hepatitis C patients who hadn't responded to drug treatments.

Typical dosage: If you have risk factors for liver disease or if you've been diagnosed with liver disease, talk to your doctor about taking 100 mg twice a day, to start—your doctor might recommend a higher dose (between 200 mg and 600 mg) if lab tests aren't improving. Milk thistle is unlikely to cause side effects, although it should be avoided if you're allergic to ragweed or one of its relatives, such as sunflower seeds or chamomile.

TURMERIC

The active ingredient in this spice, curcumin, is an exceptionally potent antioxidant that has been shown to reduce jaundice (the dark urine and/or yellowing of the skin or eyes that often occurs in liver patients).

There's also some evidence that it reduces liver scarring. A study published in Gut found that turmeric helped prevent a hepatitis-causing virus from moving from one cell to another.

Typical dosage: Between 500 mg and 1,500 mg of a turmeric supplement daily, divided into two or three doses. (Exact dose will depend on your weight, symptoms and other factors.)

Caution: Turmeric has blood-thinning properties, so it may not be best if you are on a blood thinner such as warfarin or if your liver disease is advanced and clotting of the blood is a problem.

N-ACETYLCYSTEINE (NAC)

Doctors who specialize in natural health recommend this supplement for liver patients. It reduces inflammation and increases intracellular levels of glutathione, the "master antioxidant" that is mainly produced and stored in the liver and that is depleted by liver disease.

Doctors give it to improve the viability of transplanted livers. It also is used in patients with liver damage caused by acetaminophen overdose (acetaminophen rapidly depletes glutathione).

Typical dosage: 600 mg, twice daily.

GLUTATHIONE

You don't have to take this supplement if you already are using NAC (which is converted to glutathione in the body), but I often advise my patients to take glutathione because it helps rebuild body tissues, including liver cells.

Glutathione is particularly helpful if you regularly use acetaminophen for treating arthritis or another painful condition because acetaminophen, as mentioned before, can deplete glutathione levels. Oral glutathione usually needs to be taken with cysteine, which helps glutathione get into the cells.

Follow dosing directions on the label.

COFFEE

Coffee isn't a cure for liver disease, but there's good evidence that it reduces liver inflammation and may reduce liver-related health risks, including cirrhosis and cancer.

One study found that hepatitis B patients who drank more than four cups of coffee a week were only about half as likely to develop hepatocellular carcinoma (a form of liver cancer) as those who did not drink coffee.

Another study—one that looked at 430,000 people—found that people who drank an extra two cups of coffee a day could potentially reduce their risk for cirrhosis by 44%.

WEIGHT LOSS IS CRUCIAL FOR YOUR LIVER

Non-alcoholic fatty liver disease (NAFLD) is the leading type of liver disease in the US. It affects up to 25% of all adults and is linked to obesity and metabolic syndrome (a constellation of problems that includes high blood pressure, high blood sugar and elevated triglycerides, along with obesity).

A liver is considered "fat" if more than 5% to 10% of its weight comes from fatty tissue. This serious disease can lead to severe inflammation, cirrhosis or liver failure.

You have to lose weight if you've been diagnosed with NAFLD. Studies have shown that it may be possible to eliminate the condition altogether by losing as little as 10% of your total weight.

Also helpful: Alpha lipoic acid. It's a well-researched supplement that can decrease insulin resistance and improve metabolic syndrome. I advise patients with NAFLD to take 200 mg daily, increasing the dose by 100 mg weekly until they reach a maximum dose of 400 mg to 600 mg.

If you have diabetes or are at risk for diabetes, you may need to check your blood glucose levels because alpha lipoic acid has the potential to decrease glucose levels in some individuals.

Don't Let the Flu Turn into Pneumonia

William Schaffner, MD, an infectious disease specialist at Vanderbilt University Medical Center in Nashville and medical director of the National Foundation for Infectious Diseases. NFID.org

The flu lands hundreds of thousands of people in the hospital each year and kills tens of thousands. But flu that leads to pneumonia is even deadlier.

Startling statistic: Flu-plus-pneumonia ranks eighth in leading causes of death in the US.

THE FLU/PNEUMONIA COMBO

Every year, pneumonia affects more than one million Americans—and about 50,000 die. People most susceptible to pneumonia include the elderly, especially nursing home residents and individuals who have chronic health conditions such as heart or lung disease. The flu-to-pneumonia progression isn't the only cause of pneumonia, of course, but since the combo is so deadly—and often so preventable—it's worth special attention.

Here's what happens: You get the flu, a contagious respiratory illness caused by an influenza virus. You get the typical symptoms—sore throat, cough, body aches, fever, headaches and chills. But the flu also makes your lungs more susceptible to a bacterial infection caused by *Streptococcus pneumoniae* (*S. pneumoniae*), the most common cause of pneumonia in adults.

When that happens, air sacs fill with pus and other liquid, making it harder for oxygen to reach the bloodstream and making it difficult to breathe. Death can come from organs that are starved of oxygen—or from a blood infection (sepsis).

Here's how to protect yourself…

STEP ONE: GET A FLU SHOT

If you don't get the flu, you won't be at risk for that combination of flu virus/*S. pneumoniae* that is so dangerous to susceptible people. Getting a flu shot is the best way to protect yourself. It is recommended for everyone over the age of six months. While not 100% effective, it does offer substantial protection.

Why a flu shot is so important: A bad flu year means that pneumonia cases could potentially soar.

STEP TWO: MAKE SURE YOU'RE UP TO DATE ON PNEUMONIA VACCINATION

Effective vaccines exist against *S. pneumoniae*, which, as described earlier, causes the vast majority of pneumonia cases in adults. Everyone age 65 and older should be vaccinated—yet only about 50% of healthy adults in this age group are. Some adults need protection before they turn 65—smokers and anyone with a chronic health condition (heart or lung disease, diabetes, asthma, etc.). *For the best protection, you'll need two different vaccines, spaced out over a year or more…*

- **Start with a one-time-only dose of the pneumococcal conjugate vaccine called PCV13 (Prevnar 13),** which protects against 13 types of pneumococcal bacteria.
- **One year later,** get a dose of pneumococcal polysaccharide vaccine PPSV23 (Pneumovax), which protects against 23 strains of pneumococcal bacteria. Prevnar 13 primes your immune system so that Pneumovax works better than it would if you took it by itself.
- **Based on your age and health,** your doctor may advise another dose of Pneumovax five years later.

STEP THREE: WATCH YOUR MEDS

Certain health conditions and medications can affect your susceptibility to pneumonia...

• **Steroids and other immunosuppressive drugs can make you more susceptible to pneumonia.** These drugs interfere with the immune response, so your body can't fight off infection as easily.

Low-dose steroids, even taken long term, may not increase pneumonia risk, but higher doses (such as 20 mg a day) can do so in as little as two weeks. If you need a high-dose steroid to control your condition, be especially vigilant during flu season—get vaccinated, wash your hands frequently, stay away from crowds, and call your doctor at the first sign of illness such as a sore throat.

• **Acid-suppressive medications,** such as proton pump inhibitors including *omeprazole* (Prilosec), as well as histamine-2 receptor antagonists including *ranitidine* (Zantac), inhibit the production of stomach acids. But these acids help keep harmful gut bacteria in check.

Less acid means more potential for harmful bacteria to colonize and eventually enter the lungs. Unless your doctor prescribes these on a long-term basis (a rare occurrence), use them only for short periods of time—no more than four weeks for heartburn/gastroesophageal reflux disease (GERD), for example.

• **Pneumonia occurs less often in adults who get routine dental checkups.** Routine dental visits can help decrease the overall amount of bacteria in your mouth, including those that can cause pneumonia in susceptible people.

Bonus: A healthy mouth reduces heart disease risk, too.

IF YOU DO GET THE FLU...

Since the flu shot doesn't always prevent infection, be on the lookout for symptoms including feeling feverish, chills, body aches, sore throat and fatigue. If you suspect that you have the flu, call your doctor. You may be a candidate for prescription antiviral medication such as *oseltamivir* (Tamiflu), which can shorten your illness duration and possibly decrease the odds of it progressing to pneumonia. But you need to take it within a day or two of the first symptoms for it to be effective.

MORE FROM WILLIAM SCHAFFNER, MD

Pneumonia and Your Heart

Adults hospitalized with pneumonia have a heightened risk for cardiovascular problems including sudden heart attack, often with no warning signs.

What happens: Oxygen deprivation from a bout of pneumonia can starve cardiac muscle cells so that they function less well or even die off. One study found that within the first month of pneumonia diagnosis, the risk for stroke, heart attack or death due to heart disease grew by as much as fourfold...and remained elevated for years. Patients recovering from pneumonia also are predisposed to developing it again—another good reason to prevent it in the first place.

Don't Catch Pneumonia from Your Dentures

Study titled "Denture Wearing during Sleep Doubles the Risk of Pneumonia in the Very Elderly," published in *Journal of Dental Research.*

Wearing dentures while sleeping raises pneumonia risk.

Probable reason: Bacteria that breed easily in the mouth when dentures are left in can be inhaled into the lungs and cause pneumonia. People who leave their dentures in overnight likely have other poor oral-health habits as well—a study found that they visited the dentist less often than people who removed and cleaned their dentures nightly. Always take out your dentures at night, and clean them thoroughly.

People with COPD Live Longer with Statin Drugs

Larry Lynd, PhD, is professor of pharmaceutical sciences at University of British Columbia, Vancouver, Canada.

Patients with chronic obstructive pulmonary disease (COPD) who used statins were 45% less likely to die from lung-related issues than other COPD patients and had a 21% lower risk of dying from any cause.

Possible reason: Statins, used to reduce cholesterol levels, have anti-inflammatory properties that may benefit certain people with COPD.

Sex Tips to Stay Safe from STDs

Melanie Davis, PhD, a certified sexuality educator and copresident of the Sexuality and Aging Consortium at Widener University in Chester, Pennsylvania, and founder of the website SaferSex4Seniors.org. Through Honest Exchange, LLC, she trains health-care providers, medical students and educators about sexuality and communication.

For older men and women, the fun game is no longer shuffleboard. It's sex. And that's a great thing—except that sexually transmitted diseases (STDs) are on a meteoric rise in this age group. *The latest stats...*

- **Between 2007 and 2011, chlamydia infections among Americans age 65 and over increased by 31%.**
- **Syphilis infections in this age group rose by 52% in the same period.**
- **17% of new cases of HIV infection are in people age 50 and older.**

THE NEW SEXUAL REVOLUTION

One big reason for the rise of STDs—also called "sexually transmitted infections" or STIs—is that more people continue to be sexually active well into their golden years. "The generation of people now hitting this stage of life came of age during the sexual revolution—they're healthier and fitter and expect to keep having sex," explains Melanie Davis, PhD, copresident of the Sexuality and Aging Consortium at Widener University in Chester, Pennsylvania, and founder of the website Safer Sex for Seniors.

Viagra and related erectile dysfunction (ED) drugs play a role, too. One study found that men (average age 61) who used these drugs were twice as likely to have STDs compared with men who didn't. As women become more savvy about managing sexual health after menopause, they also find sex easier to enjoy. It's also liberating for many women to be able to have sex without worrying about getting pregnant.

Being able to enjoy sex later in life, with more comfort and no worries about pregnancy, is all good. But it also opened the door to the new epidemic of STDS.

It has even become an issue in long-term-care facilities. Many STDs are asymptomatic, but most nursing homes and assisted-care facilities don't screen for them. And even if they did, all it would take is one conjugal visit with an infected nonresident for an infection to spread, according to Dr. Davis. Plus, people with chronic conditions may be more susceptible to infection, including STDs.

If you're sexually active, especially if you have recently had multiple sexual partners (or your partner has), being tested for STDs should be a regular part of your preventive medical care. It's so important for the health of seniors that Medicare now covers STD testing as a free preventive service. But as with everything related to health, prevention is always better than treatment. Here's how to stay safe—and still enjoy yourself.

HOW TO HAVE MORE FUN IN BED...SAFELY

The single best way to prevent the spread of infection during sex—heterosexual or homosexual—is to use a barrier form of protection such as an external or internal condom or dam, says Dr. Davis.

As bodies change, though, it can take new skills to use barrier protection right. For older men, for example, "the use of an external condom can be tough if he has challenges achieving a firm erection or if his erection waxes and wanes during sex," she explains.

This doesn't mean, however, that it can't be done. Nor does it mean people struggling with this issue must either consign themselves to a having a risky sex life or going back to shuffleboard. *Some tips*...

• **Hold on.** If you change position while wearing a condom during sex, either partner can reach down and keep the condom in place by holding the bottom of it (the part closest to the man's body). One slip and the protective quality of a condom goes down the drain.

• **Try an "innie."** An internal condom (aka a female condom) can be the perfect alternative to a conventional external (aka "male") one. Basically an elongated tube of pliable plastic, this disposable device has soft rings at either end. One ring is inserted into the vagina to hold that end of the condom in place. The other end stays outside the body. "It can look a little weird," says Dr. Davis, "and it takes a little practice, but it has some real advantages. The material it is made of transfers heat well, and that can feel better and more natural for both partners than an external condom," says Dr. Davis. It's fine to use an extra lubricant, but it's often not necessary. "The lubrication inside and outside of the internal condom helps with comfort," she explains. "It's pretty slippery." The female condom is more protective as well. "A conventional condom doesn't cover the base of the penis, which is where the herpes virus likes to hang out," explains Dr. Davis. "Not only does an internal condom solve that problem, it covers the entire labia, essentially providing a barrier against any other organisms as well."

• **Practice safe oral sex, too.** Pretty much any STD you can get on your genitals you also can get in your mouth, according to Dr. Davis. "Use an external condom if you're performing fellatio or an internal condom if you're performing cunnilingus," she advises.

Another option: A "dam," which uses a square of material (similar to a female condom) designed for just this purpose. Says Dr. Davis, "They make flavored condoms and dams for a reason—to be used during oral sex."

• **Lube it or leave it.** With age, vulvar and vaginal tissue gets thinner and dryer so that, even during gentle sex, it can be more easily torn—basically opening the door for a sexually transmitted organism. A woman can increase her pleasure and decrease her risk for infection by using a lubricant. Dr. Davis advises using a silicone-based lube. "It stays viscous longer than water-based lube," she explains. If dryness is a significant problem, talk to your doctor. You may benefit from a topical estrogen cream or another product that moisturizes the tissues. (A condom is still essential for protection, of course.)

• **Tinker with toys.** Safety is only one part of the satisfying senior sex equation. Men and women of a certain age also just want to have fun. "In terms of pleasure," says Dr. Davis, "adult toys are a great idea." For both genders, the older the body the more time and direct stimulation is needed for both arousal and orgasm, she explains. So don't just play it safe—it's fine to just play, too. "Small bullet-style vibrators are great for targeted stimulation of the clitoris," she explains. "Palm-sized vibrators, about the size of a computer mouse, are easy to hold against the vulva, while longer vibrators or dildos (elongated, without vibrations) are good for internal play and keeping the vaginal muscles flexible. For penises, masturbation sleeves, vibrating or not, can be pleasurable—lubricant increases comfort and sensation."

• **Try a little tenderness.** "Consider other types of 'toys' as well," says Dr. Davis. "Brushing a partner's hair is very sensual—with zero STD risk." So is a partner massage. "Massage oil can also enhance sexual experiences," she adds.

Deadly Bacteria

Aaron E. Glatt, MD, FACP, a spokesperson for the Infectious Diseases Society of America, is chairman, department of medicine, South Nassau Communities Hospital, Oceanside, New York.

The Vibrio bacteria is not well-known but deadly. The bacterium can cause deadly skin infections or gastrointestinal problems, particularly in people who have a compromised immune system or liver disease. The death rate in these patients approaches 50%. Vibrio bacteria live in warm coastal waters and get into people's bodies through unhealed cuts or if someone swallows the bacteria—which can happen when eating raw or undercooked shellfish.

The Big Mistake Most MS Patients Make

Allen C. Bowling, MD, PhD, a neurologist specializing in multiple sclerosis (MS) and a physician associate at Colorado Neurological Institute in Englewood, Colorado, and clinical professor of neurology at University of Colorado in Denver. He is author of five books on MS, including *Optimal Health with Multiple Sclerosis*. NeurologyCare.net

Medications are often a must for the roughly 400,000 Americans with multiple sclerosis (MS). Powerful disease-modifying drugs (DMDs) can reduce the development of new brain and spinal cord lesions that lead to symptoms...prevent relapses...slow the disease's progression...and delay disability.

The big mistake: For the majority of patients with MS, drugs are the only therapy used.

In my own experience treating thousands of people with MS, I have found that an integrative approach—a treatment plan that combines conventional medicine with science-supported nondrug strategies such as diet, nutritional supplements and exercise—is a much more effective way to manage symptoms and improve quality of life than medications alone.

New evidence: In a one-year study published in *Journal of the American College of Nutrition,* an integrative approach including a healthy diet, stretching, meditation and self-massage eased depression, anxiety and fatigue in people with MS and helped prevent mental decline.

Additionally, starting a healthy lifestyle when MS is diagnosed (typically between the ages of 20 and 50) can help prevent chronic, lifestyle-associated medical problems, such as obesity, arthritis, heart disease and diabetes, that may worsen disability and quality of life in those with MS.

Here are the most reliable, safest and cost-effective integrative treatments for MS patients...

DIET

I advise my MS patients to stay away from (or at least minimize) processed foods...avoid overeating...and consume a plant-based diet. This simple advice may make a huge difference in their health, especially over the long term.

What not to do: I find that extreme diets—for example, a strict Paleolithic diet or strict gluten-free diet—may be difficult to follow and may not actually be healthy for people with MS. They don't provide the variety of foods that support good health.

Bottom line: There is no one diet that is best for MS. But the worst diet for MS is the standard American diet, loaded with processed foods, fatty meats and sugar. Eliminating those foods and ingredients goes a long way toward maintaining good health.

NUTRITIONAL SUPPLEMENTS

There are two common nutritional deficiencies that I have found in people who have MS—vitamin B-12 and vitamin D. I test my patients for these two deficiencies and advise supplements if necessary, customizing the dose to the patient. A multivitamin may be considered for those with an unhealthy diet, but it is preferable to change the diet.

Recent scientific research: Dozens of studies show that low vitamin D levels or low vitamin D intake increases the risk for MS and, in those with MS, increases risk for attacks, disability progression and new brain lesions. Also, there are studies that a subgroup of people with MS are at risk for vitamin B-12 deficiency—this is of concern because many of the symptoms of vitamin B-12 deficiency are the same as those of MS.

Beware: There is a lot of hype about nutritional supplements for MS. Watch out for products asserting that a single nutritional supplement can treat many different diseases, including MS... touting one or more "secret" ingredients...or relying heavily on customer testimonials as evidence of effectiveness.

EXERCISE

Research shows that regular exercise can reduce the fatigue, muscle weakness and walking difficulties common with MS. Other symptoms that exercise may ease include anxiety, anger, depression, bowel and bladder difficulties (such as constipation, incontinence, urgency and frequency), pain, sleeping difficulties, stiffness in the arms or legs (spasticity) and cognitive decline. Exercise may even slow the progression of the disease.

New scientific research: In a six-month study of 35 people, published in *Multiple Sclerosis Journal,* researchers found that twice-a-week resistance-training slowed the rapid shrinking of the brain common in MS. Some areas of the brain even started to grow.

My advice: In addition to twice-weekly strength training (such as wall squats with or without hand weights, lunges and wall push-ups), I urge my patients to do aerobic exercise (30 minutes of medium-intensity exercise, such as stationary cycling, dancing or walking, twice weekly). Aerobic exercise has many benefits for MS patients including improved cardiovascular fitness...better bowel and bladder control...and less fatigue and depression.

Also helpful: Hydrotherapy (water exercise such as swimming and water aerobics) may be especially well-suited for people with MS who have leg weakness. And yoga is particularly good for easing spasticity. In a recent study published in the journal *Medicine & Science in Sports & Exercise,* eight weeks of water exercise or yoga improved fatigue, depression and tingling and numbness in women with MS, compared with a group that didn't exercise.

EMOTIONAL WELL-BEING

Emotional health is a crucial but often-neglected component in the treatment of MS.

New scientific research: In a study of more than 1,000 people with MS, published in *Neurology,* 44% reported their emotional well-being was worsening due to fatigue, trouble concentrating and bladder/urinary problems.

What I recommend: To improve emotional well-being, I counsel my MS patients to identify their difficult emotions—and to talk about those feelings with a spouse or friend. I have found that patients who do this not only feel happier but also dramatically reduce their feelings of stress.

Also helpful: Listening, creating or moving to music stimulates feelings and facilitates emotional processing. A professional music therapist can suggest an approach geared to your specific situation. A study published in the journal *Expert Review of Neurotherapeutics* found that music therapy improved self-acceptance and eased depression and anxiety in MS patients. To find a music therapist near you, consult the American Music Therapy Association at MusicTherapy.org.

5

Don't Die Young

These Unhealthy Habit Combos Can Be Deadly

Study titled "Traditional and Emerging Lifestyle Risk Behaviors and All-Cause Mortality in Middle-Aged and Older Adults: Evidence from a Large Population-Based Australian Cohort" by researchers at University of Sydney and George Institute for Global Health, both in Australia, and VU University Medical Centre, the Netherlands, published in *PLOS Medicine*.

Here's good news for those of us whose health habits aren't perfect. Just one bad habit isn't likely to send you to an early grave.

It's the combination that'll get you.

Do you sit for more than seven hours a day? You've surely heard by now that it's the "new smoking." There's no question that you'll be healthier if you get up and move about every hour.

But if you don't smoke—and you also eat a healthy diet, get regular exercise and sleep well—the risks of prolonged sitting are a lot less than you might imagine.

Some bad habit combos, on the other hand, are downright deadly.

WHEN YOU HAVE ONLY ONE BAD HABIT

Australian researchers started with a database of 231,000 middle-aged and older adults who had filled out questionnaires about their lifestyle habits. The researchers measured associations between risky lifestyle behaviors and mortality amongst the 15,000 subjects who died over a six-year period. Only about one-third of them lived squeaky-clean lives without any of the examined risk factors.

Some behaviors were relatively benign if the rest of the lifestyle was healthy. *Participants who...*

- **Ate a poor diet** (too few vegetables and fruit, little fish, lots of processed meats and fatty dairy foods) were 4% more likely to die over the six years than people with really healthy diets.
- **Drank more than 14 alcoholic beverages a week**...8% increased risk.
- **Slept less than seven hours a night**...9%.
- **Sat for more than seven hours a day**...15%.

Some behaviors were pretty risky even if the rest of the lifestyle was healthy. *Those who...*

- **Slept for more than nine hours a night**...44% increased risk for death. (Long sleep duration often is an indicator of underlying health problems such as depression or diabetes.)
- **Got less than 150 minutes of moderate-to-intense physical activity a week**...61%.
- **Smoked**...90%.

BAD COMPANY

When bad behaviors get together, you really have to worry...

- **Exercising too little plus drinking more than recommended**...80% increased risk for death.
- **Exercising too little plus sitting too much**...242%. (This was the most common pairing of unhealthy lifestyle behaviors in the entire study.)
- **Exercising too little plus drinking more than recommended and sitting for more than seven hours a day**...251%.
- **Sitting too much, exercising too little and sleeping less than seven hours**...259%.
- **Smoking and drinking more than is recommended**...280%.
- **Sitting too much, exercising too little and sleeping more than nine hours**...423%.
- **Smoking, drinking too much and getting too little sleep**...468%.
- **Smoking, eating a bad diet, drinking more than recommended, exercising too little and sitting for prolonged periods**...640%.
- **Smoking, drinking more than recommended, getting too little exercise, sitting for prolonged periods and sleeping more than nine hours a night**...909%. (Yes, that means you are more than nine times more likely to die over the next six years.)

HOW TO STAY HEALTHY EVEN IF YOU'RE NOT PERFECT

Like any study, this one has limitations. It shows associations, not causality. Plus, one could quibble with some of the underlying lifestyle scoring. When it comes to diet, for example, the score counted dairy fat as "bad," but new research finds that dairy fat can be part of a healthy diet. Nor should the fact that certain behaviors aren't particularly deadly be interpreted as an excuse to skip any particular healthy behavior.

In the end, we're all individuals. One person may be OK drinking more than two drinks a night, on average, for example, while another might have, say, an underlying liver problem or an alcohol addiction that turns that behavior into an individually deadly habit.

The key point is that bad habits don't just add risk—they multiply risk.

Fortunately, all of the risks measured in this study are modifiable—so you're in control. For example, if you sit all day long (as so many of us do), it's healthy to get up every hour or so and walk around—but that's even more important if you aren't getting enough regular exercise. Even better, get up from your chair and get exercise.

Too Much TV Shortens Life Span

Lennert Veerman, MD, senior research fellow, The University of Queensland, Brisbane, Australia.

Researchers studied lifestyle and health data on 11,000 adults (ages 25 and older) and found that for every hour of sedentary TV watching per day, life expectancy was reduced by 22 minutes, on average. A six-hour daily TV habit after age 25 reduced life expectancy by nearly five years.

Surprising: Watching TV may be as dangerous as cardiovascular risk factors such as smoking and obesity.

Is Your Chair Dangerous?

James A. Levine, MD, PhD, professor of medicine and director, Non-Exercise Activity Thermogenesis (NEAT) Laboratory, Mayo Clinic, Rochester, Minnesota. He is author of *Move a Little, Lose a Lot.*

Here's a surprising item to add to our list of health hazards to beware—chairs! A slew of research studies show that it's dangerous to spend too much time on your derriere—in fact, one study found a correlation between hours spent sitting and early death. On average, American adults spend more than half of their waking hours sitting. Can something so simple and commonplace really be so deadly?

Yes—but the reason why isn't as simple as you might think. Doctors are becoming aware of the magnitude of the health consequences of prolonged sitting, including not only the obvious—obesity—but also high cholesterol, diabetes, cardiovascular disease and even cancer.

DON'T SIT STILL!

Put simply, the danger in prolonged sitting is that it stalls the metabolic machinery. The body has an exquisitely designed system for trafficking fuels such as carbohydrates and fats. Serious consequences result when the muscular engine sits on "idle."

This "physiology of inactivity" results in a variety of immediate, undesirable effects. For instance, inactivity impedes the ability to metabolize fat and sugar and it also elevates triglycerides, potentially raising the risk for cardiovascular disease. Prolonged sitting weakens muscles, which can lead to back pain, arthritis and joint problems. Previous research has demonstrated that sitting for long periods suppresses lipase, an enzyme involved in fat metabolism that is produced only when leg muscles flex—low levels are associated with heart disease and other illnesses. Sex hormones, including estrogen and testosterone metabolism, also are affected.

The good news here is that just a little movement can accomplish a lot for your health. Even if you must sit for certain parts of your day, modest efforts to move your muscles—such as taking the stairs instead of the elevator...rocking in a rocking chair when you read or watch TV...standing up and moving around while talking on the phone—are meaningful. Studies have shown that even fidgeting while sitting is good for you—anything to get the blood moving! One study showed that fidgeting increased energy expenditure by 10% compared with just sitting motionless.

A simple way to be sure that you don't do damage to your body by sitting too long: For every hour you sit, get up and move around for 10 minutes—stretch, pace, do some jumping jacks. While you are seated, flex and contract your muscles from time to time...stretch...and even just shift your weight from side to side.

Also good: Turn movie and TV watching time into "moving" time—you can walk on a treadmill during your favorite show...sit on an exercise ball and rock back and forth...or make a habit of standing up and sitting down 10 times in a row every half hour.

There's not yet any data showing how much sitting is too much. But if you think you may be sitting too much, you probably are. If that sounds like you or anyone you know—the solution is simple: Get a move on!

5 DIY Tests That Could Save Your Life

David L. Katz, MD, MPH, an internist and preventive medicine specialist. He is cofounder and director of the Yale-Griffin Prevention Research Center in Derby, Connecticut, and clinical instructor at the Yale School of Medicine in New Haven, Connecticut. Dr. Katz is also president of the American College of Lifestyle Medicine and the author of *Disease-Proof: The Remarkable Truth About What Makes Us Well.*

If you're conscientious about your health, you probably see your doctor for an annual physical...or perhaps even more often if you have a chronic condition or get sick.

But if you'd like to keep tabs on your health between your doctor visits, there are some easy, do-it-yourself tests that can give you valuable information about your body. These tests can sometimes tip you off that you may have a serious medical condition even though you don't have any symptoms.

Here are self-tests that you can do at home—repeat them once every few months, and keep track of results. *See your doctor if you don't "pass" one or more of the tests...**

TEST #1: STAIRS TEST

Why this test? It helps assess basic lung and heart function.

The prop you'll need: A single flight of stairs (about eight to 12 steps).

What to do: Walk up the steps at a normal pace while continuously reciting "Mary had a little lamb" or some other simple verse.

Watch out: You should be able to talk easily while climbing the stairs and when at the top—without feeling winded. If you cannot continue to talk, or if you feel discomfort or tightness in your

*These self-tests are not a substitute for a thorough physical exam from your doctor. Use them only as a way to identify potential problem areas to discuss with your physician.

chest at any time during this test, see your doctor as soon as possible.

Beware: If the small stress of climbing one flight of stairs causes physical problems, it could be a sign of hardening of the arteries (arteriosclerosis) or heart disease.

For some individuals, being out of breath could mean that they have asthma or bronchitis...chronic obstructive pulmonary disease (COPD), including emphysema...or even lung cancer.

TEST #2: GRAVITY TEST

Why this test? It measures how well your body adapts to changes in position, which can signal a variety of health problems, ranging from anemia to medication side effects.

The prop you'll need: Either a stopwatch or clock that measures seconds.

What to do: Lie down on a bed or the floor, and rest there for a minute or two. Then, start the stopwatch and stand up at a normal pace with no pauses (it's OK to use your hands).

Watch out: If you feel dizzy, make note of this. Most people can go from lying down to standing up within five seconds—and feel perfectly normal. In a healthy person, the body responds to the change in posture by pumping blood more strongly to the head.

Beware: Dizziness can signal any of the following...

- **Low blood pressure.** With orthostatic hypotension, your body doesn't pump enough blood to counteract the effects of gravity when you stand up.
- **Medication side effects,** especially from diuretics, such as *furosemide* (Lasix)...beta-blockers, such as *atenolol* (Tenormin) or *propranolol* (Inderal)...drugs for Parkinson's disease, such as *pramipexole* (Mirapex) or *levodopa* (Sinemet)...tricyclic antidepressants, such as *imipramine* (Tofranil) or *amitriptyline*...or drugs to treat erectile dysfunction, such as *sildenafil* (Viagra) or *tadalafil* (Cialis).
- **Dehydration.**
- **Anemia.**
- **Atherosclerosis,** in which blood flow is partially blocked by fatty deposits in blood vessels, or other vascular problems.

TEST #3: PENCIL TEST

Why this test? It checks the nerve function in your feet—if abnormal, this could indicate diabetes, certain types of infections or autoimmune disease.

The prop you'll need: A pencil that is freshly sharpened at one end with a flat eraser on the other end...and a friend to help.

What to do: Sit down so that all sides of your bare feet are accessible. Close your eyes, and keep them closed throughout the test.

Have your friend lightly touch your foot with either the sharp end or the eraser end of the pencil. With each touch, say which end of the pencil you think was used.

Ask your friend to repeat the test in at least three different locations on the tops and bottoms of both feet (12 locations total). Have your friend keep track of your right and wrong answers.

Watch out: Most people can easily tell the difference between "sharp" and "dull" sensations on their sensitive feet. If you give the wrong answer for more than two or three locations on your feet, have your doctor repeat the test to determine whether you have nerve damage (neuropathy).

Beware: Neuropathy is a common sign of diabetes...certain autoimmune disorders, including lupus and Sjögren's syndrome...infection, such as Lyme disease, shingles or hepatitis C...or excessive exposure to toxins, such as pesticides or heavy metals (mercury or lead).

TEST #4: URINE TEST

Why this test? It helps evaluate the functioning of your kidneys.

The prop you'll need: A clear plastic cup or clean, disposable clear jar.

What to do: In the middle of the day (urine will be too concentrated if you do this first thing in the morning), urinate into the cup or jar until you have caught at least an inch of urine. Throughout the day, note how often you urinate (about once every three waking hours is typical).

Watch out: The urine should be a pale, straw color—not deep yellow, brown or pinkish. Urine that's discolored could indicate dehydration, abnormal kidney function or another health problem.

Next, smell the urine. It should have nothing more than a very faint urine odor (unless you recently ate asparagus).

Beware: While dark-colored or smelly urine could simply mean that you are dehydrated, there are too many other potentially serious causes to ignore the signs.

Some of the disorders that can affect urine include...

- **Kidney or bladder infection,** which can cause discolored urine and frequent urination.
- **Kidney disease,** which can cause smelly, discolored urine. Interestingly, both too frequent urination and infrequent urination are signs of kidney disease.
- **Diabetes or enlarged prostate,** which can cause frequent urination.

TEST #5: "RULE OF THUMB" TEST

Why this test? It can help identify hearing loss.

The prop you'll need: A perfectly quiet room.

What to do: Rub your right thumb and index finger together continuously to create a kind of "whisper" sound. Raise your right arm so that it's level with your ear and your arm is roughly forming a right angle. Continue rubbing your thumb and index finger together. Can you still hear the sound? If not, move your hand toward your right ear, stopping when you can just hear the sound. Repeat on the left side.

Watch out: You should be able to hear this "finger rub" when your hand is six inches or more away from your ear.

Beware: If you need to be closer than six inches to hear the sound in either ear, you may have hearing loss. See an audiologist or otolaryngologist (ear, nose and throat specialist) for an evaluation.

While many people dismiss hearing loss as a mere inconvenience, it can have serious repercussions, such as getting into a car wreck because you can't hear the sound of a car approaching from the side.

Simple Test May Reveal Longevity

Claudio Gil Soares de Araujo, MD, PhD, professor of exercise science and sports, Universidade Gama Filho, Rio de Janeiro, Brazil.

More than 2,000 healthy adults (average age 62) were scored on the number of hand, knee or other supports required to sit on the floor and then stand unaided.

Result: Those who needed the most support had up to six times greater risk for death than those who needed the least support.

Theory: These movements indicate musculoskeletal fitness, a key component of longevity.

Self-defense: If you require more than one support to sit on or rise from the floor, talk to your doctor about ways to improve your muscle strength and flexibility.

Rethinking Your Drinking

Sarah Hartz, MD, PhD, assistant professor of psychiatry at Washington University School of Medicine, St. Louis, and lead author of the study "Daily Drinking Is Associated with Increased Mortality" published in *Alcoholism: Clinical & Experimental Research.*

The studies "Alcohol Use and Burden for 195 Countries and Territories, 1990–2016: A Systematic Analysis for the Global Burden of Disease Study 2016" and "Thresholds for Alcohol Consumption: Combined Analysis of Individual-Participant Data for 599,912 Current Drinkers in 83 Prospective Studies" published in *The Lancet* and "Alcohol Consumption and Risk of Dementia: 23 Year Follow-up of Whitehall II Cohort Study" published in *The BMJ.*

Seems like there are as many conflicting studies on alcohol's effects on health as there are vineyards in France, but a recent study should have you rethinking your drinking. Researchers at Washington University School of Medicine analyzed data from more than 400,000 people ages 18 to 85 and found that, overall, those who had one to two drinks four or more times a week—what's been thought of as a moderate amount—had a 20% higher risk for premature death compared with people who drank three times a week or less. In real-life terms, this increase in death risk becomes more significant the older you are because overall death risk increases with age.

One to two drinks four times a week is roughly half the limit suggested in the *US Dietary Guidelines for Americans* of one alcoholic drink per day for women, two for men.

CUTTING THROUGH ALCOHOL CONFUSION

The Washington University study is just one piece of research making headlines. An international group of researchers reviewed 700 global studies that looked at alcohol consumption and death around the world and concluded that the safest number of drinks is zero. Death from all causes, and particularly from cancer, rose as the amount of alcohol consumed went up.

But still other research provides a mixed message, certainly in terms of the amount of alcohol that can safely be consumed. A different international study that evaluated close to 600,000 drinkers found that a much wider range—zero to 10 drinks a week—was the safest amount. (It did also find that higher amounts decreased life expectancy incrementally...as an example, 35 drinks per week cut life expectancy by four to five years.)

Studies are conflicting because alcohol's effects can vary based on many aspects of an individual's genetic makeup and environment. For example, when parsing the findings, the Washington University research found that having one to two drinks three times a week was associated with a lower risk of dying from cardiovascular disease—so if you have a strong family history of cardiovascular disease, you may benefit from drinking this amount. But they also found that any amount of drinking increased the risk of dying of cancer—so if you have a strong family history of cancer, not drinking is your safest bet.

The bottom line: There isn't one answer for everyone. But one thing is for sure—if you don't drink already, don't start with the hope of improving your health. There are no guidelines that recommend drinking if you're a nondrinker.

If you do drink and you want to continue to enjoy it (in moderation, of course), consider your personal health risks when making a decision about quantity.

Plaque: It Leads to More Than Just Tooth Trouble

Birgitta Söder, DrMedSc, PhD, professor emerita, department of dental medicine, Karolinska Institute, Stockholm, Sweden. She is the lead author of a study published in *BMJ Open.*

Plaque—that sticky mix of mucus and bacteria that coats our teeth—is known for causing dental drama, such as cavities and bad breath.

It's also been associated with major, systemic health problems, such as heart attacks.

Recent research adds yet another major health consequence to that list—premature death from cancer.

PLAQUE ATTACK

This startling study might make you want to keep a toothbrush close at hand...

Swedish researchers began the study by asking subjects to undergo one dental exam in 1985, during which the amount of dental plaque on the teeth was measured. Then, tracking up to 24 years of medical records, the researchers analyzed who went on to die from cancer within that time period—and when.

Results: People who died of cancer during that 24-year follow-up period tended to have about 27% to 40% more plaque on their teeth than those who were still alive at the end of the study. That was true even when researchers controlled for other risk factors, such as smoking and not going to the dentist regularly.

Not only were those with lots of plaque more likely to die from cancer—their cancer-related deaths, on average, were considered premature. The average ages of death from cancer—60 for the men and 61 for the women—were about nine to 13 years shorter than the average life expectancies in developed countries.

INFLAMMATION OVERLOAD

Lead author Birgitta Söder, DrMedSci, PhD, a professor emerita in the department of dental medicine at Karolinska Institute in Stockholm, said that for some people, plaque on teeth triggers a systemic inflammatory response from the immune system, and inflammation is a key feature of many chronic diseases, including cancer. So it's possible that people with lots of plaque weren't able to recover from cancer because the plaque might have led to continuing high levels of systemic inflammation.

This news reinforces the importance of proper daily dental habits such as brushing and flossing at least twice a day. And it's a good reminder to get a professional cleaning from your dental hygienist or dentist at least once every six months!

The 10 Most Toxic Skin-Care Ingredients

Sharima Rasanayagam, PhD, director of science at the Breast Cancer Fund, San Francisco.

Rick Smith, PhD, environmentalist, executive director of the Broadbent Institute in Canada and coauthor, with Bruce Lourie, of *Slow Death by Rubber Duck: The Secret Danger of Everyday Things* and *Toxin Toxout: Getting Harmful Chemicals Out of Our Bodies and Our World.*

By the time a woman steps out of her door in the morning, she's applied an average of nine personal-care products to her face, body and hair—and been exposed to about 126 different chemicals, according to Rick Smith, PhD, coauthor of *Toxin Toxout: Getting Harmful Chemicals Out of Our Bodies and Our World*. Men may use fewer products, but they get exposed to plenty of chemicals, too.

Are all of these chemicals toxic? Of course not. But there is growing evidence that exposure to certain compounds, especially hormone (endocrine) disrupting chemicals, is contributing to diseases such as diabetes, obesity, reproductive disorders, neurological conditions and cancer. There is a lot that we don't know yet, but what we're finding isn't reassuring. New laboratory research, for example, recently uncovered that parabens, once considered a weak endocrine disruptor, may be 100 times more likely to promote breast cancer tumors than originally thought.

The good news: Switching personal-care products can reduce your body's level of hormone disrupters—quickly. In a recent study, researchers at UC Berkeley School of Public Health tested urine levels of four common endocrine disrupters in teenage girls—pthalates, parabens, triclosan and oxybenzone. Then they had the young women switch to personal-care products that are free of those chemicals for just three days.

Results: Levels of endocrine disrupters went down an average of 25% to 45%. "In researching my books," says Dr. Smith, "I conducted numerous experiments on volunteers and found similar results across a range of products and chemicals."

There's no need to panic and toss out everything in your bathroom. Dr. Smith suggests replacing each product as it runs out with a healthier one. Which ones should you toss first? To get more specifics, we asked Sharima Rasanayagam, PhD, director of science at the Breast Cancer Fund, a nonprofit that works to prevent breast cancer by reducing exposure to toxic chemicals and radiation.

1. Parabens. These endocrine disrupters are so common in personal-care products that it's tough to know where to start. A recent Swedish study of mothers found levels of parabens in urine were highest in women who used more makeup, shampoo, hair-styling products, lotion, fragrance, deodorant, massage oil and nail polish.

Shopping tips: Skip any skin-care product that contains the word "paraben" by itself or as part of another chemical name, such as *ethylparaben, propylparaben, butylparaben* or *benzylparaben*. Or shop for products that specifically claim that they are "parabens free."

2. Triclosan. This antibacterial compound contributes not only to antibiotic-resistant bacteria but is also an endocrine disrupter, says Dr. Smith. "Triclosan is a registered pesticide, and extremely worrisome," he warns. It's found in soft and bar antibacterial soaps, cosmetics, shaving products, deodorants and dry shampoos, according to the Environmental Working Group's Skin Deep Cosmetics Database. The FDA is currently evaluating the ingredient based on animal studies that show that it disrupts hormones and may lead to more antibiotic-resistant bacteria, but it already emphasizes that the soaps and body washes with triclosan provide no extra health benefit to consumers.

Shopping tips: Avoid any product that contains triclosan. In particular, Dr. Smith recommends that if you have Colgate Total toothpaste, toss it immediately even though it is effective against gingivitis. Why? Exposing your gums to *triclosan* means more may be absorbed than from, for example, washing your hands with liquid soap. When shopping for face- or body-washing products, remember that plain old soap and water is highly effective at removing bacteria—if you wash long enough.

Travel tip: If you want to avoid triclosan-containing antibacterial soaps in, say, public bathrooms, carry a small bottle of alcohol-based hand sanitizer with you.

3. Polytetrafluoroethylene (PTFE), a suspected carcinogen found in some anti-aging creams. According to a recent Breast Cancer Fund study, this compound, originally used to create Teflon, often travels with a related chemical called perfluorooctanoic acid (aka PFOA or C-8).

Shopping tips: The Breast Cancer Fund study names three products to avoid—Garnier Ultra-Lift Transformer Anti-Age Skin Corrector, Garnier Ultra-Lift Anti-Wrinkle Firming Moisturizer and Cover Girl Advanced Radiance with Olay, Age Defying Pressed Powder. Read labels—in addition to PTFE, other ingredients that may mean PFOA include Polyperfluoromethylisopropyl and DEA-C8-18 Perfluoroalkylethyl. Check for products that specifically state that they are PTFE- and PFOA-free. (To learn more, see "Natural Anti-Aging Treatments for Your Skin" on page 256.)

4. Resorcinol, found in hair dyes. According to Dr. Rasanayagam, hair dyes often contain "a bunch of nasty chemicals," often derived from coal tar, but resorcinol, a potent endocrine disruptor, is the worst.

Shopping tips: Unfortunately, resorcinol is found in most hair dyes in most colors as well as certain over-the-counter acne products. Says Dr. Rasanayagam, "Hair colorings are particularly difficult to formulate without these chemicals, but some companies are working on better options."

Safer, non–coal-tar dye alternatives include temporary hair colorants and henna, which imbues a reddish tinge and is approved by the FDA as a natural dye. Indigo, which is a dark blue, is another natural nontoxic dye that may also be mixed in with henna. Other botanical-based hair dyes can also be used for lighter colors, including blond. But beware of "black henna," which may contain coal-tar–based hair dyes. The best way to approach the issue? Learn to love your gray.

5. Formaldehyde, dibutyl phthalate (DBP) and toluene, aka the "Toxic Trio," often found in nail polish. Formaldehyede is a carcinogen, DBP is an endocrine disruptor, and toluene is a toxic compound often contaminated with benzene, a carcinogen.

Shopping tips: Read labels, and shop for toxic-trio–free brands such as Honeybee Garden and Acquarella, suggests Dr. Rasanayagam.

6. Hydroquinone, found in skin lighteners and age-spot removers. Animal studies link topical use of this bleaching compound with cancer, and it can also cause a skin-darkening medical condition in some people. The US National Toxicology Program has proposed removing it from the "safe" list of ingredients—pending more studies. Meanwhile it's banned in Europe in concentrations above 1% but still legal and readily available in the US in concentrations up to 4%.

Shopping tips: Avoid any product with hydroquinone on the label. You may want to try home-remedy concoctions using food-based ingredients such as lemons, honey, oranges and/or milk that help naturally lighten skin without harsh chemicals.

7. Phthalates, commonly found in fragrances and perfumes. These are potent endocrine disrupters, and while exposure in cosmetics is dropping, one big exception is DEP, a phthalate found in fragrances. By law, companies don't have to reveal fragrance ingredients, yet many of those ingredients contain not only phthalates but also parabens and synthetic musk (another endocrine disrupter).

Shopping tips: Avoid any product that just lists "fragrance" or "parfum." Says Dr. Smith, "Because companies aren't legally obligated to disclose the presence of phthalates in their products, look for products that say 'No Phthalates' on the label."

8. Petrolatum, aka petroleum jelly, mineral oil and paraffin oil, found in many moisturizers, ointments and skin creams.

The big exception: Refined petrolatum, also called white petrolatum, has no known health concerns. That's what's in Vaseline, which is safer. But products that simply list "petroleum jelly" may be using less refined products, which may be contaminated with suspected carcinogens including polycyclic aromatic hydrocarbons (PAHs).

Shopping tips: Avoid any product that contains petroleum jelly unless it specifies white petroleum jelly or white petrolatum. Vaseline, as noted, is a safer choice. You may also want to explore moisturizers that contain botanical-based ingredients such as beeswax, coconut oil, olive oil, shea butter and coconut butter instead.

9. Oxybenzone and benzophenone found in sunscreens. How dangerous these are is still a controversy. While the Environmental Working Group warns that these are endocrine disrupters that are absorbed into the skin, the American Academy of Dermatology believes they are safe to use. According to Dr. Rasanayagam, however, you should avoid these chemicals.

Shopping tips: Avoid sunscreens with oxybenzone or benzophenone. Instead, choose cream sunscreens with zinc oxide or titanium dioxide.

10. Formaldehyde, found in hair straighteners or hair-smoothing products such as Brazilian Blowout or keratin treatments. When heated, these products can release formaldehye (a carcinogen) into the air, which can lead to eye problems, headaches, dizziness, breathing problems, nausea and rash.

Shopping tips: Avoid any product that contains formaldehyde—by FDA regulation, it must include a warning on the label. If you go to a salon, ask to look at the product they use to make sure it doesn't contain formaldehyde. However, beware of salon products that claim to be formaldehyde-free but list "methylene glycol" on the ingredient list—that's just formaldehyde by another name.

Some salons use hair-straigthening products that rely primarily on botanicals instead—Aveda makes one, called Smooth Infusion Professional Smoothing Treatment. Also consider going old school with a straight iron.

HOW TO SHOP FOR HEALTHIER PERSONAL-CARE PRODUCTS

Now that you know the ingredients that are most important to avoid, how can you start? *A few tips…*

- **Get familiar with websites.** Two sites let you search for healthy personal-care products—the GoodGuide (which also works well on your smartphone and other mobile devices) and the Environmental Working Group's Skin Deep. You can educate yourself about these issues with the Breast Cancer Fund's site, Campaign for Safe Cosmetics, as well.

- **Download an app.** The EWG has a Healthy Living app (free), and the Think Dirty app lists thousands of personal-care products. Download one on your smartphone so that you can spot-check products while shopping.

- **Decide what "healthier" means to you.** Safe Cosmetics.org addresses only long-term chronic health issues, but the Good Guide and the Skin Deep sites discourage not only products with toxic ingredients but also those that cause irritation, trigger allergies, negatively impact the environment or have been tested on animals. But if your body wash, for example, contains a possible irritant and it doesn't irritate you, you may decide to keep it anyway.

- **Don't be fooled by labels that claim a product is "All Natural" or made with "100% Natural Ingredients."** While the "organic" term is regulated on cosmetics and personal-care products, the term "natural" is not.

Surprising Dangers of Air Pollution: It Can Hurt Much More Than Your Lungs

Neil Schachter, MD, medical director of the respiratory care department at Mount Sinai Hospital and the Maurice Hexter Professor of Pulmonary Medicine at the Icahn School of Medicine at Mount Sinai, both in New York City. He is the author of *The Good Doctor's Guide to Colds and Flu* and serves on the American Lung Association's Northeast Board of Directors.

You may assume that air pollution problems in the US are a thing of the past, since environmental laws have reduced the haze that once blanketed our big cities. But that's not true. Air pollution still ranks high on the list of health threats—and not just for city dwellers.

Wake-up call: More than 40% of Americans—nearly 140 million of us—breathe unhealthy air, according to a recent report by the American Lung Association.

Even when the sky appears crystal clear, you're inhaling exhaust fumes, ground-level ozone and microscopic particles—common pollutants that can increase your risk for health problems ranging from heart disease to asthma.

Small-town living helps but not completely. Even in the wide-open spaces of the American West, drought and high summer temperatures increase levels of dust and other airborne particles that can worsen conditions such as asthma and chronic obstructive pulmonary disease (COPD).

THE BIGGEST DANGERS

You would expect bad air to threaten lung health, but there's increasing evidence showing that the risk is far more pervasive. *Examples...*

• **Heart disease.** Air pollution is ranked ninth among the most important cardiovascular risk factors—making it more harmful than lack of exercise or elevated cholesterol, according to a report in the *European Heart Journal*.

What makes air pollution so hard on the heart? Airborne particles trigger inflammation in the lungs and blood vessels that can increase atherosclerosis and the risk for clots. Even brief exposures to PM2.5—common airborne particles that are about one-fifth the size of a speck of dust—may increase cardiovascular risks. You are likely inhaling these particles if you drive to work with your car windows open, walk past a construction site or light a fire in your fireplace. In areas where particle concentrations are persistently high, such as near busy roads, there's an 11% average increased risk of dying from heart attack, heart failure or stroke.

• **Stroke.** Even if you live in a rural, "wholesome" area, you will occasionally breathe high levels of carbon monoxide and other gaseous pollutants—when you're behind a truck, for example. Such limited exposures may seem harmless, but an analysis of more than 100 studies found that intermittent spikes in air pollution caused a corresponding increase in hospitalizations and deaths from stroke.

• **Heart-rate changes.** The varying intervals between heartbeats, known as heart-rate variability, are a sign of cardiovascular health. Bad air—even inside the home—can have a harmful effect. People who frequently use air fresheners are more likely to have reduced heart-rate variability, research has found. Many air fresheners contain terpenes, chemicals that can smell like pine or citrus. They interact with other chemicals in the air and form heart-damaging compounds.

WHAT CAN YOU DO?

To help protect your health...

• **Track the Air Quality Index (AQI).** The AQI is a rating based on daily levels of major pollutants—carbon monoxide, sulfur dioxide, particle pollution, etc. When the number rises above 100, it's wise to avoid outdoor activities—particularly if you have already been diagnosed with lung or heart disease or diabetes. For an up-to-date AQI, go to AirNow.gov.

• **Exercise away from major roads.** Levels of PM2.5 particles tend to be much higher in areas with heavy traffic. If you like to walk, jog or bike, do it as close to nature as possible—and away from busy streets. Pollution is usually highest within 50 feet of roads.

Also helpful: Avoid rush-hour traffic if you can...and drive with the windows closed (see below).

- **Use the AC.** It is nice to conserve power (and save money), but don't skimp on air-conditioning. It filters incoming air and traps large particles. In fact, a study in Taiwan found that people who used home air conditioners showed none of the "cardiovascular endpoints"—such as inflammation and heart rhythm disturbances—that were apparent when they kept windows open.

In the car: Be sure to use the "recirculate" setting. Research has found that recirculating air will keep out 80% of outside air pollution.

- **Filter the air.** Dust is a major irritant for people with asthma, COPD or other lung diseases, as well as for those with cardiovascular disease. And even if it's cleaned often, the average home has a lot of dust.

My advice: If you have any of the health issues mentioned above, invest in a HEPA air purifier for any room you spend a lot of time in. Many brands are available—most of which will remove up to 99% of suspended particles in a given room. They work more effectively than electrostatic air purifiers, and they don't produce the ozone (another lung irritant) that can result from electrostatic units. HEPA filtration is also available in central ventilation systems.

Also: To keep indoor air cleaner, install solid floors (such as wood or tile)—not wall-to-wall carpet...and avoid floor-to-ceiling curtains.

- **Use natural scents.** Commercial air fresheners may smell nice, but they all contain chemical compounds. Why take chances? Natural scents smell better—and cost less.

Examples: Spritz rosewater in the air...or simmer lemon or orange peels on the stove.

CHECK YOUR AIR QUALITY

In the American Lung Association's recent report *State of the Air 2015*, six cities were ranked as having the cleanest air in the nation. They had no days when the air quality reached unhealthy levels for ozone or short-term particle pollution and had the best records for year-round particle pollution. The cities, listed alphabetically, are Bismarck, North Dakota...Cape Coral-Fort Myers-Naples, Florida... Elmira-Corning, New York...Fargo-Wahpeton, North Dakota...Rapid City-Spearfish, South Dakota ...and Salinas, California.

To check your county, go to StateoftheAir.org and enter your zip code.

Eat Less Red Meat

Study of nearly 537,000 adults led by researchers at the US National Institutes of Health, Bethesda, Maryland, published in *The BMJ.*

Red meat is linked to more than just heart disease. People who ate the most red meat had the highest risk of dying from cancer, heart disease, stroke, respiratory disease, diabetes, infections, chronic kidney disease and chronic liver disease. People who consumed more than five ounces per day of red meat had a 26% increased risk of dying during the study, versus those who ate less than five ounces per week.

Stroke: It's On the Rise Among Younger People

Brett M. Kissela, MD, professor and vice-chair of the department of neurology at the University of Cincinnati College of Medicine. He was the lead researcher of the National Institutes of Health–funded study, published in *Neurology,* that documented increasing strokes in younger adults.

Few people in their 40s or 50s can imagine having a stroke, particularly if they are generally healthy. But the risk is higher than you might think—dispelling the common belief that stroke is a risk for only the elderly.

An unexpected trend: Over the last several years, there has been an increase in strokes among adults in their 40s, 50s and 60s. What's most alarming about this development is that doctors don't expect to see strokes in these relatively young patients, so the diagnosis sometimes gets overlooked.

Important finding: One in seven young stroke patients was initially misdiagnosed as having another problem, such as a seizure or alcohol intoxication, researchers at Wayne State University–Detroit Medical Center found in a recent study.

What to do: First and foremost, be alert. Stroke can occur at any age, so it's important for all adults to pay close attention to symptoms. If you are diagnosed and treated within about four hours of having a stroke, you are far more likely to recover than someone whose diagnosis and treatment are delayed. Unfortunately, only about 20% to 30% of young patients with stroke symptoms go to the emergency room, according to research. The others are likely to shrug off the symptoms (especially if they were relatively minor and/or short-lived) and do not learn that they have suffered a stroke until a subsequent problem is detected later on.

WHAT'S CAUSING EARLIER STROKES?

Many of the so-called "age-related" diseases that greatly increase stroke risk, such as high blood pressure (hypertension), diabetes and high cholesterol, are now appearing in patients who are middle-aged or younger—primarily because so many Americans are eating more junk food, gaining too much weight and not getting enough exercise. Family history is also a risk factor for stroke.

But even if you don't have any of these conditions (or a family history of stroke), you are in good physical shape and generally eat a well-balanced diet, do not be lulled into a false sense of security. Anyone can suffer a stroke. That's why it's very important for all adults to be on the lookout for red flags that could signal a stroke.

PREVENTION WORKS

Stroke is the fourth-leading cause of death in the US. Those who survive a stroke often face a lifetime of disability, including paralysis and speech and emotional difficulties.

Fortunately, younger patients, in general, are more likely to recover than older ones because their brains have greater plasticity, the ability to regain functions after stroke-related trauma. Even so, many young stroke patients will have permanent damage.

Important: Regardless of your age, fast treatment is critical if you experience stroke symptoms. The majority of strokes are ischemic, caused by blood clots that impair circulation to the brain. Patients who are given clot-dissolving drugs, such as tissue plasminogen activator (tPA), within the first few hours after a stroke are far more likely to make a full recovery than those who are treated later.

Up to 80% of strokes can be avoided by preventing or treating the main risk factors, according to the National Stroke Association. For example, not smoking is crucial—people who smoke are twice as likely to have an ischemic stroke as nonsmokers.

Also important...

- **Do not ignore hypertension.** Like stroke, hypertension is often viewed as a problem only for the elderly. But there's been an increase in hypertension in younger patients, who often go undiagnosed.

Warning: Uncontrolled high blood pressure damages the brain—even in patients who haven't had a stroke, according to a new study published in *The Lancet Neurology*.

If your blood pressure is high (normal is below 120/80), you are two to four times more likely to have a stroke than someone with normal blood pressure.

What to do: All adults should always have their blood pressure taken during routine doctor visits (at least once every two years if your blood pressure is normal...and at least annually if you've been diagnosed with hypertension or prehypertension). You can reduce both blood pressure and the risk for stroke by maintaining a healthy body weight...eating a healthful diet...getting regular exercise...and taking medication if your blood pressure remains elevated despite lifestyle changes.

- **Manage diabetes.** It's second only to hypertension as a risk factor for stroke. Diabetes increases the risk for all cardiovascular diseases, including hypertension. People who have diabetes are up to four times more likely to have a stroke than those without the condition.

What to do: Get tested. The American Diabetes Association recommends that all adults age 45 and older get screened for diabetes every three years.

If you already have diabetes, do everything you can to keep your blood sugar stable—for example, eat properly, get exercise and lose weight, if necessary.

• **Keep an eye on your cholesterol.** It's the third most important stroke risk factor because LDL ("bad") cholesterol can accumulate in the arteries, impede circulation to the brain and increase the risk for blood clots.

What to do: Beginning at age 20, get your cholesterol tested at least every five years. If your LDL is high (less than 100 mg/dL is optimal), you'll want to get the number down by eating less saturated fat...getting more vegetables and other high-fiber foods...and possibly taking a statin medication, such as *simvastatin* (Zocor). Depending on the drug and dose, statins typically lower cholesterol by about 25% to 50%.

• **Pay attention to your alcohol consumption.** People who drink heavily (three or more alcoholic beverages daily for men and two or more for women) are more likely to have a stroke earlier in life than moderate drinkers or nondrinkers.

In fact, in a study of 540 stroke patients, French researchers found that heavy drinkers suffered their strokes at age 60, on average—14 years earlier than patients who drank less or not at all.

Warning: Heavy use of alcohol is also associated with increased risk for hemorrhagic stroke, which is caused by bleeding in the brain (rather than a blood clot). This type of stroke can occur even in patients without a history of serious health problems.

What to do: If you drink, be sure to follow the standard advice for alcohol consumption—no more than two drinks daily for men...or one for women.

SURPRISING RED FLAGS FOR STROKE

• **Stroke symptoms aren't always dramatic.** If you've had a minor stroke or a transient ischemic attack (a brief interruption of blood flow known as a "ministroke"), the symptoms might be fleeting and easy to miss.

What's more, in rare cases, symptoms may occur that you may not think of in relation to a stroke. For example, you may initially feel disoriented or experience nausea, general weakness, face or limb pain, chest pain or palpitations—all of which typically come on suddenly. Depending on the part of the brain that's affected, you may not be aware of your symptoms and must rely on someone else to call for help.

• **Don't take chances.** Get to an emergency room if you have these and/or the classic symptoms below—FAST (Face, Arm, Speech and Time) is a helpful guide.

Face: The most common stroke symptom is weakness on one side of the body, including on one side of the face. You may have difficulty smiling normally.

Arm: One-sided weakness often affects one of the arms. Hold both arms out to your sides. You could be having a stroke if one of your arms drops down.

Speech: Your words could sound slurred, or you might be unable to say a simple sentence correctly.

Time: In the past, the "window" to receive clot-dissolving medication was considered to be three hours. New research indicates that stroke patients can benefit if they get treated within 4.5 hours after having the first symptom.

Restless Legs Syndrome Linked to Higher Risk for Death

Xiang Gao, MD, PhD, research scientist, Harvard School of Public Health, assistant professor of medicine, Harvard Medical School, and associate epidemiologist, Brigham and Women's Hospital, all in Boston. His study was published in *Neurology*.

Do you ever get the annoying feeling that bugs are crawling around under the skin of your legs? Do you feel a pulling, itching or throbbing sensation in your legs along with an uncontrollable urge to move them, particularly in the evening or nighttime hours?

If so, you may have restless legs syndrome (RLS). No, that is not a made-up name for some minor annoyance. It's the actual medical term for a very real health problem...and researchers recently discovered a very scary risk associated with this disorder. The shocker: Having restless legs is linked with an increased risk for premature death.

STARTLING STUDY

Back in 1986, a group of 51,500 male healthcare professionals ages 40 to 75 enrolled in a long-term study, periodically answering questions about their medical histories, diet and lifestyles. In 2002, nearly 32,000 of those men were still alive and participating. They were mailed a questionnaire that asked the same questions posed at the start of this article. Those who answered yes to all of the questions and had symptoms at least five times per month were considered to have RLS. Men who had other disorders with symptoms that could possibly be mistaken for RLS (such as diabetes or arthritis) were excluded. This left 18,425 men in the analysis, about 4% of whom had RLS.

Over the next eight years 2,765 of the men died. Researchers ascertained the causes of death from medical records and death certificates, then analyzed the data. *What they found was startling...*

- **Men with RLS were 39% more likely to die during the eight-year study period than men without RLS.**
- **Even after researchers adjusted for numerous other risk factors** (such as body mass index, physical activity level, smoking and alcohol consumption), the death risk associated with RLS was still increased by 30%.
- **Among men who had a chronic illness, those with RLS fared far worse than those without RLS.** *Examples*: Cancer patients without RLS had a 47% increased risk for death, while cancer patients with RLS had a 97% increased risk for death...cardiovascular disease patients without RLS had a 37% increased risk, while cardiovascular disease patients with RLS had a 68% increased risk.
- **When the researchers looked only at the men who were generally healthy and did not have a chronic illness,** they found that RLS was associated with almost double the risk of dying. The more frequently the men experienced RLS symptoms, the higher their death risk was.

What did them in: Compared with men who did not have RLS, those who did have the disorder had nearly six times the risk of dying from a blood-related disease (such as anemia)...five times the risk of dying from an immune, endocrine or metabolic disease...and almost twice the risk of dying from respiratory disease.

WHAT'S BEHIND THE CONNECTION?

This study does not prove that RLS causes death, only that the disorder is associated with increased risk. *The researchers aren't sure what is behind this association, but they do have some theories...*

Sleep disruption: RLS interferes with restful sleep, and poor sleep has been linked with increased death risk in several earlier studies. One possible reason for this is that shorter sleep duration can lead to changes in levels of certain hormones than can promote the development of diabetes, obesity and cardiovascular disease.

Effect on blood pressure: RLS may contribute to nocturnal hypertension (high blood pressure at night)—and blood pressure problems increase cardiovascular risk.

Neurodegenerative disorder: Even though this study excluded people with Parkinson's disease, it is possible that RLS is an early symptom of undiagnosed Parkinson's or some other unidentified neurological disease.

Because this study included only men, we don't know whether the increased death risk also applies to women with RLS. That question certainly merits additional study, given that women actually are more likely than men to have RLS.

We also don't know whether getting treated for RLS would reduce a person's risk of dying early. But treatment certainly can help people sleep better...and the better you sleep, the better your health is likely to be.

So if you have symptoms that suggest RLS, consider this study a wake-up call—bring the matter to your doctor's attention and ask, "Could this be restless legs?" Although RLS affects an estimated 5% to 10% of the population, the vast majority of sufferers are never formally diagnosed or treated. Diet, lifestyle changes, natural therapies and/or medication can help.

The Extreme Dangers of Belly Fat

Bill Gavin, MD, an interventional cardiologist and medical director of the Heart Program at Providence St. Peter Hospital in Olympia, Washington. He is the author of *No White at Night: The Three-Rule Diet.*

Even if you're not overweight, it can significantly increase your risk for heart disease, cancer and dementia.

Everyone knows that it's unhealthy to be obese. What's surprising to many people, however, is just how serious it can be to have "belly fat."

Important recent finding: A study published in *The New England Journal of Medicine* that looked at more than 350,000 people found that a large waist can nearly double your risk of dying prematurely—even if your weight is "normal" (according to your body mass index, a measure of body fat based on height and weight).* Some people who don't exercise but generally keep their overall body weight under control, for example, may have dangerous fat deposits around the abdomen.

Why is belly fat, in particular, so dangerous? Here's what you need to know...

WHAT'S YOUR SHAPE?

It's been widely reported that about one-third of Americans are considered obese—the highest percentage of any country in the world. Though estimates vary, obesity, which is strongly linked to diabetes, heart disease, stroke and even cancer, is blamed for at least 26,000 deaths in the US each year.

Most of the body's fat—known as subcutaneous (under the skin) fat—accumulates in the thighs, buttocks and hips. This fat distribution, which leads to a so-called "pear" body shape, applies to most women—and many men.

However, belly fat—generally associated with an "apple" body shape—presents the greatest risks. Also known as visceral fat, it is stored mostly inside the abdominal cavity, where it wraps around (and sometimes invades) the internal organs, including the heart.

Long known to damage blood vessel linings, belly fat is a metabolically active tissue that secretes harmful inflammatory substances that can contribute to a variety of health problems. People with an apple body type are far more likely to die of heart attacks than those with a pear shape.

The worst of the worst: Hard belly fat (commonly known as a "beer belly") is even more dangerous than soft belly fat—perhaps because many people with hard belly fat have high levels of C-reactive-protein (CRP), an inflammation marker and risk factor for heart disease. Alcohol has been shown to slow fat metabolism by more than 30%, which is compounded by the fact that beer drinkers tend to eat high-calorie snack foods while drinking and beer itself is high in carbohydrate calories.

An increasing body of evidence is now linking belly fat to other serious health risks, such as...

- **Cancer.** Both men and women with higher percentages of belly fat are more likely to develop a variety of cancers, including malignancies of the colon, kidney and breast.
- **Dementia.** In a study of 6,583 adults, the bigger the belly, the greater the risk for dementia.

Surprising finding: Among those of normal weight who had excess belly fat, dementia risk was 1.89 times higher than for those of normal weight who did not have excess belly fat.

- **Lung problems.** Lung function is reduced in patients with higher stores of belly fat, possibly because of the higher secretion of lung-damaging inflammatory chemicals.

*To calculate your body mass index, go to NHLBI.nih.gov and search for "BMI Calculator."

•**Diabetes.** An apple-shaped fat distribution greatly increases the risk for insulin resistance (a condition in which the body's cells don't use insulin properly) and diabetes.

The risks are even higher in those who are sedentary. People who have lost muscle mass, as a result, take in less blood sugar (glucose), which is used as fuel—further increasing diabetes risk.

•**Migraines.** Researchers at Drexel University College of Medicine found that women with large amounts of belly fat were up to 30% more likely than lean women to suffer from migraine headaches.

INCHES THAT REALLY COUNT

Research has shown that waist size—even in people who aren't obviously overweight—is a key predictor of long-term health.

Important finding: In a study reported in *Circulation: Heart Failure*, researchers found that a four-inch increase in waist size raised the risk for heart disease by about 15%, even in people of normal weight. Other studies report that each five-centimeter increase in waist size (a little less than two inches) raises the risk for premature death by 13% in women and 17% in men.

My recommendation: A waist size of 35 inches or less in women and 40 inches or less in men. Even slight increases above these numbers significantly raise your health risks.

Best way to measure your waist: Place a tape measure just below your navel, exhale gently, then record the measurement.

STRATEGIES FOR WAIST LOSS

There are no proven ways to selectively reduce accumulations of visceral fat. *My advice…*

•**Strive for healthy overall weight loss.** People who follow a sensible diet, such as the American Heart Association's No-Fat Diet (Heart.org) or the Weight Watchers plan (WeightWatchers.com), lose weight proportionally—that is, they lose more weight from areas where they have the most body fat. Someone with a high percentage of visceral fat will show the effects most in the abdomen.

Another advantage of such diets is that they include large amounts of natural, wholesome foods, such as vegetables and whole grains. A plant-based diet supplies large quantities of anti-inflammatory, disease-fighting compounds.

Important: When you're trying to lose weight, avoid or eliminate most dietary sugars—not only from sweet snacks, but also from processed carbohydrates, such as white bread, snacks, beer and fruit juices. These foods have a high-glycemic index—that is, they cause a rapid spike in blood sugar that may increase the accumulation of visceral fat.

•**Drink green tea.** A study in the *Journal of Nutrition* found that obese adults who drank green tea lost about twice as much weight over 12 weeks as a control group even though people in both groups followed similar diets and exercise patterns. It's thought that compounds known as catechins in green tea increase metabolism and accelerate the breakdown of fat.

•**Focus on aerobic exercise.** This is the best way to increase metabolism, burn calories and reduce fat. Aerobic exercise is more effective than resistance workouts (such as lifting weights) because it burns more calories per hour.

There's some evidence that overweight women who engage in sustained aerobic workouts—such as 20 minutes or more of brisk walking daily—can lose up to one inch of belly fat in just four weeks.

•**Turn down the thermostat.** Researchers have recently made exciting discoveries related to so-called "brown" fat, which has been shown to burn energy to generate body heat.

This type of fat was once thought to disappear after infancy, but new studies indicate that it's present in many adults and can be activated by exposure to cool temperatures—roughly 61°F.

People who are overweight or obese may have lower brown fat activity, which could be an underlying cause of weight gain. Spending a few hours in cool temperatures—say, at night when you sleep—could potentially increase the body's energy expenditure, which, over time, could result in weight loss. More research is needed, but in the meantime, set your thermostat as low as is comfortable year-round.

Look Out for AFib

Analysis of 104 studies including more than nine million people, 590,000 of whom had A-fib, by researchers at University of Oxford, UK, and Massachusetts Institute of Technology, Boston, published in *BMJ*.

Atrial fibrillation is tied to many dangerous conditions—not just stroke, as previously believed. AFib, a common heart-rhythm disorder, is associated with heart disease, heart failure, kidney disease and sudden cardiac death—as well as death from all causes. The strongest association found was with heart failure, which was five times more likely in people with AFib.

A Charley Horse…or a Deadly Blood Clot?

Daniella Kadian-Dodov, MD, assistant professor of medicine in the department of vascular medicine at the Zena and Michael A. Wiener Cardiovascular Institute and the Marie-Josée and Henry R. Kravis Center for Cardiovascular Health at the Icahn School of Medicine at Mount Sinai Hospital in New York City.

If you've ever been stopped cold by a charley horse, you know just how excruciating these muscle spasms can be. But are you sure it's just a muscle spasm? Or is that leg pain due to something far more serious?

What can cause leg pain…

PERIPHERAL ARTERIAL DISEASE (PAD)

This is one to worry about. Even though the pain usually isn't intense, it can triple your risk of dying from a heart attack or stroke.

What it feels like: About 10% of people with PAD suffer leg cramps, leg aching and leg fatigue that occur only during physical activity involving the legs (any type of activity can trigger it—even just walking). When you rest your legs, the discomfort goes away, usually in 10 minutes or less. As PAD becomes more severe and blood circulation worsens, pain can occur during rest and result in leg ulcers and even gangrene.

What to do: See a doctor. PAD is usually caused by atherosclerosis, the same condition that leads to most heart attacks. Your doctor will compare the blood pressure in your arms to the pressure at your ankles. If there's a significant difference, that could mean that you have PAD and you'll need an ultrasound of the legs to determine the extent and location of arterial obstructions.

Next steps: The same practices that protect your heart—such as not smoking, controlling diabetes, maintaining healthy blood pressure and getting plenty of exercise—will help stop PAD from worsening and could even reverse it.

Important: You must walk—even when it hurts. Walking ultimately reduces pain and improves circulation by stimulating the growth of blood vessels that bypass the damaged ones. With your doctor's OK, walk five times a week, for 30 to 45 minutes each time. I usually advise my patients to walk fast for two blocks or until they feel moderate pain, then rest a moment and walk fast for two blocks again, repeating until the end of their workout.

DEEP VEIN THROMBOSIS (DVT)

It doesn't always cause leg pain, but if pain occurs, this warning could save your life. DVT means that you have a blood clot—most often deep in a leg vein. It can be fatal.

What it feels like: You might notice a sudden, pulsating or aching pain deep in your calf or thigh, sometimes accompanied by redness and/or swelling. DVT usually occurs after you've been immobile for a long time—you're laid up in bed after surgery, for example, or following a long car or plane trip.

What to do: Get to an emergency department or a physician's office where you can get an immediate ultrasound. The clot could break free, travel to the lungs and cause pulmonary embolism, a clot in the lungs that's fatal in up to 30% of cases.

If you have a DVT, your doctor will probably give intravenous or injectable heparin, a blood-thinning drug that prevents the clot from growing. After a day or two, you'll be switched to oral blood-thinning medication, such as *warfarin* (Coumadin) or *dabigatran* (Pradaxa). You'll need to take the medication for about six months. If the clot is not entirely dissolved after treatment, it should be monitored with ultrasound—and if you have had one clot, you might get another one. Prevention is critical.

Everyone—whether you've had a DVT or not—should flex the ankle and calf muscles for about 30 seconds every 20 or 30 minutes when sitting for longer than four hours. Stand up and move around at least every hour or so.

If you have risk factors for blood clots—you're over age 40, obese, have a family history of blood clots or use hormone replacement therapy—ask your doctor about such precautions as taking aspirin before travel and/or wearing compression stockings while you're immobile.

SCIATICA

This back condition is typically caused by a herniated spinal disk. The legs become involved because the disk exerts painful pressure on the sciatic nerve, which runs down the backs of the legs.

What it feels like: Intense, shooting and/or knifelike pains may extend through the buttocks and into one leg. Sciatica also can cause leg and/or ankle weakness.

What to do: See your doctor. If you do have sciatica, you may get better within eight weeks by doing physical therapy and using a nonsteroidal anti-inflammatory medication such as *ibuprofen* (Motrin)—90% of sciatica patients do.

Next steps: Consider surgery for a herniated disk/sciatica only when the pain is too intense to handle...you have responsibilities that don't permit extended downtime...or you're having additional symptoms such as muscle weakness or a loss of bowel/bladder control.

MORE FROM DR. KADIAN-DODOV

When It Really Is a Charley Horse

A muscle spasm, including the infamous "charley horse" of the leg, believed to have been named after a lame horse, can occur after hard exercise or for no obvious reason. It can cause sudden, localized pain (usually with sharp contractions) that often hits the calves.

If you're getting muscle spasms with any sort of regularity, see your doctor. Muscle spasms have a variety of causes—for example, you may have overworked your legs by doing yard work...you may be dehydrated (without enough water, muscle cells can spasm)...or a medication you're taking, such as a diuretic, may be the culprit.

Helpful: Because most muscle spasms are caused, in part, by tight hamstrings (the muscles in the backs of your upper legs), I recommend doing a standing hamstring stretch on a regular basis. Start in a standing position with your knees straight...bend at the waist...and reach for your toes or the floor until you feel a stretch in your hamstrings. Hold for a few seconds, and repeat a few times a day.

Sleep Apnea: Killing You While You Sleep—28 Million Americans Have This Disorder—and Most Don't Know It

Chris Meletis, ND, former chief medical officer for the National College of Naturopathic Medicine and a physician on the staff of Beaverton Naturopathic Medicine in Oregon. He is author of 18 books on health and healing, including *The Hyaluronic Acid Miracle*. DrMeletis.com

Twenty-eight million Americans have sleep apnea, a sleep disorder in which breathing repeatedly stops and starts. More than 80% of these people don't know they have it. And every year, an estimated 38,000 Americans die in their sleep because sleep apnea has exacerbated a circulatory problem, causing a fatal heart attack or stroke.

Bottom line: Diagnosing and treating sleep apnea can save your life. And now there's an exciting new treatment that's available. *What you need to know...*

THE DANGER

For people with sleep apnea, nighttime levels of blood oxygen can plummet from an optimal saturation of 100% to below 65%. This oxygen-robbing disorder can contribute to extreme daytime sleepiness, as well as high blood pressure, heart attack, stroke, congestive heart failure, type 2 diabetes, Alzheimer's disease, erectile dysfunction, depression, anxiety and gastroesophageal reflux disease (GERD). In fact, if you have sleep apnea, you have a nearly five times higher risk of dying overall.

What happens: During sleep, the muscles at the back of the throat relax, which relaxes the soft palate and the uvula, a small, triangular piece of tissue hanging from the soft palate.

When you have obstructive sleep apnea, the most common kind, this tissue doesn't just relax, it sags, plugging the airway—and breathing stops. You may snort, grunt, gasp or cough as the body rouses itself—and breathing restarts. Then you fall back to sleep, never remembering that you woke up.

This mini-suffocation and awakening can occur over and over—from as few as five times an hour (the criteria for being diagnosed with "mild" sleep apnea) to dozens of times each hour.

Risk factors for obstructive sleep apnea include snoring (a sign of a thickened soft palate), being male, being 65 or older (for women, risk rises after menopause) and obesity. But some people with sleep apnea have none of those risk factors.

DO YOU HAVE IT?

Several daytime symptoms are possible signs of sleep apnea. You might wake up with a headache and a dry mouth. You could be intensely tired during the day—even falling asleep at a red light. You might be irritable and depressed and find it hard to think clearly.

If your doctor suspects sleep apnea, he may recommend a "sleep study" conducted in a sleep disorder center. This overnight test—polysomnography—monitors and measures breathing patterns, blood oxygen levels, arm and leg movement, and heart, lung and brain activity. *But there are several downsides to a study in a sleep center...*

- **It's expensive, costing $1,500 to $2,500—** which could be out-of-pocket if your insurance has a high deductible.
- **It's inconvenient.** You're spending the night in a strange place with a video camera focused on you and personnel walking in and out.

Instead, I often recommend a sleep study at home. Using a portable device, it provides the same information as a study at a center—for a fraction of the cost ($450 to $650). It is becoming the preferred method of testing for many doctors and often is covered by insurance. I prefer the home test by SleepQuest.

For more information: SleepQuest.com.

EXCITING NEW TREATMENT

Up until now, the standard treatment for sleep apnea has been a continuous positive airway pressure (CPAP) machine. This device uses tubing and a mask worn over the nose...over the nose and mouth...or directly in the nose (via what is called a nasal pillow). The mask continuously pumps air into the airway, preventing the soft palate from sagging. But the mask often is uncomfortable. In one study, nearly half of people prescribed a CPAP device stopped using it within one to three weeks.

The exciting news is that there's a convenient treatment for sleep apnea called Provent. A small, disposable patch fits over each nostril. The treatment uses your own breathing to create expiratory positive airway pressure (EPAP)—just enough to keep the throat open.

Recent scientific evidence: In a three-month study involving 250 people with sleep apnea, 127 used Provent and 123 used a fake, look-alike device. The people using Provent had a 43% decrease in nighttime apnea events, compared with a 10% decrease for those in the fake group. Over three months, there was also a significant decrease in daytime sleepiness among Provent users.

A 30-day supply of the patches costs about $70. They are prescription-only and currently are not covered by insurance or Medicare.

My perspective: Provent is an excellent new option for many people with obstructive sleep apnea, but it is not for mouth breathers, people with nasal allergies or those with severe apnea.

Information: 888-757-9355, ProventTherapy.com.

CUSTOMIZED MOUTH GUARD

If the nasal patch is not an option for you, a customized oral appliance may be best. It moves the lower jaw forward, opening the throat. It usually is covered by insurance, either partially or totally.

I was diagnosed with severe obstructive sleep apnea six years ago—and I've had very good results with a customized oral appliance. In a recent sleep test, I used CPAP half the night and my oral appliance the other half—my blood oxygen levels were higher while using the appliance.

Red flag: Over-the-counter oral appliances for snoring are available, but for optimal results, you need an oral appliance created for your mouth and jaw by a dentist trained to make such a device.

Important: No matter which device you use, you need to get tested first and then retested after you start using the device to make sure that you are getting the oxygen you need.

LIFESTYLE CHANGES

Self-care strategies...

• **Sleep on your side.** This helps keep airways open.

• **Lose weight,** because extra pounds mean extra tissue in the throat. Just a 10% weight loss can decrease apnea events by 26%. However, thin people and children can have apnea, too.

• **Don't drink alcohol within three hours of going to bed.** It relaxes the airway.

• **Sing some vowels.** In a study by UK researchers, three months of singing lessons helped decrease snoring, which could in turn decrease apnea.

What to do: Sing the long vowel sounds a-a-a-e-e-e, taking two or three seconds to sing each vowel. Do this once or twice every day for five minutes a session.

Make-Up Sleep: How to Play Catch-Up on Weekends

Torbjörn Åkerstedt, PhD, of the Stress Research Institute of Stockholm University, senior professor in the department of clinical neuroscience at the Karolinska Institute in Stockholm, Sweden, and coauthor with researchers from Stockholm University of the study "Sleep Duration and Mortality—Does Weekend Sleep Matter?" published in *Journal of Sleep Research.*

You've tried to live by the rules when it comes to needed sleep, but going to bed and waking up at the same times every day just isn't in the cards with your hectic schedule. Unfortunately, many studies have linked an early death with getting fewer than five or six hours per night over time. So, what's the answer?

You can make up for missed slumber on the weekends and reduce your odds of premature death due to too little sleep during the week if you do it correctly. That's the reassuring finding of a new study done by psychologist Torbjörn Åkerstedt, PhD, of Sweden's Karolinska Institute.

The study: Researchers followed more than 43,000 people of all ages for a period of 13 years. They looked at the effects of many different sleep patterns—consistently getting fewer than five hours of sleep, getting more than nine hours of sleep, and the combination of shorter sleep times during the week and longer sleep times on the weekends—and compared them to a benchmark of getting seven hours on a regular basis.

True to other research, they found that people under age 65 who got five hours or less of sleep every single day of the week had a higher risk of death than those who consistently got seven hours—in this study, a 52% higher risk. Also similar to older studies, people who slept too much—typically nine hours all the time—also had a higher risk of death.

But here's the twist: Those under 65 who got five hours or less of sleep Sunday night through Thursday night but played catch-up on the weekends with nine hours of sleep Friday and Saturday nights weren't at any greater risk of dying than people who religiously got their seven hours every night of the week.

Note: For study participants aged 65 and older, weekday and weekend sleep hours did not seem to affect their mortality risk at all.

HOW TO PLAY CATCH-UP

To put this good news to work for you, you need to be consistent about your weekend makeup sleep. But you don't have to sleep all day long and give up your Saturday or Sunday to do it. Just go to sleep an hour or two earlier and wake up an hour or two later on each weekend day—the exact number depends on how many total hours you need to make up for. Compare how much sleep you got Monday through Friday to the minimum of seven hours per night—or 35 hours in all—that you needed and spread out the difference on the weekend.

Note: Makeup sleep isn't the long-term answer for sleep problems such as insomnia or trouble staying asleep. First try exercise tips and new products for getting a good night's sleep. If they don't help, or help enough, consider talking to a health professional about your sleep troubles. You may even be a good candidate for a sleep study.

Also, realize that as good as catching up on weekends is, it won't counteract how you'll feel the morning after a sleep-deprived night during the week...you'll still experience that fuzzy-headed feeling, fatigue, forgetfulness and poor decision-making that result from not getting enough shuteye.

Get Your ZZZZs—and Live Longer

L. Finn, et al., "Chronic Insomnia and All Cause Mortality in the Wisconsin Sleep Cohort Study," presented at the annual meeting of the Associated Professional Sleep Societies.

The consequences of chronic insomnia may be far worse than was previously known. Researchers at the University of Wisconsin, Madison, found that the risk of dying from any cause was three times higher in people who suffered from chronic insomnia than in those who slept through the night. Considering the potentially lethal consequences, seek help if you have any type of insomnia, including repeat awakenings or difficulty falling asleep.

Anger Addiction: How to Break Free

Robert Thurman, PhD, Jey Tsong Khapa Professor of Indo-Tibetan Buddhist Studies, department of religion, Columbia University, and president, Tibet House US, a nonprofit dedicated to the preservation of Tibetan civilization, both in New York City. He is the author or coauthor of numerous books, including (with Sharon Salzberg) *Love Your Enemies: How to Break the Anger Habit & Be a Whole Lot Happier*. BobThurman.com

A rude salesperson treats you like dung...or a conniving coworker steals your idea...or your self-absorbed sister ruins yet another gathering...and your blood begins to boil. Your indignation mounts (How dare they?), and soon a rush of anger is sweeping over you. Maybe you hold your tongue, and maybe you don't. But either way, your adrenaline is pumping and your heart is pounding...your emotions are running hot...and you experience a powerful sense of self-righteousness that's almost intoxicating.

That's right—your anger, in its own way, feels good.

If this sounds familiar, you may have an addiction problem—an addiction to anger. And like any addiction, this one can wreak havoc with your relationships, health and happiness.

How do you break free...so that anger no longer consumes you?

THE ART OF LETTING GO OF ANGER

Anger addiction is common...but there are ways to loosen its grip. I had a hot temper myself that got me into trouble, so anger is an emotion. It's when you break free of the cycle of hurt, anger and revenge that you can find inner peace.

While no one can do the work for you, here are some suggestions that will help you address your anger addiction—and the benefits are well worth the effort involved.

•**Admit that your anger hurts you more than it hurts the person you're mad at.** You are the one who's exploding so unattractively, damaging your own reputation...or getting stuck stewing inwardly, all your brainpower wasted on rehashing old or minor infractions. You can't concentrate, can't relax, can't sleep. Meanwhile, the source of your ire may be feeling equally angry with you...or he may be carrying on just fine, largely untroubled by your emotional turmoil. Either way, you gain nothing. Admit it!

•**Acknowledge anger's power to destroy you.** You may think of anger as a helpful emotion that alerts you to a situation that needs changing. Anger is seductive. It presents itself to your mind as your own helpful energy. Anger seduces you with the thought, 'This is outrageous! I should explode with fury, and my fiery energy will burn away the obstacle.' But that's not what actually happens—as with other addictions, the anger rush is followed by an inevitable crash as you realize that your words or actions did not help you (or anyone).

When you're inflamed with rage, your good sense goes out the window and you are no longer the master of your thoughts, words and actions. This kind of anger destroys all in its path, not least your own emotional balance.

For instance, if you've merely indulged in an internal rant, you may be left feeling depleted and depressed, realizing that nothing has changed. If you've exploded in front of others, you may be filled with regret for the things you said or did. And the consequences can be severe. Anger not only can interfere with professional success and ruin relationships, it also has been linked to heart disease, diabetes, cancer and premature death.

•**Pay attention to your body's anger cues.** You may think that anger surges up without warning, and that this is why you have so little control over it. But that's simply not true. Anger doesn't suddenly appear out of nowhere and explode—it arises more gradually than you may realize. The seeds of anger can be found in frustration, but many people were never taught how to catch frustration early and handle it productively before it has a chance to grow into rage.

It's not too late to learn this skill now—and an excellent way to do so is to practice mindfulness. Being mindful means training yourself to observe, moment by moment, what's happening within you and around you. To use mindfulness to overcome anger addiction, you need to pay attention to the physical sensations that accompany mounting frustration. For instance, watch for tightness in your throat and chest...stomach upset...a flush of heat. These are common indicators that anger is arising and should be dealt with before you reach the boiling point.

Why does this matter so much? Since you are not yet truly angry, you still have enough cognitive control to act effectively and influence what happens next in a positive way. In other words, while you're still at the frustration level, your brain is working well enough to allow you to look for good solutions to whatever the problem is. But once that anger rush kicks in, it takes over and your brain takes a break.

•**Analyze your level of control over the situation.** Exactly how you deal with the mounting frustration depends on whether you can influence the actual outcome. . .or whether the only aspect you can control is your own reaction to your circumstances.

Let's go back to that rude salesperson, conniving coworker or self-absorbed sister we talked about earlier. Instead of getting mad, consider what other options you might have that could improve your situation. Maybe you want to simply take your business to a different store or write a calm, carefully considered memo to your boss. Maybe you want to practice treating your sister with loving kindness, a spirit of boundless friendship. She may be so gratified when you express interest and empathy instead of irritation that she acts in a less obnoxious fashion! Think about your real goals and how to achieve them, rather than just spewing your anger all over.

Now suppose the situation is completely beyond your control—for instance, if you're stuck in traffic, so there isn't actually any particular person who is the object of your anger. In this sort of situation, what is best for you is to accept that getting angry won't help and could even lead you to do something stupid (and lead to a traffic ticket or car crash). Indulging in a road-rage tantrum only feeds your anger addiction without altering the fact that you are still stuck in traffic. In this kind of situation, defuse your anger by thinking up ways to use the time productively (here's a chance to listen to music you normally don't have much time to enjoy)...or by counting your blessings (the traffic jam could be the result of an accident, and you are not the person who's now in an ambulance). When you hone your ability to control yourself, you will no longer be a pawn to your anger addiction.

Is Your Job Physically Demanding? That's a Health Risk—and Not for the Reason You'd Think

Study titled "Do Highly Physically Active Workers Die Early?" by researchers at VU University Medical Center in Amsterdam, Netherlands and elsewhere, published in the *British Journal of Sports Medicine.*

You might think that having a job that keeps you active all day is good for your health.

That makes perfect sense given everything we're told about the benefits of physical activity.

But based on a recent research finding, it might be completely wrong—in fact, unless you take specific steps (we'll explain), being in a physically-demanding job might actually shorten your life.

Past studies have hinted at this "physical activity paradox"—one in which people who exercise during their leisure time get healthier and live longer, but those who "exercise" by working in physical jobs are harmed. To find out whether it's real or not, an international research team at the VU University Medical Center in Amsterdam gathered mountains of data from 17 studies conducted between 1960 and 2010, covering 193,696 men and women. They applied statistical techniques to weed out possible confounding variables such as chronic health conditions, body-mass index, smoking and alcohol use, so they could level the playing field between office workers and physical workers. And they didn't take into account job-related accidents—which you might reasonably assume would happen more often in highly physical jobs—because what they were studying was health, not injuries.

Eye-opening finding: Men in jobs requiring high levels of physical activity had an 18% higher risk of early death than those who were in largely inactive jobs.

In contrast, women in these kinds of jobs were no more likely to die prematurely than those in more sedentary jobs. The reasons aren't known, but one likely contributor is that even in our more gender-enlightened times, the active jobs women have tend to be different than the active jobs men have.

WORKING HARD, FROM NOT IN A HEALTHY WAY

What's so unhealthy about the kinds of labor-intensive jobs men tend to do? A leading hypothesis is that there are big differences between physical activity on the job versus during leisure hours—with very different effects on the body.

Example: A laborer who spends 40 hours a week doing manual, repetitive tasks while standing in a static position. That could easily elevate his blood pressure and heart rate—without providing the cardio-fitness benefits that come from sustained aerobic activity. In addition, he's doing these physically demanding tasks all day long—often without a sufficient recovery time. Chronic exhaustion and high blood pressure both contribute to heart disease—and thus, early death.

Contrast that with leisure time activity, whether it's walking, working out at the gym or playing golf or tennis, hiking or swimming. You're active for a shorter bout of time, engaged in aerobic activity that elevates your heart rate in a sustained way—and you have time to recover afterward. No wonder it leads to a healthier outcome.

There are exceptions, of course. Elite professional athletes, whose occupations require that they devote long hours to physical activity in the pursuit of fitness and competitive edge, tend to live longer lives than the general population, the researchers note. One could speculate that certain occupations—say, a mailman who walks his route—may be pretty healthy, too. Unfortunately, most of the studies didn't identify specific jobs but rather by exertion levels, so there's no resulting list of jobs to avoid...or seek.

But one take-away is clear: If you're in a physically demanding job—whether you're a man or a woman—you can't necessarily rely on your work-a-day activity to keep you fit and healthy. To do that the human body needs resistance (muscle) exercise, aerobic exercise and recovery time—so you might need to use your leisure time to get and stay fit, too. That's particularly important because research finds that people in physically demanding jobs tend to get less leisure time activity than those in more sedentary jobs. For the rest of us, it's more evidence that staying physically active in our leisure time is key to a healthier, longer life.

Is Your Job Giving You Atrial Fibrillation (AFib)?

Study titled "Job Strain and Atrial Fibrillation—Results From the Swedish Longitudinal Occupational Survey of Health and Meta-Analysis of Three Studies" by researchers at Jönköping University, Sweden, published in *European Journal of Preventive Cardiology.*

It's no surprise that stress—no matter what causes it—can make you more likely to have a heart attack or stroke. But you might not know that a stressful job can double your chances of developing a serious heart-rhythm disorder...one that you might not know you have because symptoms aren't always apparent.

Atrial fibrillation (AFib) is the most common type of heart arrhythmia and increases risk for stroke and early death by two to five times. Even though AFib is a major public health concern, little is known about the underlying risk factors. But researchers at Jönköping University in Sweden recently looked at what impact job stress had on risk for developing AFib.

Study: For the study, about 13,000 Swedish men and women who did not have AFib at the start of the study filled out a questionnaire that included questions about their jobs. Defining job stress as having "high demand and little control," the participants were grouped into low demand and high control...low demand and low control...high demand and high control...and high demand and low control. The participants were then followed for six years to see how many developed AFib.

Results: Of the 145 participants who developed AFib during the study period, those who had jobs with high demand and low control (highest job stress) were 48% more likely to be diagnosed with the condition than participants in all the other groups.

The researchers also compared the results of this study with two older Swedish studies that looked at work stress and AFib—one that followed 6,000 men for 17 years starting in the 1970s (436 developed AFib)...and a study that began in the 1990s and followed 10,000 men and women for 13 years (253 developed AFib). Pooling the findings from all three studies, the risk for AFib associated with high-stress work was almost 40%.

Bottom line: The study authors conclude that work stress is a significant risk factor for AFib, and they suggest that people who feel stressed at work should talk to their doctors and their employers about ways to reduce stress.

How stressful is your job? You may think you already know the answer to that, but the following questions from the demand-control questionnaire might give you more insight into just how stressful your job is...

- **Do you have to work very hard or very fast?**
- **Are there too many demands at your work?**
- **Do you have enough time to complete all the tasks of your job?**
- **Is your work very repetitious?**
- **Do you have any control over how and what you do at work?**

If you answered "yes" to any of these questions, seek out new employment options. If that is not possible, deliberately work on stress reduction through exercise, meditation or other healthful distractions. It's important to reduce stress—from your job or from any other part of your life.

6

Exercise and Fitness

Are You Walking Fast Enough to Live a Long Life?

Study titled "Self-Rated Walking Pace and All-Cause, Cardiovascular Disease and Cancer Mortality: Individual Participant Pooled Analysis of 50,225 Walkers from 11 Population British Cohorts," led by researchers at University of Sydney, Australia, published in *British Journal of Sports Medicine.*

You know walking is good for you—no, great for you. Taking a walk is a pleasant, easy, no-cost way to exercise, and it produces a bounty of well-known health benefits—from helping with weight loss to reducing stress to keeping your memory sharp and your heart healthy.

It can even help you avoid premature death—but only if you move at more than a saunter, especially as you get older, new research reveals.

The good news: While you can't just piddle along and expect walking to do all its magic, you don't have to be a speed walker like Cary Grant in *Walk Don't Run* to get these long-life benefits.

THE SPEED OF LONGEVITY

It makes logical sense that regularly walking at a brisk clip might reduce your risk of early mortality. After all, the faster heart rate from that fast clip strengthens your cardiovascular system and stimulates health-improving physiological responses throughout your body. But while the overall benefits of exercise are well documented, the role of walking speed hadn't been well studied. In fact, the new research is the first study of its kind because it teased out walking speed's impact from the rest of someone's physical activity.

Scientists at the Universities of Sydney, Cambridge, Edinburgh, Limerick and Ulster examined results from the Health Survey for England and the Scottish Health Survey, two ongoing population-based studies that have tracked more than 50,000 men and women, age 30 and up, for an average of nine years. Their goal was to measure the influence of walking speeds against mortality from all causes as well as from cardiovascular disease and cancer. The participants reported their walking speeds—slow, average or brisk/fast. They reported how much walking in particular—and physical exercise in general—they engaged in on a regular basis.

Surprising results: Average walking speed, meaning just under three miles per hour (mph), was statistically linked to nearly the same health benefits as brisk/fast walking (3.5 or 4 mph). And compared with slow walkers (around 2 mph), average-speed walkers had a 20% reduced risk of dying over those nine years. For brisk/fast walkers, the mortality risk reduction was only slightly greater: 24%. (Walking pace reduced mortality primarily by helping to prevent cardiovascular disease—there was no statistical benefit in terms of cancer prevention.)

But something much more powerful was discovered as well: The benefit of walking at an average pace—what fitness experts like to call "moderate intensity"—may get much greater as you age. For study subjects age 60 and older, walking at an average pace or faster was associated with a 46% lower rate of cardiovascular disease mortality compared with slow walkers. And brisk/fast-paced older walkers got the proverbial gold ring—a 53% reduction in cardiovascular mortality.

Now, this kind of observational study can't establish causality, so it doesn't prove that intentionally keeping up the pace in your walking style will help you avoid chronic illness or an early demise. Researchers noted the many cardiovascular benefits of walking at an average/moderate rate or faster—but they also acknowledged that some of the statistical differences in longevity between slow and average or brisk/fast walkers may come from the fact that people in declining health tend to walk slower.

In practical terms, however, the message is clear: If you can walk at a moderate pace or faster, do it! Strolling can be relaxing, but it isn't likely to do as much for your health.

HOW CAN YOU TELL IF YOUR PACE IS FAST ENOUGH?

To get the greatest potential life-extension benefits from walking, you want to make sure you walk fast enough.

An easy way to tell: Count the number of steps you take. Recent research suggests that you should aim for 100 steps a minute—a brisk pace that's easy to determine. For people with an average stride length, that pace will work out to just under three miles per hour—the "average pace" chronicled in this study.

Use your watch or a stopwatch on your phone to count how many steps you take in 10 seconds and multiply that by six, or simply count your steps for a full minute.

Tip: It's about the same as the pace of the hit 1970s disco song "Stayin' Alive" by the Bee Gees—one step per beat. Get your pace set, and then head out for at least 30 minutes of moderate-intensity walking at least five days a week—as recommended by the Centers for Disease Control & Prevention—confident that you're taking a big step towards better health and longer life.

Want to aim for a brisk pace? That's 120 to 130 steps per minute. If you can, go for it!

Be Fit, Live Long

Mark A. Stengler, NMD, naturopathic medical doctor in private practice, Encinitas, California...adjunct associate clinical professor at the National College of Natural Medicine, Portland, Oregon...author of *The Natural Physician's Healing Therapies.*

We often think that people who are thin will live longer than those who are overweight. University of South Carolina researchers found that fitness level, not weight, better predicted longevity.

Best way to improve your fitness level: Regular aerobic activity.

How Fit Are You Really?

C. Jessie Jones, PhD, professor of health science and kinesiology, director of the Fibromyalgia Research and Education Center, and former director of the Center for Successful Aging and Gerontology Programs, all based at California State University, Fullerton. She is coauthor, with Roberta E. Rikli, PhD, of *The Senior Fitness Test Manual.*

Physical inactivity is a major cause of frailty as people grow older, and more than one-third of all nursing-home admissions are prompted by mobility issues, such as balance problems or an inability to walk unassisted.

Good news: By objectively assessing your physical ability, setting goals—and then working on your weaknesses—you can improve your physical strength, flexibility and endurance to ensure that you remain active as long as possible.

BEST FITNESS TESTING

Many standardized fitness tests are designed for younger people who tend to be somewhat fit and in good health. For people over age 60, fitness assessment is tricky. A long period of time may have passed since you last exercised regularly, or you may have age-related physical limitations due to being physically inactive or a medical condition (such as arthritis or heart disease) that makes it difficult to measure your fitness level.

To address this problem, researchers at the University of California at Fullerton developed the Senior Fitness Test, which measures physical fitness parameters that are important for independent living. This assessment also is useful for people under age 60.

Before performing each test, ask a friend to help you with the measurements and to record your results. If you are in the "at risk zone," try the remedial actions suggested. Even if you easily pass, keep exercising to improve your performance! Set a goal for improving your scores and recheck yourself after a few weeks of exercising.

Important: If you have uncontrolled high blood pressure, congestive heart failure, balance problems...experience pain or dizziness...or your doctor has told you to avoid exercise, consult your physician before trying the following assessments.

30-SECOND CHAIR STAND

Why it's important: Assesses the lower-body strength needed to climb stairs...get out of chairs, the bathtub or the car...and to help stop yourself from falling when you lose your balance.

How to test yourself: Start by sitting on a straight-backed, armless chair with your feet flat on the floor. With your arms crossed over your chest, count how many times you can rise from a seated to a standing position in 30 seconds.

At risk zone: Eight times or fewer.

Actions to take: Twice a day, practice repeatedly rising from a chair (if possible, without using your hands) to the point of fatigue. When you can do this 15 times in 30 seconds, add resistance (such as holding two- to five-pound weights in your hands as you rise). Using a leg press machine (available at most gyms) is the best exercise for lower-body strength.

8-FOOT UP AND GO

Why it's important: Measures reaction time, agility and balance—all of which affect how fast you can answer the phone or doorbell...avoid a dangerous obstacle...or rush to the bathroom.

How to test yourself: From a seated position on a sturdy chair placed against a wall, see how quickly you can rise, walk around a small object (such as a wastebasket) placed eight feet away from the front edge of the chair, and return to your seated position.

At risk zone: More than nine seconds.

Actions to take: Challenge yourself occasionally to get up quickly from a seated position and to walk as fast and safely as you can for at least a short distance.

BACK SCRATCH

Why it's important: Gauges your upper-body flexibility and ability to perform tasks such as putting on overhead garments...grabbing a seat belt...or combing your hair.

How to test yourself: Reach one hand over the same shoulder while bending the other hand behind your back with the palm facing out. Try to make the fingers of both hands meet in the middle of your back.

Ask your helper to use a ruler to measure the inches between the tips of your middle fingers. If your middle fingers overlap, that's great.

At risk zone: Men should be able to get their fingertips within eight inches of each other, women four inches. Because of posture and injuries, it's not unusual to get a different score when you reverse the positions of your hands, so measure your best performance.

Actions to take: Increase your flexibility by dangling a dish towel behind you, over your shoulder, and grabbing the other end and gradually pulling the dish towel down with your lower hand, then pulling it up with your upper hand. Repeat with the towel hanging over your other shoulder.

30-SECOND ARM CURL

Why it's important: Measures upper-body strength, which is important for such tasks as carrying items, including groceries...and performing yard work, house cleaning and other such activities.

How to test yourself: Start by sitting in a straight-backed, armless chair with your feet flat on the floor. Using a hand weight (eight pounds for men and five pounds for women), count the number of times you can lift the weight, while held in your dominant hand, from the outside of your thigh to your shoulder (biceps curl) in 30 seconds. Start with your palm facing the side of your body and as you curl your arm, rotate the palm so that it is facing the front of your body. Keep your upper arm still throughout the test.

At risk zone: Fewer than 11 curls.

Actions to take: If you're too weak to work out with hand weights or can't complete at least 11 curls...or you have arthritis or osteoporosis, use elastic bands, such as Dyna-bands or Thera-bands (available at most sporting-goods stores). Stand on one end of the band. Then wrap the other end around your hand and perform biceps curls until your arm tires. When you can do 12 repetitions with each arm, get a band with more resistance and/or begin using hand weights.

How I Stay Motivated to Exercise

Ruth Heidrich, PhD, a certified fitness trainer and eight-time gold medalist in the Senior Olympics. She is cohost of the radio show "Healing and You" on KWAI-AM in Hawaii and the author of *Senior Fitness*.

I'm in my mid 70s, and I've completed more than 60 marathons (26.2-mile races) in recent decades. Today, I continue to compete frequently at shorter distances such as half-marathons. Even though I was diagnosed with breast cancer at age 47, I now have no signs of cancer in my body...my blood pressure readings are extremely healthy...my body mass index (BMI) is trim at 19...my bone density is excellent (even though I have a family history of severe osteoporosis)...and my sex life is great.

I tell you this not to brag, but to inspire you to follow the same anti-aging lifestyle that I do. As a professional health educator, I know that most of the physical decline associated with aging can be attributed to two things—disuse of our bodies (by failing to get sufficient exercise) and disease that is largely related to our diets. To counter these, I run, swim and cycle every day, and I eat a low-fat, vegan diet—meaning I consume no animal products whatsoever, including eggs and milk products.

What keeps me going? It's really quite simple—I want to remain robust and vigorous. This desire helps me overcome the excuses that many people use for not exercising. Even if you're not interested in running a marathon, my strategies work amazingly well—regardless of your current fitness level.

Five secrets that can keep your exercise program on track...

1. Visualize yourself as fit and healthy. A combination of regular aerobic exercise (such as walking or jogging)...strength training (with hand weights or exercise machines)...and stretching (including touching your toes to loosen the hamstring muscles in the back of the thigh) will increase your energy and help keep your weight down, your bones and muscles strong, and your blood vessels healthy.

But if these benefits are not enough to motivate you, try visualizing how you will look as a fit, healthy person. Close your eyes and see yourself as lean and strong, with firm, toned legs, a flat stomach and a bounce in your step. Imagine how you will move and feel once you start exercising regularly.

For best results: Do this visualization for a couple of minutes whenever you feel the need for some extra motivation.

2. Make a "rewards" list. Write down all the ways that exercise will improve your life. Don't give general answers, such as "better health." Be specific. Include rewards that will be meaningful to you, such as not needing as many (or any) medications...saving money on health-care expenses...or gaining the stamina to travel anywhere you like.

For best results: Keep this list on your desk or refrigerator where you'll see it every day.

3. Be sure that your goals are complete. Just "wanting to" start exercising is not enough of a goal. Goals must include four key parts—they must be specific, measurable and attainable—and you must create a timeline for achieving them. For example, your goal may be to "walk for 30 minutes at least three times a week for two months." Consult your doctor to ensure that your goals are appropriate and realistic.

For best results: Sign up to participate in an event that is several months away, such as a walk-a-thon or an organized bike race. Flyers for such activities are posted on the bulletin boards of many gyms, health-food stores and bookstores.

4. Get a new calendar. You say you don't have time to exercise? That's one of the oldest excuses in the book. If you decide that there's something you must do, you make an appointment—and then do it!

For best results: Find a calendar (I like the large wall calendars that are sold in office-supply stores for about $10) that has enough space for each day so that you can write not only the time that you will exercise, but also what each workout will include.

For example: For Mondays, Wednesdays and Fridays, you might write "20-minute weight workout at 8 am." For Tuesdays, Thursdays and Saturdays, it might be "30 minutes of walking at 7 am."

Also helpful: On the same monthly calendar, make a check mark next to each exercise session you complete or add a brief summary if your workout was shorter or longer. This journal will keep you honest in terms of the amount of exercise you're actually doing.

5. Share your goals. To stay motivated, share your goals with a friend, then set up regular times to exercise together. Between the support of your training partners and your desire to not let them down, your exercise program will flourish.

For best results: Join an organized exercise class or group. This can be especially helpful if the group has a coach or teacher who can help you set and reach your goals.

How to Stick to an Exercise Routine

Navin Kaushal, PhD, postdoctoral fellow in preventive medicine, Montreal Heart Institute, University of Montreal, and leader of a study published in *British Journal of Health Psychology.*

Two secrets for sticking to an exercise routine...

- **Work out at the same time on most days.** Pick a regular time for exercise, and stay with it as many days of the week as possible—workouts will become part of your regular day.
- **Use visual cues to get yourself going.** For example, lay out running clothes, shoes and headphones in a specific place so that you see them when you wake up. This also helps turn exercise into a routine that you do automatically without having to give it much thought.

4 Balance Exercises to Keep You Steady on Your Feet

Caroline DeGroot, MPT, a physical therapist at AthletiCo Physical Therapy in Bannockburn, Illinois. DeGroot founded AthletiCo's Vestibular Program, which focuses on helping people with dizziness, balance disorders and concussions.

When you are young, you can walk confidently just about anywhere without much thought—such as on an uneven sidewalk—or while chatting at the same time. As you get older, just glancing sideways at a store window while strolling can make you wobble—and fall. *Here's what's going on...and some moves that will keep you steadier on your feet...*

WHY FALLS OCCUR

One in four Americans over age 65 falls each year. One reason is that older people are more prone to medical conditions that compromise balance—such as vertigo, dizziness, arthritis-related stiffness and weakness, stroke and loss of sensation in the feet from vascular diseases. But even without major health issues, normal physical and vision changes can affect balance.

Your eyes signal the brain where you are in space relative to other objects, which helps keep you stable. Wearing bifocals or progressive lenses requires your focus to change back and forth between lenses, making it harder to notice a loose rug, sidewalk crack or pet.

The natural age-related decline in muscle strength and flexibility also makes it harder to right yourself once your center of gravity is thrown off. That's why the key to staying on your feet is to build your muscle strength and improve your flexibility and agility. *Here's how—work up to doing each move daily to get the most benefit...*

FOOT TAPS

As we age, our pace typically slows, our step length shortens and our stance widens as shifting from one leg to the other feels less secure. To keep your strides long and confident and avert a shuffling gait, you can do foot taps—an exercise that trains your body to safely shift your center of gravity left and right.

How to do it: Stand in front of a step that is four to six inches high (such as a footstool), feet hip-width apart. Slowly raise one foot to tap the step. Return that foot to the ground and then tap with the other foot. Movement should be slow and controlled. Work up to 20 taps for each foot in a session. As your stability improves, try a higher step (six to eight inches)...or try tapping the step as lightly as possible to further improve balance and increase muscle control.

Safety note: If needed, you can hold a railing or counter for support. If you use a cane for general walking assistance, hold it in the hand you usually use to hold it throughout the exercise, regardless of which foot you're tapping. If you're using a cane only while recovering from an injury or for a condition that affects your gait, such as arthritis, hold the cane on the side opposite to the injury or painful extremity.

HEAD TURNS

When you turn your head, a response called the vestibular spinal reflex (VSR) causes your brain to send messages to adjust postural muscles to keep you from being pulled in the direction your head turns. Your VSR can become less effective as you age, causing you to often stumble while turning your head. The following exercise helps train your VSR.

How to do it: Stand with your feet hip-width apart. If you need to, you can hold on to a railing, wall, sturdy piece of furniture or counter for support. Now slowly turn your head as far as you comfortably can to the right and then to the left, while maintaining upright posture. Repeat as a continuous movement for 10 repetitions.

Make sure to stay upright without leaning to one side. If you feel dizzy, pause, then continue at a slower pace.

For additional challenge: If you held on to a support, try doing the exercise without holding on to anything. Or try it with your feet only a few inches apart...or with your feet together...or with one foot in front of the other, heel-to-toe. Don't overextend your ability, though—safety first!

OVER-THE-SHOULDER WALKS

Try this exercise once you feel comfortable with standing head turns. You will look left and right as you walk—similar to what you might do when scanning shelves while grocery shopping or walking down a hallway while searching for an apartment number.

How to do it: Stand at one end of a long hallway, feet hip-width apart. Turn your head to look over your right shoulder. Maintaining that gaze, take three or four steps forward. Now turn your head to look over your left shoulder while you continue to walk forward another three or four steps. Repeat for a total of five times per side. If you feel dizzy or unsteady, stop turning your head and gaze straight ahead for a few steps. To increase the challenge, increase how quickly you turn your head.

Variation: Try head turns in a store or library. Having a stationary visual target—the items on the shelves—recruits your vision while challenging your VSR.

BALL HANDOFF

People who worry about falling often are self-conscious about walking—which is counterproductive. The more attention you pay to how you're walking, the more shuffled and fractured your gait becomes. Natural gait needs to be reflexive. This exercise uses a ball for distraction to help your gait become more fluid, increase your walking speed and improve your ability to shift weight left and right.

Safety note: This exercise is not recommended if you need to use a cane to walk.

How to do it: You'll need a partner who is comfortable walking backward and a small ball, such as a tennis ball. Start at one end of a long hallway with your partner facing you and a few feet in front of you, holding the ball. Walk forward while your partner walks backward—handing off or gently tossing the ball back and forth to each other as you go. Perform this exercise for two to three minutes or until you feel tired.

Solo variation: Stand in front of a wall, and march in place while you toss the ball at the wall and catch it as it bounces back. Repeat for 30 seconds at a time, for a total of three times.

Exercise Rejuvenates Your Brain

John J. Ratey, MD, associate clinical professor of psychiatry at Harvard University, Boston, JohnRatey.com. He is author of *Spark: The Revolutionary New Science of Exercise and the Brain.*

Staying active is a key to a vigorous, healthy body as we grow older. But exercise is just as important for mental health. Walking, biking or swimming helps keep your memory and reasoning ability sharp and your mood bright while it strengthens your heart, arteries—and muscles.

Like every organ, the brain requires a steady supply of oxygen and nutrients to maintain vigor. A sound mind needs a healthy body, and a healthy body needs exercise. Heart disease, diabetes and other illnesses can have a devastating effect on the brain, and exercise cuts the risk that you'll get them.

In recent years, scientists have learned a lot about what happens inside the brain when we think, form memories and learn new things...and what determines whether our moods are up or down. They've found solid evidence that exercise—even a modest amount—can have a positive effect on biological events within the brain cells themselves.

YOUR GROWING BRAIN

Not that long ago, everyone believed that after maturity, no new brain cells were born—your supply of several hundred billion declined gradually but inexorably with advancing years. Now we know that like other parts of the body, the brain constantly renews itself, generating blank cells that, under the right circumstances, can turn into thinking, functioning tissue.

At work are naturally occurring chemicals called growth factors. They are produced by the brain itself and by blood vessels and muscles. They act like fertilizer on a flowerbed, stimulating new brain cells to grow and new blood vessels to support them.

Brain cells are constantly dying, succumbing to a mix of toxins and overstimulation called molecular stress. With age, the balance shifts—growth factors decline, along with the cells' ability to withstand stress. After age 40, we lose 5% of our brain cells per decade, on average. The network of capillaries feeding the brain withers.

Nothing can stop the effects aging has on the brain, but exercise can dramatically slow it down. Animal experiments have shown that exercise boosts growth factors and the number of new brain cells produced. Other studies found that when animals were active, their brains worked better—exercise increased their ability to learn new things.

KEEP YOUR MENTAL EDGE

There's evidence that just a modest amount of exercise can have a powerful anti-aging effect on the human brain.

A study at the University of Illinois divided 59 sedentary people aged 60 to 79 into groups that did one hour of stretching three times a week, or had sessions of aerobic exercise (activity that gets your heart rate up and keeps it up) for the same amount of time. After six months, magnetic resonance imaging scans found that brain volume had increased in the aerobic exercisers—the frontal and temporal lobes, which are involved in thinking, decision-making and learning, had actually grown bigger.

These results "suggest a strong biological basis for the role of aerobic fitness in maintaining and enhancing central nervous system health and cognitive functioning in older adults," the researchers concluded.

Looking at actual performance on tests of mental ability, scientists have found that a regular aerobic program can apparently push back age-linked decline in brain function by seven to 10 years.

Exercise also protects against the worst brain-killers of all—diseases such as Alzheimer's and Parkinson's. Besides generally strengthening brain circuits, it helps keep arteries healthy and blood sugar under control, cutting the risk for dementia.

IMPROVE YOUR MOOD

Low moods can strike no matter how old you are, but the stresses and losses that frequently come with age—illness, ending a career, retiring to an unfamiliar place—make depression a special danger. Biology also plays a role. The neurotransmitters that carry messages between brain cells dwindle as the years pass. Low levels of these chemicals—serotonin, dopamine and norepinephrine—are associated with depression, and antidepressants appear to work by raising them.

Exercise stimulates neurotransmitter production and can battle depression as effectively as medication. In a Duke University study, an aerobic program proved as potent as the antidepressant Zoloft in relieving depressive symptoms.

You needn't be clinically depressed to benefit. The neurotransmitter boost of exercise raises mood, increases motivation and can charge up anyone's zest for life.

AEROBICS AND BEYOND

Your goal should be to get some physical activity nearly every day. But, especially if you've been sedentary, get there slowly. The good news is that noticeable benefits start at a much lower level—with as little as an hour a week of exercise.

Important: Check with your doctor before starting any exercise program.

Aerobic exercise appears to be the most beneficial to the brain. Swimming, biking and jogging are good, but for most, brisk walking is perfect.

How hard you should work out: To calculate your "maximum heart rate," subtract your age from 220. Your goal is walking (or doing another activity) strenuously enough to get your pulse up to 60% to 65% of maximum. Vary your workouts from 30 minutes to an hour, four days a week.

After you've become used to exercising, pick up the pace—go for 70% to 75% of maximum for 20 to 30 minutes, then back down to 60% to 65%—during two of the four workouts.

Keep it interesting. Many find that walking is more stimulating out of doors. Team up with a friend so that you can motivate each other and add the pleasures and benefits of social interaction. Variety spices up routine. If you have access to a health club or gym, try the treadmill, exercise bike or elliptical trainer.

Strength training: The brain benefits of strength training (with weights or resistance machines) haven't been researched as thoroughly as those of aerobics, but it's well worth the effort anyway—to counter the muscle deterioration that otherwise comes with age. Try to include strength training in your workouts twice a week. If you're new to it, have a personal trainer design a program for you.

---

5 Exercises That Make Everyday Life Better...and Keep Your Body Younger

Beth and Lee Jordan, both certified American Council on Exercise (ACE) health coaches and personal trainers based in Jacksonville Beach, Florida.

What are your fitness goals? Amazing endurance? Extraordinary strength? Lightning speed? If so, more power to you—literally. But many of us just want to stay healthy so we can keep doing the activities we need to do...and activities we love to do...for a good long time.

Try this test: Can you put your socks on standing up? Can you stand up from a chair without using your arms, sit back down, and repeat another 11 times within 30 seconds? Can you stand on one foot for 30 seconds? These are tests of functional fitness, sometimes called neuromotor or neuromuscular fitness.

The good news is that you can improve your functional fitness level with simple exercises. The goal is to increase your ability to do the activities that you need to do every day at home, at work and during recreational fun...such as lifting work files or children or grandchildren...carrying the laundry down to the basement and back...bending down to garden...keeping your balance getting in and out of the tub and when you're out for a nice hike. It's a combination of balance and power.

"Functional fitness exercises combine upper- and lower-body movements into what are known as compound exercises, while emphasizing core stability," explain Lee and Beth Jordan, a husband-and-wife team of personal trainers with the American Council on Exercise (ACE). "They often mimic real everyday movements."

These exercises are especially important as you age, when your muscles weaken and simple activities can feel more difficult. All the things you used to barely give a thought to can become challenging if you don't give those muscles some extra attention.

Get started with these five functional exercises designed to help you keep living the active life you enjoy...for a long, long time.

BENT-OVER DUMBBELL ROW

What it helps you do: Bend over to reach things...and pick up an object such as a laundry basket, package of mulch or bag of groceries.

How to do it: Use a dumbbell with a weight that challenges you but that you can lift repeatedly. Stand next to a bench or chair and, holding the dumbbell in your right hand, bend at a 90-degree angle so that your back is parallel to the floor. Brace your left hand and left knee on the bench or chair. You weight will be on your right foot, and your right hand should hang down directly under your shoulder, holding the weight. Keeping your back straight, head in line with your spine and abdominal muscles taut, pull the dumbbell up toward your shoulder as far as you can. Your elbow should remain higher than the dumbbell. Then lower the weight by straightening your arm toward the floor. Repeat several reps and then switch sides.

SINGLE-LEG SQUAT

What it helps you do: Control and balance your own weight when walking on unstable ground, going up and down stairs, getting out of bed and getting up out of a chair.

How to do it: Start by standing with your feet hip-width apart, one foot several inches in front of the other, with feet parallel. Slowly squat down as far as you're able to, without losing balance and keeping your bent knee of the leg in front behind your toes. Your hands can be on your hips or your arms can be extended straight out in front of you. Rise to your starting position. Perform several reps and then switch legs.

FORWARD LUNGE

What it helps you do: Move with ease during activities such as yard work, vacuuming and putting groceries in your cupboard.

How to do it: Start in a standing position. Keeping one leg in place, step your other foot out in front of you and bend your knees—your ultimate goal is for them to both reach 90-degree angles. (Once you get good at this, your front thigh and back shin should be parallel to the floor.) Push off with your front leg to return to your starting position. Maintain a straight spine and taut abdominals throughout the movement, keeping your arms at your sides or your hands on

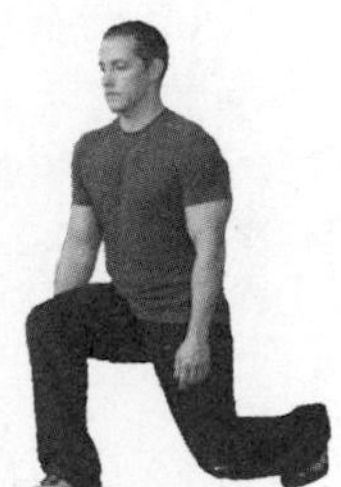

your hips. Perform several reps, alternating legs with each lunge. (Once you're comfortable with the forward lunge, try side lunges and walking lunges with twists.)

SUPERMANS

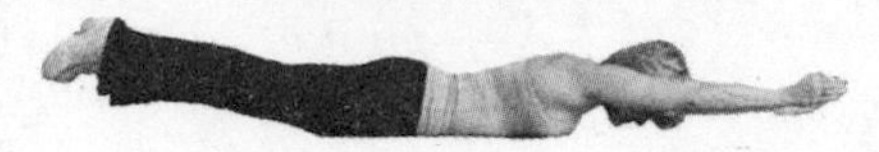

What it helps you do: Maintain a healthy posture while sitting, standing and walking.

How to do it: Lie on your stomach, facing straight down, with your head in line with your spine, legs extended straight, toes pointing, and your arms extended straight out in front of you, palms facing each other. Simultaneously, lift both your arms and your legs a few inches off the floor. Make sure your head stays aligned with your spine during the entire movement, and avoid arching your back or lifting your head. Hold the lift for a few seconds, and then gently return your arms and legs to the starting position. Perform several reps.

FARMER'S WALK

What it helps you do: Increase your grip strength and improve coordination when walking and carrying items at the same time.

How to do it: You'll need to walk during this exercise. Don't worry if you don't have much space—this is fun if you have a lawn, driveway or walkway to use, but you can also just go in circles inside. Start in a standing position with a dumbbell beside each foot. (Choose a weight that's challenging for you but not so heavy that you can't lift it.) Keeping your back straight, squat down and grip the handles of the weights, lifting them as you stand back up, keeping your weight on your heels. Then take short, quick steps as you walk for up to 100 feet. Remember to breathe throughout the walk. Set the weights back down on the floor. Rest and repeat.

GETTING STARTED WITH A FUNCTIONAL FITNESS ROUTINE

How often should you do these exercises? The American College of Sports Medicine recommends about two or three 20 to 30-minute sessions each week. You'll still want to keep up a regular routine of aerobics, strength training and flexibility exercises, too.

As with any new exercise routine, it's always a good idea to check with your doctor before getting started...and that's especially true if you have any joint problems or other physical challenges. And as with any physical activity, if it starts to hurt, stop.

Are these five exercises the only way to improve functional fitness? Of course not. Yoga and tai chi are also great, and they "count" toward the recommendations. You can even do functional exercises with a paper towel tube.

But if you're looking for a streamlined routine, the five exercises above all work together to improve your ability to do the things that matter every day.

Note: The images in this story that demonstrate each exercise are used with permission, courtesy of the American Council on Exercise. You can see more in their Exercise Library.

Add a Mini-Workout to Your Workday...and Live Longer

James A. Levine, MD, PhD, is a professor of medicine in the division of endocrinology and director of the Non-Exercise Activity Thermogenesis Laboratory, both at the Mayo Clinic in Rochester, Minnesota. He is also the coauthor of *Move a Little, Lose a Lot.*

Catrine Tudor-Locke, PhD, is an associate professor and director of the Walking Behavior Laboratory at Pennington Biomedical Research Center in Baton Rouge.

For those of us with desk jobs, it was a big bummer to learn that sitting on our bums for hours on end can increase our mortality risk—even if we get regular exercise!—according to a recent article in *Current Opinion in Cardiology.* What's more, research has shown that the extreme dangers of prolonged sitting include an increased risk for cardiovascular disease...colorectal cancer...obesity...diabetes...and potentially deadly blood clots in the lungs.

Given that more than 80% of jobs in the US are now sedentary (compared with just 50% five decades ago), day-in-day-out sitting represents a huge and growing health problem. But there is good news—because breaking up sedentary time with spurts of activity has been shown to help offset the health risks of sitting. So, even when we're stuck at the office, we can protect ourselves with some creative get-up-and-go strategies and a few nifty gadgets sold at sporting-goods stores and/or online.

For specifics, we consulted two renowned exercise experts and research collaborators, James A. Levine, MD, PhD, a Mayo Clinic professor in Rochester, Minnesota, and coauthor of *Move a Little, Lose a Lot*...and Catrine Tudor-Locke, PhD, director of the Walking Behavior Laboratory at Pennington Biomedical Research Center in Baton Rouge. *Their suggestions...*

- **Stand up when you can.** Using the muscles necessary to stand activates substances that have good effects on how the body uses and stores sugars and fats. Plus, standing burns three times as many calories as sitting, Dr. Levine pointed out.

Automatically get to your feet whenever a coworker stops by to talk.

When on the phone, stand and rise up onto your toes, then lower your heels back to the ground...repeat these heel lifts as many times as you can.

- **Get an adjustable-height computer workstation.** Raise it so you can see the screen and reach your keyboard while standing...lower it when you want to sit down. (Avoid prolonged standing if you have back problems, Dr. Tudor-Locke cautioned.)

- **Step on it.** "Standing is better than sitting, but walking is even better than standing," said Dr. Levine.

Walk fast to the restroom (and take the stairs to one on a different floor), then do an extra lap around the office before heading back to your desk.

Helpful: Drink plenty of water throughout the day, Dr. Tudor-Locke suggested—this forces you to take more frequent bathroom breaks (as well as promoting good hydration).

Rather than meeting with a colleague or two in your office or a conference room, have a "walking meeting" in the corridor.

If you have enough space and the whir of a machine won't bother coworkers, try a treadmill desk (a treadmill with a flat surface at the front). You don't have to use it all day or even go fast—walking for one hour at a leisurely pace burns 100 to 200 calories more than sitting for the same period of time, Dr. Levine said. Or use a mini-stepper—a small device with two footpads that lets you step in place against resistance—when standing at your adjustable-height workstation.

- **When you must sit, move some muscles.** "You're not trying to 'feel the burn' with an intense workout—the idea is just to move as much as you can," said Dr. Tudor-Locke.

- **Sit on a stability ball (a large inflatable plastic ball).** The continuous tiny adjustments necessary to stay upright on the ball will engage many more muscles (especially the abs, back and pelvis) than sitting on a chair, Dr. Levine noted. An average-height woman needs a 21-inch-diameter ball...use a 17-inch ball if you are shorter than five feet...use a 25-inch ball if taller than five feet, seven inches.

- **When waiting for a report to print, do some seated biceps curls or shoulder presses with five-pound hand weights.** Or use a resistance band (a three-foot-long strip of latex) for some seated row exercises or triceps toners (for instructions, go to BottomLineInc.com and search "3 Resistance Band Exercises Everyone Should Learn.")

- **March in place as you read your e-mail,** raising your knees as high as you can without hitting the underside of your desk.

- **Put a portable mini-cycle (a diminutive version of a stationary bicycle) beneath your desk and pedal while you work.**

Helpful: Encourage your coworkers—especially your boss—to join in your "deskercise" movement. Dr. Levine said, "If workday physical activities are frowned upon or laughed at, they fail quickly. But when everyone is into them, you get a sense of merriment in the workplace—and then people are quite happy to get moving."

What Older Athletes Can Teach Us About Staying Young

Vonda Wright, MD, director of the Performance and Research Initiative for Master Athletes (PRIMA) at the University of Pittsburgh Medical Center. She is author of *Fitness After 40: How to Stay Strong at Any Age.* VondaWright.com

Olympic swimmer Dara Torres won three silver medals in Beijing in 2008 and set an American record in the women's 50-meter freestyle. At 41 years old, she was nearly twice the age of many of her competitors.

Torres is not the first athlete to compete at an elite level after age 40. Baseball Hall of Famer Nolan Ryan threw a no-hitter at age 44...golfer Jack Nicklaus won the Masters Tournament at age 46...quarterback George Blanda remained in the NFL until age 48...tennis star Martina Navratilova won a US Open mixed doubles title at 49...and hockey player Gordie Howe played professional hockey until he was 52.

Here's what older athletes can teach us all about remaining physically active into middle age and beyond...

• **Fight the real enemy.** The enemy isn't age—it's inactivity. The widely held belief that physical decline is inevitable once we pass 30 is a myth. There is no scientific reason why we cannot continue to perform at or near our peaks into our 50s. Serious declines often can be staved off until our late 70s.

Most people over age 40 experience more precipitous physical declines not because their bodies fail them, but because they fail their bodies. The vast majority of Americans get less and less exercise as they age. This inactive lifestyle, not the passage of time, is the single greatest cause of their physical deterioration.

• **Push hard, but not all the time.** Older athletes must make a few concessions to their advancing age, but easing up on the throttle during workouts is not one of them. Don't just go for a walk...go for a jog. Don't just try to repeat the same performance in each exercise session...shoot for faster times and additional reps. (Always check with your doctor before starting an exercise program.)

People over age 40 should not attempt to go all out all the time, however. Older bodies take longer to recover from strenuous workouts than younger bodies. Schedule a rest day without guilt after a physically challenging day.

Example: If you plan a weeklong hiking trip with the grandkids, schedule challenging hikes only every other day, with days off for relaxing at campsites in between.

If you can't see yourself taking a day off from exercise, at least select an activity that challenges a different muscle group.

• **Try to never get out of shape.** Getting back in shape is good, but never getting out of shape is better. Athletes who remain physically competitive after age 40 usually don't have to worry about getting back in shape—most of them have never allowed themselves to get out of shape.

Example: Dara Torres was swimming competitively just three weeks after giving birth.

For those who are in great shape, staying in shape is like taking a well-tuned sports car out for a spin. But for those who are out of shape, exercising is like pushing a broken car up a hill. Their hearts and lungs are inefficient, and their muscles are weak. Exercise is unpleasant, so they avoid it.

The psychological challenge of getting back in shape can be equally daunting. Once middle-aged people let their fitness levels slide, they tend to assume that this decline is natural and inevitable, which makes it easy for them to surrender to the process. Those who never get out of shape continue to think of good health and physical fitness as their natural state and exercise as a natural part of their lives.

As difficult as rebounding from a period of inactivity can be, it will only become more difficult the longer this inactivity lasts. If you are out of shape, the best time to begin your return to fitness is today.

• **Ignore advancing age.** Successful older athletes don't think of their age as a disadvantage—most don't even think of themselves as old. They feel young, think young and react with surprise when others suggest that competing at their age is unnatural.

Example: NHL hockey player Chris Chelios was still active at age 47. When asked how someone so old managed to stay in the league, he said, "I don't feel old."

When successful older athletes think about their age at all, they tend to focus on its advantages—decades of experience and improved technique. They believe that their younger competitors are at the disadvantage.

• **Work on injury-prevention muscles, not cosmetic muscles.** Leave the bulging biceps to the younger athletes. The muscles that matter the most to those over 40 are the ones that help us avoid aches and injuries. *Among the most important...*

• Rotator cuff muscles. Injuries of the rotator cuff (the muscles and tendons inside your shoulder) are extremely common among those over 40. These injuries make it painful to swim, swing a golf club or tennis racket, throw a baseball or do virtually anything else that involves the shoulder. To strengthen the rotator cuff, use an exercise band, placing one end under your right foot and the other end in your right hand. Raise the band slowly in front of your body, keeping your elbow straight. Do one set of eight to 10 reps. Work up to two sets. Repeat on the left side.

• Abdominals and pelvic muscles. The secret to a healthy back is a healthy front. Keep your abs and pelvic muscles toned, and back pain is less likely. A key exercise is the plank. Lie on your stomach, hold in your abs and raise your body on your elbows and toes. Begin by holding for 30 seconds, and work up to two minutes.

• Quads. Knee pain is not always caused by a problem with the joint itself. Strengthening the four large quad muscles on the front of your thighs can make your knees feel as good as new. Quad exercise: Place your back against a wall with your feet about 18 inches in front of the wall. Place two rolled towels between your knees, and squeeze them with your knees. Then lower your back down the wall until your knees are bent about 60 degrees. Hold for 10 to 30 seconds, and work up to doing it 10 times. Keep your stomach pulled in.

• **Don't forget flexibility and balance.** Successful older athletes almost invariably understand that stretching and "equilibrium training" are just as important as aerobic exercise and strength training.

Our muscles become shorter and stiffer as we age. This shortens our stride when we run and makes full, fluid 360-degree shoulder motion difficult when we swim, golf or play tennis. Daily stretching can allow us to move as we did when we were young.

Stretch the major muscle groups for 30 seconds every day, not just before physical activity. After age 65, double this stretching time to 60 seconds per stretch per muscle group.

Our natural equilibrium begins to decline in our 30s, but most people do not realize that their balance is slowly failing until they start to fall down, typically in their 60s or 70s.

The best way to slow equilibrium loss is to practice balancing every day.

An easy way: Stand on one foot as long as you can while doing the dishes or brushing your teeth, then switch.

Go Ahead and Pound (On) Your Aging Bones

Vonda Wright, MD, assistant professor, department of orthopaedic surgery, University of Pittsburgh School of Medicine, and orthopedic surgeon at the University of Pittsburgh Medical Center. She is author of *Fitness After 40: How to Stay Strong at Any Age*. VondaWright.com

---

You can't turn back the clock, but according to some very interesting research, you can—and perhaps should—act as young as you feel when you play sports. The conventional wisdom has been that older folks should avoid high-impact sports like running due to the risk for fracture or other debilitating injury. But this research demonstrates that older individuals would benefit from more challenging exercise...and those who do work out hard build up their bone mineral density, resulting in stronger bones that are less likely to break.

Researchers at the University of Pittsburgh Medical Center used ultrasound scans to examine the bones of 560 male and female athletes, ages 50 to 93, who were in town to participate in the 2005 National Senior Games. Scans revealed that the athletes competing in high-impact sports had substantially higher bone mineral density than those who were there for low-impact events such as swimming and shuffleboard.

POUND THE PAVEMENT

Vonda Wright, MD, an orthopedic surgeon and the study's lead researcher, says these findings can be put to use by the rest of us. "We want you to pound your bones!" exclaims Dr. Wright.

Though conventional wisdom says older folks should accept that they can't do all that they used to do, she says that it's fine—even smart—to participate in the types of activities, including track-and-field and sports like volleyball, squash and basketball, where you bang your hands and feet fast and hard against balls or the ground. Jogging, running and jumping rope fit into this category, while walking or playing golf (even though the ball gets hit with some force) do not, because they involve a softer surface and/or a more leisurely pace.

Dr. Wright agreed that low-impact sports —such as swimming or pedaling a stationary bicycle—are beneficial for building strong muscles and a healthy cardiovascular system, but she noted that high-impact sports confer these same benefits and the advantage of increasing bone density.

WHY IS THIS GOOD?

Our bones are made of organic and inorganic matter—the latter being crystalline, which literally sparks upon compression. Decades-old research has established that hard, quick impact creates a type of electrical current (called piezoelectric) that helps preserve bone density and, surprisingly, actually speeds the healing of fractures.

Dr. Wright offered this advice to people who want to maintain strong bones...

- **Give high-impact exercise a try...but check with your doctor first, especially if you already know that you have low bone density.** Those who can't or don't want to do high-impact exercise should still engage in brisk walking, which is also of benefit.
- **Don't become discouraged if it hurts a bit (though be aware that severe pain is—as always—to be paid attention to).** Generally speaking, it's okay to work through an ache such as the burned-out feeling of muscle you've worked hard... but if you experience sharp or acute pain, it's better to stop. Dr. Wright said that enduring a bit of soreness is a "relatively small price to pay for avoiding a fractured bone in the future."
- **Don't be a hero.** Start slow and easy and assess how your body is taking to your new regimen. A good way to get started is with short bursts of activity—a day on and a day off.
- **Don't let age deter you from participating in high-impact sports even if your performance isn't as good as you'd wish.** As Dr. Wright says, "Even at age 85, there's no evidence that our bodies are not capable of jogging—even if at that age it might look more like shuffling!"

Make Exercise Safer and Much More Comfortable

Colin Milner, CEO of the International Council on Active Aging, a Vancouver, British Columbia–based organization dedicated to improving fitness and quality-of-life issues in older adults. Milner serves on the World Economic Forum's Global Agenda Council on Aging, is a contributor to the US Department of Health and Human Services' "Be Active Your Way" blog and is a recipient of the Canadian Fitness Professional Association's Lifetime Achievement Award.

Let's face it. Exercise sometimes hurts. So when we fear that our bodies might rebel, we're tempted to put off exercise or even skip it.

That's a shame because it doesn't make sense to deprive ourselves of exercise—it's hands-down the most powerful health protector there is. So what's the solution?

By choosing the right workout aids, you can dramatically ease the discomfort of key exercise routines. Here's what works best for...

STRETCHING

Who among us isn't just a little—or a lot—stiff and achy at times? Stretching is perhaps the best exercise you can do to loosen up those tight, inflexible muscles. It will help limber you up and improve your range of motion—both of which make it easier to do day-to-day activities such as grabbing groceries off a high shelf.

But if you're not very flexible to begin with, stretching is likely to cause some discomfort.

What helps: Gaiam Multi-Grip Stretch Strap ($10.38, Gaiam.com). With multiple handholds along the strap, this product allows you to ease into your stretches with greater control than you could on your own or if you relied on a regular strap without handholds.

WALKING

Walking is the easiest, most approachable workout there is. But if you've got pain due to arthritis, back problems or a hip or other joint replacement... or balance problems, even walking can be difficult.

Adding walking poles helps reduce impact on your joints, normalize your gait and improve your balance. The addition of poles also helps to boost your cardio endurance and increase your caloric burn—with poles, your heart rate will be 10% to 15% higher compared with traditional walking, and you'll burn about 400 calories per hour versus 280 calories.

What helps: ACTIVATOR Poles ($109.99 per pair, UrbanPoling.com). These aren't just any old walking poles. They feature bell-shaped, rubber tips for added grip and reduced vibration. With a doctor's prescription, this product may be covered by insurance.

Also: For people with peripheral neuropathy, a type of nerve damage that leads to numbness, tingling and/or weakness in the feet and other limbs, it can be tough to rely on walking as a form of exercise.

What helps: WalkJoy ($3,495 per pair, WalkJoy.com). This device is attached with straps worn below the knees. Sensors in the device signal healthy nerves around the knees (which are unaffected by peripheral neuropathy), letting your brain know that one foot has hit the ground and it's time to lift the toes of the opposite foot for another step. WalkJoy is FDA-approved and available by prescription.

SWIMMING

Swimming is a great low-impact, whole-body exercise for people who are watching their weight, building cardio strength or looking for relief from arthritis pain.

For the average recreational swimmer, however, efficient breathing can be challenging. Many swimmers feel like they're struggling for air...or their necks tire or become painful from constantly twisting and lifting.

What helps: Finis Swimmer's Snorkel ($29.99, FinisInc.com). Unlike many snorkels, which are designed for scuba divers, this product was created specifically for swimmers. Its adjustable head bracket lets you wear it with a swim cap and/or goggles while allowing you to keep your head in a fixed position so that you don't have to remove your mouth from the water to breathe.

CYCLING

Riding a bicycle is another great low-impact exercise. It has been shown to improve muscle strength and promote lung and heart health. The problem is, traditional bike saddles (on both stationary and road bikes) place a lot of pressure on the perineum (the area between the genitals and the anus). This contributes to pain and erectile dysfunction in men and numbness in women.

What helps: ISM Comfort Saddles ($50 to $70, ISMSeat.com). This is a noseless saddle, which directly supports your "sits" bones (at the base of the buttocks) while easing pressure on the perineum. Research has found that no-nose saddles reduce most perineal pressure in male riders and improve penile blood flow when compared with traditional bike seats. No-nose saddles also reduce numbness in women.

6 Common Stretching Mistakes That Can Hurt You

Karl Knopf, EdD, director of fitness therapy and senior fitness for the International Sports Sciences Association and retired director of adaptive fitness at Foothill College in Los Altos Hills, California. He is author of many fitness books including *Stretching for 50+* and a board member of Sit and Be Fit, a nonprofit organization dedicated to healthy aging.

We now know that stretching is key to staying limber and flexible. But did you know that it also could be dangerous?

Many people stretch improperly, overstressing muscles and even tendons in ways that lead to strains and sprains. An injury can come on gradually as a result of cumulative "insults" from performing a stretch a certain way over and over again. You don't know you're hurting yourself...until you're really hurt.

Other people don't stretch wrong—they just don't stretch at all or only once in a while. Many people focus more on cardiovascular exercise and weight training, yet often neglect stretching—until they get hurt. To benefit from a flexibility program, you need to practice it regularly, ideally every day.

As we age, stretching becomes even more important. Our bodies undergo changes that result in lack of elasticity. Women tend to be more flexible than men, but starting in their 50s, both genders start to lose flexibility and range of motion, especially in the shoulders and low back, which can lead to shoulder and back issues. The good news is that this age-related decline can be slowed through a regular stretching program.

By learning to stretch properly, you'll maximize your mobility...greatly reduce the risk for pain and injury...perform better at any sport you engage in...and look younger. (*One caution*: If you've had a recent fracture, sprain, injury or surgery, or if you suspect that you have osteoporosis, speak to your doctor/physical therapist first.)

Here are common stretching mistakes that can hurt you—and how to steer clear of them...

HOLDING YOUR BREATH

One common stretching mistake is holding your breath as you hold a stretch. Muscles need oxygen throughout a stretch—plus, holding your breath can elevate your blood pressure. Breathe slowly and consistently throughout each phase of a stretch—especially when you're holding one.

Simple stretches, such as shoulder rolls (see "Safe, Effective Stretches You Can Do Anywhere" on the next page), don't require that you hold them. But most do. These stretches should be held for at least 20 seconds—and recent studies suggest that for older adults, 60 seconds is even better. Breathe throughout.

STRETCHING COLD

Not that long ago, we were instructed to stretch before playing sports when our muscles were "cold." Now we know that's a bad idea. Think of your muscles and tendons as taffy. Then imagine trying to stretch and bend cold taffy. It can snap. On a micro level, that's like stretching a cold, tight muscle. Ouch!

Much better: Warm up for five minutes or more first, before you do any stretch that you hold. Try light running...a few minutes in a steam room or sauna...or, if you're home, a warm bath.

GETTING INTENSE

Too many people follow the old paradigm that the more intense the exercise, the better. They overdo it with weights, aerobics—and stretching. In my opinion, no pain, no gain is...insane. If you feel sore a few hours after exercising, you overdid it.

Much better: When stretching, move slowly and gently, and stay within your comfort zone. You should feel mild tension in your muscles and joints. Don't push past it. Listen to your body, especially your neck, back, shoulders and knees. If you have tightness or joint pain, take some time off. If it continues, see your doctor or a physical therapist before it turns into a real issue.

GOING OLD SCHOOL—FAST AND BOUNCY

If you played a sport in high school, it's time to unlearn some things you learned, including bouncing toe touches. These moves weren't safe then, and they are even riskier now that you're older. Those neck circles you started every gym class with? Terrible! They strain supporting ligaments and can lead to pinched nerves.

That hurdler stretch where you sit with one leg out in front of you and the other bent behind you? It stresses the meniscus and the medial collateral ligament of your knee—an injury in the making. Windmill toe touches? No! Bending and rotating at the same time is a recipe for trouble.

Red flag: Avoid stretches such as the hurdler that make your knees twist or move in an unnatural position. Be careful about back bends that call for you to raise both hands over your head and lean back. That can pinch the facet joints of the spine.

Much better: Always keep knees "soft" (slightly bent) when stretching. When turning, move your body slowly, as a unit, and pivot your feet.

STRETCHING ONLY WHEN YOU EXERCISE

Chances are that if you stretch, you do so only before working out or playing a sport. Big mistake! To maintain flexibility, your muscles need to be worked just about every day.

Much better: Think of stretching as part of your daily routine, like brushing your teeth. You don't need a designated area or even to wear gym clothes. Spend a few minutes doing a body-flexibility session daily, especially in high-risk areas such as the hamstrings, shoulders and lower back.

NOT BEING WELL-BALANCED

The body is designed with opposing muscle groups, and each group needs to be worked equally. Weight training can unbalance muscles, so you need stretching to get you back into balance. Example: If you do a movement such as a bench press that rolls your shoulders forward, you should do a stretch that pulls them back. My golden rule is, Do unto the front as you do unto the back, and do unto the left as you do unto the right.

Conversely, being too flexible can be a problem, especially if you don't have muscles that are strong enough to support your joints. I once taught a dancer who kept dislocating her shoulder joints because her muscles weren't strong enough to keep her shoulders in place. It's all about balance.

One final tip—enjoy your stretching session. It's a great time to integrate the mind and the body.

SAFE, EFFECTIVE STRETCHES YOU CAN DO ANYWHERE

Here are two different kinds of stretches—no-hold stretches that you can do anywhere anytime and standard stretches for which you warm up for five minutes and then hold for at least 20 seconds, ideally 60.

Together, these stretches work on your upper and lower body. Repeat each one at least three times.

UPPER-BODY NO-HOLD STRETCHES...

- **Elbow touches (for the chest).** Place your hands on your shoulders (left on left, right on right), elbows pointing forward as much as possible. Slowly move your elbows out to the side as far as is comfortable, pinching the shoulder blades together, and hold for just a few seconds. Bring your elbows back to the starting position and repeat.
- **Shoulder rolls (for the upper back).** With your arms hanging down naturally, shrug your shoulders up and squeeze them back, as if attempting to touch them together...then relax them.
- **Apple pickers (for the shoulders).** Place your hands on your shoulders (left hand on left, right on right). Then slowly raise your right hand as high up as is comfortable—reach for that apple! Return to the start position, and repeat with the left hand. Keep good posture throughout.

THESE ARE STANDARD "HOLD 'EM" STRETCHES...

- **Chest stretch (for the chest and shoulders).** Stand facing a corner. Place one hand on each side wall, with your elbows in a push-up position. Lean gently into the corner until you feel a stretch across your upper chest. Hold for at least 20 seconds.
- **Seated knee to chest (for the lower back and gluteal muscles/butt).** Sit on a stable chair with your feet flat on the floor. Clasp your hands beneath your left leg. Pull your left knee toward your chest with your hands and hold for at least 20 seconds, feeling the stretch in the gluteal and low-back area. Return to start position, and repeat with other leg.
- **Rear calf stretch (for your calves).** Stand facing a wall, with both hands on the wall at shoulder height. Your knees should be slightly bent.

Keeping the heel down, slide your right leg back until you feel the stretch in the calf area. Hold for at least 20 seconds. Switch sides and repeat.

Weak Hands = Weak Lungs

Study titled "Relationship Between Handgrip Strength and Pulmonary Function in Apparently Healthy Older Women" by researchers at Yonsei University College of Medicine, South Korea, published in *Journal of the American Geriatrics Society.*

Getting older sometimes means getting help with ketchup bottles and pickle jars that used to be easy to open. We might not be happy about it, but it's not surprising. But did you know that the reason you struggle with jar lids can also affect your breathing? Here's why...and what you absolutely should do about it.

Losing muscle strength and mass is a natural process of aging called sarcopenia. How much you lose depends on your health, genetics and lifestyle. Many people think of age-related muscle loss as affecting their arms, legs, torso, etc. But sarcopenia affects all the muscles in the body, including the muscles that control respiration, such as the diaphragm.

Because measuring hand strength is a proven way to infer muscle strength in the rest of the body, researchers at Yonsei University in Korea wondered whether hand strength could predict pulmonary function—how efficiently a person's lungs work. Early detection of impaired lung function can help avert episodic respiratory problems such as bronchitis and pneumonia and help avert cardiovascular disease, chronic obstructive pulmonary disease (COPD), heart failure and early death.

Study: The researchers analyzed data from a health survey of 1,773 healthy women ages 65 to 79. The survey included physical examinations that measured handgrip strength and pulmonary function.

Results: The stronger her hands, the more likely a woman was to have a well-functioning respiratory system—and the weaker her hands, the more likely to have impaired lung function.

Although the study was small and involved only women, and the researchers did comment that research on men is needed, other research has found that grip strength in men is associated with better overall health, including better quality of life and lower risk of dying of from heart disease.

While we can't entirely avoid losing muscle as we age, our lifestyle can minimize the loss. Exercise, both aerobic and resistance, and a healthy diet that includes adequate protein are key. There also are things you can do to keep your lungs in top working order, such as breathing exercises, playing a harmonica or even blowing through a straw.

Strong Hands, Long Life

Elaine LaLanne, wife of the late Jack LaLanne, is the author or coauthor of numerous books on exercise and health, including the classic *Fitness After 50 Workout*. JackLalanne.com

Can our ability to open a jar of pickles or wring out a washcloth give us a greater chance of living longer? That's an implication of recent research published in *British Medical Journal (BMJ)*.

Scientists in the UK analyzed data on more than 53,000 people from 14 separate studies, ranking them into four groups based on the strength of their grips.

Findings: Compared with the group that had the strongest hands, those with the weakest grips were 67% more likely to die during the study periods (which ranged from less than five years to more than 20 years). The link between grip strength and longevity was seen not only among seniors, but also in studies in which participants were younger than 60 years old, on average.

This research doesn't necessarily prove that strengthening our hands will prolong our lives—but it well might. Besides, strong hands certainly do make countless daily tasks easier.

Jack LaLanne, often called the "godfather of fitness," passed away at age 96. According to his widow and coauthor, Elaine LaLanne, "Jack did hand exercises every single morning for strength, coordination, dexterity and flexibility."

Here's the LaLanne daily hand workout, which takes about 10 to 15 minutes. All exercises can be done standing or sitting. Why not try them for yourself? (As with any exercise program, get your doctor's OK before beginning. These particular hand exercises may not be appropriate for people with certain medical conditions—for example, carpal tunnel syndrome.)

• **Big squeeze.** Use a rubber ball that fits easily into your palm. Grasp ball with all five fingers of right hand and squeeze as tightly as possible…hold for a count of three…release. Do 10 repetitions (reps), then switch hands. Work your way up to three sets.

• **Hand flexes.** Extend arms straight out in front of you at mid-chest height, palms up, fingers spread. Quickly clench hands into fists, then open again. Do 10 reps as rapidly as possible…then repeat with palms facing down. Work up to three sets.

• **Shake-a-hand.** Hold hands out in front of you and shake them, moving arms all around in whatever manner you like. Continue for one minute… work up to two minutes.

• **Newspaper roll.** Unfold a section of newspaper (try four full sheets to start—if that proves too easy, use eight to 10 sheets). With both hands, grasp the newspaper at one end so that hands are shoulder-width apart. Elbows straight, extend arms in front of you at chest height, palms facing down. Begin rolling up the newspaper, twisting as if wringing out a towel…when you reach the end, reverse the motion to unroll newspaper. Work up to 10 sets.

• **Five to four.** Hold hands in front of you at shoulder height, elbows comfortably bent, palms facing forward, fingers spread wide (as if each hand were indicating the number five). Then bring thumbs across palms (as if indicating the number four)…then extend thumbs again. Do 10 reps at a moderately fast pace. Work up to three sets.

• **Knuckle sandwich.** Hold hands in front of you at shoulder height, elbows comfortably bent, palms facing forward, fingers together and pointing up. Without making a full fist or bending wrists, curl fingers until fingertips touch tops of palms…hold for a count of five…then uncurl fingers. Do 10 reps. Work up to three sets.

• **Spread 'em.** Place hands flat on a desktop or tabletop in front of you, fingers spread as wide as possible. Press down firmly for 10 seconds, then relax. Do three reps.

How Much to Jog to Live Longer

Peter Schnohr, MD, chief cardiologist, Copenhagen City Heart Study, Bispebjerg University Hospital, Copenhagen.

Lacing up your sneakers and going for a run has long been considered a smart way to boost overall health—and a recent Danish study takes that idea even further, showing that jogging a certain amount per week at a certain pace may add six whole years to your life.

Living six extra years is great—but is it worth it if you have to jog long and hard for hours every day? Would you? The good news is that you don't have to turn yourself into a jogging machine.

If you enjoy jogging, but you don't like to push yourself too hard, you're going to be pleasantly surprised by how little jogging you have to do to extend your life!

RUN FOR YOUR LIFE

This news is so promising that it'll make you want to lace up your sneakers right now!

In this large study, researchers followed 20,000 adult men and women over a maximum of 35 years, comparing the overall mortality of outdoor joggers to nonjoggers. The results? Jogging was associated with an average increase in life span of 6.2 years in men and 5.6 years in women. This held true after researchers adjusted for all known variables associated with mortality.

The best part: The biggest benefit didn't come from running the most or the hardest. Though all runners had longer life expectancies, compared with nonrunners, those who had the longest life expectancies ran just one to 2.5 hours a week total (spaced out over two to three workouts a week)... and they ran at a slow-to-average pace!

It's obvious why running, in general, can help you live longer. It improves oxygen uptake, cardiac function and bone density and helps you maintain a healthy weight and improve mental health, among other things. But why did moderate runners fare the best? Would jogging indoors on a treadmill have a similar effect? And would moderate types of other aerobic activities, such as biking or swimming, similarly extend your life? More research is needed to find out what's best for all forms of exercise.

STEP TO IT

It's very inspiring to hear that we can gain so many extra years of life from as little as one total hour of running a week. Think about that for a moment—if you split up the time, that's just three 20-minute jogs per week at a pace that leaves you a little breathless but not totally out of breath. You can do that!

You Can Exercise Less and Be Just as Healthy

Barry A. Franklin, PhD, director of preventive cardiology/cardiac rehabilitation at William Beaumont Hospital in Royal Oak, Michigan. He is a past president of the American Association of Cardiovascular and Pulmonary Rehabilitation and the American College of Sports Medicine. He is also coauthor, with Joseph C. Piscatella, of *109 Things You Can Do to Prevent, Halt & Reverse Heart Disease*.

Do you struggle to fit the recommended amount of exercise into your busy schedule? Well, what if we told you that the amount of exercise needed to reap health benefits might be less than you think? Maybe you could free up some of your workout time for other activities that are important to you and beneficial to your health—like playing with your kids or grandkids, volunteering for a favorite charity or cooking healthful meals.

THE LATEST IN EXERCISE RESEARCH

A recent study published in the *Journal of the American College of Cardiology* found that people lived longest when they ran, on average, for 30 minutes or more, five days a week. Surprisingly, that research also showed that people who jogged at an easy pace for as little as five to 10 minutes a day had virtually the same survival benefits as those who pushed themselves harder or longer.

Also surprising: A study recently done at Oregon State University found that one- and two-minute bouts of activity that add up to 30 minutes or more per day, such as pacing while talking on the telephone, doing housework or doing sit-ups during TV commercials, may reduce blood pressure and cholesterol and improve health as effectively as a structured exercise program.

HOW TO EXERCISE SMARTER, NOT HARDER

Here are four strategies to help you exercise more efficiently...

- **Recognize that some exercise is always better than none.** Even though exercise guidelines from the Centers for Disease Control and Prevention (CDC) call for at least 150 minutes of moderate exercise each week, you'll do well even at lower levels.

A *Lancet* study found that people who walked for just 15 minutes a day had a 14% reduction in death over an average of eight years. Good daily exercises include not only walking but working in the yard, swimming, riding a bike, etc.

If you're among the multitudes of Americans who have been sedentary in recent years, you'll actually gain the most. Simply making the transition from horrible fitness to below average can reduce your overall risk for premature death by 20% to 40%.

- **Go for a run instead of a walk.** The intensity, or associated energy cost, of running is greater than walking. Therefore, running (or walking up a grade or incline) is better for the heart than walking—and it's easier to work into a busy day because you can get equal benefits in less time.

For cardiovascular health, a five-minute run (5.5 mph to 8 mph) is equal to a 15-minute walk (2 mph to 3.5 mph)...and a 25-minute run equals a 105-minute walk.

A 2014 study of runners found that their risk of dying from heart disease was 45% lower than non-runners over a 15-year follow-up. In fact, running can add, on average, three extra years to your life.

Caution: If you take running seriously, you still should limit your daily workouts to 60 minutes or less, no more than five days a week. (See below for the dangers of overdoing it.) People with heart symptoms or severely compromised heart function should avoid running. If you have joint problems, check with your doctor.

- **Ease into running.** Don't launch into a running program until you're used to exercise. Make it progressive. Start by walking slowly—say, at about 2 mph. Gradually increase it to 3 mph...then to 3.5 mph, etc. After two or three months, if you are symptom-free during fast walking, you can start to run (slowly at first).

- **Aim for the "upper-middle."** I do not recommend high-intensity workouts for most adults. Strive to exercise at a level you would rate between "fairly light" and "somewhat hard."

How to tell: Check your breathing. It will be slightly labored when you're at a good level of exertion. Nevertheless, you should still be able to carry on a conversation.

Important: Get your doctor's OK before starting vigorous exercise—and don't ignore potential warning symptoms. It's normal to be somewhat winded or to have a little leg discomfort. However, you should never feel dizzy, experience chest pain or have extreme shortness of breath. If you have any of these symptoms, stop exercise immediately, and see your doctor before resuming activity.

TOO MUCH OF A GOOD THING?

Most people who run for more than an hour a day, five days a week, are in very good shape. Would they be healthier if they doubled the distance—or pushed themselves even harder? Not necessarily. *Risks linked to distance running include...*

- **Acute right-heart overload.** Researchers at William Beaumont Hospital who looked at distance runners before and immediately after marathon running found that they often had transient decreases in the pumping ability of the right ventricle and elevations of the same enzymes (such as troponin) that increase during a heart attack.

- **Atrial fibrillation.** People who exercise intensely for more than five hours a week may be more likely to develop atrial fibrillation, a heart-rhythm disturbance that can trigger a stroke.

- **Coronary plaque.** Despite their favorable coronary risk factor profiles, distance runners can have increased amounts of coronary artery calcium and plaque as compared with their less active counterparts.

Watch out: Many hard-core runners love marathons, triathlons and other competitive events. Be careful. The emotional rush from competition increases levels of epinephrine and other "stress" hormones. These hormones, combined with hard exertion, can transiently increase heart risks.

Of course, all this doesn't mean that you shouldn't enjoy a daily run...or a few long ones—just don't overdo it!

Are You Tough Enough for Tai Chi?

Peter M. Wayne, PhD, an assistant professor of medicine at Harvard Medical School and research director of the Osher Center for Integrative Medicine, jointly based at Harvard Medical School and Brigham and Women's Hospital, both in Boston. He has trained in tai chi for more than 35 years and is the author, with Mark L. Fuerst, of *The Harvard Medical School Guide to Tai Chi.*

Perhaps you've seen people performing the graceful, seemingly slow-motion movements of tai chi in a nearby park. If you've never tried it before, you may think that this form of exercise is easy to do and provides little more than a mild workout.

The truth: Even though tai chi consists of slow, gentle movements, this exercise is no pushover. Long known for its stress-reducing benefits, it also gives you an aerobic workout that's as intense as walking at a moderate pace...increases muscle strength and flexibility...improves breathing... improves posture and balance (to help prevent falls)...and focuses the mind.

What's new: Tai chi, which was developed centuries ago in China as a means of self-defense, is now linked to a number of new health benefits, including improved cardiovascular health and bone density...and reduced back and neck pain.

Even better: Tai chi is safer than many forms of exercise because of its 70% rule: You never move your joints or exert yourself beyond 70% of your maximum potential.

Recently discovered benefits...

BETTER BREATHING

Many Eastern-based practices, including yoga, meditation and tai chi, emphasize diaphragmatic breathing, in which the muscles of the diaphragm (rather than the chest) are used to take in more oxygen. This style of breathing not only helps the lungs to move with less effort but also allows more oxygen to pass into the bloodstream.

Efficient breathing is more important than you might think. Multiple studies indicate that healthy breathing—as measured by "forced expiratory volume," the amount of air that you can exhale in one second—may help you live longer.

LOWER BLOOD PRESSURE

The stress relief that can come from tai chi, along with improved breathing and other factors, make it an ideal exercise for lowering blood pressure. In fact, research suggests that tai chi is at least as effective for lowering blood pressure as lifestyle changes that are usually recommended, such as losing weight and cutting back on sodium.

A Johns Hopkins study found that light-intensity tai chi improved blood pressure almost as much as moderate-intensity aerobic exercise.

PERIPHERAL NEUROPATHY

Millions of people with diabetes and other conditions have peripheral neuropathy, nerve damage in the hands and/or feet that causes numbness, tingling or pain. The condition is particularly troublesome because reduced sensations in the feet can impair balance and increase the risk of falling.

Research has found that people with peripheral neuropathy who practiced tai chi had improved sensitivity in the soles of the feet. They also had better balance and walking speed.

STRONGER BONES

You don't need to lift weights to increase bone strength and reduce risk for osteoporosis. Researchers in Hong Kong found that women who did tai chi three times per week had increased bone density within 12 months.

IT'S EASY TO GET STARTED

Tai chi classes are commonly offered at health clubs, YMCAs and even some hospitals. Classes are particularly useful because of the feedback given by the instructor and the group support, which helps keep you motivated.

Good goal: Two one-hour tai chi classes a week—plus at-home practice for at least 30 minutes, three times a week.

You can find a tai chi expert in your area at AmericanTaiChi.net.

A TASTE OF TAI CHI

Tai chi consists of dozens of different moves. Here's one called "Tai Chi Pouring"...

What to do: Stand with your feet shoulder-width apart. Slightly bend one knee and allow your weight to shift to that side. Briefly pause, and then gently bend your other knee and shift your weight in that direction. Pause again. "Pour" your weight back and forth for a few minutes while breathing deeply and feeling a relaxed flow connecting your whole body.

How to Make Yoga Safe for Every Body

Carol Krucoff, C-IAYT, E-RYT, a yoga therapist and codirector of the Integrative Yoga for Seniors Professional Training at Duke Integrative Medicine, Durham, North Carolina. She is coauthor of, most recently, *Relax into Yoga for Seniors: A Six-Week Program for Strength, Balance, Flexibility and Pain Relief.* HealingMoves.com

---

I'd love to try yoga, but... It's a common lament of people with arthritis, osteoporosis or other chronic health problems. But yoga doesn't have to be off-limits if you have one of these conditions.

With a few precautions and a tailored approach, yoga is a wonderfully effective, research-backed method of improving strength, balance and flexibility...easing pain...and relieving the anxiety and depression that are often associated with chronic health complaints.

For anyone with one or more painful and/or limiting chronic conditions, the relaxation breathing and mindfulness that are central to yoga also can be exceptionally helpful.

Note: Older adults and people with health challenges should look for a class called "Gentle Yoga" or one geared to their needs, such as "Yoga Over 50" or "Yoga for Creaky Bodies." *Follow these steps to ensure that you stay safe if you have...*

ARTHRITIS

Decades ago, people with osteoarthritis and rheumatoid arthritis were advised to rest and "save their joints." Now we know that inactivity can actually cause stiff joints. Yoga relieves pain and stiffness, improves range of motion and sleep, and boosts energy levels and overall mood. *If you have arthritis, be sure to...*

- **Avoid putting excessive pressure on arthritic joints.** Arthritis in your left knee? Keep the toes of your right foot on the ground in single-leg balance poses like Tree Pose. If you have arthritis in both knees, you can relieve the load on your joints by lightly touching a wall or chair.

- **Understand the meaning of different types of pain.** Sharp, immediate pain—especially in a joint—is a sign to ease up. If you have dull pain in your muscles the day after a yoga session, that's likely delayed-onset muscle soreness after using your muscles in new ways—a sign that you're getting stronger! It generally goes away in a few days.

- **Don't overstretch.** This is especially true for people with rheumatoid arthritis, which can render joints loose and unstable. To tell whether it's a good or risky stretch: Check your breath. If your breath is compromised in any way, back off.

- **Avoid chin-to-chest poses that place pressure on your head.** Poses, such as Plow, place undue pressure on vulnerable cervical spine joints.

- **Turn certain poses around to "take a load" off.** If a pose is bothering an affected joint, try turning it upside down or sideways, taking weight off the joint and letting gravity do the work for you. Child's Pose, for example, can be done while lying on your back in bed.

Caution: Hot, red and/or swollen joints indicate active inflammation. Stick with rest or gentle range-of-motion activities for that joint. Talk with your health-care provider about appropriate treatment.

OSTEOPOROSIS

Yoga is an effective way to improve strength, balance and flexibility in people with osteoporosis. And because yoga improves your balance and strengthens bone, it may help lower your risk of falling and breaking a bone. *If you have osteoporosis, be sure to...*

- **Avoid rounding your spine when sitting or standing, since this position increases the risk for vertebral fracture.** In yoga poses—and in daily life—keep your spine long and hinge forward at your hips, rather than bending at your waist.

- **Don't twist your spine to its end range of rotation.** Instructors may encourage their students to twist as far as possible, using their hands to move even deeper into the twist. This is called end-range rotation and can increase fracture risk in people with osteoporosis. Keep any twists in the midrange, as you would when turning to look over your shoulder while driving. Move slowly, don't round your back and keep your spine elongated.

- **Avoid loading body weight on your neck and/or shoulders** as occurs during such poses as Shoulder Stand and Plow.

- **Keep your head on the ground during supine (face-up) poses.** Lifting your head when lying on the ground creates the forward-flexing, "abdominal crunch" action that can be dangerous because it places excess pressure on vertebral bodies and can lead to compression fractures. Yoga poses that can create this "crunch" are not necessarily supine—they include Standing Forward Bend and Seated Forward Bend. To perform these poses safely, hinge at the hips and keep your spine in neutral (don't round your back).

The Best Anti-Aging Exercise for Your Muscles

Study titled "Enhanced Protein Translation Underlies Improved Metabolic and Physical Adaptations to Different Exercise Training Modes in Young and Old Humans" by researchers at Mayo Clinic, Rochester, Minnesota, published in *Cell Metabolism*.

Exercise benefits the body at any age, but a certain kind of exercise, research finds, is particularly effective at counteracting the effects of aging on your muscles. It stimulates literally hundreds of genes that enhance the ability of muscle cells to convert nutrients into energy—an essential function that tends to decline with age. For younger people, this form of exercise is a good way to get fitter and healthier.

If you're older, it's a great way.

Background: There's no question that exercise is key to aging gracefully—being fit and strong fights age-related risks for disease and disability. As we age, our muscle mass decreases—and our muscles become less efficient at turning oxygen and nutrients into energy. Exercise counters both trends. But little has been known about what kind of exercise is most effective at keeping older muscles younger.

Study: Researchers from Mayo Clinic in Rochester, Minnesota, enrolled healthy men and women in a study that looked at the effects of three different types of exercise. The first was resistance (strength) training. The second was high-intensity aerobic interval training (HIIT), during which the exerciser pushes all-out for a brief spurt and then recovers while exercising at a reduced pace, and then repeats the process. The third was a combination of moderate-intensity aerobic exercise plus less intense resistance training. The researchers evaluated various markers of health.

Unlike similar studies, however, this one was conducted on two groups of people in very different stages of life. The younger group was 18 to 30 years old...the older group, 65 to 80. Baseline laboratory tests and muscle biopsies were conducted at the beginning of the study and after it ended 12 weeks later.

Results: All three exercise types improved insulin sensitivity, a key way that exercise helps prevent diabetes. Both HIIT and combined aerobic/resistance training led to improvements in aerobic capacity. Resistance training increased muscle mass. None of these results was surprising—and the effects were similar in both age groups.

But HIIT was really a hit for the older set in the way it increased the activity of genes that are thought to improve mitochondrial function. Mitochondria are tiny power plants inside every cell. As we age, the mitochondria in our cells diminish in both quantity and quality...and that leads to reduced ability to convert oxygen and nutrients into energy.

In the older study group, muscle biopsies showed that nearly 400 genes that affect mitochondria became more active with HIIT. In the younger group, 274 such genes became more active. In the older exercisers, HIIT was particularly effective at reversing low activity levels of 11 genes that are known decline with age.

Bottom Line: HIIT is a great approach to fitness, especially if you're older. *Here's the program that was used in the study...*

- **Three days a week, exercisers pedaled stationary bikes**—fast and hard for four minutes, followed by a three-minute interval of slow pedaling. They repeated that cycle for a total of four times.

•**Twice a week, on other days, they ran on a treadmill at 70% of capacity for 45 minutes.** That's not interval training, but it rounded out the weekly aerobic program.

If this program seems intense, that is because it is! Although the study didn't look at less intense intervals, do what you are comfortable doing and work your way up. You may not reap the same benefit of the study participants right off the bat, but you will be on the right track. A good place to start is with this guidance from The American Council on Exercise (go to ACEFitness.org and search HIIT).

The Easy Way to Do HIIT

Robert Zembroski, DC, DACNB, a functional medicine physician, board-certified chiropractic neurologist, clinical nutritionist and director of the Darien Center for Functional Medicine in Connecticut. He is author of *Rebuild: Five Proven Steps to Move from Diagnosis to Recovery and Be Healthier Than Before*.

High-intensity interval training (HIIT) is one of the most exciting trends in fitness, but the word "intensity" can scare away all but the most committed. Exercise is already hard, you may be thinking, and now experts want to make it harder?

Actually, it's the opposite. Most people find HIIT easier than traditional cardio workouts, such as jogging, swimming or even shoveling snow. Compared with cardio training, HIIT more effectively improves your metabolic rate (for burning calories)...and improves your VO2 max—a parameter associated with cardiovascular health—according to research. In addition, it strengthens the immune system.

What most people don't realize: Even though HIIT alternates periods of all-out exertion with periods of lower-intensity exercise, the intense segments of the workout don't have to be too grueling. *Facts you need to know to get started with HIIT...*

THE MAGIC OF HIIT

With HIIT, you exercise as hard as you can for 30 seconds to a minute. (The actual exertion level and duration of the "burst" will vary from person to person.) Then you slow down to a lower intensity for a minute or two...then repeat the hard-easy sequence a few more times. The total length of the workout depends on your fitness level and physical abilities.

It's the "explosive" part of the workout that creates what can only be called "magic." People who engage in HIIT have better cardiovascular health—including improved cholesterol profiles and less insulin resistance—than those who do conventional endurance workouts, according to research published in *Experimental Gerontology*.

EASE INTO HIIT

HIIT is a safe form of exercise, which poses no more risk for sprain/strain injuries than any other exercise regimen. As with any new workout, however, it's a good idea to get the go-ahead from your doctor before starting HIIT.

I tell people who are elderly or have physical limitations—or are merely new to exercise—to start with a low-intensity version of HIIT.

Example: If you're a 65-year-old who has mainly been sedentary, you might start out with a slow walk (the easy part of the exercise at up to 3 mph), then pick up your speed—walking at around 4 mph to 5 mph while swinging your arms for the hard part. After 30 seconds or a minute of fast-walking/arm-swinging, you'd drop back to a stroll for a minute or two, then maintain the cycle for four to five rounds. *To get started...*

•**Choose your sport.** With HIIT, it doesn't matter which activity you choose. You can do the exercise/rest cycles in a swimming pool or on a treadmill or an exercise bike—or using your own two feet. All that matters is that the activity allows you to go all-out for a brief period of time...drop down to a slower level...then go all-out once again. For most people, four of these intervals are enough to get an excellent workout.

•**Don't exercise on an empty stomach.** If you don't have enough blood sugar when you exercise, your body will pull sugar from the muscles first. That's the opposite of what you want to happen. To improve body composition, you want to preserve muscle and burn fat. The best way to do this is to exercise within one to three hours after having a small meal.

Good pre-workout meal choices: A couple of scrambled eggs with a few slivers of avocado and a side of veggies. Or a healthful protein bar such as RXBAR, Oatmega or SimplyProtein Whey Bar.

• **Work with your limitations.** Many of my patients have some physical limitations. They might be overweight...out of shape...or deal with arthritis, leg pain or other minor (or not so minor) disabilities. You can still engage in HIIT—you just have to find what works for you. A personal trainer can offer advice.

• **Go low and slow.** To start, I recommend doing an HIIT workout three days a week, for about 10 minutes each time. You'll slowly increase the total time—by increasing the number of intervals and/or the duration of the exertion/rest components—as you get stronger. Aim to work up to 20 to 30 minutes for each session.

• **Don't forget the warm-up and cooldown.** When you start your workout, whether it's biking, jogging or using a StairMaster, slowly go through these movements for the first few minutes...and shift into low intensity of the same exercise for a few minutes of cooldown at the end of the workout.

Each week, you'll find that you can gradually increase the duration and intensity of the workouts.

4 Easy Exercises for Better Posture and Better Health

Steven Weiniger, DC, managing partner and instructor at BodyZone.com, an organization devoted to improving posture as a way to promote health and longevity. Dr. Weiniger is also the author of *Stand Taller–Live Longer: An Anti-Aging Strategy* and developer of the new app PostureZone.

Once you move out of your mother's house, probably no one reminds you to stand up straight. But good posture is not only important for looking your best, it's also essential for good health!

Why: As human beings, our bodies are designed to stand upright, a position that helps us maintain balance. When your shoulders are hunched, you have an increased risk for falls. Plus, hunching causes other parts of your body to compensate to restore balance, which can result in upper and lower back pain, neck pain, headaches and other aches. Additionally, some research has linked bad posture to reduced lung function, poor circulation, digestive issues and much more.

WHY WE HUNCH

Let's face it—hunching is easier than standing up straight. Over the years, your body settles into its most comfortable position, and that becomes your "normal." The problem with this comfortable position is that it contributes to atrophy of the hip, shoulder, upper back and core muscles because they aren't being used to hold your body in alignment. Year by year, this muscle atrophy makes slumping more exaggerated and can lead to the health problems mentioned above.

Modern life also contributes to hunching. According to a 2016 Nielsen report, we spend an average of three hours each day hunched over a smartphone, computer or tablet...and another four hours slouched in front of a TV.

HELP FOR THE HUNCH

To develop good posture and lose the hunch, you need to strengthen the muscles mentioned earlier that help make standing up straight second nature. This simple routine takes no more than about four minutes to complete. If you do the exercises daily, you will start showing results in as little as two weeks.

EXERCISE 1—STABILIZE SHOULDERS DOWN

• **Lie flat on your back on a mat on the floor, legs extended or knees bent** (whatever is most comfortable), with your arms in a "T" position (elbows should be in line with your shoulders). Your face needs to be parallel to the ceiling.

• **Bend your elbows so that your fingers point toward the ceiling and your palms face your feet.**

• **Keeping your elbows on the floor, pull your shoulders down toward your feet.** Then bring your palms toward the floor as far as you comfortably can while keeping your shoulders down. Hold the position for three to five breaths (see below for the proper breathing technique).

EXERCISE 2—OPEN CHEST UP

• **Lie flat on your back and bend your elbows so that your fingers point toward the ceiling and your palms face your feet as in Exercise 1.**

• **Bring your hands backward toward the floor as far as you comfortably can.** Your arms will be in a "goalpost" position. Important: Keep your shoulders down as in Exercise 1. Do not shrug them.

• **Do this three to five times.** Inhale as you point your fingers to the ceiling, and exhale as you bring your hands toward the floor.

EXERCISE 3—FLOOR ANGELS

• **Lie flat on your back as above but with your arms flat on the floor in a goalpost position.**

• **Keeping your forearms parallel and your shoulders on the floor, slide your arms up and down on the floor.** Again, do not shrug your shoulders while performing this exercise.

• **Do this three to five times.** Inhale as you slide your arms up; exhale as you slide your arms down.

Once you master this, make the exercise more challenging by holding and stretching an elastic exercise band between your hands as you move your arms up and down.

EXERCISE 4—PINKIE TOUCH

• **Lie facedown on the floor, with your forehead resting on the floor.** Your arms should be straight at your sides with palms facing down.

• **Keeping shoulders down and elbows straight, move your hands together beneath your torso so that your pinkie fingers are touching.** (You'll have to raise your hips a bit to give your hands room to move.) Hold this position for three to five breaths.

BETTER BREATHING

As you perform these exercises, it's important to breathe from the belly, not the chest.

Why: When you breathe from the chest, your shoulders naturally hunch...but when you breathe from the belly, your shoulders stay in place.

To get the hang of belly breathing: Stretch an elastic exercise band across your lower back, with an end in each hand. Then crisscross the band in front of you, across your waist, about the level of your navel (you will need to exchange the band ends in your hands). Keeping your elbows bent at your sides, make the band snug but not tight. If you are breathing correctly, as you inhale, you will feel your belly pressing against the band, while your chest remains still. Exhale through pursed lips as your belly deflates.

HOW TO MONITOR YOUR POSTURE

To track changes in your posture, ask a friend to take an annual photo of you from the front and side. Or use PostureZone, a free app.

Self-test for hunching: Even people who don't think that they hunch their shoulders probably slump to some degree. *Try this simple exercise to find out if you're slumping (you can do this while standing or sitting)...*

• **First, bring your shoulders forward and in toward your chest, and then bring them up toward your ears.** This is an exaggerated hunch.

• **Next, pull your shoulders back and down toward your feet.** This is how your shoulders should be positioned for good posture. If this position feels uncomfortable or painful, you may have a hunching problem.

The Surprising Way To Get More From Your Exercise

Paul A. Estabrooks, PhD, behavioral scientist, professor and Harold M. Maurer Distinguished Chair of the department of health promotions at University of Nebraska Medical Center in Omaha. His research has been published in *Annals of Behavioral Medicine, American Journal of Preventive Medicine* and other professional journals. He is an author of "Group-Based Physical Activity for Older Adults Randomized Controlled Trial," recently published in *Health Psychology*.

If you're skeptical that group workouts could offer more than an intense solitary jog on your treadmill, there's a body of research that gives some convincing reasons why going solo may not be the best approach. *Compared with solo exercise, group workouts are linked to...*

• **Less pain.** When adults exercised for 45 minutes on rowing machines, those who had rowed in groups demonstrated a higher pain tolerance versus solitary rowers, according to research published in *International Journal of Sport and Exercise Psychology*. Researchers theorize that physically syncing up with others stimulates a release of feel-good endorphins.

• **Greater motivation to push harder.** A phenomenon called the Köhler effect motivates people to strive harder when working in a group. Research conducted at Kansas State University found that this phenomenon really kicks into high gear when you exercise with people you perceive as stronger than yourself, inspiring exercisers to work out nearly 200% longer and harder than when working out alone.

Caveat: Simply being in a room with other people isn't enough to reap all of these great benefits. The key is finding what researchers call a "true group class."

THE MAGIC OF A TRUE GROUP CLASS

A true group class is one in which the instructor takes steps to promote bonding among participants and a collective goal. For example, your instructor might start class by saying, "Over the next 45 minutes, we are going to collectively walk the equivalent of three laps around the Parthenon."

Important: Typically, group-based fitness classes are more effective than solo workouts only when they use these types of group dynamic strategies. In a meta-analysis published in Sport & Exercise Psychology Review, researchers compared the benefits of home workouts, standard exercise classes and true group classes. Result: True group classes were deemed the most beneficial—mainly because people stick with exercise longer when they are working out in these groups. Solo exercise at home ranked last.

The special ingredient seems to be the bonding that takes place in these classes. Feeling like you belong to a group is a very basic human need...one that research has linked with improved health and longevity—especially as one ages.

WHAT TO LOOK FOR

To find a class with this dynamic...

• **Find an instructor you love.** If you feel inspired and challenged by the instructor, the rest of the class likely feels the same way. This creates a sense of connection among participants and gives everyone something to chat about in the locker room.

• **Exercise with people your age.** A study of 627 adults published in Health Psychology found that being in a class with other people your own age improves the chances that you will stick with your exercise plan—more so than being among classmates of the same gender. Look for a class with members who are within about five years of your own age.

• **Look for a class with competition built in.** Boot camps and boutique fitness classes—such as those offered by Orangetheory Fitness, a nationwide fitness franchise, and Flywheel Sports, which offers cycling studios at 42 locations across the US and an app for on-demand cycling workouts you can do at home (with purchase of the Fly bike)—encourage friendly competition by allowing participants to compare their performance results.

• **Experiment with virtual group classes.** No class available? You can still reap the benefits of a collective workout with a virtual group class, such as those offered by Peloton, which provides cycling workouts you can do while streaming live and on-demand fitness classes with instructors and fellow participants.

Note: While on-demand classes offer the benefit of friendly competition, they do not provide the positive effects associated with bonding.

7

Feel Young Forever

The End of "Old Age"—Change Your View to Live Longer

Marc E. Agronin, MD, a geriatric psychiatrist at Miami Jewish Health in Florida. He is author of *How We Age: A Doctor's Journey into the Heart of Growing Old* and *The End of Old Age: Living a Longer, More Purposeful Life* (MarcAgronin.com). Dr. Agronin recently recorded a series of podcasts for Bottom Line's Conversations with the Experts. Bottomlineinc.com/podcast-playlist/marc-agronin

"Old age" has long gotten a bad rap. The conventional thinking has been that it's a time for rocking chairs, fading memory, illness and decrepitude.

Now: As an increasing number of Americans are living—and thriving—into their 80s and beyond, it's more important than ever to cast aside those outdated and harmful attitudes.

What the new thinking can mean for you: Older adults who see aging as a positive stage of life have fewer cardiovascular problems and actually outlive those with gloomier self-perceptions by more than seven years, according to landmark research conducted at Yale University.

So what are you waiting for? There are simple steps you can take to make sure that you aren't missing out on the richness of aging—and this uniquely positive life stage.

THE GIFTS OF AGE

As a geriatric psychiatrist, I have worked with hundreds of older adults who have developed life skills and perspectives that, in many ways, enable them to live more successfully than younger adults.

Of course, we can't kid ourselves. Old age does bring some challenges. We become more susceptible to disease. Our brains and bodies slow down. Daily life gets harder in many ways. The flip side is that some of the traits that come with age make us more adept at dealing with adversity and finding purpose in our lives.

Don't believe the myth that older adults get stuck in the past and can't handle new challenges. For example, research has shown that many older adults excel at divergent thinking, the ability to generate different solutions to particular problems. A lifetime of experiences helps them sort through complexities and explore novel ideas.

Other significant benefits that come with growing older—and what you can do to cultivate them in your own life...

•**A reserve of wisdom.** You can be smart and capable at any age, but wisdom is something different. It's an amalgam of all the knowledge, skill and attitudes that you've gained over time.

Wisdom is a trait that we often attribute to the world's great thinkers, but it also has a smaller, day-to-day scope.

Example: Mary, a woman in her 90s, had no earth-shattering life experiences. She wasn't known by anyone outside her small circle of family and friends. But within that circle, she had tremendous influence.

She had two Sunday rituals that gave her a sense of purpose—Catholic Mass in the morning and a family dinner in the afternoon. Her son-in-law would take her to church. After that, she would spend hours with her daughter and other family members preparing a multicourse Italian meal. She was the glue that held the family together—the one who shared recipes...passed along family stories...and overflowed with love. These are powerful forms of wisdom.

My advice: People sometimes ask, "How do I achieve wisdom?" The answer: You already have it. Think of wisdom as your life's résumé. It might consist of knowledge from previous careers...military experience...being a good listener...a tolerance for different ideas, etc.

•**Resilience.** Hurricane Katrina, which devastated the Gulf Coast, was one of the deadliest hurricanes in history. Older adults were among the most vulnerable and suffered disproportionately. Thousands lost their homes, support networks and even their lives.

Yet subsequent research found that many of them coped just as well with the chaos as younger adults—and, in many cases, even better. Decades of experience increased their stores of resilience, the ability to manage life's obstacles without feeling helpless.

Examples: They didn't sweat the storm-related loss of cell-phone service or the Internet because they tended to view these things as luxuries, not necessities. Shortages of food and water? People who have lived through tough times know how to be resourceful when things are scarce. They could see beyond the chaos and find glimmers of acceptance and hope.

Resilience has physical benefits, as well. Not getting overwrought about difficulties allows the body to quickly recover from stress-related changes—muscle tension, increased heart rate, elevated stress hormones, etc.

Remarkable finding: A study of hundreds of older victims after the storm found that they often had the emotional and psychological strength to deal with the widespread loss of electricity and other basic services. In a way, it's not surprising—these were the same people who went through the Great Depression and World War II. Unlike younger victims, they already knew how to be resourceful in these types of situations.

My advice: Even resilient adults will eventually hit what I call an "age point," in which their resources and coping skills are temporarily overwhelmed. It's important to get help—from a therapist and/or friends and family members—when you suffer such a potentially serious setback. The ultimate resolution can bring growth and greater resilience.

For example, one of my elderly patients had a blood test that indicated abnormal liver enzymes. She was convinced that she had a terminal disease and would be unable to care for her husband who had Alzheimer's disease. Her emotional state started to rapidly deteriorate.

Along with therapy, I treated her with a short-acting tranquilizer, which allowed her to get out of bed, leave the house and function more normally overall. She eventually recovered and was able to go off the medication—and, in some ways, grew stronger.

After further tests showed that she was fine, she recognized that she'd had a turning point that clarified what she wanted from life. She felt that she had been given a second chance to do what really mattered—to care for her husband, be a guide for her son, be active in the community and form a close network of friends.

•**Reinvention.** Older adults can do some of their best work late in life. After a serious illness, the French painter Henri Matisse turned his attention, in his 70s and 80s, to the paper cutouts that appeared in the influential book *Jazz* and eventually revolutionized the world of art. He brought a lifetime of experience to the new medium, along with a sense of freedom that's often missing in the young.

Gene Cohen, MD, a well-known psychiatrist, describes an encore phase that starts in the late 70s and continues until the end of life. People often take up new activities during this phase. It can be artistic endeavors...more reading...landscape design...or even real estate investing!

Important: You can reinvent yourself even if you're dealing with physical/cognitive issues. In fact, these issues mean that you should reinvent. You can shape your interests to circumvent otherwise detrimental changes.

My advice: Start small. Manage your expectations to match your current reality.

For example, one of my clients, a retired professor, suffered from memory loss that made it difficult to keep up with the high-powered, distinguished people she had always spent a lot of time with. She was deeply depressed.

We decided that she should find new intellectual opportunities that didn't require her to be on stage or to "compete." She started taking art and adult-education classes. Family members helped her get used to a computer and an iPad. She was able to pursue her intellectual interests in new (and more comfortable) ways. The opportunities are endless!

Happy Older People Live Longer

Study by researchers at Duke-NUS Medical School, Singapore, published in *Age and Ageing*.

Among men and women ages 60 and older who said that they felt happy about their lives and the future, 15% died over a six-year period. Among those who did not say that they felt happy, 20% died during the same period.

Aging Myths Debunked

Marc E. Agronin, MD, a geriatric psychiatrist at Miami Jewish Health in Florida. He is author of *How We Age: A Doctor's Journey into the Heart of Growing Old* and *The End of Old Age: Living a Longer, More Purposeful Life* (MarcAgronin.com). Dr. Agronin recently recorded a series of podcasts for Bottom Line's Conversations with the Experts. Bottomlineinc.com/podcast-playlist/marc-agronin

Old age is often portrayed as a time of loneliness, depression and significant cognitive decline. But most research shows that the opposite is true for most people. *Among the common myths about getting older...*

***MYTH #1:* Depression hits.** No one loves the physical changes of age, let alone the likelihood of dealing with age-related illnesses. But the emotional prospects are better than you think. The rates of major depression, for example, actually go down with age. A recent study that tracked participants for about 10 years found that their feelings of well-being increased until they reached their 70s. The feelings plateaued at that point but still didn't fall.

People who develop serious medical problems or experience traumatic life events (such as the death of a spouse) obviously will be more likely to suffer from depression than those who have an easier path. But even in the face of adversity, older people are resilient—they've accumulated enough wisdom to help them through hard times.

***MYTH #2:* You'll be lonely.** One of the inevitabilities of aging is the loss of friends and family members. Older people do spend more time alone. But that's not the same as feeling lonely or isolated.

A number of studies have shown that the quality of relationships improves with age. You may have fewer close friends in your 70s than you did in your 50s, but you'll probably find that the connections have matured and become richer and more fulfilling.

Remember your earlier relationships—how often were they tumultuous and emotionally fraught? Studies have shown that older adults tend to be more positive about their relationships and less likely to experience social tensions.

MYTH #3: **Your mind slips.** Yes, it will, in some ways—but the typical "slips" that most people experience will be offset by improvements in other mental areas.

Take memory and the ability to concentrate. Both start to decline by middle age. You won't be as quick at math, and your verbal skills won't be quite as sharp. You'll retain the ability to learn, but new information will take longer to sink in.

At the same time, you'll notice improvements in other mental abilities. You'll have a lot of accrued knowledge, along with an edge in reasoning and creative thinking. You won't keep up with the youngsters on cognitive tests, but you may perform better in real-world situations.

To keep your mind active, take up painting or other hobbies. Read challenging novels. Learn another language, or learn to play a musical instrument. People who stretch themselves mentally can improve memory and cognitive skills and possibly slow the rate of subsequent declines.

MYTH #4: **No more sex.** In surveys, older adults often report more sexual satisfaction than is reported by their younger counterparts. They might have sex less often, but they tend to enjoy it more.

A national survey of sexual attitudes, published in *The New England Journal of Medicine*, found that, on average, the frequency of sexual activity declines only slightly from the 50s to the 70s.

And the sexual attitudes among seniors are sufficiently frisky to make their grandchildren blush. About 50% of people ages 57 to 75 reported engaging in oral sex. More than half of men and about 25% of women masturbated.

Good health (and an available partner) are among the best predictors of a robust sex life. Sex-specific disorders—such as erectile dysfunction in men and vaginal dryness in women—now can be overcome with a variety of aids and treatments. Even when sexual activity does decline (or disappear), older adults enjoy cuddling and other intimacies.

MYTH #5: **Falls are normal.** Falls are never a normal part of aging...and they're not merely accidents. Anyone who is unsteady on his/her feet has a health problem that needs to be addressed. It could be osteoporosis, reduced muscle strength, impaired vision, disturbed sleep or side effects from medications.

Warning: Falls are the main cause of more than 90% of hip fractures and a leading cause of emergency room visits and deaths.

People who get any kind of exercise—a daily walk, working around the house, digging in the garden—are much less likely to fall or to suffer serious injuries should they have a misstep.

Important: A good night's sleep. We've found that people who don't sleep well tend to have more disorientation and balance problems, particularly if they happen to be taking sleep medications that contain the antihistamine diphenhydramine.

Practice good sleep hygiene—go to bed and get up at the same times each day...avoid sleep distractions (such as watching TV in bed)...don't drink caffeinated beverages late in the day...and drink a soothing cup of warm milk or chamomile tea at bedtime.

Your Mind—The Most Powerful Tool for a Longer and Healthier Life

Ellen J. Langer, PhD, professor of psychology at Harvard University and author of numerous books, including the recently published *Counterclockwise: Mindful Health and the Power of Possibility.* EllenLanger.com

---

Remember the cliché "You're only as old as you feel"? A significant body of scientific evidence shows that it may be more accurate to say, "You're only as old as you think."

THE POWER OF THE MIND

Much of what we call aging is shaped by mental and cultural cues. Our bodies obviously undergo changes, but many of the "typical" characteristics of age, such as achy joints or memory lapses, are often triggered more by self-perception than by physical changes.

Key lessons in using your thoughts to optimize your health...

***Lesson #1:* Change your vocabulary.** Our medical system promotes the use of labels. If you have diabetes, for example, you are a "diabetic." If you are ill, you are a "patient." Such labels encourage us to see ourselves as always being sick.

People who are diagnosed with "chronic" pain are also affected by labeling. Some expect to always be in pain, so they don't notice the times when the pain is absent or less severe. If they did, they might try to figure out why and find a way to control their pain. The chronic pain label can become a detrimental self-fulfilling prophecy, leading those in pain to act as if their lives are only about pain.

Advice: Focus on the healthy parts of your life. Someone with asthma, for example, can enjoy walks when his/her lungs are feeling strong. Someone with arthritis can play nine holes of golf instead of 18, or one hole instead of nine. If you have chronic pain—or any other condition with symptoms that come and go—use the times of day when you are basically pain-free to feel good and do the things that you want.

***Lesson #2:* Remember what's important.** Our world is filled with negative stereotypes about aging. Most of us assume, for example, that older adults are forgetful. (Young people forget things all the time, but this doesn't get noticed.) However, the reason we may not remember certain things is that we didn't care to learn the information in the first place.

Scientific evidence: In a three-week study, one group of nursing-home residents were given incentives to remember information—chips that could be exchanged for prizes whenever they recalled certain information, such as nurses' names and when certain activities were scheduled. Comparison groups were not awarded prizes for this task.

In tests of cognitive ability at the end of the study, the "prize group" outperformed the other groups. And in a follow-up study, the death rate was more than four times higher in the comparison groups than in the prize group.

Advice: Get involved so that you care about things. When something has meaning to you, you are more likely to remember it than to recall information that is not relevant to your daily life.

***Lesson #3:* Live mindfully.** Being mindful simply means noticing new things. It doesn't matter what they are, as long as they are novel. This entails being engaged in life...cultivating a sense of personal responsibility and control...and staying alert to new experiences and information.

Advice: Stay engaged. People who pursue new interests, make their own decisions and live life on their terms are the ones who live best—and, in many cases, longest.

***Lesson #4:* Expect good health.** Nearly everyone can live longer and feel better by being active. Yet about 250,000 deaths annually in the US can be attributed to a sedentary lifestyle. How you think about exercise makes a difference.

Important research: In a study of hotel maids, it was explained to one group that the work they did met the standard recommendations for an "active" lifestyle, while the second group was not given this information.

Result: After four weeks, maids who recognized that their work was good exercise lost an average of two pounds, had a significant reduction in body fat and an average drop in blood pressure of 10 points systolic (top number) and five points diastolic (bottom number). Women in the other group did not get these benefits.

Advice: When striving for a physiological result, engage your mind. People who expect to feel good are more likely to feel good.

Whatever the goal, take the smallest step necessary to get you started. If you've failed to lose 20 pounds, try to lose two pounds...or one pound... or an ounce. You'll feel a greater sense of control once you realize that small changes make a big difference over time.

Feel Younger by Taking Control

Study titled "Feeling Young and in Control: Daily Control Beliefs Are Associated with Younger Subjective Ages" by researchers at North Carolina State University in Raleigh and Friedrich Schiller University in Jena, Germany, published in *The Journals of Gerontology: Series B.*

Feel younger, live longer. It's a simple prescription for longevity and one that is backed up by research. For older people, feeling younger than your chronological age is strongly linked with better memory, better health and improved longevity, studies show.

But what is the secret to feeling younger?

After all, there are many reasons why people feel older than their actual age—including health issues. But now new research has found a powerful factor in how young we feel—and it's one you can do something about. For older adults, the study finds, how young you feel has a lot to do your sense of control.

HOW OLD DO YOU FEEL DAY TO DAY?

Previous research has found that how old we feel (our subjective age), as well as how in control, both fluctuate from day to day as events and encounters with others influence our perceptions and mood. This new study was designed to investigate how those fluctuations might be linked in both older and younger adults.

Researchers at North Carolina State University in Raleigh and at Friedrich Schiller University in Jena, Germany, recruited 116 men and women ages 60 to 90 and another 106 men and women ages 18 to 36. In the older group, 55% were still working and 45% were retired.

In daily surveys over nine days, participants were asked eight questions that tapped into their sense of control—to what extent they felt they could influence the events in their lives—and were also asked how old they felt that day. In addition, both groups submitted information about daily stressors they encountered such as disagreements or potential disagreements as well as stressful events at work, home or among friends. They also logged daily physical symptoms they experienced from a checklist of 28 (such as allergies, fatigue, joint pain, cough).

WHAT MATTERS OVER AGE 60

For both the younger and older groups, subjective age varied day to day. But among the older participants, these variations were keenly tied to their sense of control.

Key finding: On the days when they felt more in control, they tended to feel younger. (For the younger participants, the number of stressors and physical symptoms made a difference, but their sense of control didn't.)

Given the challenges of growing older, it's easy to feel out of control some days. But the more you feel in control on a daily basis, the less likely you are to overreact to stress. In addition to physical health benefits of reduced stress, your cognitive abilities—how well your brain performs—benefit, too.

The findings have implications for elderly caregiving, the researchers note. In nursing homes, for example, letting residents have more choices in their daily lives—choices as simple as how the furniture is arranged, how they spend time with friends, even who takes care of the houseplants—have been shown to improve well-being.

For the rest of us who are in our 50s, 60s and older, there's no one-size-fits-all solution to feeling more in control. Setting priorities, finding time to disconnect from devices and spending time with friends are common advice. But one activity may be particularly effective—exercise.

Everyone knows that exercise is key to lifelong health. But one of the ways that it benefits us is by giving us a sense that we have a little more control over how the day goes. A regular exercise habit—something as simple as a daily walk—has been shown to improve mood, reduce anxiety, boost self-esteem...and increase a sense of control. In a separate pilot study from the group at the University of North Carolina, previously sedentary men and women aged 35 to 69 who started exercising regularly reported that they felt—you guessed it—younger.

Age Gracefully, Not Grumpily

Judy Kuriansky, PhD, clinical psychologist, sex therapist and adjunct faculty, Columbia University Teachers College, New York City. She is the author of five books, including *The Complete Idiot's Guide to a Healthy Relationship*. DrJudy.com

In our youth-obsessed culture, it can be tough to face the fact of getting older. Many men and women find themselves bemoaning their deepening wrinkles and rounder bellies...resenting those who still have the vigor of the young...and falling deeper into depression or dread with each passing birthday.

What a waste of years! Aging doesn't have to be awful. No matter how much you don't like getting older, there are ways to make an attitude adjustment...let go of resentment...age with grace and good humor...and find joy, peace and well-being in the process. *Suggestions...*

• **Give some thought to time-honored words of wisdom about aging.** Some sayings passed down through generations may sound trite on the surface but actually provide valuable insights. If you are willing to open your mind and reconsider them, they will help you.

What to do: Take at least two minutes each day to ponder the truths behind common adages about aging and really take them to heart. For instance, with the phrase, "You're not getting older, you're getting better," you may recognize that a certain kind of wisdom or life-enhancing enlightenment comes only with years of experience. If you have a longtime partner, you can think about poet Robert Browning's lines, "Grow old along with me! The best is yet to be," letting them inspire you to better appreciate how decades of shared history make possible a uniquely close and loving future. For a smile, consider one of my favorite quotations from Mark Twain—"Age is an issue of mind over matter. If you don't mind, it doesn't matter." Need more inspiration? Check out quotations about aging on websites such as BrainyQuote, Bartleby and Quotations Page.

Caution: Resist the urge to repeat negative phrases, either aloud or to yourself. Saying, "I'm having another senior moment" (even if you think it's funny), or, "This old body is a wreck," imprints negativity in your own mind and in the minds of others about your capabilities.

• **Focus on your accomplishments, not on your regrets.** When you're feeling blue about getting older, take a moment to say, "After 40 years of experience as a [parent/accountant/artist or whatever], I can say with confidence that—" and then fill in the blank with some highlights from your life to remind yourself that you have the right to feel proud. What if no proud declaration comes to mind? You don't have to set the world on fire to feel justifiably good about your accomplishments. For example, as a parent, you might finish the phrase with, "I did a good job raising kids who turned out to be good people." As an accountant, you might say, "I've helped a lot of people get their finances in order despite very tough times."

If you do have regrets about lost opportunities, make a list of things you never had time for before (touring Italy, say, or playing a musical instrument well) and formulate concrete plans to do those things now. If you assume that you can never again achieve something wonderful, you are selling yourself short.

Here's just one example of a "late bloomer" who was recently in the news. The legendary blues guitarist/singer T-Model Ford, who died recently in his 90s, had no musical experience until he learned to play the guitar in his late 50s and didn't release a record until he was in his 70s—yet he toured as a successful musician into his ninth decade. Think about all the vibrant years he might have missed if he had said, "I'm too old to start something new."

Even if a certain door truly has closed, you can find related ways to satisfy at least part of that ambition. For instance, you do have to accept that you'll never compete in the Olympics, but it's never too late to support a current Olympic hopeful or get involved with the National Senior Games Association.

• **Be inspired by role models.** Actress/comedienne Betty White and singer Tony Bennett both enjoyed renewed popularity and career success well into their 90s.

What you can do: Make a list of your favorite 70-plus public figures...consider what it is about their attitudes and actions that you find so admirable or interesting...and then seek to emulate those qualities.

A role model who will help you be a happier older person needn't be a celebrity at all. You can admire and be inspired by the way an octogenarian neighbor still cuts his own grass with a hand mower...or by the fact that your older sister still dresses in her finest and goes out to late-night cabarets rather than crawling into bed by 9:00 pm.

• **Spend time with younger people.** Instead of wasting psychic energy envying the young, make young people an active part your life. Their vitality may rub off on you...and you'll have the satisfaction of sharing your knowledge with them. You might mentor young students in your field of expertise, teaching them what you know while keeping your own mind sharp as you learn from them about new advances in the industry you love. If today's technology befuddles you, take a class (which will probably be taught by a younger person) on how to use an iPad, the latest apps, Instagram, Pinterest and Twitter. The more you involve yourself with the younger generations, the less resentful you're likely to feel.

• **Smile.** Frowning furrows your brow and imprints your face with an unpleasant expression that can add years to your appearance—and it makes you feel bad. In contrast, a smile—while it may add crinkle lines—also brightens your eyes, plumps your cheeks, makes your whole face shine and makes you feel better. Dr. Kuriansky said, "When you smile, you actually become more beautiful because people stop noticing your age lines and instead focus on your inner glow...which makes you and everyone around you feel more joyful."

What You Talk About Affects Your Happiness

Matthias R. Mehl, PhD, assistant professor of psychology, University of Arizona, Tucson, and **Simine Vazire, PhD,** assistant professor of psychology, Washington University, St. Louis. They are coauthors of a study published in *Psychological Science*.

The happiest people (in a recent study) had twice as many substantive conversations or discussions about meaningful information (such as philosophy and current affairs) and one-third as much small talk (discussions about trivial information, such as the weather) as the unhappiest people. Also, happy people spend less time alone and more time talking to others than unhappy people.

The Dementia Gene—Here's How to Beat It

Study titled "Positive Age Beliefs Protect Against Dementia Even Among Elders with High-risk Gene," by researchers at Yale University and the National Institute on Aging, published in *PLOS One*.

You might already know that your attitude about aging has a powerful effect on your health. *Example:* People with a positive view of aging are less likely to develop heart disease—and more likely to live longer—than people with a gloomier outlook. They also perform better on cognitive tests.

But what if your DNA, the essence of what makes you who you are, makes you particularly susceptible to dementia? What if, because of your DNA, your chance of developing dementia is nearly one in two? Can attitudes be so powerful that they can protect you from your own genetic predisposition? That's what researchers at Yale University and the National Institute on Aging (NIA) set out to discover.

THE DEMENTIA GENE

One of the strongest risk factors for dementia (including Alzheimer's, one form) is having the APOE e4 gene variant. One-quarter of people have this variant, and nearly half (47%) of those people will develop dementia.

No one knows why the other 53% of people with the APOE e4 variant remain unaffected. The Yale-NIA researchers decided to explore whether having positive beliefs about aging, which we tend to absorb from the culture around us from an early age, might help explain why some people with the APOE e4 variant don't wind up with dementia.

They also explored how attitudes affect the rest of us who don't carry such a risky gene.

They selected 4,765 men and women, average age 72, all free of dementia, who had already participated in the Health and Retirement Study, a biennial survey of nationally representative older Americans, and followed them for four years. The participants provided saliva samples at the outset to determine whether or not they had the APOE e4 variant, and just as expected, about one-quarter (26%) were found to have it.

To learn the participants' attitudes, they were given validated psychological tests. (Sample test statement, which they were asked to rate on a sliding scale: "The older I get, the more useless I feel.") After two years, and again at the end of the study, they were given cognitive tests, which included measures of both short-term and delayed recall as well as math skills, to see whether they had developed dementia. In addition, the researchers weighed the possible effects of other factors that have been associated with dementia including age, education, gender, race and incidence of cardiovascular disease or diabetes.

Results: While studies like this can't show cause and effect, positive attitudes about aging were strongly associated with less risk of developing dementia...

Among participants without the "dementia gene," 2.6% of those with positive attitudes developed dementia—compared with 4.6% of those with negative attitudes.

Among participants with the gene variant, 2.7% of those with positive attitudes about aging developed dementia—but 6.2% of those with negative attitudes developed dementia.

In short, people with a very high genetic dementia risk were able to have an almost-normal level of risk during the study period if they had positive attitudes about aging. A negative attitude was particularly risky for those people already at high genetic risk.

How can a positive outlook be so powerful? The researchers suggest it might affect the same pathway that leads to the increased genetic risk from APOE e4. This is referred to as an epigenetic effect—a nongenetic influence that nevertheless affects genes. In other words, these participants were able to halt the expression of their dementia gene.

NEGATIVE ATTITUDES, STRESS AND DEMENTIA

What could cause gene expression to change? In a word, stress. Other studies have found that chronic stress may contribute to the development of dementia. And holding negative attitudes about aging—that it makes you feeble, incompetent, over-the-hill, useless—has been found to ratchet up stress. On the other hand, having positive views—such as that aging makes you wiser, kinder, more skillful and empathetic—has been shown to help buffer the harmful effects of stress.

If you're concerned that your own views on aging could use a makeover, rest assured that you can transform negative into positive beliefs. Here are four tips adapted from the "Reframing Aging" initiative, a consortium of nonprofit organizations dedicated to helping individuals and society change attitudes toward aging:

- **Choose to focus on what's positive in your life.** Whenever you find yourself zeroing in on what's going wrong—that pain in your knee, your accumulating wrinkles—catch yourself and refocus on what's going right.

Examples: Your grandkids think you're funny... you own your home free and clear...your garden produced beautiful tomatoes this year.

- **Embrace new images.** Instead of dwelling on those scary/depressing ads for AFib drugs or TV shows that mock older people to a laugh track, choose to watch shows like *Grace and Frankie* and movies like *Book Club* or *The Old Man and the Gun* that celebrate the lives and creativity of older people.
- **Post positive words.** Make a list of words that say "aging well" to you and write "I am fill-in-the-blank" on sticky notes that you post where you can see them. Suggestions: "wise," "strong," "fit," "resourceful," "creative."
- **Remind yourself of people who break the age "mold."** There are plenty of pioneering older people, including Jane Goodall (84) and Carl Reiner (96)...and probably someone you know personally.
- **Speak up and engage with others.** Our culture has stereotypical views of aging that need to be changed. You'll feel more positive and empowered if

you encourage others to be more respectful of older people and to include them as peers rather than to talk down to them or ignore them.

Don't Make Aging a Disease!

John La Puma, MD, a board-certified specialist in internal medicine. Dr. La Puma and Michael Roizen, MD, are the first physicians to teach cooking and nutrition in a US medical school. A trained chef with a private nutritional medical practice in Santa Barbara, California, Dr. La Puma is a cofounder of the popular ChefMD video series and author of *Refuel: A 24-Day Eating Plan to Shed Fat, Boost Testosterone, and Pump Up Strength and Stamina*. DrJohnLaPuma.com

Male aging is now a disease—at least that's what the pharmaceutical companies are telling us. They're trying to convince men that the natural consequences of aging—such as tiring faster than you used to and reduced sex drive—are signs of a medical problem, namely low testosterone levels. Not surprisingly, the pharmaceutical companies also claim to have the solution—prescription testosterone. Such prescriptions have tripled since 2001 and now earn the pharmaceutical industry billions of dollars of revenue each year.

But "low T," as the condition is called, isn't nearly as common as the drug ads would have you believe. There are many potential causes of fatigue, and erectile dysfunction is nearly always a blood flow issue that testosterone won't cure, warns internist John La Puma, MD, author of *Refuel: A 24-Day Eating Plan to Shed Fat, Boost Testosterone, and Pump Up Strength and Stamina*.

Worse, several studies have suggested that taking prescription testosterone increases a man's risk for heart attack, especially for men age 65 and older.

Fortunately, there are safer ways for men to combat age-related testosterone loss. One is to lose weight. A 2012 study found that obese men can increase their testosterone levels by 15% by shedding just 17 pounds. Also, ask your doctor to check your vitamin D level. If it is below 50 nanograms per milliliter (ng/mL), your testosterone levels likely would benefit from taking up to 2,000 international units of vitamin D-3 per day.

How Estrogen Helps Men Stay Manly

Study titled "Gonadal Steroids and Body Composition, Strength, and Sexual Function in Men," published in *The New England Journal of Medicine*.

You probably consider testosterone the "male hormone" and estrogen the "female hormone," and for good reason. Men's bodies do make and use more testosterone, while women's bodies make and use more estrogen.

But it's not quite that simple. Both genders need both hormones to varying degrees. And now new research shows that estrogen plays a very important role in keeping men fit and virile!

TESTING TESTOSTERONE

When a male patient complains of low energy, loss of strength and a diminished sex drive, his doctor may have him tested for a condition called male hypogonadism, in which the body doesn't produce enough testosterone. If results show that the man's testosterone level is below a certain threshold, he'll likely be given a prescription for testosterone—which, it's hoped, will bring back his manly vigor.

Even though millions of men now are on testosterone therapy for just this reason, not a lot is known about the effects of different doses. So researchers at Massachusetts General Hospital in Boston designed a study to evaluate the effects of varying doses. And since men with low testosterone also tend to have low estradiol, a form of estrogen that in men is a by-product of testosterone, they also measured what happened when estradiol production was blocked.

The study included 400 healthy men between the ages of 20 and 50. All took a medication to suppress their natural production of testosterone. The men were divided into groups and received a daily dose of topical testosterone gel—1.25 grams (g), 2.5 g, 5.0 g or 10 g—or a placebo gel. Additionally, some men also were given a drug to prevent testosterone from being turned into estradiol, allowing the researchers to separately compare their effects.

The participants came in every four weeks for blood tests and an evaluation of their health status, including physical function and sexual function (as assessed by patients' own reports on sexual desire and erectile function). At the beginning and end of the 16-week study, the researchers measured each man's overall body fat, abdominal fat, lean muscle mass and strength.

THE BIG SURPRISE

As expected, the men who had been given the placebo gel—meaning nothing to replace their greatly diminished testosterone levels—gained fat, lost strength and muscle mass, and reported problems with libido and erections.

In the men who received varying levels of testosterone and whose production of estradiol was not blocked, results varied widely depending on the testosterone dosage...

- **Overall body fat increased in men** receiving anything less than 5.0 grams of testosterone.
- **Abdominal fat didn't change** in men receiving any dose of testosterone.
- **Lean muscle mass decreased** in men who received less than 2.5 grams of testosterone.
- **Strength did not change** in men receiving any dose of testosterone.
- **Sexual function decreased in all the men**—and the smaller the testosterone dosage, the worse the sex problems were.

Then came the group of men who had received varying doses of testosterone but whose production of estradiol had been blocked. Though lean muscle mass and strength were not affected by estradiol, there were some big surprises in other areas...

- **All of the men with blocked estradiol** had significant increases in body fat.
- **All of the men had increases in abdominal fat**—and the higher their testosterone dosage was, the more this fat increased.
- **Sexual desire and erectile function decreased** significantly in all the men.

That these changes happened across the board suggested that it wasn't only the lack of testosterone that caused problems—but also the lack of estradiol.

What this means for patients: Going forward, in treating men who are found to have low testosterone, doctors may closely monitor their patients' estrogen levels as well and prescribe medications to keep estrogen within the normal range.

In the meantime: If you are being treated for low testosterone, it would be wise to talk with your doctor about how low estradiol could be contributing to your increased body fat and sexual problems... and to review your testosterone dosage, given that in this study the amount of testosterone required to maintain muscle mass, strength and sexual function varied widely.

Women: To Control Hot Flashes, Keep This Diary

JoAnn E. Manson, MD, MPH, DrPH, chief, division of preventive medicine, interim executive director, Connors Center for Women's Health and Gender Biology, Brigham and Women's Hospital and professor of medicine and Michael and Lee Bell Professor of Women's Health, Harvard Medical School, Boston. She is the author of *Hot Flashes, Hormones & Your Health*.

If you're experiencing hot flashes, the hallmark symptom of menopause, you're eager—OK, maybe desperate—to find ways to make them stop. Maybe you're wondering if you should consider supplements, a change in diet, breathing exercises, hypnosis or even hormone therapy.

But there is an effective approach you may have overlooked entirely.

You.

Understanding your own response to factors in your daily life that can bring hot flashes is the first step to minimizing them. It's also a good way to figure out whether anything you're doing is helping. All you have to do is live your life the way you already are—and jot down certain things that happen to you. Below are the exact steps to take—and we've even created a downloadable tracker to get you started.

HOT FLASH TRIGGERS ARE PERSONAL... SO GET TO KNOW YOURS

Hot flashes seemingly come out of the blue, often at inopportune times—in a meeting at work, at a family event, in the middle of the night (waking you up). In reality, though, many hot flashes occur in response to a trigger.

Drinking a hot beverage or sleeping in a warm room are common triggers, but there are many others, according to JoAnn Manson, MD, an endocrinologist at Brigham and Women's Hospital and professor of medicine and women's health at Harvard Medical School. Other commonly reported triggers include spicy food, smoking, hot weather, alcohol, caffeine, exercising vigorously, becoming dehydrated and even using a hair dryer or curling iron.

But here's the rub: Not every woman is affected by any particular trigger...and your set of triggers could be unique to you.

One woman may have hot flashes after drinking wine—while another is fine with wine but coffee sets her off. A nice warm bath? That's an invitation to an internal furnace for one woman, while for another it's a relaxing, soothing—even cooling—ritual.

Although there is little rigorous research on the role of "triggers," many are common sense and women are able to identify them quickly, explains Dr. Manson. If you can identify the foods, actions and scenarios that set off hot flashes for you, you can learn to avoid them. Presto—fewer flashes.

THE TRACKING EDGE

The best way to identify your triggers? Keep a hot flash diary. In addition to helping you notice physical triggers such as eating hot soup or sitting in an overheated room—which make immediate sense when you think about it—tracking can help uncover the less obvious triggers that you might not have imagined are setting you off, including other foods, activities and the powerful effect of emotional stress. Women can feel a hot flash coming on when they hear upsetting news or sometimes when they are preparing to speak in front of a group of people. Indeed, anything that stresses you, even the most mundane hassles, could be a trigger. And, once again, women don't all react to different stresses the same way—so learning how to deal with your stress triggers can be a "cool" thing.

Tracking your hot flashes is also a great way to monitor the effects of any actions that you take to minimize symptoms—to see if what you're trying is working. Maybe you'll try nutritional approaches such as soy and flax seeds or mind-body methods such as hypnosis, paced breathing or cognitive behavioral therapy. By tracking your flashes before you start and for a few weeks afterward, you'll know whether any new approach is helping.

Got an appointment with your health-care provider? Bring in your diary to inspire constructive discussion about what may help you, and continue using it if you start on a new medical treatment such as an antidepressant or hormone therapy.

How long should you track? It depends on how frequent your hot flashes are. If you get one or more every day, tracking for just a week or so should give you a good idea. If flashes come only a few times a week or even less, you may need to track for a month.

Women should feel empowered to play a role in managing their menopause symptoms, emphasizes Dr. Manson. She does offer a reality check, however. While many flashes occur because of triggers, others are simply physiological responses to fluctuating estrogen levels. So don't expect zero flashes. But if you're bothered by hot flashes, finding a safe and easy way to have fewer is always a good idea.

Love Your Looks...No Matter What Your Age

Pamela D. Blair, PhD, holistic therapist in private practice, life coach and motivational speaker in Shelburne, Vermont. She coordinated the Institute for Spiritual Development at Wainwright House, a learning center in Rye, New York.

Do you catch your reflection in a mirror and feel shock when you see an "old woman" gazing back, because inside you still feel so young?

Coping with our changing appearance requires looking inward. Coming to rely on who we are rather than what we look like yields profound confidence, strength and self-assurance that often elude younger people. Paradoxically, that self-knowledge creates a magnetism that also is deeply attractive. *To nourish healthy self-acceptance...*

• **Savor each day.** Perhaps more than any other quality, being able to take pleasure in life makes a woman beautiful.

• **Pay attention to your senses.** Really taste the food you eat. Feel the fresh air on your skin as you walk outdoors. Relish the touch of a loved one. Some attractive qualities we tend to associate with youth—eagerness, curiosity, openness—can become stronger with age if we take time to appreciate the world around us.

• **Reexamine your goals.** Does your life now reflect your true values? Or are you investing time in relationships that are no longer fulfilling...activities that are no longer interesting...surroundings that no longer meet your needs?

Each morning, try this affirmation exercise. Say, "I am a woman who..." 10 times, and finish the sentence with a different ending each time, specifying goals you are striving for.

Examples: "I am a woman who is free of back pain...likes a gentle, relaxed pace to her life...has all the financial rewards she wants and needs... takes pleasure in her work."

After several weeks, notice what has shifted in your life. Even if these dreams have not yet come true for you, the power of positive thought can help bring about profound changes in the choices you make and in the way you live.

Example: If I am a woman who is free of back pain, I will choose not to lift that heavy box, and I will ask for help instead. I will choose not to skip yoga class. I will take actions that support who I want to be.

• **Reclaim beauty.** We all know that the media promotes an impossible standard of beauty. A recent study at the University of Missouri-Columbia found that women felt worse about their bodies after viewing photos of models in ads.

We do not need to accept the media's definition of beauty. I've stopped reading magazines that show only young, implausibly perfect models in their articles and ads. These pictures are not real. My former husband was an art director for a major fashion magazine, so I often saw the "before" photos of models with wrinkles, crooked noses and large hips—all of which were airbrushed away.

I am learning to be proud of my wrinkles. They represent laughter, conversation, concern for others and the hard work to become a good writer, mother, therapist, gardener. They are symbols of a beautiful life.

Find role models who exemplify a more enlightened beauty. My idol is the actress Tyne Daly—a little overweight, gray-haired, strong-willed, absolutely beautiful and unapologetically not "young." Many European actresses, such as Helen Mirren and Judi Dench, proudly look their age and remain elegant and desirable. I enjoy watching their films and reading about their personal and professional successes. If they can pursue their dreams and not be ashamed of their aging faces, then so can I.

• **Revisit your beauty rituals.** Valuing inner beauty doesn't mean ignoring your appearance. Decide which maintenance routines are worth keeping and which ones you can let go. By fighting the aging process a little less, you gain time and energy that you can put into other fulfilling pursuits. You also will become more relaxed, which is an attractive quality.

Example: I get manicures and pedicures because they make me feel pampered and cared for. They are a source of energy for me, rather than an energy drain. On the other hand, this past year I chose to stop dying my hair. I have gained many hours, and my skin looks better, too—the natural gray provides a softer contrast than the dyed color did. My choice wouldn't work for everyone. Someone who loves dying her hair should keep doing it.

Also experiment with new styles and products that acknowledge your changing body.

Helpful: Make an appointment with an image consultant to find out which clothing styles and colors complement your skin, hair and body shape now. Find a consultant through the Association of

Image Consultants International (651-290-7468, AICI.org).

Cost: $75 to $350 per hour, depending on your location and the extent of services provided.

Alternative: Get a free makeover at a department store cosmetics counter.

Example: I learned to switch to a lighter-consistency foundation and to stop using powder, which can emphasize imperfections in skin. My image consultant also suggested V-necklines to draw attention away from my filled-out chin...and pants that drop gently from my wider hips. I look and feel more elegant.

• **Pace yourself to allow for physical changes.** Your strength may be slightly less, your reaction time a bit longer. I have been doing Pilates exercises, which have increased my muscle strength, bone density and energy as well as decreased my arthritis pain.

• **Increase your serenity by taking a meditative approach.** Before you start your day, sit quietly and visualize what you need to accomplish that day. Pick no more than three major tasks, and go about them with full attention.

Once you've completed those tasks, you can add one or two more. Notice how much calmer and more graceful you feel than when you race around trying to cross 20 items off your to-do list yet give them all short shrift. Enjoy the alertness that comes from being fully present with one task at a time. Your increasing serenity will radiate outward, assuredly making you feel and look more beautiful.

Depression Treatment Boosts Longevity

Joseph J. Gallo, MD, MPH, associate professor of family medicine and community health, University of Pennsylvania, Philadelphia.

In a study of 1,226 people, those with clinical depression whose treatment involved a depression care manager (a nurse, social worker or psychologist who oversees psychotherapy and/or antidepressant use) were 45% less likely to die over a five-year period than those who received primary-care treatment without this additional resource.

If you've been diagnosed with clinical depression: Ask your doctor about all your treatment options.

Worrying Helps You Live Longer

Howard S. Friedman, PhD, distinguished professor of psychology at University of California, Riverside, and lead researcher of the most extensive study on longevity ever conducted. He is author, with Leslie R. Martin, PhD, of *The Longevity Project: Surprising Discoveries for Health and Long Life from the Landmark Eight-Decade Study*. HowardSFriedman.com/longevityproject

Much of the common advice about living a long life—chill out and don't work too much—is wrong. These surprising findings emerged from a groundbreaking eight-decade study that followed 1,528 Americans from early childhood until their deaths. The study, which began in 1921, gathered information from interviews conducted every five to 10 years. It looked at nearly 10 million pieces of data, including work habits, exercise routines, social relations and personality traits.

The study revealed that people who plan and worry tend to stay healthier and live longer than those who don't—and that hard work and the accompanying stress actually are good for you.

Here's what really does extend life...

CONSCIENTIOUSNESS

People who are detail-oriented, responsible and organized live longer than those who aren't. By about the year 2000, 70% of the men and 51% of the women in the study had died. The majority of deaths occurred among those with low conscientiousness scores.

Conscientious people are more prudent in their personal habits. They're less likely to smoke or consume excessive amounts of alcohol. They have healthier, more stable relationships and better work lives.

Scientists speculate that conscientious people have higher levels of serotonin and/or other neurotransmitters that curb impulsive, risk-taking behavior—and so they have a biological tendency toward being prudent and staying healthy.

The good news is that you can become more conscientious. A number of the study participants originally tested in the bottom 25% for conscientiousness. A decade or more later, as they became less impulsive, more mature and more motivated, they scored in the upper 25% and lived long, healthy lives.

WORRY IS GOOD

It's a myth that people who are really cheerful tend to be healthier and live longer than those who view the world through a darker lens. In the study, children who were described by their parents as being unusually cheerful and worry-free tended to die sooner than their less optimistic counterparts.

Those with an excess of optimism may feel so invincible that they don't take reasonable precautions. They might ignore medical advice, for example.

Better: A personality trait known as "realistic optimism." People with this trait are optimistic at the right times...and they worry when they should.

Example: Someone with troublesome health symptoms doesn't just ignore them but makes an appointment to see his/her doctor.

A separate study of Medicare patients found that those who were somewhat neurotic—and worried too much at times—tended to be healthier than those who worried less.

BUT DON'T BE A CHICKEN LITTLE

Too much optimism isn't good, but neither is too much pessimism. People who think that the sky is falling tend to die sooner than those who are more optimistic. They're especially more likely to die from accidents and violence (including suicide), as well as from diseases such as cancer.

You don't have to suffer from persistent negative thinking. The first step is to understand that thoughts, including negative thoughts, are only thoughts—and thoughts can be changed.

Cognitive therapy teaches patients how to recognize negative, harmful thoughts and then replace them with more sensible ones.

Example: Someone who tells himself that all my friends hate me can learn to recognize how distorted that is. He will be taught to replace the negative thought with one that is more realistic, such as I had dinner with John last night, and we had a wonderful time, even though we disagree about politics.

STAY BUSY

Starting in the 1980s, we followed study participants who were by then over the age of 70. Over the next 20 years, those who stayed productive in some fashion lived much longer than those who took it easy.

That's partly because people who are busy and productive tend to have healthier habits. They have things to look forward to and to get them out of their chairs. They also tend to have stable relationships—good partners and/or friends.

Older people often are told to "take it easy" and "avoid stress." Our study shows that this is rotten advice. Productivity and pressure are signs of healthy engagement. Productive people strive to achieve goals and then set new goals when the old ones are reached.

MORE FRIENDS

It's true that steadily married men tend to live longer than single or remarried men, and much longer than divorced men. However, women who are divorced or those who never married live just about as long as women who were steadily married. The difference is due to relationships—women usually find it easier than men to have fulfilling social relationships outside of marriage.

The best social networks are those that involve helping others. Being loved makes people happy, but it doesn't prolong their lives. Those who help others are the ones who live longest.

A Little Bit of Exercise Helps Depression a Lot

Samuel Harvey, PhD, associate professor, School of Psychiatry, University of New South Wales, Sydney, Australia, and leader of an analysis of a Norwegian survey of nearly 34,000 adults, published in *American Journal of Psychiatry*.

Just one hour of exercise weekly can reduce depression risk. People who do one hour a week of any type of exercise, at any intensity level, have a 44% lower risk of developing depression over a decade than people who do not exercise at all. More exercise or more intense exercise is not better from a mental-health standpoint. Any type of physical activity, including simple walking, had the same benefit.

Don't Let Stress Harm Your Health

Irene Louise Dejak, MD, an internal medicine specialist who focuses on preventive health, including counseling patients on the dangers of chronic stress. She is a clinical assistant professor at the Cleveland Clinic Lerner College of Medicine of Case Western Reserve University in Cleveland and an associate staff member at the Cleveland Clinic Family Health Center in Strongsville, Ohio.

It's widely known that acute stress can damage the heart. For example, the risk for sudden cardiac death is, on average, twice as high on Mondays as on other days of the week, presumably because of stress many people feel about going back to work after the weekend. People also experience more heart attacks in the morning because of increased levels of cortisol and other stress hormones.

Important research: In a study of almost 1,000 adult men, those who had three or more major stressful life events in a single year, such as the death of a spouse, had a 50% higher risk of dying over a 30-year period.

But even low-level, ongoing stress, such as that from a demanding job, marriage or other family conflicts, financial worries or chronic health problems, can increase inflammation in the arteries. This damages the inner lining of the blood vessels, promotes the accumulation of cholesterol and increases risk for clots, the cause of most heart attacks.

Among the recently discovered physical effects of stress...

- **Increased blood sugar.** The body releases blood sugar (glucose) during physical and emotional stress. It's a survival mechanism that, in the past, gave people a jolt of energy when they faced a life-threatening emergency.

However, the same response is dangerous when stress occurs daily. It subjects the body to constantly elevated glucose, which damages blood vessels and increases the risk for insulin resistance (a condition that precedes diabetes) as well as heart disease.

What helps: Get regular exercise, which decreases levels of stress hormones.

- **More pain.** Studies have shown that people who are stressed tend to be more sensitive to pain, regardless of its cause. In fact, imaging studies show what's known as stress-induced hyperalgesia, an increase in activity in areas of the brain associated with pain. Similarly, patients with depression seem to experience more pain—and pain that's more intense—than those who are mentally healthy.

What helps: To help curb physical pain, find a distraction. One study found that postsurgical patients who had rooms with views of trees needed less pain medication than those who had no views. On a practical level, you can listen to music. Read a lighthearted book. Paint. Knit. These steps will also help relieve any stress that may be exacerbating your pain.

Also helpful: If you have a lot of pain that isn't well-controlled with medication, ask your doctor if you might be suffering from anxiety or depression. If so, you may benefit from taking an antidepressant, such as *duloxetine* (Cymbalta) or *venlafaxine* (Effexor), which can help reduce pain along with depression.

- **Impaired memory.** After just a few weeks of stress, nerves in the part of the brain associated with memory shrink and lose connections with other nerve cells, according to laboratory studies.

Result: You might find that you're forgetting names or where you put things. These lapses are often due to distraction—people who are stressed and always busy find it difficult to store new information in the brain. This type of memory loss is rarely a sign of dementia unless it's getting progressively worse.

What helps: Use memory tools to make your life easier. When you meet someone, say that person's name out loud to embed it in your memory. Put your keys in the same place every day.

Also: Make a conscious effort to pay attention. It's the only way to ensure that new information is stored. Sometimes the guidance of a counselor is necessary to help you learn how to manage stress. Self-help materials, such as tapes and books, may also be good tools.

- **Weight gain.** The fast-paced American lifestyle may be part of the reason why two-thirds of adults in this country are overweight or obese. People who are stressed tend to eat more—and the "comfort" foods they choose often promote weight gain. Some people eat less during stressful times, but they're in the minority.

What helps: If you tend to snack or eat larger servings when you're anxious, stressed or depressed, talk to a therapist. People who binge on "stress calories" usually have done so for decades—it's difficult to stop without professional help.

Also helpful: Pay attention when you find yourself reaching for a high-calorie snack even though you're not really hungry.

Healthy zero-calorie snack: Ice chips.

Low-calorie options: Grapes, carrots and celery sticks. Once you start noticing the pattern, you can make a conscious effort to replace eating with nonfood activities—working on a hobby, taking a quick walk, etc.

STRESS-FIGHTING PLAN

There are a number of ways to determine whether you are chronically stressed—you may feel short-tempered, anxious most of the time, have heart palpitations or suffer from insomnia.

In general, it helps to...

- **Get organized.** Much of the stress that we experience comes from feeling overwhelmed. You can overcome this by organizing your life.

Examples: Use a day calendar to keep your activities and responsibilities on-track, and put reminder notes on the refrigerator.

- **Ask for help.** You don't have to become overwhelmed. If you're struggling at work, ask a mentor for advice. Tell your partner/spouse that you need help with the shopping or housework.

Taking charge of your life is among the best ways to reduce stress—and asking for help is one of the smartest ways to do this.

- **Write about your worries.** The anxieties and stresses floating around in our heads often dissipate, or at least seem more manageable, once we write them down.
- **Sleep for eight hours.** No one who is sleep-deprived can cope with stress effectively.

Hidden Harms of Long-Ago Trauma: It's Never Too Late to Get Help

Vincent J. Felitti, MD, clinical professor of medicine at University of California, San Diego, and an expert on how childhood trauma affects adults. Dr. Felitti is coprincipal investigator of the Adverse Childhood Experiences (ACE) Study, one of the largest investigations of childhood abuse and neglect and later-life health and well-being.

If you've ever suffered physical, sexual or emotional abuse, you might think that psychological scars are the only long-lasting damage. But that couldn't be further from the truth.

A lingering threat: Volumes of scientific evidence show that these negative experiences also increase risk for chronic disease and early death...even when the incidents occurred several years earlier.

THE SHOCKING STATISTICS

The veil of secrecy regarding abuse has slowly lifted as more people have recently opened up about their past. With sexual abuse, in particular, recent allegations lodged against film producer Harvey Weinstein, actor and comedian Bill Cosby and others have prompted a renewed interest in the harmful effects of such experiences—whether the victim is a child or an adult.

Even though sexual abuse in adulthood has been linked to physical health problems, such as headaches, digestive disorders and other chronic ailments, the most extensive research has focused on the long-term effects when mistreatment occurs during childhood.

Landmark investigation: The Adverse Childhood Experiences (ACE) Study, a massive collaborative research project cosponsored by the Centers for Disease Control and Prevention, looked at the backgrounds of 17,000 adults, beginning in 1995 at Kaiser Permanente in San Diego. With more than 20 years of follow-up, the study offers crucial insights into the physical effects of abuse and mistreatment.

In the original research, two-thirds of the study's middle-class participants reported at least one incident of childhood trauma or neglect. More specifically, 28% reported physical abuse...and 21% said they were abused sexually. More than one in five people reported three or more categories of adverse childhood experiences, or ACEs. (To determine your own ACE score, see the next page.)

THE HEALTH RISKS ARE REAL

The ACE Study determined that the more of these experiences a person has suffered, the higher his/her risk is for a range of mental and physical health conditions.

For example, compared with participants who did not experience any abuses or mistreatment, those who reported four categories of adverse childhood experiences were twice as likely to be diagnosed with lung cancer and/or depression as adults. They also had a fourfold increase in chronic lung disease, such as chronic obstructive pulmonary disease (COPD), and a sevenfold increase in alcoholism. A person with six or more categories of ACEs had their life expectancy shortened by nearly 20 years.

WHY PHYSICAL HEALTH SUFFERS

It's easy to imagine how trauma would affect a person's mental health. But why would it also impact physical health? *Long-term research has identified such factors as...*

- **Coping mechanisms.** Trauma victims are more likely to use self-soothing habits, such as smoking, drinking, overeating and drug abuse, which are helpful in the short term but are known risk factors in the long term for many chronic health problems.

- **Complex brain-mediated effects.** Chronic stress due to ACEs can distort the function of brain networks, resulting in immune system suppression, which in turn can lead to a variety of diseases. In addition, it causes the release of pro-inflammatory chemicals that are responsible for additional diseases such as heart disease, pulmonary fibrosis, etc.

WHAT HELPS MOST

If you experienced trauma as a child, it is never too late to get help to reverse or at least moderate the negative physical and/or emotional effects of ACEs. *The strategies below, which tend to yield positive results more quickly than psychotherapy and/or antidepressants, are likely to also be helpful for those who experienced trauma as an adult...*

- **Tell a trusted person.** People who have experienced childhood trauma often carry the secret into adulthood. Victims of abuse feel shame and assume that they did something wrong to deserve the abuse. By simply telling someone, and having that person continue to accept you, the shame dissipates.

- **Try eye movement desensitization and reprocessing (EMDR).** The American Psychiatric Association recognizes this therapy as an effective treatment for trauma. Studies have found that trauma victims no longer had signs of posttraumatic stress disorder after as few as three 90-minute EMDR sessions.

How it works: During EMDR, a clinician asks the patient to hold a traumatic memory in mind while the therapist moves one or two fingers from side to side, or diagonally, in front of the patient's eyes. This guides the eyes to move as they do during the rapid eye movement (REM) sleep phase, during which the most active dreaming occurs. Dreaming can help process trauma and move it to long-term memory, enabling the patient to feel as if it is now resolved and only in the past.

The therapist repeats the process multiple times as needed, until the distress related to the targeted memory is gone and a positive belief replaces it. For example, a rape victim shifts from feeling horror and self-disgust to feeling empowered—I survived it and I am strong.

To find an EMDR clinician near you, visit the website of the EMDR Institute at EMDR.com. Check with your health insurer to see if your policy covers the treatment.

• **Consider clinical hypnosis.** This method helps patients identify past events or experiences that are causing problems. With hypnotherapy, a trained practitioner uses imagery and presents ideas or suggestions during a state of concentrated attention that helps bring about desired changes in thinking.

To find a certified hypnosis professional in your area, visit the website of the American Society of Clinical Hypnosis at ASCH.net. Check with your health insurer to see if clinical hypnosis is covered.

HOW TRAUMATIC WAS YOUR CHILDHOOD?

For each of the following questions, give yourself one point for every "yes" answer. *During your first 18 years of life...*

1. **Did a parent or other adult in the household often swear at you, insult you, put you down or humiliate you?** Or act in a way that made you afraid that you might be physically hurt?

2. **Did a parent or other adult in the household often push, grab, slap or throw something at you?** Or ever hit you so hard that you had marks or were injured?

3. **Did an adult or person at least five years older than you ever touch or fondle you or have you touch his/her body in a sexual way?** Or try to or actually have oral, anal or vaginal sex with you?

4. **Did you often feel that no one in your family loved you or thought you were important or special?** Or that your family didn't look out for one another, feel close to one another or support one another?

5. **Did you often feel that you didn't have enough to eat, had to wear dirty clothes and had no one to protect you?** Or that your parents were too drunk or high to take care of you or take you to the doctor if you needed it?

6. **Were your parents ever separated or divorced?**

7. **Was your mother or stepmother often pushed, grabbed or slapped?** Or did she often have something thrown at her? Or was she sometimes or often kicked, bitten, hit with a fist or hit with something hard? Or ever repeatedly hit for at least a few minutes or threatened with a gun or knife?

8. **Did you live with anyone who was a problem drinker or an alcoholic or who used street drugs?**

9. **Was a household member depressed or mentally ill, or did a household member attempt suicide?**

10. **Did a household member go to prison?**

Takeaway: If you score a four or higher, tell your doctor about your history of abuse and follow the recommendations in the main article. If these steps don't help, consult a trained therapist.

Don't Repress Anger

Ernest Harburg, PhD, research scientist emeritus, department of psychology, University of Michigan School of Public Health, Ann Arbor, and leader of a study of 192 married couples, published in *Journal of Family Communication.*

Husbands and wives who repress their anger tend to die earlier than spouses who express it, according to a recent study. Conflict in marriage is inevitable—but couples who air their differences and try to solve them stay healthier and live longer than ones who hold in their resentments.

Possible reason: Repressing anger leads to increased stress, which can shorten life.

Drinking Wine Guards Against Depression

Study of more than 5,500 people ages 55 to 80 led by researchers at University of Navarra, Pamplona, Spain, published online in *BMC Medicine*.

People who drank two to seven small glasses of wine each week were 30% less likely to develop depression than nondrinkers.

Possible reason: A compound found in grapes helps protect parts of the brain from inflammation that is linked to depression.

Power of Positive Thoughts

BMC Medicine.

Researchers have found that heart patients who were encouraged to be optimistic about post-surgical outcomes did better at six months than those who weren't encouraged to expect the best.

Kirtan Kriya Meditation: 12-Minute Brain Boost for Stressed-Out People

Helen Lavretsky, MD, psychiatrist and professor, department of psychiatry, University of California, Los Angeles. Her study was published in *International Journal of Geriatric Psychiatry*.

Are you ready to pull your hair out? Does a 12-minute, stress-relieving break sound appealing? We are not going to use those 12 minutes to get junk food from the vending machine, vent to a friend or stick pins into voodoo dolls. Instead, we're going to practice a simple technique that promotes relaxation...improves brain function...fights depression...and even helps counteract stress-induced chromosomal damage, right down at the cellular level!

What is this technique? It's a form of meditation called kirtan kriya (pronounced KEER-tun KREE-uh). According to a recent study, it showed remarkable benefits for family caregivers—people who typically are under constant stress as they struggle to take care of ill loved ones. If the technique can help people with that high level of chronic stress, surely it can help the average stressed-out human.

12 MINUTES TO CALM

Earlier research has shown that kirtan kriya meditation improves brain function and mood in people with mild cognitive impairment or mild-to-moderate Alzheimer's disease. For the more recent study, researchers wanted to see whether kirtan kriya could help stressed-out caregivers rather than patients themselves. Why? Because roughly 50% of family caregivers develop clinical depression... and that, of course, can negatively affect their own health and well-being.

At the start of the study, all participants completed tests that assessed their level of depression... overall mental health...and cognitive functioning (attention, verbal memory, information-processing speed, etc.).

They also had blood tests that measured the activity of telomerase, an enzyme responsible for maintaining telomeres. A telomere is the section at the end of each chromosome, and it helps protect the chromosome from damage. Studies suggest that telomeres and telomerase are affected by chronic stress and can be used as biomarkers of cellular aging—with shortened telomere length and reduced telomerase activity being linked to increased risk for various diseases and premature death.

Next, participants were randomly divided into two groups and instructed to practice their assigned stress-reducing technique for 12 minutes per day, at the same time each day, for a total of eight weeks.

Group one: These participants practiced kirtan kriya meditation, which involves repeating a mantra consisting of four syllables—Saa, Taa, Naa, Maa—while doing simple finger movements. The mantra is first chanted aloud...then said in a whisper...then repeated silently in one's mind...

then whispered again...and then chanted aloud again. During the meditation, eyes are closed and one imagines a light shining through the center of one's head.

Group two: These participants de-stressed in a basic way that many of us instinctively do—they listened to soothing instrumental music while relaxing in a quiet place with eyes closed.

IMPRESSIVE RESULTS

After eight weeks, all the assessment tests were repeated. Basically, both stress-reducing techniques helped—but kirtan kriya helped much more. *Here's how participants fared with regard to...*

- **Depression.** A 50% or greater improvement in depressive symptoms was seen in 65% of the kirtan kriya group—compared with just 31% of the basic relaxation group.
- **Mental health.** A 50% or greater improvement in overall mental health scores was experienced by 52% of participants in the kirtan kriya group...but by only 19% in the relaxation group.
- **Cognitive function.** The kirtan kriya group showed significant improvement on various tests of cognitive function...the relaxation group did not.
- **Telomerase activity.** Here was actual physical proof of kirtan kriya's benefits, with the meditators showing a 43% improvement in telomerase activity—compared with only a 4% improvement in the relaxation group.

How does it work? The researchers theorized that the chanting and finger movements of kirtan kriya add a "brain fitness" effect to the meditation technique's stress-reducing benefits.

DO TRY THIS AT HOME!

If you are a family caregiver, you have a particularly good reason to take note of these encouraging findings...but even for people who are not caregivers, stress reduction is very good for emotional and physical health. And we now have scientific proof that kirtan kriya meditation is a very powerful stress reducer. So why not try devoting just 12 minutes per day to kirtan kriya to see whether it helps you feel and function better?

Kick Your Bucket List

Marc E. Agronin, MD, a geriatric psychiatrist at Miami Jewish Health in Florida. He is author of *How We Age: A Doctor's Journey into the Heart of Growing Old* and *The End of Old Age: Living a Longer, More Purposeful Life* (MarcAgronin.com). Dr. Agronin recently recorded a series of podcasts for Bottom Line's Conversations with the Experts. Bottomlineinc.com/podcast-playlist/marc-agronin

Maybe it's time for bucket lists to kick the bucket. People who create bucket lists often dedicate huge amounts of time and money to crossing off entry after entry—visit China...learn to hang glide...see the Northern Lights. It becomes an addiction, pulling people away from things that matter more.

"They pursue what they imagine will be the thrills of a lifetime, but in the process, they trade away close connections to family, friends and community," says Marc Agronin, MD, a geriatric psychiatrist and author of *The Dementia Caregiver*. "There is nothing inherently wrong with going on adventures, but I've had many seniors who spend their retirements doing these things complain that their lives feel empty." *What to do...*

- **Seek balance between exciting adventures and existing connections.** Before pursuing a bucket-list goal, ask yourself whether you likely would be happier spending that time with people and projects that matter most to you.
- **Combine bucket-list adventures with your greater goals.** If your number-one priority is your grandchildren, for example, maybe you could invite a grandkid or two along on each bucket-list trip. If your top priority is leaving the world better than you found it, perhaps you could do volunteer work in an exotic location rather than just sightsee.
- **Consider taking longer trips.** Rather than go on lots of short trips to exotic destinations, schedule a smaller number of visits for a month or longer. The longer you spend in a location, the greater the odds that you will form deep, meaningful connections to people and communities there—but only if you go where the locals go rather than just to touristy sites.

Practice Compassion for a Long, Pain-Free Life

Emma Seppälä, PhD, science director, Center for Compassion and Altruism Research and Education, Stanford University School of Medicine, California, and author of *The Happiness Track: How to Apply the Science of Happiness to Accelerate Your Success.*

If you suffer from chronic pain, and perhaps the angry emotions that may result, there's a drug-free treatment that takes only 15 minutes a day and can bring real relief.

It's called compassion meditation. It's not like "regular" meditation. Rather than simply calming your mind, you actively direct your thoughts—toward kindness and altruism. Don't believe this could relieve your pain? Rigorous scientific studies have found that it can—and it may even help you live longer.

THE SCIENCE OF KINDNESS

At the Center for Compassion and Altruism Research and Education at Stanford University School of Medicine, we study the health effects of compassion and altruistic behavior. *Recent research at our center and other institutions has found that compassion meditation helps...*

- **Chronic pain—and anger.** Among people with chronic pain, a nine-week compassion meditation program at Stanford University led to significantly reduced pain severity and greater pain acceptance by the end of the program.

One benefit was that it reduced levels of anger, based on self-evaluations of the patients. Anger has been shown to be an important predictor of chronic pain symptoms, and cultivating compassion has been shown to positively influence how we process emotions, reducing the tendency toward negativity, including anger.

- **Posttraumatic stress disorder (PTSD) symptoms.** In a study at the Veterans Administration's Puget Sound Health Care System in Seattle, researchers found that when veterans with PTSD practiced loving-kindness meditation (a form of compassion meditation) for 12 weeks, they experienced a reduction in PTSD symptoms and depression. The benefits were still evident three months later.

- **Migraines.** A study from the University of Massachusetts Medical School in Worcester found that migraine sufferers who learned loving-kindness meditation in a single session experienced a 33% decrease in pain and a 43% reduction in emotional tension.

- **Longevity.** While there's certainly no conclusive evidence that learning to be compassionate to yourself and to others will help you live longer, there are intriguing clues that it might.

The connection: Telomeres, which are "caps" on the tips of each strand of DNA on your chromosomes.

A study from Massachusetts General Hospital and Harvard Medical School found that people experienced in practicing loving-kindness meditation had longer telomeres, which are associated with greater longevity.

HOW TO PRACTICE COMPASSION MEDITATION

Compassion meditation aims to strengthen feelings of compassion and empathy toward yourself and other people—to generate feelings of kindness toward yourself and others. It's different from the well-known "mindfulness" meditation, which is mostly focused on calming the mind and increasing awareness. In compassion meditation, rather than letting your thoughts come and go without judgment, you focus your attention in specific ways as you silently repeat benevolent phrases or visualize kind wishes.

The goal is to express your intention to move from judgment or dislike to caring, compassion, acceptance and understanding. Compassion meditation involves bringing to mind people you know and love, feeling their love and spreading caring feelings toward strangers or even people you find challenging.

It isn't hard to do.

What to do: Sit quietly, close your eyes, breathe gently and silently repeat a phrase designed to evoke a feeling of goodwill toward yourself, such as "May I be happy, healthy and strong." Then, extend the good wishes to someone you feel thankful for, then to someone you're indifferent toward, then to someone you find challenging and finally to the world at large.

Practicing loving-kindness or compassion meditation is a way to stretch the "muscles" of kindness, caring and empathy toward everyone and to remember our common humanity. The key is to give your "compassion muscles" a workout by practicing regularly, just as you might any other skill. Doing so will help you cultivate more loving relationships, greater happiness and better health...and could noticeably reduce your chronic pain.

Ready to do it now? You can use my YouTube video, "A Gift of Loving Kindness Meditation," which runs for less than 15 minutes. Close your eyes and follow the prompts. Once you know it by heart, you can do it in your own time and voice.

Simple Sleep Habits for a Long Life

Michael J. Breus, PhD, clinical psychologist, Los Angeles, and a fellow of The American Academy of Sleep Medicine. He is author of *The Power of When: Discover Your Chronotype—and the Best Time to Eat Lunch, Ask for a Raise, Have Sex, Write a Novel, Take Your Meds, and More*. TheSleepDoctor.com

---

You know that drinking too much can mean a bad night's sleep, but just one glass of wine or a nip of bourbon before bed won't hurt you, will it?

It will. You may fall asleep fine, but as little as one drink can impair sleep quality. The alcohol can interfere with the deep, restful stage of sleep that lets you wake up feeling rejuvenated, according to sleep expert Michael J. Breus, PhD.

The idea that one drink at bedtime is harmless is just one of the sleep "myths" that might be robbing you of quality sleep—and therefore reducing your energy and mental focus, too. (If you don't wake thoroughly refreshed on most mornings, here's what Dr. Breus suggests—for each alcoholic drink you consume on a given day, stop drinking at least that many hours before bed.)

Here are eight more sleep myths that Dr. Breus regularly encounters and that might be harming your sleep...

Myth: Thomas Edison, Leonardo da Vinci and Mozart excelled on only a few hours of sleep, so I can, too?

Truth: Some people, maybe including those above, have a rare genetic abnormality that lets them do well on little sleep. If you had that anomaly, you would know it—you would wake every morning feeling refreshed after perhaps three to five hours of sleep.

What to do: When your schedule permits—for example, during a vacation—let yourself fall asleep at whatever time you feel tired in the evening and rise whenever you awake refreshed. Don't set an alarm. Do this for a week or more. The amount of sleep you get on these nights likely is the amount that your body needs—for most people, that will be between six-and-a-half and eight hours.

Myth: People require less sleep as they age.

Truth: We do tend to sleep less deeply and wake up sooner as we age—but that's because we have more trouble sleeping. The result can be less alertness and focus and unintentional "napping" while watching TV or reading.

What to do: If you can't get sufficient sleep at night, schedule early-afternoon naps to avoid poorly timed unplanned naps or loss of mental sharpness.

Myth: I don't sleep at all some nights!

Truth: People sometimes imagine that they have lain in bed all night without getting a wink of sleep—but they're usually wrong. Most likely, you drifted off at least once or twice but woke up within a few hours each time. People who wake during the early stages of sleep often believe that they never fell asleep at all.

What to do: If you want to find out how much you really are sleeping—and perhaps, reassure yourself—wear a sleep-tracking device to bed. Most wearable fitness trackers include a sleep-tracking function. (*Note:* If you find that after using a tracker you sleep fewer than five hours in total over 24 hours, wake up for more than 30 seconds more than twice an hour and wake up feeling unrefreshed, you should see a sleep specialist about possible clinical insomnia.)

Myth: Sleeping in on the weekends can help me live longer.

That's how a lot of news articles covered a new study published in *Journal of Sleep Research*. It's technically true—but only compared with people who always sleep five hours or less a night on weeknights. They were helped by sleeping in on weekends.

Truth: Unless you get very little sleep throughout the week, regularly oversleeping on weekends is bad for your health. The truth is, you can't entirely "make up" for sleep lost during the week—research shows that you'll still have worse reaction time (behind the driver's wheel, for example) and mental focus. Plus, too much weekend sleep can throw off your sleep/wake schedule so that it's hard to fall asleep early enough on Sunday night—messing up another week's schedule. That's called "social jet lag." In fact, studies find that a pattern of sleeping more than two extra hours on weekends is linked to a rise in blood fats (triglycerides), increased risk for diabetes, weight gain and depressed mood. Sleeping in up to an hour or so on a Saturday or Sunday, though, is fine.

Myth: When I can't fall asleep, the best thing I can do is stay in bed.

Truth: Chances are you'll get frustrated—which makes it even harder to fall asleep.

What to do: If you've been lying in bed for 25 minutes or longer and you sense your frustration rising, get out of bed and do something you find relaxing until you feel sleepy, such as reading a book or magazine (not your smartphone or tablet) in a chair.

Exception: If you feel relaxed, not frustrated, continue lying there until you drift off.

Myth: Counting sheep is a time-tested strategy for falling asleep.

Truth: It's time to put the sheep back in the barn—counting them won't reduce the time you need to fall asleep, according to research at Oxford University. Counting sheep (or counting anything else you might imagine instead) requires so little brainpower that you still can ruminate about the other matters that are probably keeping you awake.

What to do: Engaging your brain as a distraction can help you fall asleep faster, but it needs to be something more involving.

Example: Try counting backward by threes starting at 300. That's boring enough to promote drowsiness but requires sufficient brainpower to deter your mind from wandering to other matters.

Myth: A warm, cozy bedroom is conducive to sleep.

Truth: When the body is warm, it produces less melatonin, a hormone that helps us enter the sleep cycle.

Exception: There is some evidence that keeping the feet warm—wearing socks, for instance—can encourage sleepiness.

What to do: Set your bedroom temperature to between 65°F and 75°F at night. The optimal temperature for most people is 68°F to 72°F. When you have trouble falling asleep, try lowering it a few degrees at a time to see whether that helps.

Myth: A glass of warm milk will help me fall asleep.

Milk contains tryptophan, an amino acid that can be conducive to sleep—but you would have to drink a gallon and a half of milk to have any significant sleep benefit. People may feel sleepy when they drink warm milk because they associate the beverage with comforting memories of a loved one putting them to bed in childhood.

What to do: If drinking warm milk helps you fall asleep, go ahead and drink warm milk—the sleep benefits are purely psychological, but that doesn't mean they're not real. The good news is that if you're lactose-intolerant, warm soy milk or almond milk should work just as well—it's the feeling of comfort, not the milk itself, that matters.

8

Food, Nutrition and Diet

The Secret Anti-Aging Agent You Should Be Eating

Paul Robbins, PhD, associate director of the Institute on the Biology of Aging and Metabolism at University of Minnesota, Minneapolis, and co-senior author of "Fisetin Is a Senotherapeutic That Extends Health and Lifespan" published in *EBioMedicine*.

Move over, vitamin C. Step aside, collagen. There's a new micronutrient stealing center stage. It's the flavonoid fisetin, and it's starting to get its share of attention as a promising way to slow down aging.

Yes, that's what we said. Previously, lab studies on animals and on human cells had found that fisetin can reduce diabetes complications, protect against stroke and enhance memory. Fisetin also has been shown to relieve allergic reactions by inhibiting cytokine production.

But now we can add one more benefit: Slowing down the aging process and increasing the prime-of-life years. When researchers from University of Minnesota and Mayo Clinic gave fisetin to older mice, the animals experienced a rejuvenation and longer-than-average span of time during which they were healthy (before any chronic diseases set in)—what researchers call their healthspan. The study looked at 10 flavonoids in all, each with the potential to stop the aging process, but it was fisetin that stood out as the most potent.

FISETIN: FIGHTING CELL DAMAGE

In our bodies, cells go through an aging process known as cellular senescence, in which the cell stops dividing. These types of cells have been linked to many age-related diseases. Certain flavonoids have been shown to help the body remove these cells, with fisetin being the most effective.

So where can you get it and how much do you need? Clinical trials are under way to help find the best human dosages for fisetin's different benefits—it's likely that a higher amount is needed for anti-aging than for enhancing memory, for instance. It's found naturally in (in order of richness) strawberries, apples, persimmons, lotus root, onions, grapes, kiwis, peaches and cucumbers, but current thinking is that it will take more food than you can comfortably eat every day to get enough fisetin to fully reap its anti-aging benefits. You can already buy concentrated fisetin supplements, generally in 100 mg tablets, but there are no guidelines stating whether that's the ideal amount. To give an idea of what that amount translates to in food, you'd need to eat a pound of strawberries to get 100 mg of fisetin—but at just 150 calories, that could be a wise choice.

In fact, despite the open questions on dosing, there's no reason not to choose fisetin-rich foods to get your recommended five to seven servings of fruits and vegetables each day...you'll also get the benefits of the many other nutrients in these foods.

---

5 Surprising Foods to Help You Live Longer

Bonnie Taub-Dix, RD, a registered dietitian and owner of BTD Nutrition Consultants located in New York City. A nationally recognized nutrition expert and the author of *Read It Before You Eat It*, she has advised patients on the best ways to control diabetes for more than three decades. BonnieTaubDix.com

---

Whether your blood sugar (glucose) levels are normal and you want to keep them that way...or you have diabetes and glucose control is your mantra...it is smart to eat a well-balanced diet to help keep your glucose readings healthy. In fact, maintaining healthy glucose levels may even help you live longer by avoiding diabetes—one of the leading causes of death in the US.

Most people already know that cinnamon is an excellent choice for blood sugar control. Consuming just one-half teaspoon to three teaspoons a day can reduce glucose levels by up to 24%. Cinnamon is great on cereals, vegetables, cottage cheese and snacks (think fresh apple slices sprinkled with cinnamon).

Other smart food choices...*

GLUCOSE-CONTROLLING FOOD #1: BLACK BEANS.

Beans, in general, are the most underrated food in the supermarket.

Beans are high in protein as well as soluble and insoluble fiber. Soluble fiber helps you feel fuller longer, and insoluble fiber helps prevent constipation. Beans also break down slowly during digestion, which means more stable blood sugar levels.

Black beans, however, are particularly healthful because of their especially high fiber content. For example, one cup of cooked black beans contains 15 g of fiber, while a cup of pink beans has just 9 g.

*If you take diabetes medication, consult your doctor before making significant changes to your diet—drug dosages may need to be adjusted.

Bonus: Beans protect the heart by lowering cholesterol and reducing damage from free radicals. For example, one study showed that you can lower your total and LDL ("bad") cholesterol by about 8% simply by eating one-half cup of cooked pinto beans every day.

Helpful: To shorten cooking times, use canned beans instead of dried beans. They are equally nutritious, and you can reduce the sodium in salted canned beans by about 40% by rinsing them.

Another healthful way to use beans: Hummus. In the Middle East, people eat this chickpea (garbanzo bean) spread as often as Americans eat bread. It is much healthier than bread because it contains both protein and olive oil—important for slowing the absorption of carbohydrate sugars and preventing blood sugar "spikes."

Hummus is a good weight-loss dish because it is high in fiber (about 15 g per cup) as well as protein (about 19 g). Ample amounts of protein and fiber allow you to satisfy your appetite with smaller portions of food.

Hummus is made with mashed chickpeas, tahini (a sesame seed paste), lemon juice, garlic, salt and a little olive oil. Stick to the serving size on the label, which is typically two to four tablespoons.

GLUCOSE-CONTROLLING FOOD #2: COCOA.

The flavanols in cocoa are potent antioxidants that not only fight heart disease but also help guard against diabetes. In recent studies, cocoa improved insulin sensitivity, the body's ability to transport sugar out of the bloodstream. It's wise for people with diabetes or high blood sugar to choose unsweetened cocoa and add a small amount of sugar or sugar substitute.

Cinnamon hot cocoa combines two glucose-controlling ingredients in one delicious recipe.

To prepare: Mix one-quarter cup of baking cocoa, one tablespoon of sugar (or Truvia to taste) and a pinch of salt. Gradually add one-quarter cup of boiling water and blend well. Add one cup of skim or 1% low-fat milk and a cinnamon stick. While stirring occasionally, heat on low for 10 minutes. Remove the cinnamon stick and enjoy!

GLUCOSE-CONTROLLING FOOD #3: DATES.

These little fruits are sweet enough to qualify as dessert but have more antioxidants per serving than oranges, grapes and even broccoli. The antioxidants can help prevent heart disease as well as neuropathy—nerve damage that frequently occurs in people who have diabetes.

A single serving (for example, seven deglet noor dates) has 4 g of fiber for better blood sugar management.

Be careful: Seven dates also have 140 calories and 32 g of sugar, so this must be added to your total daily carbohydrate intake, especially if you have diabetes. Dates, in general, have a low glycemic index, so they don't spike glucose levels. Medjool dates, however, are not an ideal choice. They have significantly more sugar and calories per serving than deglet noor dates.

GLUCOSE-CONTROLLING FOOD #4: SARDINES.

Many people know about the heart-healthy benefits of cold-water fish, such as salmon and mackerel. An analysis of studies involving hundreds of thousands of adults found that just one to two fish servings a week reduced the risk of dying from heart disease by more than one-third.

What's less well-known is that the high concentration of omega-3 fatty acids in cold-water fish also helps prevent a too-rapid rise in blood sugar. Besides being low on the glycemic index, fish contains protein, which blunts blood sugar levels.

Best for helping to prevent high blood sugar: In addition to salmon and mackerel, sardines are an excellent choice (when canned with bones, they also are a good source of calcium). Tuna, to a somewhat lesser extent, offers omega-3s (choose canned light—albacore white has higher levels of mercury). Also avoid large fish, such as king mackerel and swordfish, which have more mercury than smaller fish. Aim for a 3.5-ounce serving two or three times a week.

GLUCOSE-CONTROLLING FOOD #5: ALMONDS.

High in fiber, protein and beneficial fats, nuts can significantly lower glucose levels. In fact, women who ate a one-ounce serving of nuts at least five times a week were nearly 30% less likely to develop diabetes than women who rarely or never ate nuts, according to one study.

The poly- and monounsaturated fats in nuts improve the body's ability to use insulin. Nuts also help with cholesterol control—important because diabetes increases risk for heart disease.

All nuts are beneficial, but almonds contain more fiber, calcium and protein than most nuts (and are best for blood sugar control). Walnuts are highest in antioxidants and omega-3 fatty acids. Avoid salted nuts—they have too much sodium.

Excellent way to add nuts to your diet: Nut butters. Almost everyone likes peanut butter, and it is healthier than you might think. Like butters made from almonds, cashews or other nuts, the fats it contains are mostly monounsaturated, which are good for the heart. The fiber in nut butters (about 1 g to 2 g per tablespoon, depending on the nut) can help lower blood sugar.

Good choice for blood sugar control: One serving (one to two tablespoons) of almond butter (rich in potassium, vitamin E and calcium) several times a week. Look for nut butters that have a short list of ingredients—they are the most nutritious.

A SIMPLE BLOOD SUGAR BUSTER

Taking two tablespoons of apple-cider vinegar in eight ounces of water with meals or before bedtime can slow the absorption of sugar into the blood—vinegar helps to block the digestive enzymes that change carbs to sugar.

The Ultimate Superfoods

Steven Pratt, MD, FACS, ABIHM, world-renowned authority on the role of nutrition and lifestyle in the prevention of disease and optimization of health. Dr. Pratt is the author of the best-selling *Superfoods* books, including *Bottom Line's SuperFoods Rx* and *SuperHealth: Six Simple Steps, Six Easy Weeks, One Longer, Healthier Life*.

Odds are you know that nutrient-packed blueberries and broccoli are among the most healthful foods available. But does your daily diet include the widest possible variety of the other nutritional powerhouse foods? Many such "superfoods" are overlooked—even by people who are health-conscious.

Latest development: My new "SuperHealth" pyramid gives you advice on foods that have the greatest nutritional value and how much you should aim to eat each day.

Bonus: In addition to fighting heart disease, cancer, diabetes and other chronic ailments, these foods also help many people overcome the lack of vitality that is so often associated with aging. *Superfoods you shouldn't miss out on...*

VEGETABLES

As a phytonutrient-rich cruciferous vegetable, ever-popular broccoli has been shown to reduce risk for heart disease, certain types of cancer (such as bladder, prostate and ovarian) and cataracts.

• **Don't overlook—Broccoli sprouts.** Developed by scientists at Johns Hopkins University, these three-day-old sprouts are grown from seeds that yield the highest levels of sulforaphane glucosinolate, a natural compound that stimulates enzymes in the body to boost its own antioxidant defenses. Broccoli sprouts contain 20 to 100 times more cancer-fighting substances than mature broccoli, according to research.

Broccoli sprouts, which can be used in salads or as a garnish on sandwiches, look and taste similar to alfalfa sprouts. Broccoli sprouts are available at many supermarkets. As an alternative, you can buy the seeds and grow your own sprouts at home.

Daily recommendation: In addition to consuming broccoli sprouts, aim to get at least five one-half to one-cup servings of vegetables daily, including cruciferous varieties such as cauliflower and brussels sprouts. Frozen or canned vegetables are fine as long as they do not contain added salt.

FRUITS

Blueberries top most superfood lists—primarily because they are rich in polyphenol antioxidants, substances that reduce inflammation and appear to stop cancer-producing genes from "turning on."

• **Don't overlook—Purple grapes.** They provide most of the same health benefits as blueberries.

Daily recommendation: In addition to consuming purple grapes (or some type of berry), eat three to five one-half to one-cup servings of fruits daily.

Helpful: If purple grape juice is more convenient, drink two half-cup servings daily with meals. Choose 100% Concord grape juice—it has no added sugar.

WHOLE GRAINS AND FIBER

When it comes to whole grains, oats are a favorite of many people who are health-savvy.

• **Don't overlook—Wheat bran and ground flaxseed.** Both provide valuable vitamins and minerals and are rich sources of fiber, which helps us achieve and maintain an optimal body weight. A healthy weight helps prevent or control diabetes and reduces blood pressure.

Daily recommendation: As an alternative to traditional whole grains (five to seven servings daily), get 10 g to 20 g of fiber daily. Include two tablespoons of wheat bran or ground flaxseed—use on cold or hot cereals...stir into yogurt...and/or add to casseroles.

PROTEIN

Protein (from either animal or vegetable sources) helps us maintain muscle strength and our bodies' immune and hormone functions.

• **Don't overlook—Skinless turkey breast.** For people who are tired of fish (or never really liked it), skinless turkey breast is a great protein alternative. (Skinless turkey breast typically contains 0.2 g of saturated fat per three-ounce serving.) The minerals selenium and zinc in turkey help fight inflammation, which can lead to cancer, stroke, heart disease and diabetes.

Smart idea: Use 97% to 99% fat-free ground turkey breast instead of ground beef in burgers. Organic turkey is best—it limits your exposure to antibiotics and growth hormones.

Weekly recommendation: Four servings of fish per week or as much skinless turkey breast as you like. One serving of fish or turkey is about the size of a deck of cards.

• **Don't overlook—Soy foods.** They are a good source of protein and also contain phytochemicals that have a weak estrogenic effect. This effect helps block environmental toxins, such as those found in pesticides and many common household cleaners (such as mold and mildew removers), from attaching to cells where they can cause damage or even cancer.

Important: If you have had breast cancer, consult your doctor before adding soy foods to your diet—some animal research suggests that the foods' estrogenic effects may stimulate cancer growth in some individuals. Daily recommendation: One to three half-cup cooked servings of high-protein vegetables.

Example: Legumes (such as pinto, kidney or black beans). Your protein intake may include 10 g to 15 g of soy protein daily—for example, one cup of soymilk…or one-half cup of soybeans (edamame).

BONE-BUILDING FOODS

People who choose whole milk and/or high-fat cheeses as sources of bone-building calcium run the risk of getting too much potentially harmful saturated fat.

•**Don't overlook—Nonfat organic yogurt.** Six ounces of nonfat organic yogurt typically provides about 25% of the Daily Value (DV) of calcium and ample supplies of probiotics—the "friendly" bacteria your gastrointestinal system needs to digest foods properly.

Daily recommendation: At least one six- to eight-ounce serving daily of nonfat organic yogurt…and at least one serving daily of tofu, canned wild salmon (with bones) or dark green, leafy vegetables.

HEALTHFUL FATS

Extra-virgin olive oil is well-known for its healthful fats.

•**Don't overlook—Soybean oil.** It is low in saturated fat and high in healthful polyunsaturated fat.

Daily recommendation: In addition to using one tablespoon of soybean oil (or some other healthful oil such as extra-virgin olive, canola or peanut oil) on most days, consume at least one handful of nuts (walnuts, almonds or pistachios) or seeds (sesame, sunflower or pumpkin) five times a week.

HEALTHFUL TREATS

Dark chocolate has become a superfood favorite ever since studies found that its antioxidant flavonoids help reduce blood pressure.

•**Don't overlook—Buckwheat honey (a type of dark honey).** The darker the honey, the more flavonoids it contains. Preliminary research shows that honey may help lower total cholesterol levels.

Daily recommendation: 100 calories daily of a healthful treat, such as dark chocolate (with at least 70% cocoa)…or one to two teaspoons of buckwheat honey daily in such foods as cereal, oatmeal or plain yogurt or in tea.

Also important: Whenever possible, use spices (as much as you like).

Among the best choices: Nutmeg (for its anti-inflammatory and anticancer effects)…oregano (for its antioxidant, antifungal and antibacterial effects)…and turmeric (for its curcumin, which has been linked to the prevention of heart disease and cancer).

SUPERHEALTH FOOD PYRAMID

What to eat daily…

•**Fruits.** 3–5 servings. Try to eat some type of berry every day.

•**Vegetables.** Unlimited. Aim for at least 5 servings.

•**Whole grains and fiber.** 5–7 servings of whole grains (such as whole-grain cereal) or 10 g to 20 g of fiber (such as wheat bran and ground flaxseed).

•**Protein.** Fish (such as wild salmon, sardines or herring) 4 times a week or as much skinless turkey breast as you like (one serving is about the size of a deck of cards)…and 1–3 half-cup servings daily of high-protein vegetables such as legumes (pinto, kidney or black beans).

•**Bone-building foods.** 1 serving of nonfat organic yogurt and at least 1 serving of sardines, canned salmon (with bones) and/or dark green, leafy vegetables. such as legumes (pinto, kidney or black beans).

•**Spices.** Use plenty.

•**Healthful fats.** One tablespoon of extra-virgin olive, soybean or canola oil on most days. One handful of nuts (such as walnuts or almonds) or seeds (such as sesame or pumpkin).

- **Healthful treats.** 100 calories.

  Examples: Dark chocolate, buckwheat honey.

The Superfood You've Never Heard Of—Spirulina Slows Aging

Jennifer Adler, MS, CN, a certified nutritionist, natural foods chef and adjunct faculty member at Bastyr University, Seattle. She is the founder and owner of Passionate Nutrition, a nutrition practice with offices in eight locations in the Puget Sound area, and cofounder of the International Eating Disorders Institute. PassionateNutrition.com

When you think of a superfood, you probably think of salmon or blueberries—not the algae that floats on the surfaces of lakes, ponds and reservoirs.

But there's a type of blue-green algae that has been used for food and medicine in developing countries for centuries...that NASA has recommended as an ideal food for long-term space missions...that is loaded with health-giving nutrients...and that might be a key component in a diet aimed at staying healthy, reversing chronic disease and slowing the aging process.

That algae is spirulina.

Spirulina grows mainly in subtropical and tropical countries, where there is year-round heat and sunlight. It is high in protein (up to 70%), rich in antioxidants and loaded with vitamins and minerals, particularly iron and vitamin B-12. And it has no cellulose—the cell wall of green plants—so its nutrients are easy for the body to digest and absorb.

GREEN MEDICINE

Dried into a powder, spirulina can be added to food or taken as a tablet or capsule. And ingested regularly, spirulina can do you a lot of good. *Scientific research shows there are many health problems that spirulina might help prevent or treat...*

- **Anemia.** Researchers from the University of California at Davis studied 40 people age 50 and older who had been diagnosed with anemia (iron deficiency), giving them a spirulina supplement every day for three months. The study participants had a steady rise in levels of hemoglobin, the iron-carrying component of red blood cells, along with several other factors that indicated increased levels of iron.

- **Weakened immunity.** In the UC Davis study mentioned above, most of the participants ages 61 to 70 also had increases in infection-fighting white blood cells and in an enzyme that is a marker for increased immune activity—in effect, reversing immunosenescence, the age-related weakening of the immune system. Immunosenescence is linked not only to a higher risk for infectious diseases such as the flu but also to chronic diseases with an inflammatory component, such as heart disease, Alzheimer's and cancer.

- **Allergies.** Spirulina has anti-inflammatory properties and can prevent the release of histamine and other inflammatory factors that trigger and worsen allergic symptoms. Studies also show that spirulina can boost levels of IgA, an antibody that defends against allergic reactions. In one study, people with allergies who took spirulina had less nasal discharge, sneezing, nasal congestion and itching.

- **Cataracts and age-related macular degeneration.** Taking spirulina can double blood levels of zeaxanthin, an antioxidant linked to a reduced risk for cataracts and age-related macular degeneration, reported researchers in *British Medical Journal.*

- **Diabetes.** In several studies, researchers found that adding spirulina to the diets of people with type 2 diabetes significantly decreased blood sugar levels.

  Caution: Spirulina has not been approved by the FDA for treating diabetes, so consult your doctor before taking.

- **Lack of endurance.** In a small study, men who took spirulina for one month were able to run more than 30% longer on a treadmill before having to stop because of fatigue, reported Greek researchers in *Medicine & Science in Sports & Exercise.*

•**Heart disease.** Nearly a dozen studies have looked at the effect of spirulina intake on risk factors for heart disease, both in healthy people and people with heart disease. Most of the studies found significant decreases in negative factors (such as LDL cholesterol, total cholesterol, triglycerides, apolipoprotein B and blood pressure) and increases in positive factors (such as HDL cholesterol and apolipoprotein A1).

IDEAL DOSE

A preventive daily dose of spirulina is one teaspoon. A therapeutic dose, to control or reverse disease, is 10 grams, or one tablespoon.

Spirulina has been on the market for more than a decade, and it's among the substances listed by the FDA as "Generally Recognized as Safe" (GRAS).

Caution: If you have an autoimmune disease, such as multiple sclerosis, rheumatoid arthritis or lupus, talk to your doctor. Spirulina could stimulate the immune system, making the condition worse.

BEST PRODUCTS

Like many products, the quality of spirulina varies. *What to look for...*

•**Clean taste.** Top-quality spirulina tastes fresh. If spirulina tastes fishy or "swampy" or has a lingering aftertaste, it's probably not a good product.

•**Bright color.** Spirulina should have a vibrant, bright blue-green appearance (more green than blue). If spirulina is olive-green, it's probably inferior.

•**Cost.** You get what you pay for—and good spirulina can be somewhat pricey.

Example: Spirulina Pacifica, from Nutrex Hawaii—grown on the Kona coast of Hawaii since 1984 and regarded by many health experts as one of the most nutritious and purest spirulina products on the market—costs $50 for a 16-ounce, 454-gram jar of powder. (Available at Amazon.com.) Store it in the refrigerator. Also in tablet form.

•**Growing location.** The best spirulina is grown in clean water in a nonindustrialized setting, as far away as possible from an urban, polluted environment. If you can, find out the growing location of the product you're considering buying.

HOW TO ADD IT TO FOOD

There are many ways to include spirulina in your daily diet...

•**Put it in smoothies.** Add between one teaspoon and one tablespoon to any smoothie or shake.

•**Add to juice.** Add one teaspoon or tablespoon to an eight-ounce glass of juice or water, shake it up and drink it.

•**Sprinkle it on food.** Try spirulina popcorn, for instance—a great conversation starter at a potluck. To a bowl of popcorn, add one to two tablespoons of spirulina powder, three to four tablespoons of grated Parmesan cheese, two or three tablespoons of olive oil, one-half teaspoon of salt and one-eighth teaspoon of cayenne pepper.

•**Add it to condiments.** Put one-quarter teaspoon in a small jar of ketchup, barbecue sauce, mustard or salad dressing. This way you'll get a little each time you use these products.

Studies Say Berries Are More Powerful Than Drugs!

Bill Gottlieb, CHC, a health coach certified by the American Association of Drugless Practitioners and former editor in chief of Rodale Books and Prevention Magazine Health Books. He is author of 16 health books including *Bottom Line's Speed Healing*. BillGottliebHealth.com

---

If you were asked to make a list of "superfoods"—nutrient-loaded foods that effectively fight disease—you'd probably include items such as kale, beans, walnuts, broccoli, green tea, wild-caught salmon...and berries.

What few people realize: As a superfood, berries—blueberries, strawberries, raspberries, blackberries, cranberries and the like—are in a class by themselves. They can be more health-giving than medications or supplements, according to experts at Harvard Medical School and Harvard T.H. Chan School of Public Health. The antioxidants in berries—anthocyanins, the compounds that give these fruits their lustrous colors—deliver a pure dose of prevention and healing to the brain, heart and every other system and cell in the body. And you don't have to eat a bushelful to get the benefits.

Here's what you need to know about the amazing power of berries...

BERRIES AND YOUR BRAIN

For more than a decade, scientists at the Jean Mayer USDA Human Nutrition Research Center on Aging at Tufts University have been studying the effect of berries on the brain—in cells and in laboratory animals. They have found that regular ingestion of blueberries, strawberries and/or blackberries can help improve "plasticity," the ability of brain cells to form new connections with one another...generate new brain cells...stop inflammation and oxidation from damaging brain cells...ease the destructive effect of stress on the brain...prevent and reverse age-related memory loss, particularly short-term, or "working," memory...and protect against amyloid-beta, the plaques in the brain that cause Alzheimer's disease. Now research has shown that blueberries can help rejuvenate the aging human brain...

Startling new findings: The researchers from Tufts studied 37 people, ages 60 to 75, dividing them into two groups—one group consumed one ounce of freeze-dried blueberries every day (the equivalent of one cup of fresh blueberries)...the other a blueberry placebo. At the beginning, middle and end of the three-month study, the participants took tests measuring learning and memory. By the end of the study, those in the blueberry group had a 20% improvement in their scores on a memory test compared with those in a placebo group.

- **Strawberries are good, too.** The Tufts researchers gave participants either freeze-dried strawberry powder (the equivalent of two cups of fresh strawberries) or a placebo. After three months of daily intake, the strawberry group had much greater improvements in memory than the placebo group.

What to do: Eat one cup of blueberries or strawberries daily, either fresh or frozen. Choose organic. Every year, the Environmental Working Group announces its "Dirty Dozen," a list of the produce with the most pesticides. In 2017, strawberries topped the list and blueberries ranked number 17.

BERRIES AND YOUR HEART

Hundreds of studies show that anthocyanins battle oxidation and inflammation, the evil twins of chronic disease—including heart disease. *Berries can...*

- **Reduce high blood pressure**—the number-one risk factor for heart attack and stroke. Researchers from Florida State University studied 48 postmenopausal women with high blood pressure, giving them either one-third cup of freeze-dried blueberry powder daily or a placebo. After two months, the women getting the blueberry powder had a drop in systolic blood pressure (the upper number in a blood pressure reading) of 5.1% and a drop in diastolic blood pressure (the lower reading) of 6.3%—decreasing the risk for heart attack and stroke. Their arteries were also more flexible. There were no changes in the placebo group.

- **Reduce other risk factors for heart disease.** The cranberry is no slouch when it comes to guarding the heart. Scientists from the USDA's Human Nutrition Research Center studied 56 people, average age 50. Half drank two eight-ounce glasses of no-sugar-added cranberry juice daily...the other half made no changes to their diets. After two weeks, the scientists measured several risk factors for heart disease. Those drinking the juice had lower levels of C-reactive protein (CRP), a biomarker for heart-damaging inflammation...lower levels of triglycerides, a heart-hurting blood fat...and lower levels of blood sugar.

Bottom line: More berries, fewer heart attacks. In a study published in *Circulation*, researchers examined 18 years of health data from 93,600 women and found that those who ate three or more servings of blueberries and strawberries per week (one serving is one-half cup) had a 34% lower risk for heart attack, compared with women who ate them less than three times weekly.

What to do: If you have heart disease or any risk factors for heart disease (high blood pressure, high LDL cholesterol, high blood sugar, high CRP, a family history of heart disease), eat three cups of blueberries or strawberries per week.

BERRIES AND CANCER

Cellular research and animal research have shown that berries can fight just about every kind of cancer.

Example: A scientific paper recently published by researchers from the Medical College of Wisconsin in *Antioxidants* shows that cranberries can help fight 17 different cancers, including bladder, blood, brain, breast, colon, esophageal, oral, prostate and stomach cancers.

But the real test of berries' anticancer power is whether berries can help people with cancer. *Research published in 2016 shows that they can...*

- **Oral cancer.** Researchers at The Ohio State University Comprehensive Cancer Center gave lozenges of freeze-dried black raspberry powder (which contains very high levels of anthocyanins) to people with oral cancer for two weeks. Analyzing the tumors, they found that several genetic markers of cancer severity—prosurvival genes and proinflammatory genes—were significantly reduced by up to 21%.

In an earlier study, researchers at University of North Carolina and three other universities gave a "bioadhesive" black raspberry gel or a placebo to 40 people with premalignant oral lesions (neoplasia), which often progress to oral cancer. After four months, the lesions of those using black raspberry had shrunk in size and were less likely to advance to cancer.

- **Colon cancer.** In several studies on colon cancer at the National Cancer Institute and other institutions, daily intake of 60 grams of black raspberry powder (the equivalent of 15 servings of black raspberries) reversed dozens of biomarkers of the disease. These studies showed that the powder can kill cancer cells, block the growth of new blood vessels to tumors (angiogenesis), kill cancer cells (apoptosis) and stop cancer cells from dividing and growing (proliferation).

What to do: If you are at risk for oral or colon cancer...or are being treated for one of those diseases...or are a survivor of any of them—talk with your doctor about adding black raspberry powder to a daily smoothie. (You could never eat enough black raspberries to get the cancer-reversing effect.)

Good product: Freeze-dried black raspberry powder from BerriHealth (BerriHealth.com).

For preventing cancer, eat five or more servings of fruits and vegetables every day—including berries.

Eat Nuts, Live Longer—Now There's Proof

Ying Bao, MD, ScD, associate epidemiologist, Brigham and Women's Hospital, Boston.

In a study of nearly 119,000 adults, those who ate one ounce of any kind of nuts each day were 20% less likely to die of any cause over a 30-year period than those who didn't eat nuts.

Reason: Nutrient-rich peanuts and tree nuts such as walnuts, cashews and pecans help ward off cancer, heart disease and respiratory conditions.

To boost your overall health: Eat a handful of raw or dry-roasted, unsalted nuts every day.

Time-Tested Anti-Aging Food and Drinks

Mao Shing Ni, LaC, DOM, PhD, a Santa Monica, California–based licensed acupuncturist and doctor of oriental medicine, TaoOfWellness.com. He is cofounder of Yo San University, an accredited graduate school of Traditional Chinese Medicine in Los Angeles, and author of *Secrets of Longevity*.

We all know that a nutritious diet is one of the keys to living a long, healthy life.

Problem: Even health-conscious individuals get stuck in a rut of consuming the same foods and drinks all the time.

Solution: Traditional Chinese Medicine (TCM) offers a wide variety of healthful, delicious foods and drinks that have been consumed for their disease-fighting properties for thousands of years.

Best anti-aging food...

• **Orange peel for cholesterol.** As we age, LDL "bad" cholesterol often accumulates in the arteries, leading to heart disease and stroke. Orange peel actually may lower cholesterol better than some medications, such as statin drugs, without the side effects.

Studies show that compounds called polymethoxsylated flavones (PMFs), found in pigments of oranges and tangerines, can reduce bad cholesterol—without decreasing the level of HDL "good" cholesterol.

My advice: Grate or chop the peel of an orange or tangerine (preferably organic to avoid potentially toxic pesticides). If cooking a 12-ounce serving of meat or chicken, use the whole rind. As an alternative, use low-sugar marmalade, which contains orange rind, in your sauce.

• **Papaya to fight inflammation and allergies.** Papaya is rich in the enzyme bromelain and has long been used by the Chinese to help reduce the inflammatory process that promotes allergic reactions. Other bromelain-rich foods include pineapple and kiwifruit.

My advice: Try eating two to three cups of the bromelain-rich fruits mentioned above daily—and add cherries and grapes (all types), which are rich in phytochemicals that also fight the inflammation that results from the body's immune response to allergens. Bromelain is also available in supplement form. If you suffer from hay fever or other allergies, take 200 mg daily. Do not take bromelain if you have a bleeding disorder, high blood pressure, or liver or kidney disease or if you have food allergies, especially to pineapple. Talk to your doctor first if you are taking antibiotics, blood thinners or sedatives, since bromelain may interact with these drugs.

My favorite anti-aging beverages…

• **Chicory for heart health.** Chicory, an herb that is popular in China and parts of Europe, contains a compound called inulin that helps strengthen the heart muscle—and may even be useful in treating congestive heart failure (a condition that causes inadequate pumping action of the heart).

One study found that chicory helps regulate an irregular heartbeat—a potentially dangerous condition that can lead to heart failure. Other research shows that chicory helps lower cholesterol levels and may slow the progression of hardening of the arteries.

My advice: In the US, chicory root is most often roasted for use as a brewed coffee substitute that can be found in most organic food markets. For heart health, drink one to two cups daily of chicory coffee substitute. Don't use chicory if you have gallstones or are allergic to plants in the ragweed family.

My favorite: Teeccino Mediterranean Java Herbal Coffee. Radicchio, a type of leafy chicory, is also widely available. Eat it two to three times weekly (in salads, for example).

• **Chinese asparagus root for increased energy and brain function.** This close cousin to the asparagus found on Western dinner tables contains many phytonutrients, including quercetin, an antioxidant and anti-inflammatory compound. It has been used in China to promote longevity for more than 2,000 years. Chinese asparagus root can be found online, in health-food stores and at the offices of TCM practitioners.

My advice: Consume as a brewed tea (one to two cups daily) or in capsule form (300 mg to 500 mg daily).

• **White willow bark tea for pain relief and blood-thinning properties.** This herb contains salicin, a compound found in aspirin. Aspirin was originally discovered in—and extracted from—this bark. Besides its pain-relieving properties, white willow bark acts as an anticoagulant, which helps prevent the formation of blood clots and thickening of blood that can lead to heart attacks and strokes.

My advice: If you have pain caused by arthritis, muscle strain or tendinitis (tendon inflammation) or are at increased risk for heart disease or ischemic stroke (from a blockage)—due to family history, high blood pressure or smoking—drink one to two cups of white willow bark tea daily. If you take daily aspirin therapy for heart attack and/or stroke prevention, ask your doctor about taking supplemental white willow bark (100 mg daily) instead.

Caution: If you have a bleeding disorder...take a blood thinner, such as *warfarin* (Coumadin) or a beta-blocker...or are allergic to aspirin, do not use white willow bark.

The Pizza That Fights Heart Disease (Cancer, Too)

John La Puma, MD, a board-certified specialist in internal medicine who has a private nutritional medical practice in Santa Barbara, California. He is a cofounder of the popular ChefMD video series airing on PBS nationwide and author of *Refuel: A 24-Day Eating Plan to Shed Fat, Boost Testosterone,* and *Pump Up Strength and Stamina.* He and Michael Roizen, MD, are the first physicians to teach cooking and nutrition in a US medical school. DrJohnLaPuma.com

Americans love their pizza! On any given day, about one in eight of us has a slice or two. And pizza eaters get up to one-third of their daily calories from their favorite pies.

Unfortunately, a typical slice of pizza is loaded with fat, sugar and salt and is low in fiber and nutrients. But pizza doesn't have to be bad for you. In fact, you can turn it into a food that is really good for you. It can even help prevent heart disease (cancer, too). The secret is to make the pizza yourself.

Homemade pizza is different. It can satisfy your cravings without jamming up your arteries. And you can make it in about the same amount of time that it would take to phone in an order and drive across town for your favorite pie.

What, exactly, does a healthy pizza look like? *It depends on the ingredients...*

FULL-FAT CHEESE (BUT NOT TOO MUCH)

New research suggests that saturated fat—and particularly the saturated fat found in cheese and other dairy foods—isn't the cardiovascular demon that doctors once thought. Saturated fat actually can improve HDL "good" cholesterol and may reduce triglyceride levels.

You can't have good pizza without good cheese. Don't bother with pregrated cheeses that come in a can or a bag. They have almost no flavor, and they often are spiked with extra sodium.

My advice: Use high-quality mozzarella, Romano, Parmesan, goat or gouda—or a combination of your favorites. A 12-inch pie needs about two to four ounces of cheese—the equivalent of one-half to one cup of grated cheese.

PLENTY OF TOMATOES

Tomatoes are one of the main ingredients in a heart-healthy Mediterranean diet. The lycopene in tomatoes—along with beta-carotene and other carotenoids—has been linked to lower rates of heart disease and cancer. Lycopene is particularly important for men because studies suggest that it could reduce the risk for prostate cancer.

My advice: Processed tomatoes may have more lycopene than fresh, but fresh tomatoes have fiber in the skin and seeds—so use both. Look for low-sodium, no-added-sugar tomato sauce. Layer sliced fresh tomatoes (or cherry tomatoes) over a base of the tomato sauce.

WHITE ANCHOVIES

The American Heart Association advises everyone to eat fatty fish at least twice a week. The omega-3 fatty acids in fish have been shown to lower triglyceride levels and reduce dangerous heartbeat irregularities (arrhythmias).

The especially healthy thing about anchovies—unlike, say, albacore tuna or other fatty fish—is that they contain little mercury while being rich in omega-3s.

My advice: Try white anchovies. They have a "meatier" texture and better flavor than other canned or jarred anchovies. They also are lower in salt.

Kitchen tip: You can remove much of the salt from any kind of canned or jarred anchovies by soaking them in water for a half hour. Or soak them in milk. It softens the texture and reduces the fishy flavor while removing sodium.

ONIONS, GARLIC AND CHILE PEPPERS

These vegetables contain a variety of anti-inflammatory compounds that protect the arteries and reduce the risk for heart disease. One large study found that men who consumed the most flavonoids (a class of antioxidants found in onions, garlic and other vegetables and fruits) had a 68% reduced risk for cardiovascular disease.

Capsaicin, the chemical compound that puts the "bite" in jalapeños and other chile peppers, may have similar effects. It is a potent antioxidant that's been linked to lower cholesterol and blood pressure.

My advice: Lightly cook onions, garlic and chile peppers before you add them to pizza. You can't count on fully baking raw ingredients placed on raw pizza dough. The extra cooking time will give them a fuller flavor and a softer texture.

Kitchen tip: Before I add onions to pizza, I caramelize them in a sauté pan by slowly cooking them in a little olive oil until they are browned. It makes them sweeter and richer. Or if you prefer, you can microwave them for 30 seconds. That won't caramelize the sugars, but it will blunt the sharp flavors.

ARUGULA

This peppery salad green is one of my favorite pizza toppings. It has a strong, "bright" flavor that can hold its own with other pungent toppings.

Arugula, along with broccoli and Brussels sprouts, is a cruciferous vegetable that lowers inflammation and may reduce the risk for heart disease. It also is a detoxifying agent. When researchers looked at previous studies, they found that about 70% of the studies confirmed the link between cruciferous vegetables and lower cancer risk. The report was published in *Journal of the American Dietetic Association*.

My advice: After washing and slicing arugula into bite-size pieces, toss it lightly in a little olive oil before adding it to the pizza. The oil brings out the flavor and prevents the leaves from crisping during cooking. Oil also helps you absorb fat-soluble vitamins such as vitamin A and vitamin K.

PERFECT DOUGH

You can buy ready-to-go pizza crusts, but generally I don't recommend them because many contain too much sugar and fat and chemicals.

Better: Fresh whole-wheat dough that's ready for rolling. You can buy both white and whole-wheat varieties at Whole Foods, Trader Joe's and other markets.

If you're not bound by tradition, you also can use crust substitutes. I often use corn tortillas for pizza.

FENNEL, CUMIN OR SESAME SEEDS

When rolling out pizza dough, don't use too much flour on it. In fact, you don't have to use any flour to prevent the dough from sticking.

You can make your dough healthier (and better-tasting) by using crushed seeds or cornmeal instead of the flour you might sprinkle on the board. Try fennel seeds for an Italian pizza or cumin seeds for a Mexican-style pie. Sesame seeds are another tasty choice.

Helpful: Buy a pizza peel, a broad wooden or metal paddle that makes it easy to shift the pizza from the counter to the oven and from the oven to the table. If you like, you can roll out the dough on top of the peel, which saves having to shift the dough from the counter. Or roll it out on a pizza stone, which can be put directly in the oven.

MORE HEART HELPERS

Here are other ingredients you can add to your pizza for flavor and heart-helping benefits. *All can be added before putting the pizza in the oven (or on the grill)...*

- **Cooked, sliced beets.** Beets contain nutrients that help to naturally reduce blood pressure.
- **Avocado slices contain heart-healthy monounsaturated fats.**
- **Chopped walnuts and almonds, rich in plant sterols, prevent the absorption of cholesterol.**
- **Dried herbs and spices.** Their anti-inflammatory, heart-helping antioxidant value is concentrated. Sprinkle on oregano, sumac, cumin, rosemary, basil, thyme or pepper.

FOUR STEPS TO PERFECT PIZZA

Pizza really is quite simple to make, especially if you use prepared dough. You can even cook it on the grill.

Here are four easy steps for making pizza in your kitchen...

1. Preheat your oven to 450°F.

2. Roll out your crust thinly, to about one-quarter-inch thickness on a cornmealed or seeded surface.

3. Ladle the sauce...layer the tomatoes...scatter the onions, garlic and chiles...sprinkle on the arugula and cheese (and anchovies if using).

4. Bake until golden, about 10 minutes. Let cool for five minutes before slicing.

Chocolate: Yummy and Healthful

Janet Bond Brill, PhD, RDN, FAND, is a registered dietitian nutritionist, a fellow of the Academy of Nutrition and Dietetics and a nationally recognized nutrition, health and fitness expert who specializes in cardiovascular disease prevention. Based in Allentown, Pennsylvania, Dr. Brill is author of *Blood Pressure DOWN, Cholesterol DOWN* and *Prevent a Second Heart Attack*. DrJanet.com

---

Dark chocolate—with a high content of cocoa—is now considered a bona fide health food and a guilt-free superfood! You may have heard that it can be good for your heart. It's been linked to reduced arterial inflammation, for example, and lowered blood pressure, particularly in people who have hypertension. To get the heart benefits, the recommended "dose" of dark chocolate is approximately 30 g to 60 g per day (roughly one to two ounces, or one to two squares). But those aren't the only salutary effects from dark chocolate. An increasing body of evidence shows an even broader range of potential health benefits—from improving short-term memory and alertness by increasing blood flow to the brain...to curbing diabetes risk by improving the body's response to insulin.

What is the magic ingredient in dark chocolate? Flavonoids—the powerful, disease-fighting subclass of polyphenols (plant chemicals) that pervade the plant kingdom. And cocoa contains lots of them. In fact, dark chocolate has such a highly concentrated amount of flavonoids that it beats out tea and red wine, ounce for ounce, and has almost five times the amount of these miraculous plant chemicals than an apple. *Here is one of my favorite dark chocolate recipes...*

EUROPEAN TO-DIE-FOR DECADENT HOT CHOCOLATE

1½ cups 1% milk
½ cup soy creamer
1 packet Splenda (or sweetener of choice)
1 teaspoon instant coffee
8.8-ounce Trader Joe's Pound Plus 72% Cacao Dark Chocolate bar (half the bar), chopped into small pieces
Fat-free whipped cream

Directions: Over medium heat, whisk together in a medium saucepan the milk, creamer, sweetener and instant coffee until small bubbles form around the edge (but don't let the mixture boil). Add the chopped chocolate pieces. Stir until melted, about five minutes. Serve in espresso cups (one-quarter cup is rich enough to satisfy any chocoholic) and top with a squirt of fat-free whipped cream. Makes eight servings (one-quarter cup each).

Nutrition information per serving: Calories, 190...fat, 15 g...cholesterol, 5 mg...carbohydrates, 18 g...sugar, 11 g...protein, 4 g...sodium, 40 mg.

Shopping for chocolate: To ensure that you're getting enough cocoa and not too much sugar, always opt for dark chocolate—not milk. To start, do a quick check of the label to make sure that the first ingredient on your chocolate bar is chocolate or cacao and not sugar.

Note: All chocolate products are made from the beans of the cacao tree. Also, pay close attention to the percentage number on the wrapper. This indicates the percentage of the bar's weight that comes from the cacao bean. (Aim for at least 65%.) The higher the percentage of cocoa, the lower the sugar content.

Important: If you're using cocoa powder, skip the "alkalized" or "Dutch-processed" varieties—two flavonoid-robbing manufacturing procedures.

Good product: Natural, unsweetened Hershey's 100% Cocoa.

And remember that chocolate is highly caloric, so be sure to eat it by the piece and not by the pound!

The Best Cinnamon

Bonnie Taub-Dix, MA, RDN, CDN, author of *Read It Before You Eat It* and nutrition expert in New York City. BetterThanDieting.com

Cinnamon is a delicious spice with antioxidant properties. To receive the biggest health boost, choose Ceylon cinnamon, also known as "true" cinnamon. It's available at specialty-food stores and online. The other, more common type is Chinese or Saigon cinnamon (also called cassia), which is the less expensive kind typically found in supermarket cinnamon brands. Both have healthy antioxidants, but Ceylon cinnamon is more potent. Cassia also has coumarin, a blood thinner that can interact with blood-thinning drugs. However, it's unlikely that consuming this type of cinnamon will cause health risks, since you would have to eat at least 6 g (nearly three jars) of it! Use a teaspoon of cinnamon daily in hot cereal or yogurt.

Foods That Are Good for Your Gut

Roundup of experts on foods that are good for the gut, reported at Health.com.

Foods that are good for the gut because they nourish the helpful intestinal bacteria: Oatmeal, which contains a fiber that may help protect the colon against damage and can help control cholesterol…Jerusalem artichokes, root vegetables filled with beneficial prebiotic fiber…leftover pasta develops resistant starch that helpful bacteria convert to an anti-inflammatory compound…walnuts, which, if eaten regularly, may increase levels of bacteria associated with reduced inflammation and improved insulin sensitivity…freekeh, a form of wheat with very high fiber content, which helps to feed the good bacteria and also helps to keep you feeling full longer…kefir, a fermented milk drink typically containing at least 10 strains of healthful probiotics.

Live Longer by Taking Oatmeal to a Whole New Level

Qi Sun, MD, ScD, assistant professor, department of nutrition, HarvardSchool of Public Health and assistant professor of medicine, Channing Division of Network Medicine, Brigham and Women's Hospital, both in Boston. His study appeared in *JAMA Internal Medicine.*

Sam Stephens, Quaker Oats chief creative oatmeal officer and owner of OatMeals Restaurant in New York City.

Did you know that more than 40% of Americans never eat whole grains? No wonder the US population is plagued by heart disease, diabetes and obesity. Meanwhile, research continues to accumulate that regular consumption of whole grains—at least three servings a day—can reduce cholesterol and blood sugar levels, lower the risk of type 2 diabetes and cardiovascular disease, boost immunity and improve your digestion and bowel function. And because they're chock-full of fiber and make you feel full longer, they can also help you lose weight.

Bottom line—whole grains can extend your life. This was recently proven by researchers from Harvard University. They followed more than 100,000 people for more than 24 years to confirm that a higher intake of whole grains was associated with a lower risk of premature death from cardiovascular disease. Compared with people who rarely ate whole grains, people who ate the equivalent of just one bowl of oatmeal daily reduced their risk of early death by 9% and their risk of death from heart disease by 15%. Each additional ounce of whole grains per day reduced risk of early death by another 5% and risk of death from cardiovascular disease by another 9%.

Maybe you're not crazy about the taste of a bowl of oatmeal? Then try the recipes below!

EXOTIC OATMEAL MAKEOVERS

To get more whole grains in your diet, think beyond breakfast. Of course, you can opt for whole-grain sandwich bread or whole-grain pasta or serve cornmeal polenta or a whole-grain pilaf instead of white rice or potatoes—but why not try something really different and adventurous? Do something really creative and scrumptious with oatmeal...

Here are two hearty and exotically flavorful recipes from chef Sam Stephens, owner of OatMeals Restaurant in New York City. One recipe puts a Latin twist on oatmeal, the other an Asian one. The main ingredient in both is steel-cut oats, which are more flavorful, chewier (in a good way) and less processed than rolled oats. Many people who don't like rolled oats find that they love steel-cut oats—so give these a try.

CUBAN-STYLE BLACK BEANS AND PLANTAINS OVER OATMEAL

Ingredients for four servings:
1 cup steel-cut oats
2 tablespoons olive oil
2 firm, ripe plantains, peeled and sliced lengthwise into 2-inch pieces
1 whole large onion, diced
1 whole green pepper, diced
2 15-oz. cans of black beans, rinsed and drained
½ cup chicken broth/stock
1 teaspoon cumin
1 pinch of salt and pepper to taste
Fresh cilantro leaves (optional)
Fresh sliced avocado (optional)
Queso fresco cheese (optional)

Cook the oats according to the package directions, and set aside but keep warm.

Heat 1 tablespoon of olive oil in a medium skillet over medium heat, and sauté the sliced plantains in it for four to five minutes until they are golden and slightly browned.

Remove them from the pan, and then heat the remaining tablespoon of olive oil and sauté the diced onion and green pepper for five to seven minutes until the onion is translucent and beginning to brown.

Add the beans, chicken stock, cumin, salt and pepper to the pan, and cook for another five to eight minutes until the beans are heated.

Divide the oatmeal into four servings, and top with the black beans and the plantains. If desired, garnish the dish with fresh cilantro, sliced avocado and cheese.

THAILAND SMILES (FOR PEANUT LOVERS)

Ingredients per serving:
¼ cup steel-cut oats
2 tablespoons flaked coconut
1 tablespoon chopped peanuts (roasted and salted)
¼ cup diced or crushed pineapple (canned or fresh)
1 tablespoon creamy peanut butter
1½ teaspoons hot sauce
1 lime wedge
1 tablespoon chopped fresh cilantro

Cook the oatmeal according to package directions, and set aside but keep warm.

Toss the coconut, peanuts and pineapple together.

Blend the peanut butter and hot sauce.

Top the oatmeal with the coconut, peanuts and pineapple, and drizzle with the peanut butter and hot sauce mixture.

Garnish with a wedge of lime and fresh cilantro.

Whole Grains to the Rescue

Holly Lucille, ND, RN, a naturopathic doctor based in West Hollywood, California. She is the author of *Creating and Maintaining Balance: A Woman's Guide to Safe, Natural Hormone Health* and serves on the board of directors for the Institute for Natural Medicine. DrHollyLucille.com

Everyone knows that eating ample amounts of fruits and vegetables can lower cholesterol, promote weight control and help prevent heart attack, stroke, diabetes and some types of cancer. But few people realize that whole grains are just as good as fruits and vegetables—and sometimes even better—at fighting many of these serious illnesses.

Fiber gets most of the credit for the healthful properties of whole grains, but studies have found that the phytochemicals, antioxidants, vitamins and minerals found in whole grains, which contain all parts of the grain, are just as important.

*The whole grains described below can be found at most health-food stores and many grocery stores...**

AMARANTH

What it's good for: This tiny grain with an earthy, faintly grassy taste may protect against heart disease and cancer. It is also an excellent source of complete protein—that is, one that contains all eight essential amino acids.

Major effective ingredients: Vitamins E and B. Amaranth is also rich in calcium, phosphorus and iron.

How to add it to your diet: As it cooks, amaranth releases a glutinous starch that adds body to soups and stews.

BROWN RICE

What it's good for: Helps fight eye disease (macular degeneration) and certain cancers, including lung cancer.

Major effective ingredients: Vitamin E and other antioxidants.

How to add it to your diet: Season brown rice as you would white rice, or it can be added to soups, casseroles, stir-fry dishes and salads.

CORN

What it's good for: Helps fight heart disease and cancer... and may guard against cataracts.

Major effective ingredients: Of all the grains, whole-grain corn is the richest source of antioxidants. It's also a good source of insoluble fiber, which cannot be digested but adds bulk to the stool.

How to add it to your diet: Choose whole-grain corn-based cereals, whole-grain cornmeal breads and cornmeal tortillas.

OATS AND BARLEY

What they are good for: Lowering cholesterol.

Major effective ingredient: Soluble fiber. When soluble fiber is digested, it changes to a gummy consistency that lowers blood cholesterol. The exact mechanism of this effect is not yet known.

*For recipes using whole grains, read *Whole Grains Every Day Every Way* by Lorna Sass or visit the website of the Whole Grains Council, WholeGrainsCouncil.org.

How to add oats to your diet: Choose an oat cereal or oatmeal or make oatmeal cookies.

How to add barley to your diet: Use it to thicken soups and make creamy risottos, or cook it with carrots.

RYE

What it's good for: Protects against heart disease and hormone-dependent cancers, such as breast and prostate malignancies.

Major effective ingredient: Rye is a rich source of lignans, a class of phytoestrogens (plant compounds that help protect against the harmful effects of excess estrogen).

How to add it to your diet: Use whole-grain rye bread or whole-grain rye crackers.

WHEAT

What it's good for: It has a laxative effect that aids digestion and also is high in vitamins, minerals and antioxidants.

Major effective ingredient: Insoluble fiber.

How to add it to your diet: Replace white bread with whole-wheat bread...and highly processed cereals with whole-grain cereals.

Helpful: To ensure that a bread product contains whole grain, the label must include the word "whole."

Example: For whole wheat, look for whole-wheat flour or whole-wheat grain. Breads that contain seven, 12 or even 15 grains are not necessarily whole-grain breads.

Chili Pepper for Long Life

Study of more than 16,000 adults by researchers at University of Vermont, Burlington, published in *PLOS One*.

A chili pepper a day may help you live longer. In a recent study, those who consumed chili peppers on a regular basis had a lower risk for death, especially from heart attack and stroke.

Eat Your Way to Low Cholesterol

Kenneth H. Cooper, MD, MPH, founder of The Cooper Clinic and The Cooper Institute for Aerobics Research, both in Dallas. A leading expert on preventive medicine and the health benefits of exercise, he is author of *Controlling Cholesterol the Natural Way*. CooperAerobics.com

Surprising superfood cuts heart attack risk 35%. If you have high cholesterol, your primary objective should be to find a way to lower it without drugs and their side effects. The good news is that just eating the right foods often can reduce cholesterol by 50 points or more.

Most people know to eat a low-fat diet, but there are certain foods that can help lower cholesterol that may surprise you...

MACADAMIA NUTS

Macadamia nuts are among the fattiest plant foods on the planet, about 76% total fat by weight. However, nearly all of the fat is monounsaturated. This type of fat is ideal because it lowers LDL (bad) cholesterol without depressing HDL (good) cholesterol.

A team at Hawaii University found that study participants who added macadamia nuts to their diets for just one month had total cholesterol levels of 191 mg/dL, compared with those eating the typical American diet (201 mg/dL). The greatest effect was on LDL cholesterol.

Macadamia nuts are higher than other nuts in monounsaturated fat, but all nuts are high in vitamin E, omega-3 fatty acids and other antioxidants. Data from the Harvard Nurses' Health Study found that people who ate at least five ounces of any kind of nut weekly were 35% less likely to suffer heart attacks than those who ate less than one ounce per month.

Caution: Moderation is important because nuts—macadamia nuts, in particular—are high in calories. Limit servings to between one and two ounces daily—about a small handful a day.

RHUBARB

Rhubarb is ideal for both digestive health and lowering cholesterol because it contains a mix of soluble (see "Oats" on the next page) and insoluble fibers.

A study reported in *Journal of the American College of Nutrition* found that participants who ate a little less than three ounces of rhubarb daily for four weeks had an average drop in LDL cholesterol of 9%.

This tart-tasting vegetable isn't only an ingredient in pies. You can cut and simmer the stalks and serve rhubarb as a nutritious side dish (add some low-calorie strawberry jam for a touch of sweetness).

RICE BRAN

It's not as well-known for lowering cholesterol as oats and oat bran, but rice bran is just about as effective and some people enjoy it more. A six-week study at University of California, Davis Medical Center found that people who ate three ounces daily of a product with rice bran had drops in total cholesterol of 8.3% and a reduction in LDL of 13.7%.

You can buy rice bran in most supermarkets—it's prepared like oatmeal. Or you can try prepared rice-bran breakfast cereals, such as Quaker Rice Bran Cereal and Kenmei Rice Bran.

RED YEAST RICE

Made from a yeast that grows on rice, red yeast rice contains monacolins, compounds that inhibit the body's production of cholesterol.

One study found that people who took red yeast rice supplements and did nothing else had drops in LDL of 23%. When the supplements were combined with healthy lifestyle changes, their LDL dropped by about 42%.

Red yeast rice may be less likely than statins to cause the side effect myopathy (a painful muscle disease).

Recommended dose: 600 milligrams (mg), twice daily. It is available online and at health-food stores.

GREEN TEA

Green tea is a concentrated source of polyphenols, which are among the most potent antioxidants. It can lower LDL cholesterol and prevent it from turning into plaque deposits in blood vessels. In one study, men who drank five cups of green tea daily had total cholesterol levels that were nine points lower than men who didn't drink green tea.

Three to five cups daily are probably optimal. Black tea also contains polyphenols but in lower concentrations than green tea.

VITAMINS C AND E

These vitamins help prevent cholesterol in the blood from oxidizing. Oxidized cholesterol is more likely to cling to artery walls and promote the development of atherosclerosis, the cause of most heart attacks.

I advise patients with high cholesterol to take at least 400 international units (IU) of d-alpha-tocopherol, the natural form of vitamin E, daily. You might need more if you engage in activities that increase oxidation, such as smoking.

For vitamin C, take 1,000 mg daily. People who get the most vitamin C are from 25% to 50% less likely to die from cardiovascular disease than those who get smaller amounts.

THE BIG THREE

In addition to the above, some foods have long been known to reduce cholesterol, but they are so helpful that they bear repeating again…

- **Cholesterol-lowering margarines.** I use Benecol every day. It's a margarine that contains stanol esters, cholesterol-lowering compounds that are extracted from plants such as soy and pine trees. About 30 grams (g) of Benecol (the equivalent of about three to four pats of butter) daily will lower LDL by about 14%.

Similar products, such as Promise Buttery Spread, contain sterol esters. Like stanols, they help block the passage of cholesterol from the digestive tract into the bloodstream. We used to think that sterols weren't as effective as stanols for lowering cholesterol, but they appear to have comparable benefits.

- **Oats.** They are among the most potent nutraceuticals, natural foods with medicine-like properties. Both oat bran and oatmeal are high in soluble fiber. This type of fiber dissolves and forms a gel-like material in the intestine. The gel binds to cholesterol molecules, which prevents them from entering the bloodstream.

A Harvard study that analyzed the results of 67 scientific trials found that even a small amount of soluble fiber daily lowered total cholesterol by five points. People who eat a total of 7 g to 8 g of soluble fiber daily typically see drops of up to 10%. One and a half cups of cooked oatmeal provides 6 g of fiber. If you don't like oatmeal, try homemade oat bran muffins. Soluble fiber also is found in such foods as kidney beans, apples, pears, barley and prunes.

Also helpful: Psyllium, a grain that's used in some breakfast cereals, such as Kellogg's All-Bran Bran Buds, and in products such as Metamucil. As little as 3 g to 4 g of psyllium daily can lower LDL by up to 20%.

- **Fish.** People who eat two to three servings of fish a week will have significant drops in both LDL and triglycerides, another marker for cardiac risk. One large study found that people who ate fish as little as once a week reduced their risk for a sudden, fatal heart attack by 52%.

I eat salmon, tuna, herring and sardines. Other good sources of omega-3 fatty acids include walnuts, ground flaxseed, tofu and canola oil.

Fish-oil supplements may provide similar protection, but they are not as effective as the natural food, which contains other beneficial nutrients as well.

Fiber Helps You Live Longer

Yikyung Park, ScD, staff scientist, National Cancer Institute, Bethesda, Maryland, and leader of a study of more than 388,000 people, published in *Archives of Internal Medicine*.

In a recent study, researchers followed more than 388,000 volunteers, ages 50 to 71, and found that men and women who consumed the most fiber were 24% to 59% less likely to die from infections, heart disease or respiratory illness than those who did not.

Possible reason: Fiber may steady blood sugar, lower blood lipids and control inflammation.

Recommended: 21 to 25 grams of fiber daily for women and 30 to 38 grams for men from naturally occurring plant-based sources, such as grains, legumes, vegetables and fruits. Commercially made foods that are fortified with fiber were not studied.

Good and Easy...Eating the Mediterranean Way

Wendy Kohatsu, MD, assistant clinical professor of family medicine at the University of California, San Francisco, and director of the Integrative Medicine Fellowship at the Santa Rosa Family Medicine Residency Program in Santa Rosa, California. Dr. Kohatsu is also a graduate of the Oregon Culinary Institute.

There is abundant scientific evidence on the health benefits of the so-called Mediterranean diet, which promotes the traditional eating habits of long-lived people in such countries as Greece and Italy.

Landmark research: Among the most compelling evidence is one long-term European study of healthy men and women ages 70 to 90.

It found that following the Mediterranean diet as part of an overall healthful lifestyle, including regular exercise, was associated with a more than 50% lower rate of death from all causes over a decade. Numerous studies have associated this type of eating with reduced risk for heart disease, cancer, cognitive decline, diabetes and obesity.

But many Americans are reluctant to try the Mediterranean diet for fear that it will be difficult or costly to follow because it emphasizes such foods as omega-3–rich fish, vegetables and nuts.

Surprising findings: Mediterranean eating does not increase food costs, according to a recent study—and this style of eating need not be complicated.

Below, Wendy Kohatsu, MD, an assistant clinical professor of family medicine at the University of California, San Francisco, and a chef who conducts cooking demonstrations for patients and doctors, explains the best ways to incorporate Mediterranean eating into your daily diet...

EASY WAYS TO GET STARTED

To effectively tap into the Mediterranean diet's powerful health benefits, it's important to know exactly which foods should be eaten—and in what quantities.

Start by getting four to five daily servings of whole grains (one serving equals one-half cup of cooked quinoa, brown rice or whole-wheat pasta, for example, or one slice of whole-wheat bread) and two to three daily servings of low- or nonfat dairy products (such as yogurt, cottage cheese or milk), which are an important source of bone-protecting calcium. *In addition, be sure to consume...*

- **Oily fish.** This high-quality protein contains abundant omega-3 fatty acids, which help fight the inflammation that plays a role in cardiovascular disease, Alzheimer's disease and asthma.

Best choices: Follow the acronym SMASH—salmon (wild)...mackerel (Spanish, not king, which tends to have higher levels of mercury)...anchovies...sardines...and herring.

How much: Three ounces (the size of a deck of cards), twice a week.

Chef's secret: Drain canned sardines (the large size), grill briefly, sprinkle with fresh lemon juice and chopped parsley.

Beware: Some fish—such as shark, swordfish, golden bass (tilefish), king mackerel and albacore tuna—can be high in mercury. Avoid these. If you eat tuna, choose the "light" version, which contains less mercury than albacore tuna does.

If you don't like fish: Take a fish oil supplement (1,000 mg daily). Choose a brand that guarantees that no lead or mercury is present.

My favorite brands: Carlson's and Nordic Naturals.

Vegetarians can get omega-3s from flaxseed, walnuts and other nonfish sources. However, nonfish food sources of omega-3s are largely in the form of alpha-linolenic acid (ALA), which is not as potent as the more biologically powerful fatty acids found in fish. Algae-derived docosahexaenoic acid (DHA) capsules contain the omega-3s found in fish. The recommended dose of DHA capsules is 1,000 mg daily.

What most people don't know: A small but important study shows that eating oily fish with beans, such as lentils and chickpeas (also known as garbanzo beans), improves absorption of the iron found in beans.

- **Olive oil.** Olive oil contains about 77% healthful monounsaturated fats. Olive oil is also high in sterols, plant extracts that help reduce LDL "bad" cholesterol and increase HDL "good" cholesterol.

Best choice: Look for extra-virgin (or "first-press") olive oil. ("Extra virgin" means that the oil is derived from the first pressing of the olives.)

How much: Use olive oil as your primary fat—in salad dressings, marinades and sautées. To minimize your total daily intake of fat, do not exceed 18 g to 20 g of saturated fat and 0 g of trans fat from all food sources.

Chef's secret: If you dislike the "grassy" taste of some extra-virgin olive oils, look for Spanish and Moroccan versions, which tend to be more mellow. One good choice is olive oil made from the arbequina olive, which has a buttery taste.

What most people don't know: Nutrients in extra-virgin olive oil may offer some pain-relieving qualities over the long term.

•**Nuts.** Like extra-virgin olive oil, nuts are high in healthful monounsaturated fats. In fact, a recent Spanish study found that a Mediterranean diet that included walnuts significantly lowered risk for heart disease.

What kinds: Besides walnuts, best choices include almonds and peanuts. Choose plain raw nuts—not salted or honey-roasted.

How much: One-quarter cup daily.

Beware: A quarter cup of nuts contains about 200 calories. Eat only a small handful daily—for example, about 23 almonds or 35 peanuts. If you're allergic to nuts, try pumpkin, sunflower or sesame seeds instead.

Chef's secret: Store nuts in your freezer to prevent them from going rancid.

•**Fruits and vegetables.** Many of the most healthful vegetables—including those of the brassica family, such as cabbage, kale, broccoli and cauliflower—originated in the Mediterranean area.

What kinds: Choose brightly colored fruit, such as citrus and berries, and vegetables, such as spinach, watercress, beets, carrots and broccoli.

How much: Five to nine servings daily. (A serving is one-half cup of cooked vegetables, one cup of leafy greens, one medium orange or one-half cup of berries.)

Contrary to popular belief, frozen vegetables, which are often far less costly than fresh produce, are just as nutritious—if not more so because they're frozen at their peak level of freshness and don't spoil in the freezer.

Chef's secret: Cooking tomatoes in olive oil concentrates the tomatoes' levels of lycopene, a powerful antioxidant that has been associated with a decreased risk for prostate, lung and stomach cancers.

PQQ: The Nutrient You've Never Heard Of

Karen R. Jonscher, PhD, associate professor, department of anesthesiology, University of Colorado Anschutz Medical Campus, Denver, and lead author of study titled "Pyrroloquinoline Quinone Prevents Developmental Programming of Microbial Dysbiosis and Macrophage Polarization to Attenuate Liver Fibrosis in Offspring of Obese Mice," published in *Hepatology Communications*.

It's not likely that you've heard of PQQ, or pyrroloquinoline quinone (say that three times fast!), but research is showing that this antioxidant with a funny name has the potential for wide-ranging benefits on many health fronts...

LIVER HEALTH

NAFLD or nonalcoholic fatty liver disease (too much fat in the liver, not from excessive drinking) is a growing epidemic that affects approximately three times as many American adults as diabetes. Unchecked, it can progress to cirrhosis and liver cancer and is predicted to become the leading cause of liver failure and death due to liver disease within the next two decades. Now, research at the University of Colorado Anschutz Medical Campus has found that PQQ can prevent the progression of NAFLD in mice and could hold the potential for stemming the disease in people.

BRAIN HEALTH

A small clinical trial done in Japan showed that elderly participants who were given PQQ had better blood flow in the brain, so it's possible that PQQ could help prevent the decrease in memory and attention that often comes with age.

CHOLESTEROL LEVELS

A separate Japanese study found that PQQ decreased the LDL ("bad") cholesterol levels in middle-aged participants (40 to 57 years old) whose cholesterol levels were in the normal-to-moderately high range.

BONE HEALTH

Osteoporosis is not limited to women—it's also a health concern for older men. Researchers at the Nanjing Medical University in China showed that in the lab, PQQ holds the possibility of helping prevent osteoporosis in male mice caused by low testosterone (levels of the hormone naturally decline with age)—it helped prevent DNA damage and stimulated bone cell formation.

PQQ: WHAT'S NEXT

Despite all this research, study of PQQ is still in the early stage. All of these studies used supplements and were either lab tests involving mice (and very high doses of PQQ) or very small human clinical trials. That means that large, controlled studies on people are needed before experts can draw sweeping conclusions about PQQ's effects on the human body. If these results continue to prove out, we might learn that adding PQQ to our diets could very well help protect the liver, keep bones and joints healthy, and improve brain function, said Karen Jonscher, PhD, associate professor at the University of Colorado and lead author of the study.

What about the PQQ supplements already on store shelves? Dr. Jonscher said that, according to GRAS (generally regarded as safe) notices from the FDA, commercially available PQQ taken once a day in a 10- to 20-milligram pill is well within the safe range—human studies have tested doses up to 60 mg per day short-term and 20 mg per day for 2 years with no adverse effects.

Even so, whenever you are considering taking a new supplement, particularly if you take any other medications or supplements, you should discuss it with your physician and even a pharmacist to learn of any known potential interactions or other concerns, Dr. Jonscher cautioned. And definitely do so if you're interested in consuming higher levels of PQQ to fight a disease such as NAFLD.

GETTING YOUR PQQS FROM FOOD

Until we learn more about the most effective supplement dose of PQQ, eating foods high in the antioxidant can give you access to its potential benefits.

Good-for-you-foods that are also naturally high in PQQ include...

- **Green peppers**
- **Spinach**
- **Parsley**
- **Kiwi**
- **Papaya**
- **Fermented soybeans (natto)**
- **Tofu**
- **Oolong and green tea**

Foods That Jump-Start Metabolism

Roundup of experts in nutrition and fitness, reported in *Health.*

Foods that boost metabolism and help you burn more calories...

Egg whites, which are rich in amino acids that stoke metabolism...lean meat, which contains iron (deficiencies in the mineral can slow metabolism)...cold water, which forces your body to use calories to warm up and keeps you hydrated...chili peppers, which contain the metabolism-boosting chemical capsaicin...caffeinated coffee...green tea, which contains a compound that promotes fat burning...and milk, which contains calcium that can help you metabolize fat more efficiently.

Ketogenic Diet: More Than a Weight-Loss Fad

Tanya J. W. McDonald, MD, PhD, a practicing epileptologist and assistant professor of neurology in the department of neurology at the Johns Hopkins University School of Medicine in Baltimore. Her research interests include dietary therapies for adults with epilepsy, evaluations for seizure surgery and epilepsy in women. She is lead author of "The Expanding Role of Ketogenic Diets in Adult Neurological Disorders," a review article published in *Brain Sciences*.

The ketogenic diet has shaped up as the biggest weight-loss trend of the last few years.

What's not being talked about: Even though there are positive anecdotal reports on using this high-fat, very-low-carbohydrate diet for weight loss—and research is promising (see below)—few people know about its current and potential uses for neurological conditions and other chronic diseases...

NEUROLOGICAL CONDITIONS

• **Epilepsy.** Diet therapy was a common epilepsy treatment until the development of antiseizure drugs in the 1930s. Now researchers are taking a second look at the ketogenic diet because some patients with epilepsy are drug-resistant—that is, they have failed to respond to two different medications...and have less than a 5% chance of becoming seizure-free with the use of additional drugs.

Scientific evidence: Research has confirmed that 40% to 50% of adults with epilepsy will improve on the diet with the most benefits seen in patients who stick with it.

Among the many possible mechanisms, the diet is thought to dampen the brain-cell "excitability" that's associated with seizures. It also improves the balance of intestinal bacteria, which appears to provide seizure protection.

The ketogenic diet doesn't replace anti-epilepsy drugs—most patients will continue to take medication, although many will require fewer drugs and/or a lower dose. I advise a variety of epilepsy patients to try the diet for at least three months. If it's effective, they stick with it. If not, they slowly resume their consumption of carbohydrates, under the supervision of a medical professional or nutritionist.

• **Brain cancer.** Glioblastoma, a type of malignant glioma, is the most frequently diagnosed primary brain tumor. Early research suggests that a ketogenic diet could help patients with this type of cancer, particularly when combined with radiation and/or other treatments.

In laboratory studies, animals given a ketogenic-like diet showed improved survival times of 20% to 30%. Small studies—many of them case reports (descriptions of individual patients)—have shown improvements in disease progression and survival.

The diet may help because the cells that fuel cancer depend on glucose as an energy source. When you take away glucose with a ketogenic diet, cancer cells may lose the ability to proliferate.

My advice: If you or a loved one has been diagnosed with this type of cancer, ask your doctor if a ketogenic diet might help—and if he/she recommends participating in one of the clinical trials listed at ClinicalTrials.gov. (There are also trials that focus on the use of this diet for other types of cancer.)

• **Alzheimer's disease.** Like the cancer cells described above, the amyloid deposits that are the hallmark of Alzheimer's may depend on high levels of glucose in the blood.

In laboratory studies, animals given extracts that put their bodies into a ketosis-like state (see "How the Diet Works" on next page) showed improved learning and memory. Studies involving Alzheimer's patients or those with mild cognitive impairment have shown that people given similar extracts had improvements in working memory and visual attention.

My advice: Because the research is too preliminary to conclude that the diet is—or isn't—effective for this purpose, I wouldn't advise Alzheimer's patients to try the diet without close medical supervision. But if you've been diagnosed with Alzheimer's—or have a high risk of developing it—you might want to discuss it with your doctor.

OTHER USES

• **Weight loss.** The ketogenic diet is a far cry from the plant-rich diets that most experts recommend for weight loss. In its most restrictive form, it limits many vegetables, fruits, beans and grains—all of the foods that can help you lose weight.

Yet people who switch to a ketogenic diet (the plans for weight loss are somewhat less restrictive than those used for some of the conditions described above) do lose weight—and they lose it quickly.

Caveats: Most experts agree that people who follow the diet can lose weight. But it doesn't appear to be any more effective than other, more conventional diets, and the drop-out rate is probably much higher.

• **Diabetes.** People with diabetes are usually advised to eat less fat because weight loss and a lower-fat diet have been thought to go hand in hand. But experts are taking another look at the ketogenic diet for diabetes control.

Reasons: Not only can the diet promote weight loss, but there's some evidence that it improves insulin sensitivity and lowers blood sugar.

Caution: People with diabetes who follow a ketogenic diet have an increased risk for diabetic ketoacidosis, a life-threatening condition due to elevated blood sugar and blood acids (ketones).

MORE FROM DR. MCDONALD

How the Diet Works

The term "ketogenic" has become a catchall phrase for any high-fat, low-carbohydrate diet. But in the medical community, the diet calls for a severe restriction of carbohydrates and high amounts of fat. The requirements are so rigorous that the diet should be attempted only with the supervision of a doctor, as with any medical therapy.

How it works: Normally, blood sugar (glucose) from carbohydrates is your main source of energy. But when glucose is restricted, your body starts breaking down fat, a process that releases ketone bodies into the bloodstream. Cells use ketone bodies as an alternative fuel source until you start eating carbohydrates again.

If you stay on the diet long enough, the body enters ketosis. (You experience a mild form of ketosis when you've gone all night without food.) Ketosis mimics a starvation state—it triggers metabolic changes, including those that promote weight loss and improve insulin sensitivity.

The diet emphasizes foods high in fat, moderate in protein and low in carbohydrates (eggs, cheese, avocados, butter, olive oil, cream, bacon, steak, salmon, sardines, nuts, seeds, etc.).

Intermittent Fasting: Easier Than a Diet... and Great for Health

Tina Marinaccio, RDN, integrative registered dietitian nutritionist and adjunct professor in clinical nutrition and food studies at Montclair State University in New Jersey. She leads the nutrition element of Dr. Dean Ornish's Program for Reversing Heart Disease. TinaMarinaccio.com

I am the first to admit that fasting sounds even worse than dieting. But some kinds of fasting can be easier than dieting—and have benefits that go well beyond weight loss. In fact, even people who are not overweight can get amazing benefits from fasting, including healthier hearts, stronger muscles and clearer thinking.

The technical term for what I'm talking about is "intermittent fasting," which means fasting for short periods—sometimes, just 12 hours—on a regular basis. Most intermittent-fast techniques are not daily, and many allow for some calories even on "fast" days. This is definitely not a hunger strike! Some researchers believe that these intermittent fasts are easier to maintain than daily "caloric restriction"—aka traditional dieting, which basically requires that you eat less than you want every single day forever. Intrigued? *Here's more on the benefits of intermittent fasting and how you could easily try it...*

WHY INTERMITTENT FASTING IS SO HEALTHY

Studies have shown that intermittent fasting can help people lose weight without losing muscle. Maintaining muscle is key to keeping weight off and healthy aging. People on intermittent fasts find it easier to control their appetite even on nonfasting days.

One reason: They are producing less insulin, a key "hunger hormone."

But there are many more benefits. These kinds of fasts have been shown to reduce blood pressure... reduce blood glucose levels and improve insulin sensitivity...reduce levels of triglycerides (blood fats) and improve the cholesterol profile...reduce inflammation...enhance muscle endurance...and even improve learning and memory. In animal studies, intermittent fasting can reverse type 2 diabetes, slow the progression of cardiovascular disease and prolong life.

Why is this kind of fasting so good for the body? One hypothesis is that our gut biome—the mix of gastrointestinal bacteria that's key to health—needs a rest to function optimally. In addition, fasting has been shown to help the body get rid of damaged cells and regenerate healthy new ones. Humans likely evolved eating this way—food was scarce, and we couldn't spend every day eating and snacking every few hours like we can now. Periodic fasting respects—maybe even resets—our internal body clocks.

CHOOSING A WAY TO FAST

The best fast is the one that fits into your lifestyle. *Here are three options supported by scientific evidence...*

- **Time-restricted eating.** This is the easiest fast to pull off. Every day, you simply restrict eating to a specific stretch of the day. You'll get the most benefits by limiting yourself to eating during just an eight-hour stretch—say, 10 am to 6 pm. But time-restricted eating is something you can ease into—for example, by restricting your eating to 12 hours... and then gradually scaling back to eight hours.

Eating at night, in particular, interferes with the body's natural day-night cycle, disrupting hormones in a way that favors weight gain. And there's psychology—choosing an endpoint to the day's eating helps eliminate nighttime eating.

Let's face it: No one is sitting in front of the TV at night eating carrot sticks. It's more likely to be ice cream or chips.

Tip: Get most of your calories early in the day, meaning you eat a big breakfast and a smaller lunch and dinner. It's fine to eat breakfast several hours after you wake up—that's healthy as long as it's not paired with late-night eating.

- **Periodic fasting.** On two consecutive days, you cut way back on calories—by 75%. The rest of the week, you eat in a normal fashion. The popular 5:2 Diet is an example of this approach.

- **Alternate-day fasting.** In this approach, you alternate days when you restrict calories—to perhaps 500 calories for the day—with days when you eat a normal, healthy diet. This way of fasting is one day on, one day off. It's effective, but some people find that they are too hungry on fasting days to sustain it.

Tip for periodic or alternate-day fasting: To meet your calorie goal and assure good nutrition on partial-fast days, make protein shakes with fruit and some form of healthy fat, such as ground flax or a no-sugar-added nut butter. A low-sugar plant-protein powder serves as the base. Two brands I like are Vega and Kashi GoLean (I'm fond of the Vanilla Vinyasa flavor).

Caution: Before you start any fast, discuss it with your health-care provider. That's especially important if you have a medical condition. For example, although fasting may help improve diabetes, people who take blood sugar–lowering agents need to be especially careful about low blood sugar. Plus, some medications need to be taken with food.

More tips for successful intermittent fasting...

- **See a registered dietitian (RD).** An RD can help you determine which of the eating patterns—if any—makes sense for you and help you put a plan into place. He/she can help you choose the most nutritious foods (especially important on days when you don't eat as much as you normally do)...and, if you need them, recommend nutritional supplements.

Be extra wary when you eat out on partial-fasting days. Restaurants use more fat and sugar than you would at home, and portions are huge. It's easier to eat at home so that you know what you're taking in.

- **Consider professional metabolic testing.** How can you know what to eat to cut calories by, say, 75%? You start by calculating the calories you burn at rest—your resting metabolic rate, aka RMR—and then add everyday activities plus physical exercise. Online RMR calculators are notably inaccurate.

Better: An FDA-approved calorimeter, which measures your RMR when you breathe into it. These instruments are too expensive to make it worth buying one for home use, but many RDs have them in their offices.

- **"Cheat" with nonstarchy vegetables.** If you find yourself extra-hungry on a fasting day, don't suffer too much. The best way to "cheat" is with low-glycemic vegetables, many of which have lots of filling fiber and all of which have very little effect on blood sugar or insulin levels.

Examples: Salad greens, cruciferous vegetables (broccoli, cabbage, cauliflower, etc.), radishes, zucchini, summer squash, eggplant, tomatoes and mushrooms.

Bonus: These types of vegetables are especially good at feeding beneficial gut bacteria.

One caution, though: Don't pile on potatoes, winter squashes, corn, peas and the like—these are starchy vegetables that you shouldn't cheat with.

The One-Week Detox Diet

The late **Shari Lieberman, PhD, CNS, FACN,** a nutrition scientist in Hillsboro Beach, Florida, who was in private practice for more than 25 years. She was a board member of the Certification Board for Nutrition Specialists, fellow of the American College of Nutrition and coauthor of *User's Guide to Detoxification.*

Every minute of your life, your body is detoxifying—breaking down hundreds of hazardous chemicals that you breathe in or ingest. To do this, your body relies on specific nutrients. Yet even if your everyday diet is reasonably healthful, your body faces an enormous toxic load.

Problem: The world is filled with synthetic toxins—industrial pollutants and car exhaust... fumes from copy machines and dry cleaning... foods grown with pesticides or processed with potentially harmful additives. Chemicals in tobacco and alcohol increase the liver's burden.

Theory: Toxins in the body may lead to cell damage, increasing the risk for disease.

Solution: A one-week detoxification diet, followed four times a year, can give your body a break from the toxic onslaught...replenish healthful nutrients...alleviate cell-damaging inflammation...combat disease...even slow the aging process.

Get your doctor's approval before beginning the one-week detox diet. This regimen may not be appropriate for people with certain chronic health conditions, such as heart disease, a kidney disorder, cancer or anemia. Do not follow the detox diet if you are pregnant or breast-feeding or if you have diabetes or hypoglycemia.

WHAT TO EAT

The majority of the body's self-cleansing takes place in the liver, which uses enzymes to break down hazardous toxins. The dual goal of a one-week detox is to boost intake of nutrients that these enzymes may need...and to lighten the liver's workload by limiting ingestion of additional toxins.

Choose a week when you don't expect to be under stress or eating out a lot. Plan on three meals a day plus two snacks. Eat until satisfied—there's no need to go hungry.

Important: The main components of the detox diet are vegetables and fruits. Buy organic to avoid pesticides that make the liver work harder.

- **Eat a variety of vegetables.** These are loaded with antioxidants and may fuel liver enzymes. Choose any veggies you like—carrots, cucumbers, eggplant, mushrooms, peppers, salad greens, spinach, sprouts, tomatoes. Include sulfur-rich vegetables—asparagus, broccoli, brussels sprouts, cabbage, cauliflower, garlic, onions—which are especially supportive of detoxification enzymes.

Fresh is best, but frozen or canned vegetables are all right if they have nothing added. Eat vegetables raw, steamed or sautéed in a bit of olive oil. Try a salad or crudité platter for lunch...and a medley of cooked vegetables for dinner.

• **Focus on fruit.** Most fruits are rich in antioxidants. Try something new—boysenberries, guavas, kumquats, passion fruit—plus familiar favorites, such as apples, blueberries, cherries and raspberries. Mix up a fruit salad for breakfast...have a pear or an orange as a snack...drink juice with lunch or dinner. Choose fresh or frozen fruits and juices with no added sugar or syrup.

• **Enhance flavor.** Many ready-made salad dressings, dips and sauces contain unhealthful oils and too much sugar and salt.

Better: Make your own using monounsaturated oil, herbs and other healthful ingredients.

For salads: Toss greens with one teaspoon each of olive oil and balsamic vinegar plus a pinch of oregano...or one teaspoon of olive oil plus a splash of lemon juice.

For dipping: Try hummus, made from chickpeas and tahini (ground sesame seeds)...and baba ghanoush, made from eggplant and tahini.

For cooked vegetables: Sprinkle with clove, turmeric or other spices.

• **Add a little protein for energy.** Many people feel energized during a detox week, but others feel tired because they are eating less protein than usual. Nuts and seeds are excellent sources of protein. Choose unsalted varieties to avoid bloating. If energy remains low after the first three days, once or twice a day have a poached or hard-boiled organic egg...four ounces of fish, such as wild Alaskan salmon (try it poached with dill)...or four ounces of baked or broiled free-range chicken.

• **Have eight glasses of filtered water daily.** Staying hydrated helps your body excrete toxins.

• **Drink tea.** Green and white teas are rich in antioxidants. Drink tea hot or over ice. Add a wedge of lemon or lime—this improves absorption of antioxidants.

• **Try "green drinks."** Typically these are made from powdered dehydrated wheatgrass, green barley, vegetables and herbs. Some include the naturally sweet and calorie-free herb stevia. Once a day, stir the label-recommended amount of green drink mix into one cup of water or unsweetened diluted juice.

WHAT NOT TO EAT

Throughout your detox week, avoid foods with a high glycemic index (GI). The GI is a ranking system that indicates a food's potential to cause rapid spikes in blood sugar and insulin levels, which in turn promote cell-damaging inflammation and hinder detoxification.

Helpful: To find the GI of various foods, see GlycemicIndex.com.

Sugar has a very high GI—so avoid foods such as cakes, cookies, donuts, honey, soda and syrup. Other potentially high-GI foods include those made with white flour (bread, crackers) and all types of rice.

Even some vegetables and fruits have a high GI. Avoid or limit consumption of beets, parsnips, potatoes and pumpkin...as well as watermelon, raisins and dates.

Also stay away from dairy foods. Milk contains sugars and proteins that can be difficult to digest.

Many people do not realize that they are sensitive to gluten, a protein found in wheat, rye, barley and many other grains. During detox week, stick to gluten-free grains that have a relatively low GI, such as quinoa and buckwheat.

Avoid alcohol, preservatives and artificial colorings and sweeteners. These can tax the liver.

DETOX SUPPLEMENTS

Throughout your weeklong detox, continue taking whatever supplements you normally take. Also take the three supplements below to enhance detoxification activity (continuing even after the detox week, if desired)...

• **Alpha-lipoic acid.** This antioxidant may help maintain normal liver function and improve glucose metabolism.

Dosage: 100 mg daily. Avoid if you have thyroid problems.

• **Milk thistle extract.** Studies show that this herb protects the liver from toxins...and can lower blood sugar levels.

Dosage: 100 mg to 200 mg daily.

• **N-acetylcysteine (NAC).** This antioxidant is so effective at protecting the liver that hospitals use it to treat overdoses of acetaminophen (Tylenol), which can cause liver failure.

New finding: NAC may help the body excrete mercury, often found in fish.

Dosage: 500 mg daily.

When detox week is over, gradually reintroduce whole grains, lean beef and other healthful foods into your diet, while continuing to eat lots of organic fruits and vegetables. Your liver will benefit—and your whole body will, too.

To Live Longer, Cook This Way

Helen Vlassara, MD, endocrinologist and a coauthor, with Sandra Woodruff, MS, RD, and Gary E. Striker, MD, of *Dr. Vlassara's AGE-Less Diet: How Chemicals in the Foods We Eat Promote Disease, Obesity and Aging, and the Steps We Can Take to Stop It.* TheAge-LessWay.com

When it comes to our health, we often focus on what to eat and what not to eat. But just as important is how we prepare the foods we eat. Certain cooking methods can unleash chemical by-products that have been linked to heart disease, diabetes, Alzheimer's and other chronic diseases.

GLYCOTOXINS

Sugar is a clingy molecule that attaches to amino acids and fats and changes their structures—a process known as glycation. This triggers a complex chemical reaction that culminates in the production of advanced glycation end products (AGEs). They're sometimes called "glycotoxins" because they trigger inflammation and can lead to cell injury and cell death.

Almost all foods contain AGEs. They're naturally produced by the body as well. But their number vastly increases during food preparation, particularly when you cook with dry, high heat.

Small amounts of AGEs aren't a problem—most are excreted through the kidneys. But the foods that many people prefer—particularly those that are high in sugar and fat and are cooked certain ways—are teeming with AGEs. The body can't cope with the excess, so the AGEs pile up over time. *This leads to...*

• **More heart disease.** AGE-modified proteins and fats can accumulate in blood vessel walls and stimulate clots—the cause of most heart attacks.

• **Uncontrolled diabetes.** The high blood glucose (blood sugar) that is the hallmark of diabetes provides fuel for AGE formation. AGEs damage pancreatic cells (resulting in less insulin)...make insulin less effective...and increase diabetes complications, including nerve and blood vessel damage.

• **More cognitive decline.** AGEs damage the protective barrier that insulates the brain from the rest of the body. This allows AGEs to damage brain-specific proteins and produce amyloid plaques—the deposits that occur with Alzheimer's disease. In laboratory studies, animals given a high-AGE diet were much more likely to experience harmful brain changes than those given healthier foods.

• **More kidney disease.** AGEs can injure the blood vessels and other parts of the kidneys. Studies have shown that patients with chronic kidney disease who are treated with a low-AGE diet have a decrease in circulating AGEs, as well as in levels of markers of inflammation and oxidative stress.

The inflammation from excessive AGEs has been linked to many other conditions, including arthritis, obesity, vision problems and even skin wrinkles.

CUT AGEs IN HALF

You can reduce your AGE levels by 50% in as little as one month. *Best steps...*

• **Add moisture, and reduce the heat.** Any form of high-heat cooking—mainly grilling, broiling, frying and roasting—greatly increases AGEs.

Examples: The 500 kilounits (kU) in one serving of raw meat might increase to 5,000 kU after broiling. Moist-heat cooking methods—such as poaching, stewing and braising—are ideal. Consider one serving of chicken. It will contain 600 kU to 1,000 kU when it is stewed or braised, but up to 6,000 kU when it's roasted or grilled.

It is fine to have roasted or grilled food now and then. What's Thanksgiving without roast turkey! But try to limit how often you have these foods.

• **Marinate.** This is a good solution for meat lovers. The acidic ingredients in most marinades—such as lemon juice, wine, tomato juice and vinegar—greatly inhibit AGE formation even when meat is grilled. Depending on the meat's thickness, marinating it for one to two hours will reduce AGEs by up to 50%.

• **Choose lower-AGE foods.** In general, this means eating less meat, cheese and fat and more produce (see the list at right). Beef, poultry and pork have the highest levels of AGEs.

Important: Fatty meats tend to have more AGEs than leaner cuts, but even lean meats will readily produce AGEs when they're prepared with dry heat.

• **Eat minimally processed cheeses.** They aren't cooked, so why are some cheeses so high in AGEs? It is because they're heated during processing and because aging and the removal of liquids during cheese-making increase AGE formation.

My advice: Avoid Parmesan cheese (2,500 kU) and American cheese (2,600 kU).

• **Get more flavonoids.** These are naturally occurring compounds that appear to activate enzymes that deactivate AGEs, inhibit AGE-related oxidation and trap the molecules that can increase AGE formation.

Good sources: Apples, chili peppers, berries, broccoli, kale and green or black tea. Spices and herbs that have similar effects include turmeric, cinnamon, parsley, rosemary and sage.

• **Go easy on the sweets.** Even though sugar and other sweeteners don't contain a lot of AGEs, levels increase when they're heated—when you're baking, for example, or during the factory production of breakfast cereals. High-sugar foods often contain fats and proteins, which increase the potential for harmful chemical reactions.

Warning: The fructose in many soft drinks and processed foods causes a 10-fold greater rate of glycation than simple glucose. Dark-colored soft drinks (such as colas) are particularly bad because the color comes from caramelized (dry-heated) sugars. Diet colas contain nearly the same amount of AGEs as their sweetened counterparts.

MORE FROM HELEN VLASSARA, MD

AGE Counts

• **Very low (100 kU/serv or less)**—Bread; Eggs (poached, scrambled, boiled); Fruits (fresh); Grains (boiled, steamed); Milk; Soy milk; Vegetables (fresh, steamed) and Yogurt.

• **Low (101–500 kU/serv)**—Avocado; Fruits (dried, roasted, grilled); Legumes (cooked, canned); Olive oil; Olives; Pasta; Vegetables (roasted, grilled).

• **Medium (501–1,000 kU/serv)**—Cheese (reduced-fat); Chicken (poached, steamed, stewed, braised); Chocolate (dark); Fish (poached, steamed); Sunflower and pumpkin seeds (raw); Tofu (raw) and Tuna or salmon (canned.)

• **High (1,001–3,000 kU/serv)**—Beef or pork (stewed, braised); Butter; Cheese (full-fat and processed varieties); Fish (grilled, broiled, baked); French fries and Sweets (donuts, pastries, etc.).

• **Very high (3,001–5,000 kU/serv)**—Chicken (skinless, broiled, grilled, roasted); Fish (breaded and fried); Pork chops (pan-fried); Single cheeseburger (fast food); Grilled cheese sandwich; Tofu (broiled, sautéed) and Turkey (roasted)

• **Highest (5,001 kU/serv or more)**—Bacon (fried); Beef (roasted, grilled, broiled, well-done); Chicken with skin (broiled, grilled, roasted); Chicken (fried, fast-food nuggets); Double cheeseburger (fast food); Fish sandwich (fast food); Hot dog; Sausage and Pizza.

Eat This Plus That!

Tonia Reinhard, MS, RD, registered dietitian and professor at Wayne State University, Detroit. She is author of *Superfoods: The Healthiest Foods on the Planet* and *Superjuicing: More Than 100 Nutritious Vegetable and Fruit Recipes*.

Well-chosen food pairings do more than just excite your taste buds. Consuming certain food combos or food and drink combos creates a synergy that increases the absorption of important nutrients and phytochemicals. *Here are four supercharged combinations...*

FISH + WINE

The American Heart Association recommends eating fish at least twice a week. The omega-3 fatty acids in fish have been shown to reduce triglycerides, irregular heartbeats and blood pressure and slow the growth of arterial plaques. It turns out that wine can boost those omega-3 levels.

A large European study looked at the dietary habits and alcohol consumption of more than 1,600 people. The participants underwent comprehensive medical exams and gave blood samples that were used to measure omega-3 levels. Their amount of "marine food intake," defined as the total intake of fish, shellfish, cuttlefish, squid, octopus, shrimp and crab, was also measured.

The researchers found that people who drank moderate amounts of alcohol (one daily drink for women and two for men) had higher concentrations of omega-3s than nondrinkers, despite consuming similar amounts of marine food. Wine drinkers had the biggest gains, but people who drank beer or spirits (such as Scotch) also showed an increase in omega-3s.

Important caveat: The study found that heavy drinkers had lower amounts of omega-3s.

LEMON + TEA

Both black and green teas contain catechins, a group of antioxidants that are surprisingly good for cardiovascular health. A study published in *Stroke,* which looked at more than 83,000 Japanese adults, found that those who drank two to three cups of green tea daily were 14% less likely to have a stroke than those who rarely drank tea.

Tea has been found to reduce cholesterol and reduce the risk for cancer, diabetes and heart disease. But there's a catch—the catechins in tea aren't very durable. They tend to break down during digestion, leaving behind less than 20% of the active compounds.

Tasty solution: Add a squeeze of lemon to your tea. A laboratory study published in *Molecular Nutrition & Food Research* found that combining lemon juice with tea allowed 80% of the catechins to "survive" post-digestion. Orange, lime and grapefruit juices also stabilized the compounds, although not as much as the lemon.

If you prefer bottled to brewed tea, you'll get a similar effect by picking a product that includes vitamin C—listed as ascorbic acid on the label.

CITRUS + IRON-RICH FOODS

Low iron is common in people who take acid-suppressing drugs for GERD and in people who have gastrointestinal problems in which inflammation and bleeding occur (such as inflammatory bowel disease and bleeding ulcers).

Many foods contain iron. Iron-rich animal foods include beef, liver, oysters and sardines. Iron-rich plant foods include dark leafy greens such as spinach, kale and collard greens...beans...lentils... whole grains...and nuts. But iron is not the easiest mineral to absorb. The body can absorb only 2% to 20% of the non-heme iron in plant foods. The absorption of the heme iron from meats and fish/shellfish is better but still not great—typically between 15% and 35%. And certain supplements such as calcium can interfere with iron absorption.

How can you boost absorption of iron? By eating citrus fruits or other vitamin C–rich foods such as strawberries and yellow and red peppers with heme or non-heme foods.

Examples: Add orange slices to your kale salad...or yellow peppers to your beef stew. One study found that consuming as little as 63 mg of vitamin C (a little more than the amount in one orange) nearly tripled the absorption of non-heme iron.

FAT + SALAD

Salads are rich in carotenoids—antioxidants such as lutein, lycopene and beta-carotene that reduce your risk for cancer and heart disease, preserve bone density and prevent macular degeneration. A fat-based salad dressing can maximize the absorption of these carotenoids (so avoid fat-free salad dressings). Researchers at Purdue University served participants salads with dressings made from a monounsaturated fat (canola oil)...a polyunsaturated fat (soybean oil)...or a saturated fat (butter). All the fats boosted absorption of the carotenoids, but the monounsaturated fat required the least amount of fat to get the most carotenoid absorption. Another monounsaturated fat often found in salad dressings is olive oil.

You can get similar benefits by adding hard-boiled eggs to your salad. The fat from the yolks will increase your absorption of carotenoids. In a Purdue University study published in *The American Journal of Nutrition*, participants who ate a salad with one-and-a-half eggs had double the carotenoid absorption of people who had a salad with no eggs.

Move Over Olive Oil!

Torey Armul, MS, RD, LD, a registered dietitian in private practice in Columbus, Ohio, media spokesperson for the Academy of Nutrition & Dietetics and author of *Bun Appétit: A Simple Guide to Eating Right During Pregnancy*.

You've heard that olive oil is best for health. But is it best for all different cooking methods? And what if you want a subtler flavor?

You may be surprised to learn that there are other tasty and nutritious choices. This doesn't mean it's time to ditch your olive oil, but these four oils deserve shelf space for their versatility as well as their health benefits.

Note: Healthy oils play an important role in satiety and flavor of food, but they are still calorie-dense, so portion control counts. Aim for a daily total of one to two tablespoons and maximize their nutritional impact by using a variety of oils.

- **Avocado oil.** Pressed from creamy avocados, avocado oil stands out because of its slightly buttery flavor—great for smoothies, sauces and baked goods.

It's also a top choice for high-heat cooking. That's because it has the highest smoke point of all oils, at 520°F. Smoke point is the temperature an oil can withstand before breaking down. Oil heated beyond its smoke point loses nutritional value and may create harmful carcinogens. (As a point of reference, generic olive oil in general has a medium smoke point of 320°F, which makes it best for sautéing and cooking at low heat. Extra-virgin olive oil's smoke point, however, is higher at 405°F.)

Choose avocado oil for high-heat cooking methods like searing, roasting, barbecuing and frying.

Health benefits: Avocado oil is high in healthy monounsaturated fats, especially oleic acid. These improve blood cholesterol levels, which can reduce the risk for heart disease. Avocado oil's anti-inflammatory nutrients also may help ease inflammation, joint pain and stiffness from arthritis.

- **Sesame oil.** Sesame oil, pressed from sesame seeds, is very versatile. Just read labels carefully. "Pure" sesame oil has a light, nutty flavor and, with a medium-high smoke point of 350°F, can be used for light sautéing. "Toasted" sesame oil, on the other hand, has a very bold taste and is used as a seasoning, not as a cooking oil, to complement the flavors of Indian, African and Asian dishes.

Health benefits: Sesame oil is equally rich in polyunsaturated and monounsaturated fats. Although the ideal amount to have in your diet is not yet known, research shows it can promote heart health by decreasing LDL cholesterol and reducing blood pressure.

- **Flaxseed oil.** Flaxseed oil has a smooth and slightly nutty taste. With a very low smoke point of 225°F, it's most suitable for cold preparations such as salad dressings and dips or as an addition to smoothies and precooked foods.

Health benefits: Flaxseed oil is the best vegetarian source of alpha-linolenic acid (ALA), one of the omega-3 fats known for improving cholesterol levels, lowering triglyceride levels and blood pressure, reducing inflammation and decreasing the risk for certain types of cancer. (Fatty fish contain the other omega-3s—EPA and DHA.) Just one tablespoon provides at least four times the daily recommended amount of ALA.

- **Walnut oil.** Walnut oil is another excellent source of ALA—one tablespoon provides the recommended daily amount. Unrefined walnut oil has a medium smoke point of 320°F. It becomes slightly bitter when heated, so use it for salad dressings or for adding flavor to cooked pasta, poultry, fish or even smoothies.

Health benefits: According to research published in *Journal of the American College of Nutrition*, healthy men and women who substituted 1.3 ounces of walnuts and one tablespoon of walnut oil for other fats in their diets for six weeks had lower resting blood pressure and lower stress-induced blood pressure than those who ate a more typical American diet, despite their calorie intakes being equal.

COOKING OIL TIPS

Look for cold-pressed or unrefined oils. While more expensive, this method extracts oil by putting the fruits or seeds through a press. Refined oils are usually processed with chemicals and undergo bleaching and/or deodorizing. Store flaxseed and sesame oils in the fridge. The other oils may be kept in the fridge or in a dark cabinet, away from heat. Let refrigerated oils come to room temperature before using. All of these oils should be stored in dark, airtight containers.

Recipe for Youth: A Pinch of Basil, an Ancient Herb for Anti-Aging

Vaibhav Shinde, MPharm, lecturer, department of pharmacognosy, Poona College of Pharmacy, Bharati Vidyapeeth University.

Recent research adds more evidence to what practitioners of Ayurvedic natural medicine have believed for thousands of years—Indian basil has anti-aging properties. Popularly known as holy basil (*Ocimum sanctum*) or tulsi, Indian basil was studied by researchers at the Poona College of Pharmacy in Pune, India, and the results were reported at the recent British Pharmaceutical Conference, "Pharmacy in the 21st Century: Adding Years to Life and Life to Years," in Manchester, United Kingdom.

While there are more than 40 varieties of basil (all members of the mint family), holy basil in particular has tremendous cultural importance in India and Nepal and is among the most important herbs in the Ayurvedic tradition. It is used to treat a wide variety of conditions, including stress, heart and respiratory problems, diabetes, digestive and skin disorders, inflammation and pain. In this study, researchers set out to substantiate traditional Ayurvedic beliefs in holy basil's antioxidant and rejuvenation properties.

HOLY BASIL HAS ANTIOXIDANT EFFECT

Experimental groups of mice received either no extract of holy basil or one of three different doses. The findings showed cellular antioxidant effects. Holy basil is highly protective against oxidative damage, with a multidimensional role—it scavenges free radicals, balances the antioxidant enzyme system, and stimulates metabolism of oxidative waste products.

Holy basil is typically ingested in one of two ways...the traditional Ayurvedic method is to boil fresh leaves and water until the water reduces to half. Then you can either drink the resulting "tea" or eat the crushed herb when it cools. However, since it is difficult to find the fresh leaves in the US, you can also use dried holy basil. It is also available as an ingredient in commercially available herbal teas.

Holy basil has a clove-like fragrance and a sharper, spicier taste than the more familiar sweet basil (*Ocimum basilicum*) commonly used in Italian, Asian and American cooking, though the two are closely related. Holy basil can be found online and in health food stores as a supplement and the fresh leaves are available in many Thai and Vietnamese markets. Generally speaking, however, it is more valued for cultural and healing purposes than for cooking.

Great Reasons to Eat More Mushrooms

Men's Health.

Mushrooms are packed with potassium, which helps to keep your blood pressure under control. One cup of cooked white mushrooms contains about 10% of the daily recommended 4,700 milligrams of potassium. They are the only vegetable source of vitamin D, which is linked to a lower risk for cancer, diabetes and hypertension. They have high levels of two powerful antioxidants—ergothioneine and glutathione. They are low in calories but satisfying—a half dozen large white mushrooms contains only 30 calories but are more filling than many other vegetables. So a diet rich in mushrooms could help you lose weight.

Chamomile for Longevity

Bret Howrey, PhD, assistant professor of family medicine, The University of Texas Medical Branch at Galveston.

The popular tea and herbal remedy was linked to a 33% lower risk for death in women, but it had no similar effect on men, according to a recent study of nearly 1,700 adults age 65 and older. Chamomile's beneficial effects may be due to its antioxidant and anti-inflammatory properties, combined with its ability to help reduce anxiety and depression. Women may benefit from drinking chamomile tea daily (but avoid it if you're allergic to ragweed).

Coffee Drinkers Live Longer

Neal D. Freedman, PhD, MPH, cancer prevention fellow, division of cancer epidemiology and genetics, National Cancer Institute, Rockville, Maryland.

Coffee has already been shown by numerous studies to do plenty of wonderful things for your body.

For example, it's well-known that coffee boosts concentration and reduces the risk for heart disease, type 2 diabetes, liver disease, Parkinson's disease, depression and Alzheimer's disease.

Recent research takes this good news a step further, showing that coffee lowers the risk for death from a wide variety of major diseases. In fact, it's the largest study to ever look at the link between coffee and health.

But how many cups do you really have to drink to potentially tack on years to your life? Is it a practical amount...or one of those absurd laboratory amounts that you often see in studies?

BREWING HEALTH BENEFITS

At the start of the study, researchers at the National Cancer Institute in Rockville, Maryland, gave questionnaires to more than 400,000 men and women ages 50 to 71 and asked them to report their coffee intake. They noted whether they drank mostly caffeinated or decaf coffee, what type (regular ground, instant, espresso, etc.) and whether they added products such as cream or sugar.

Results: Regardless of the drink's caffeine content, the way the coffee was made or how much milk and/or sugar was used, the more coffee that people drank—up to about five cups a day—the lower their risk for death at the end of the 13-year study from health problems including heart disease, respiratory conditions, diabetes, stroke and infection. *Check out this chart...*

Coffee per day (ounces)	Reduced risk of dying
8	5% to 6%
16 to 24	10% to 13%
32 to 40	12% to 16%
48 more	10% to 15%

Alas—no association was seen between coffee and death from cancer.

Results differed a little bit between men and women, with the association being slightly stronger for women than men.

MO' JOE, ANYONE?

Coffee's association with a lower death risk doesn't mean that a cause-and-effect relationship between the two was established.

And it's impossible, at this point, to know exactly what properties of coffee may be helpful in preventing death. Coffee's most famous constituent is caffeine, of course, but in reality coffee contains more than 1,000 compounds, including antioxidants and many others. Any of these could play a role.

Back in the mid-1990s, when the study began, a typical cup of coffee out on the street was actually a cup—about eight ounces. But with the rise of specialty coffee shops, today's "cup" is more like two or three cups. (Starbucks' "venti" large size for a hot beverage, for example, is 20 ounces or two and one-half cups—and for a cold beverage, it's 24 ounces or three cups.) So if you're downing a few of today's "mega-cups" of coffee each day, you're getting more ounces than you might realize. But that seems fine. In some people, lots of coffee can lead to side effects, such as the jitters and insomnia—but this study suggests that there's perhaps also a fantastic benefit to America's big coffee habit.

High-Fat Foods Help You Live Longer

Study of 135,335 people, ages 35 to 70, in 18 countries, led by researchers at McMaster University, Ontario, Canada, published in *The Lancet.*

High-fat foods help you live longer, while high-carb intake is linked to increased risk for death.

Recent finding: People who had the highest carbohydrate consumption were 28% more likely to die than those who ate the least amount of carbs.

But the opposite was true for high-fat foods: Those with the highest total fat intake, averaging about 35% of calories from fat, were 23% less likely to die than those with the lowest intake. Higher-fat diets also were associated with lower stroke risk. Increased intake of all types of fat—saturated, polyunsaturated and monounsaturated—was associated with a lower risk for death.

I'm Kicking the Sugar Habit!

Patricia K. Farris, MD, author of the best-seller *The Sugar Detox.* SanovaDermatology.com/locations/old-metairie/

The average American consumes 32 teaspoons of added sugar per day. That's right—32 teaspoons a day.

We all know that sugar can lead to weight gain, but that's just the beginning. People who eat a lot of sugar have nearly double the risk for heart disease as those who eat less, according to data from the Harvard Nurses' Health Study. They're more likely to develop insulin resistance and diabetes. They also tend to look older because sugar triggers the production of advanced glycation end-products (AGEs), chemical compounds that accelerate skin aging.

If you want to avoid these problems, you may want to kick the sugar habit with an easy-to-follow sugar detox. *Here's how...*

- **It's not enough to merely cut back on sugar.** In my experience, patients need to eliminate it from their diets—at least at the beginning—just like addicts have to eliminate drugs from their lives. In fact, a study showed that sugar cravings actually are more intense than the cravings for cocaine.

- **You don't have to give up sugar indefinitely.** Once the cravings are gone, you can enjoy sweet foods again—although you probably will be happy consuming far less than before. After a sugar-free "washing out" period, you'll be more sensitive to sweet tastes. You won't want as much.

Bonus: Some people who have completed the four-week diet and stayed on the maintenance program for four or five months lost 35 pounds or more.

FIRST STEP: THREE-DAY SUGAR FIX

For sugar lovers, three days without sweet stuff can seem like forever. But it's an essential part of the sugar detox diet because when you go three days without any sugar, your palate readjusts. When you eat an apple after the three-day period, you'll think it's the sweetest thing you've ever tasted. You'll even notice the natural sweetness in a glass of whole or 2% milk (which contains about three teaspoons of naturally occurring sugar).

You may experience withdrawal symptoms during the first three days. These can include fatigue, headache, fogginess and irritability, but soon you'll feel better than you have in years.

Caution: If you have any type of blood sugar problem, including hypoglycemia, insulin resistance or diabetes, you must consult your physician before starting any type of diet, including the sugar detox diet. In addition, if you are on insulin or an oral medication to control blood sugar, it is likely that your dosage will need to be adjusted if you lower your daily sugar intake. *During the three days...*

- **No foods or drinks with added sugar.** No candy, cookies, cake, doughnuts, etc.—not even a teaspoon of sugar in your morning coffee.

- **No artificial sweeteners of any kind, including diet soft drinks.** Artificial sweeteners contribute to the sweetness overload that diminishes our ability to taste sugar.

- **No starches.** This includes pasta, cereal, crackers, bread, potatoes and rice.

- **No fruit,** except a little lemon or lime for cooking or to flavor a glass of water or tea. I hesitate to discourage people from eating fruit because it's such a healthy food, but it provides too much sugar when you're detoxing.

- **No dairy.** No milk, cream, yogurt or cheese. You can have a little (one to two teaspoons) butter for cooking.

- **Plenty of protein,** including lean red meat, chicken, fish, tofu and eggs.

- **Most vegetables,** such as asparagus, broccoli, cauliflower, celery, peppers, kale, lettuce and more—but no corn, potatoes, sweet potatoes, winter squash, beets or other starchy vegetables.

- **Nuts—two one-ounce servings a day.** Almonds, walnuts, cashews and other nuts are high in protein and fat, both of which will help you feel full. Nuts also will keep your hands (and mouth) busy when you're craving a sugary snack.

- **Lots of water, but no alcohol.** It's a carbohydrate that contains more sugar than you might think. You can drink alcohol later.

NEXT STEP: A FOUR-WEEK PLAN

This is the fun part. During the three-day sugar "fix," you focused on not eating certain foods. Now you'll spend a month adding tasty but nutritious foods back into your diet. You'll continue to avoid overly sweet foods—and you'll use no added sugar—but you can begin eating whole grains, dairy and fresh fruits.

WEEK 1: **Wine and cheese.** You'll continue to eat healthy foods, but you now can add one apple a day and one daily serving of dairy, in addition to having a splash of milk or cream in your coffee or tea if you like. A serving of dairy could consist of one ounce of cheese...five ounces of plain yogurt...or one-half cup of cottage cheese. You also can have one serving a day of high-fiber crackers, such as Finn Crisp Hi-Fibre or Triscuit Whole Grain Crackers.

You also can start drinking red wine if you wish—up to three four-ounce servings during the first week. Other alcoholic beverages such as white wine, beer and liquor should be avoided. Red wine is allowed because it is high in resveratrol and other antioxidants.

WEEK 2: **More dairy, plus fruit.** This is when you really start adding natural sugar back into your diet. You can have two servings of dairy daily if you wish and one serving of fruit in addition to an apple a day. You can have one-half cup of blackberries, blueberries, cantaloupe, raspberries or strawberries each day. Or you can have a grapefruit half. You'll be surprised how sweet fruit really is. You also are allowed one small sweet potato or yam (one-half cup cubed) daily.

WEEKS 3 AND 4: **Whole grains and more.** The third and fourth weeks are very satisfying because you can start eating grains again. But make sure it's whole grain. Whole grains are high in fiber and nutrients and won't give the sugar kick that you would get from processed grains.

Examples: A daily serving of barley, buckwheat, oatmeal (not instant), quinoa, whole-grain pasta, whole-wheat bread or brown rice.

You might find yourself craving something that's deliciously sweet. Indulge yourself with a small daily serving (one ounce) of dark chocolate.

9

Healthy Heart

14 Little Things You Can Do for a Healthier Heart

Joel K. Kahn, MD, clinical professor of medicine at Wayne State University School of Medicine, Detroit, and founder of The Kahn Center for Cardiac Longevity. He is author of *The Whole Heart Solution: Halt Heart Disease Now with the Best Alternative and Traditional Medicine*. DrJoelKahn.com

Heart disease is America's number-one killer. But just because it's a major health risk does not necessarily mean that you must make major lifestyle changes to avoid it. *Here are 14 simple and inexpensive ways to have a healthier heart...*

DOABLE DIET TIPS

1. Don't eat in the evening. Research suggests that the heart (and digestive system) benefits greatly from taking an 11-to-12-hour break from food every night. One study found that men who indulge in midnight snacks are 55% more likely to suffer from heart disease than men who don't. So if you plan to eat breakfast at 7 am, consider your kitchen closed after 7 or 8 pm.

Warning: You cannot produce the same health benefits by snacking at night and then skipping breakfast. This might create an 11-to-12-hour break from eating, but skipping breakfast actually increases the risk for heart attack and/or death—by 27%, according to one study. Our bodies and minds often are under considerable stress in the morning—that's when heart attack risk is greatest. Skipping the morning meal only adds to this stress.

2. Use apple pie spice as a topping on oatmeal and fruit. Some people enjoy it in coffee, too. This spice combo, which contains cinnamon, cloves, nutmeg and allspice, has been shown to reduce blood pressure, improve cholesterol levels and lower the risk for heart disease.

3. Take your time with your tea. Tea contains compounds called flavonoids that have been shown to significantly reduce the risk for heart disease—green tea is best of all. But you get the full benefits only if you have the patience to let the tea leaves steep—that is, soak in hot water—for at least three to five minutes before drinking.

4. Fill up on salad. It's no secret that being overweight is bad for the heart. But most people don't realize that they can lose weight without going hungry. Salad can make the stomach feel full without a lot of calories. But don't add nonvegetable ingredients such as cheese, meat and egg to salads...and opt for balsamic or red wine vinegar dressing—they are rich in nutrients, including artery-healing resveratrol.

As a bonus, vegetables...and fruits...contain nutrients that are great for the heart regardless of your weight—so great that eating a plant-rich diet could improve your blood pressure just as much as taking blood pressure medication. In fact, one study found that increasing consumption of fruits and vegetables from 1.5 to eight servings per day decreases the risk for heart attack or stroke by 30%.

One strategy: Become a vegetarian for breakfast and lunch. That way you still can enjoy meat at dinner, but your overall vegetable consumption will be increased.

5. Marinate meat before grilling it. Grilling meat triggers a dramatic increase in its "advanced glycation end products" (AGEs), which stiffen blood vessels and raise blood pressure, among other health drawbacks. If you're not willing to give up your grill, marinate meat for at least 30 minutes before cooking it. Marinating helps keep meat moist, which can slash AGE levels in half. An effective marinade for this purpose is beer, though lemon juice or vinegar works well, too. You can add herbs and oil if you wish.

6. Sprinkle Italian seasoning mix onto salads, potatoes and soups. This zesty mix contains antioxidant-rich herbs such as oregano, sage, rosemary and thyme, which studies suggest reduce the risk for heart disease and cancer.

7. Avoid foods that contain dangerous additives. There are so many food additives that it's virtually impossible to keep track of them all. Focus on avoiding foods that list any of the following seven among their ingredients—each carries heart-related health risks. The seven are aspartame...BHA (butylated hydroxyanisole)...BHT (butylated hydroxytoluene)...saccharin...sodium nitrate...sodium sulfate...and monosodium glutamate (MSG).

8. Savor the first three bites of everything you eat. When people eat too fast, they also tend to eat too much. One way to slow down your eating is to force yourself to pay close attention to what you are eating. If you cannot do this for an entire meal or snack, at least do it for the first three mouthfuls of each food you consume. Chew these initial bites slowly and thoroughly. Give the food and its flavor your undivided attention, and you will end up eating less.

9. Prepare your lunch the night before if you won't be home for your midday meal. People who intend to make their lunch in the morning often are in too much of a rush to do so...then wind up resorting to fast food.

10. Buy organic when it counts. Higher pesticide levels in the blood predict higher cholesterol levels as well as cardiovascular disease. Organic food is free of pesticide—but it can be expensive. The smart compromise is to buy organic when it counts most—when traditionally grown produce is most likely to contain pesticide residue. According to the Environmental Working Group, the foods most likely to contain pesticide residue are apples, celery, cherry tomatoes, collard greens, cucumbers, grapes, hot peppers, kale, nectarines, peaches, potatoes, spinach, strawberries, summer squash and sweet bell peppers.

Important: If your options are eating conventionally farmed fruits and vegetables or not eating fruits and vegetables at all, definitely consume the conventionally grown produce. The health risks from small amounts of pesticide residue are much lower than the health risks from not eating produce.

EASY LIFESTYLE HABITS

11. Stand two to five minutes each hour. Recent research suggests that sitting for extended periods is horrible for your heart. Sitting slows your metabolism and reduces your ability to process glucose and cholesterol. But standing for as little as two to five minutes each hour seems to significantly reduce these health consequences (more standing is even better). Stand while making phone calls or during commercials. Buy a "standing desk," then stand when you use your computer.

12. Take walks after meals. Walking is good anytime, but walks after meals have special health benefits, particularly after rich desserts. A 20-minute postmeal stroll significantly improves the body's ability to manage blood sugar. Maintaining healthful blood sugar levels reduces risk for coronary artery blockage.

13. Exercise in brief but intense bursts. Research suggests that exercising as intensely as possible for 20 seconds...resting for 10 seconds...then repeating this seven more times provides nearly the same benefits for the heart as a far longer but less intense workout. Try this with an exercise bike, rowing machine, elliptical machine or any other form of exercise. Do an Internet search for "Tabata training" to learn more. There are free apps that can help you time these intervals. Download Tabata Stopwatch in the iTunes store if you use an Apple device...or Tabata Timer for HIIT from Google Play if you use an Android device.

Caution: Talk to your doctor. High-intensity training could be dangerous if you have a preexisting health condition.

14. Get sufficient sleep. One study found that the rates of heart disease for people who get seven to eight hours of sleep a night are nearly half those of people who get too little or too much sleep.

5 Surprising Ways to Prevent a Heart Attack

Barry A. Franklin, PhD, director of preventive cardiology and cardiac rehabilitation at William Beaumont Hospital, Royal Oak, Michigan. Dr. Franklin has served as president of the American Association of Cardiovascular and Pulmonary Rehabilitation and the American College of Sports Medicine. He is also coeditor of *The Heart-Healthy Handbook,* available at HealthyLearning.com.

There are hopeful signs that Americans are increasingly embracing a heart-healthy lifestyle. The percentage of smokers has plunged to approximately 15% over the last decade. Many people are eating better and doing a better job of controlling high blood pressure and elevated cholesterol.

But despite these gains, cardiovascular disease still accounts for one out of three deaths in the US. Much of the blame goes to the obvious culprits that fuel heart disease—cigarette smoking, elevated blood cholesterol, high blood pressure, obesity, diabetes and a lack of exercise, to name a few. But others might surprise you.

SMALL CHANGES COUNT

Research shows that our daily habits account for 40% to 50% of all deaths caused by cardiovascular disease. The good news is that even small lifestyle choices may offer big benefits. *Five little things you can do to reduce heart attack risk...*

***SECRET #1:* Avoid secondhand smoke.** Most people associate secondhand smoke with lung disease—but the danger to the heart is worse than you may realize.

Here's why: Exposure to cigarette smoke—from smoking yourself or from secondhand smoke—increases arterial inflammation and impairs the ability of arteries to dilate and constrict normally. It also makes blood more likely to coagulate, the major cause of heart attacks.

If you live with an indoor smoker or spend time in other smoke-filled environments, your risk for a heart attack is 30% higher than in someone without this exposure. Cities (and countries) that have adopted public-smoking bans have reported reductions in heart attacks of 20% to 40%—with most of the reductions occurring in nonsmokers.

***SECRET #2:* Know your family genes.** If you have inherited gene variants known to increase the risk for heart disease, your risk of developing coronary disease and having a cardiac event is higher than you probably think. In an important new study, researchers from Massachusetts General Hospital followed more than 55,000 participants for up to 20 years, analyzing genetic variants and lifestyle data. Conclusion: People with a genetic predisposition for heart disease had nearly double the risk of developing it themselves.

But bad genes don't have to be destiny. The same study found that people who made positive changes in two or three out of four common areas known to negatively impact heart health—smoking, obesity, lack of regular exercise and an unhealthful diet—were able to reduce their cardiovascular risks by nearly 50%.

***SECRET #3:* Get a flu shot.** The flu can be deadly, yet fewer than half of at-risk Americans (including those with chronic health conditions, such as cardiovascular and/or lung disease) get an annual vaccination.

Why it matters: The fever, dehydration and pneumonia that often accompany the flu can be devastating for people who have cardiovascular disease. The flu can worsen preexisting conditions such as heart failure or diabetes or trigger an asthma attack or heart attack in some people.

A 2013 *JAMA* study that looked at more than 6,700 patients (mean age, 67 years) found that those who got a flu vaccination were 36% less likely to suffer cardiovascular events (such as heart attacks) during the following year than those who weren't vaccinated. When researchers looked only at patients who had recent cardiac events, they found that vaccination cut the risk by 55%.

Recommended: An annual flu shot for everyone age 50 or older...and for anyone who has been diagnosed with cardiovascular disease. Adults age 65 and older should discuss the pros and cons of the high-dose flu vaccine with their physicians—it's reported to be about 24% more effective than standard vaccines but may have greater side effects.

SECRET #4: **Don't stop taking a beta-blocker drug abruptly.** Used for treating high blood pressure, irregular heartbeats, rapid heart rates and many other conditions, beta-blockers are among the most commonly prescribed drugs in the US.

Drugs in this class—*propranolol* (such as Inderal), *atenolol* (Tenormin) and many others—are generally safe but may cause side effects including fatigue, light-headedness and even impotence. As a result, patients sometimes decide on their own to stop taking these drugs.

The danger: If these drugs are suddenly stopped, the patient can have a dangerous upsurge in adrenaline activity, which can cause a faster heart rate, heavy sweating, spikes in blood pressure and an increased risk for heart attack and stroke. People who want to stop taking a beta-blocker are advised to slowly decrease the dose over 10 to 14 days.

Important: If you believe that you need to stop taking any prescribed medication, be sure to first check with your doctor. If side effects are a problem, you can probably switch to another drug or a dose that's easier to tolerate.

SECRET #5: **Lower your resting pulse.** When you increase your heart rate during aerobic exercise, you're helping to prevent a heart attack or stroke—this signifies that you're getting the cardiovascular benefits of moderate-to-vigorous exercise. Paradoxically, a slower resting heart rate is also protective.

Here's why: In general, a slower resting rate means a longer life—probably because a slower heart rate exerts less stress on blood vessel walls. Studies have shown that healthy men and women with lower resting heart rates (less than 60 beats per minute) have fewer cardiac events and a lower risk of dying from cardiovascular disease than those with faster rates (greater than 80 beats per minute).

A study of heart patients taking beta-blockers found that each 10-beat reduction in resting heart rate reduced the risk for cardiac death by 30%. For example, if someone with a resting heart rate of 80 beats per minute is given a beta-blocker to slow the rate to 60, the risk for cardiac death will drop by 60%.

Recommended: A resting heart rate of 50 to 70, depending on your cardiac history and typical physical activity level. Regular exercise...quitting smoking...maintaining a healthy weight...and avoiding high doses of caffeine can slow the resting heart rate.

Also important: Your recovery heart rate, the time that it takes your pulse to approach its resting rate after exercise. The fitter you get, the more quickly your heartbeat will return to a resting rate.

Heart Rate: Why It Matters More Than You Might Think

Wayne Westcott, PhD, a certified strength and conditioning specialist, is the fitness research director and an instructor of exercise science at Quincy College, in Quincy, Massachusetts. He is the author or coauthor of 24 books on fitness and an advisory board member for HealthyWoman from Bottom Line.

Most of us grew up in the days before gym teachers talked about resting heart rates and target heart rates. When coaches at school wanted us to work harder, they would just yell, "Hustle!" When we overdid it, we would flop down onto the ground for a few minutes until we felt better.

But now that we're older, the whole heart rate business is not something we can ignore. *Recent research reveals the reasons...*

A study of 50,088 adults found that for women under age 70, every increase of 10 beats per minute (bpm) in resting heart rate (number of heartbeats per minute while at rest) boosted the risk of dying from a heart attack by 18%. (No such association was found among women 70 or older.)

In a study of 129,135 postmenopausal women, those whose resting heart rate was above 76 bpm were 26% more likely to have or to die from a heart attack than those whose resting heart rate was below 63 bpm.

A strong heart pumps blood more efficiently, so it doesn't need to beat as fast. Regular aerobic exercise can lower your resting heart rate—but only if you work out at the right intensity. According to Wayne Westcott, PhD, a Quincy College exercise science instructor, if you go too easy during workouts, you miss out on cardiovascular benefits…but if you push too hard, you might experience lightheadedness, nausea and a higher-than-normal rise in blood pressure that could dangerously overwork your heart if you have hypertension. *Here's how to gauge the right workout intensity for you…*

- **Find out your current resting heart rate.** First thing when you wake up, take your pulse at your wrist or neck for one minute.

What resting heart rate suggests about fitness level for women in midlife and beyond…

Excellent	Below 60 bpm
Very good	60 to 65 bpm
Good	66 to 70 bpm
Average	71 to 75 bpm
Worse than average	Above 75 bpm

- **Plan to do a cardio workout at least three times per week.** Good options include brisk walking, running, dancing, cycling and swimming, Dr. Westcott said. (Get your doctor's OK before beginning or intensifying any exercise regimen.)

- **Determine your target heart rate.** Your ideal heart rate while exercising depends on two factors—your age and current fitness level. Dr. Westcott explained that the problem with the target heart rate charts often seen online or at gyms is that they generally are based only on age, not on fitness level, so you could wind up working out too hard or not hard enough. And though one target heart rate formula (called the Karvonen method) does account for resting heart rate, it requires more complicated calculations and, in Dr. Westcott's opinion, yields guidelines that may be too high.

Better: Follow the guidelines in the charts below. To track heart rate during your workout, use a heart rate monitor (about $100 at sporting-goods stores).

Remember: Your warm-up and cool-down do not count as time in your target range.

If your resting heart rate currently is above 70 bpm…

In your…	Your target heart rate is…	Your cardio workout should last…
40s	120 to 130 bpm	15 to 20 minutes
50s	110 to 120 bpm	15 to 20 minutes
60s	105 to 115 bpm	15 to 20 minutes
70s	95 to 105 bpm	15 to 20 minutes
80s	80 to 90 bpm	15 to 20 minutes

If your resting heart rate is 60 to 70 bpm…

In your…	Your target heart rate is…	Your cardio workout should last…
40s	130 to 140 bpm	20 to 25 minutes
50s	120 to 130 bpm	20 to 25 minutes
60s	115 to 125 bpm	20 to 25 minutes
70s	105 to 115 bpm	20 to 25 minutes
80s	90 to 100 bpm	20 to 25 minutes

If your resting heart rate is below 60 bpm…

In your…	Your target heart rate is…	Your cardio workout should last…
40s	135 to 145 bpm	25 to 30 minutes
50s	125 to 135 bpm	25 to 30 minutes
60s	120 to 130 bpm	20 to 25 minutes
70s	110 to 120 bpm	20 to 25 minutes
80s	95 to 105 bpm	20 to 25 minutes

Adjust your workout intensity as needed. Check your resting heart rate monthly—as it improves, intensify your workouts according to the guidelines above.

For safety: Reduce workout intensity and/or duration if you feel exhausted rather than invigorated after exercising…your muscles feel sore for more than a day after working out...you are recovering from an illness...you feel stressed...or the pollen count or air pollution index is high.

Quick Self-Test Signals Stiff Arteries

Kenta Yamamoto, PhD, research fellow, department of integrative physiology, University of North Texas Health Science Center, Fort Worth, and leader of a study of 526 people.

Physical fitness has been shown to delay age-related arterial stiffness, a risk factor for cardiovascular disease.

New study: Participants sat on the floor, legs straight, then bent forward at the waist to see how far they could reach toward or past their toes. Among middle-aged and older adults, the least flexible people generally had the stiffest arteries, as measured by a test called pulse wave velocity. Researchers theorize that stretching exercises may prompt physiological reactions that slow age-related arterial stiffening.

Best: Incorporate flexibility exercises, such as stretching, yoga and Pilates, into your regular workouts.

Why a Creased Earlobe May Kill You and Other Hidden Signs of Heart Problems

Anne Tybjaerg-Hansen, MD, DMSc, professor of clinical biochemistry, University of Copenhagen, and chief physician in the department of clinical biochemistry at Copenhagen University Hospital, Denmark.

When it comes to your cardiovascular health, you might think that if you don't have any typical risk factors for heart attack or coronary artery disease, such as obesity, high blood pressure or high cholesterol, then your heart is in good shape.

But a new study may make you think twice.

It may sound crazy, but how you look—as in, whether you look young or old for your age—can actually affect your risk for certain cardiovascular problems.

In fact, researchers have pinpointed four specific physical traits.

So check out what the four traits are and then take a look in the mirror...

THE HEART OF THE MATTER

After studying 35 years of data from nearly 11,000 male and female volunteers, Danish researchers found that two of the traits are fairly common and easy to recognize—a receding hairline and a bald spot on the head. (If a participant was mostly or completely bald, that person was put into the "bald spot" group.) The association of baldness and cardiovascular risk was seen among both men and women, though baldness was much less common in women.

The third trait is a little more obscure—a crease in one or both earlobes. And the fourth is having small, lumpy, yellow deposits on, above, below or next to the eyelids, a condition called xanthelasma that's caused by excess cholesterol under the skin. (For photos of the last two traits, see the next page.)

The study showed that the more of these traits a person had, the higher his or her chance of having a heart attack or developing coronary artery disease. For example, the researchers discovered that for people with three or four of these traits, the chances of suffering a heart attack are 57% greater and the chances of developing coronary artery disease are 39% greater, on average, than for people who have none of these traits.

What's remarkable is that these elevated risks held true even when researchers controlled for other common risk factors for cardiovascular problems, such as age, high blood pressure, high cholesterol, excess weight, poor nutrition, smoking, not exercising, gender and a family history of heart disease.

Why are these traits associated with these serious cardiovascular problems—and what might your doctor be able to do to help treat each trait? *Lead author of the study, Anne Tybjaerg-Hansen, MD, DMSc, explained what she and her colleagues found...*

• **Xanthelasma.** This condition remains a mystery to medical science. One potential cause of these fatty eyelid deposits is a diet that includes too much saturated fat—because saturated fat can raise your cholesterol levels. A doctor may advise you to eat a healthier diet and get more exercise, which may help lower your cholesterol numbers and, in turn, prevent more fatty deposits from appearing. But it's possible to have a normal cholesterol level and still have xanthelasma. Other potential causes of xanthelasma are diabetes, certain cancers and cirrhosis of the liver. You can have the deposits surgically removed, but unless the underlying cause is treated, the deposits may return and your cardiovascular risk would not be reduced.

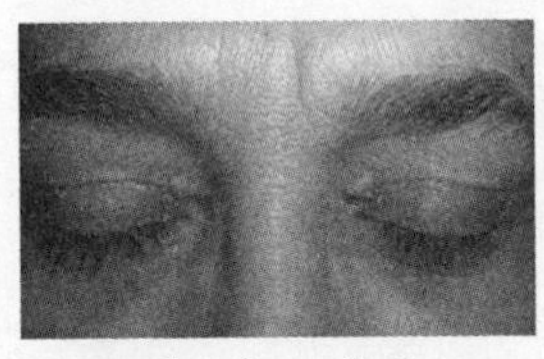

Example of xanthelasma around the eyes.

Credit: Klaus D. Peter

• **Hair loss.** There are a wide variety of potential causes for hair loss. It could be due to genetics (male pattern baldness)...a hormone imbalance...a drug (for instance, some medications that treat cancer, arthritis, depression and high blood pressure are associated with hair loss)...a thyroid problem...the disease alopecia, in which the immune system destroys hair follicles...a scalp infection...a skin disorder (such as lichen planus or lupus)...emotional or physical shock (due to, say, a death in the family or sudden weight loss)...anxiety (certain mental disorders make people want to pull hair from their heads)...a certain hairstyle (pulling hair too tightly can cause it to break and fall out)...overusing hair products (when hair gets too brittle, it can break and fall out)...or improper nutrition (a lack of iron and protein can cause hair to thin). If you have a treatable condition that's causing your hair loss, treating the condition may or may not have a positive effect on your cardiovascular risk factors—we don't know.

• **Earlobe crease.** This is a tricky trait. You might have an earlobe crease if the trait is passed down genetically through your family. As far as what else may cause this, that's up for debate. One theory suggests that it could be due to impaired circulation leading to a collapsed blood vessel near the earlobe. Another theory, which comes from a dermatologist, is that it may develop from a combination of aging and sleeping on one particular side of your body. But the cause is hard to pin down and there aren't any current treatments for it.

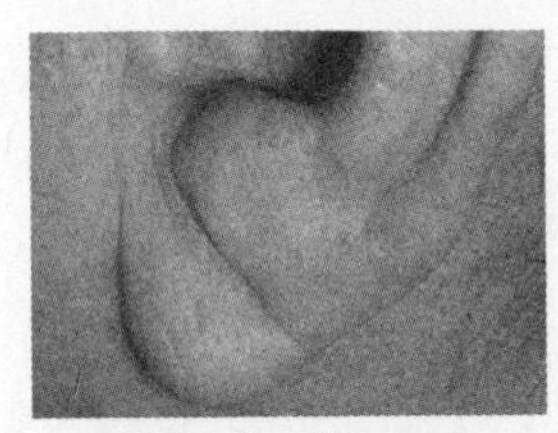

Example of earlobe crease.

Reprinted from *Dermatology Nursing*, 2010, Volume 22, Number 3 by permission of the publisher, Janetti Publications, Inc.

So all in all, it's not entirely clear why these traits are associated with certain increased cardiovascular risks and it's not yet known how to counteract these increased risks. But if you have at least one of these traits, Dr. Tybjaerg-Hansen said it probably wouldn't hurt to talk to your doctor about making more aggressive lifestyle changes, even if you're already eating some healthy foods and exercising a little. Your test results may lead you to believe that you're in the clear, but these findings show that you're not! It's possible that you'll need to make more of an effort than most people to protect your heart health.

How to Avoid a Heart Attack in Extreme Weather

Barry A. Franklin, PhD, director of preventive cardiology and rehabilitation at William Beaumont Hospital in Royal Oak, Michigan. He has served as president of the American Association of Cardiovascular and Pulmonary Rehabilitation and the American College of Sports Medicine. Dr. Franklin is coauthor of *109 Things You Can Do to Prevent, Halt & Reverse Heart Disease.*

The arctic blast that brought tundralike temperatures to much of the country this winter has left behind more than frozen pipes and frost-nipped noses. During a typical winter, there are up to 36% more circulatory-related deaths than during warmer months.

And it's not just cold weather that puts you at risk. Researchers have identified other types of weather—throughout the year—that trigger spikes in hospitalizations and death.

For details on the effects that weather can have on your heart, we spoke to Barry A. Franklin, PhD, a leading expert in cardiac rehabilitation.

We hear a lot about cold weather being hard on the heart. At what temperature does this really become an issue?

When it's cold enough to wear a winter jacket, it is cold enough to think about the health of your heart. In fact, research that was recently presented at the European Society of Cardiology Congress 2013 shows that the risk of having a heart attack increases by 7% for every 18°F drop below 73°F.

Why exactly is cold weather so dangerous?

Cold temperatures cause blood vessels throughout the body to temporarily constrict, raising blood pressure. Since the arteries that supply the heart are only about the thickness of cooked spaghetti, even a slight narrowing can cause reduced blood flow.

Winter temperatures aren't generally a problem if you are young and active. But risk rises as you hit middle age and beyond. The risk is highest for adults who are ages 65 and older, particularly those with underlying health problems, such as diabetes, obesity or preexisting heart disease. For people in these groups, spending even a few minutes in below-freezing temperatures can trigger a 20- to 50-point rise in blood pressure.

That's why I advise older adults, in particular, to stay indoors on the coldest days if possible. When you do go outdoors, don't depend on a light jacket—you should really bundle up by wearing a hat and gloves and dressing in multiple loose layers under your coat. Each layer traps air that's been heated by the body and serves as insulation.

And what about hot weather—does it harm the heart?

Actually, heat kills more people every year than any other type of weather.

High temperatures, generally above 80°F, but especially greater than 90°F, can cause heat syncope (sudden dizziness and/or fainting)...heat edema (swelling in the feet/ankles)...and heat stroke, in which the body's core temperature can rise above 104°F. People with atrial fibrillation or dementia are at a 6% to 8% increased risk of dying on hot days. Dementia affects the brain's ability to regulate the body's heat response.

Why is strenuous exertion so dangerous for many people during weather extremes?

Snow shoveling provides a good example. This activity creates a "perfect storm" of demands on the heart. With snow shoveling, the real danger—particularly for those who are older and/or sedentary—is the exertion itself.

Moving snow is hard work. Each shovelful weighs about 16 pounds (including the weight of the shovel). If you lift the shovel once every five seconds and continue for 10 minutes, you'll have moved nearly one ton of snow. This exertion can have adverse effects on the heart.

Here's why: Snow shoveling involves isometric exercise and unaccustomed muscle tension, which increases heart rate and blood pressure. Your legs may stay "planted" when you shovel, which allows blood to pool and reduces circulation to the heart.

Also, people tend to hold their breath (this is known as a Valsalva maneuver, and it often occurs when people are straining to lift heavy loads) when they are wielding a shovel, which causes a further rise in heart rate and blood pressure. That's why every year, we read or hear about people who dropped dead while shoveling snow.

Is there any way to reduce the risk associated with snow shoveling?

If you have or suspect you have heart disease, I suggest that you don't shovel your own snow. Hire someone to do it for you.

If you are in good shape and want to shovel your own snow, it may be safer in the afternoon. In general, most heart attacks occur between 6 am and 10 am, when heart rate and blood pressure tend to be higher. You're also more likely to form blood clots early in the day.

Then be sure to shovel slowly...work for only a few minutes at a time...and keep your legs moving to circulate blood. And remember, it's best to push snow rather than lift it. This helps keep your legs moving and takes less exertion than lifting. There are snow shovels designed for pushing snow.

What types of exertion are especially dangerous during hot weather?

Racket sports, water skiing, marathon running and certain highly competitive sports seem to be associated with a greater incidence of cardiac events in hot, humid weather. Why? Heart rates are disproportionately increased. Electrolytes, such as sodium and potassium, also are lost, which can lead to dangerous heart rhythms.

What steps should people take to protect themselves in hot weather?

Everyone knows to drink water when it's hot. But even people who are consciously trying to stay hydrated often do not drink enough. Drink plenty of cool liquids before, during and after heat exposure. If you're sweating a lot, you might want to drink an electrolyte-rich sports drink such as Gatorade or Powerade. And be sure to wear lightweight, loose-fitting clothing when you go outdoors.

In addition, think about any medications you may be taking. Many common drugs, including certain antihistamines and antidepressants, have anticholinergic effects—they inhibit your body's ability to cool off.

To help your body adapt to heat and humidity: As the weather grows hotter, gradually increase your daily exposure to the heat. The body's circulation and cooling efficiency increases, generally in eight to 14 days. Afterward, the body is better able to cope with extremes in heat and humidity.

Forehead Wrinkles Warning

Yolande Esquirol, MD, PhD, associate professor of occupational health, Centre Hospitalier Universitaire de Toulouse, France.

People with the most and deepest horizontal forehead wrinkles had nearly 10 times the risk of dying from heart disease as those with no wrinkles, according to a 20-year study of 3,200 adults ages 32 to 62.

Theory: Some of the factors that lead to premature skin aging and wrinkles also are linked to aging of the arteries and atherosclerosis.

'Tis the Season...For Heart Attacks

Robert A. Kloner, MD, PhD, professor of medicine in the cardiovascular division, Keck School of Medicine at the University of Southern California in Los Angeles, director of research at the Heart Institute of Good Samaritan Hospital in Los Angeles.

Thanksgiving to New Year's is the time of year for family...festivities...good eating—and heart attacks!

Sobering landmark finding: When researchers analyzed 25 years of data, they found that there were four times more deaths from heart attack or heart failure during the holiday period than at any other time of year. The grim numbers were highest on December 25, December 26 and January 1.

Who is most at risk: You're more likely to have a holiday heart attack if you've had a previous heart attack or stroke...or if you have a risk factor for heart disease, such as high blood pressure, inactivity, smoking or a family history of heart disease. Studies show that 49% of Americans have one or more of these risk factors.

6 CRUCIAL DANGERS

Cold weather is a well-known threat to people who have—or are at risk for—heart disease.

What else increases heart attack risk during the holidays...

Holiday heart risk: **The flu.** The fever and nasal congestion of the flu are hard on the heart—speeding heart rate and decreasing blood oxygen (the less oxygen available, the harder the heart has to work).

Research has shown that patients with heart disease who got flu vaccinations reduced their risk of dying from cardiovascular disease by nearly 40%, compared with similar patients who did not get flu shots.

What to do: If you have not done so already, ask your doctor about getting a flu shot now—it takes approximately two weeks after vaccination for antibodies to develop. In the US, flu activity typically peaks between December and February.

***Holiday heart risk:* The fireplace.** The tiny particles generated when you burn wood can inflame and damage blood vessels and may even trigger arrhythmias (abnormal heartbeats associated with heart attack) within hours.

What to do: The best strategy is to not light a fire in the fireplace if you have coronary artery disease or are at risk for lung or heart disease. As an alternative, sit as far away from the fire as possible. Using a HEPA air purifier also helps. Research shows that these machines can improve arterial health in people who live in communities with a lot of wood-burning stoves.

***Holiday heart risk:* Overeating.** Huge, high-fat meals impede functioning of arteries, making them less likely to dilate, which reduces blood flow.

What to do: Use your common sense. Never eat to the point of discomfort, particularly if you've already had a heart attack or stroke or have known risk factors for heart disease. When you start to feel full, walk away from the table.

Also: Eating a high-salt meal can be risky because too much salt causes water retention and can raise blood pressure. Whenever possible, use salt substitutes, such as spices and fresh lemon juice.

***Holiday heart risk:* Having one too many.** Drinking too much alcohol can increase arrhythmias and spike blood pressure—both of which are bad for the heart.

What to do: As with food, practice moderation—that's no more than one drink a day for women and no more than one to two drinks a day for men. (A drink is five ounces of wine...12 ounces of beer...or 1.5 ounces of spirits.) Avoid alcoholic drinks made with high-fat ingredients, such as eggnog.

***Holiday heart risk:* Anger, anxiety and depression.** The holidays leave many people feeling angered by difficult relatives...anxious about finances...and/or depressed about the absence of loved ones who have died.

Anger, anxiety and depression are all proven risk factors for heart attack. Here's why: Anger and anxiety can raise blood pressure and heart rate, increasing the load on the heart, reducing oxygen levels and contributing to the rupture of plaque in coronary arteries. Depression can imbalance the nervous system, increasing the risk for arrhythmias.

What to do: During the holidays, be sure to use stress-reduction techniques. If you're angry, for example, count to 10 before acting or remove yourself from the tense situation. Whenever you feel anxious, take three or four deep breaths. If you're depressed, go for a five- or 10-minute walk—studies show that walking is as effective as antidepressants for mild-to-moderate depression.

***Holiday heart risk:* Not going to the ER.** If you're not sure whether you're having a heart attack, don't worry about embarrassing yourself or inconveniencing holiday guests.

What to do: If you have any heart attack symptoms, call an ambulance. Symptoms can include chest pain...pressure, squeezing or fullness in the center of the chest...pain or discomfort in one or both arms, the back, neck, jaw or stomach...shortness of breath...breaking out in a cold sweat...nausea...and/or light-headedness.

MORE FROM DR. KLONER

TV Sports Can Kill You, Too

Planning to watch some football games during the holidays?

I've conducted research that analyzed death certificate data in a city whose team lost a Super Bowl and again when the team won the Super Bowl. In the two weeks after the losing game, there were 20% more heart attack deaths than in the winning year or when the team was not in the Super Bowl. Emotional stress may have contributed to these deaths. The same type of risk could very likely occur during holiday college bowl games.

What to do: You can't control a sporting event or an intense reaction to it, but you can try to stay calm by taking slow, deep breaths. If you have heart disease, also make sure that you take all the medications your doctor has prescribed, such as a heart-slowing beta-blocker or blood-thinning aspirin, to help minimize your holiday heart risks.

When Your Heart Needs a Jump-Start

Jeffrey L. Williams, MD, medical director of electrophysiology at The Good Samaritan Hospital, with a private practice in cardiology and heart-rhythm disorders at Lebanon Cardiology Associates, both in Lebanon, Pennsylvania. He is the author of *What Is a Pacemaker? A Cardiologist's Guide for Patients and Care Providers.*

You might think that you'd never be a candidate for a pacemaker. Perhaps your doctor has told you that your cholesterol levels are good. Maybe your blood pressure readings are normal, too. But these facts don't mean that the electrical components of your heart, which control the speed and rhythm of your heartbeats, are firing on all cylinders.

Common misconceptions: Many people assume that pacemakers are needed only by individuals who have serious cardiovascular disease or are approaching the end of their lives. Neither assumption is true.

It can be common for someone who needs a pacemaker to be otherwise healthy—in these cases, the heart just needs help to generate the signals that make it pump efficiently. And even though people who get pacemakers usually are over age 60, a person of any age may need the device, which is about the size of two poker chips stacked on top of one another. Those with cardiovascular disease also are more likely to need a pacemaker.

WHAT CAN GO WRONG

The heart normally beats 60 to 100 times a minute. The rate and rhythm of the heart are set by a natural pacemaker—a cluster of cells known as the sinoatrial, or SA, node.

What can go wrong: Electrical signals that are delayed or interrupted, due to conditions such as those described later in this article, cause the heart to beat too slowly (a condition known as bradycardia)...or to pump insufficient amounts of blood (a condition known as heart failure).

These problems can lead to unexplained symptoms, such as dizziness, shortness of breath, fatigue and/or episodes of syncope (a sudden loss of consciousness). More subtle symptoms include chest pain, swelling, coughing, difficulty walking and weight gain.

When such symptoms occur, doctors routinely recommend an EKG and/or use of a Holter monitor, a device that's worn at home to record the heart's electrical activity over 24 to 48 hours. An echocardiogram (an ultrasound test that shows how well the heart is working) and/or an intracardiac electrophysiology study (to pinpoint where the heart's electrical system is damaged) also may be needed.

Note: Many heart failure patients need defibrillators, which are different from pacemakers. If a potentially fatal arrhythmia is detected by the device, it can give the patient a lifesaving shock. Pacemakers do not have this ability.

WHEN THE HEART NEEDS HELP

After certain problems are ruled out, you may be advised to get a pacemaker for these conditions...*

- **SA-node dysfunction.** It's common for these electricity-producing cells to slow with age. The heart might beat as little as 30 to 40 times a minute—not allowing the heart to circulate enough of the blood the body needs, particularly during exercise. A pacemaker can help the heart beat more quickly and prevent patients from suffering such symptoms as dizziness and fatigue.

What doctors check before suggesting a pacemaker: Patients with angina (chest pain caused by reduced blood flow to the heart) may be advised to take a beta-blocker drug, such as *atenolol* (Tenormin), to reduce the heart's demand for oxygen. But this type of medication may slow the heart too much and cause bradycardia. Calcium channel blockers, such as *diltiazem* (Cardizem), or other

*Doctors should follow the American College of Cardiology's evidence-based guidelines when deciding whether a patient needs a pacemaker. To read these guidelines, go to ACC.org.

anti-arrhythmics, such as *amiodarone* (Pacerone), also can slow heart rates.

What to try first: If a drug you're taking is causing bradycardia, it's possible that changing the drug and/or dose will help. Be sure to discuss this option with your doctor. If a different drug and/or dose doesn't help within several weeks, you may need a pacemaker.

- **Acquired AV (atrioventricular) block.** The AV node is an area of heart tissue that conducts electrical impulses from the upper heart chambers, atria, to the lower chambers, ventricles. AV block occurs when there's an electrical conduction delay between the heart's upper and lower chambers—or, in more serious cases, when there's a complete electrical block. The heart still beats but in a disorganized fashion.

What doctors check before suggesting a pacemaker: In some cases, an AV block is temporary—for example, due to Lyme disease or a potassium deficiency.

What to try first: If your doctor says that you are experiencing an AV block, ask about blood tests to check your electrolytes (including potassium) and to ensure that you don't have Lyme disease, which can lead to forms of AV block that usually resolve on their own when the underlying condition is treated.

A "third-degree" AV block is potentially the most serious. It can occur with aging and may even follow a heart attack because the interruption in circulation from a blood clot can damage the AV node.

Important: The AV node usually recovers on its own within a day or two after a heart attack is treated. If the node recovers, you won't need a pacemaker...if symptoms continue, a pacemaker is almost always needed.

- **Atrial fibrillation (AF).** This common rhythm disturbance causes the atria to beat very fast and send a signal to the ventricles to beat very fast. Most AF patients need medication to control the fast heartbeat (tachycardia), which can lead to bradycardia when normal rhythm returns. This is called tachycardia-bradycardia syndrome, and these patients may benefit from a pacemaker.

Other conditions that can cause a slow and irregular heartbeat that may require a pacemaker include congestive heart failure, neuromuscular diseases (such as Parkinson's disease) and carotid sinus hypersensitivity.

A SPECIAL TRAVEL PRECAUTION

If you have a pacemaker, it's safe to pass through freestanding security systems at airports. But ask security officers to avoid holding a metal-detecting wand near the pacemaker area for more than a second or two because the magnet inside the wand may affect the operation of the pacemaker. Always carry your pacemaker ID card.

Heart-Saving Snack

Study by researchers at Technion-Israel Institute of Technology, led by Professor Michael Aviram of the Rappaport Faculty of Medicine and Rambam Medical Center, Haifa, Israel, published in *Food & Function.*

Israeli researchers found that four ounces of pure pomegranate juice (not sweetened) and three dates (no added sugar), eaten together once a day, is hugely protective of heart health. It reduced oxidative stress in the arterial walls by as much as 33% while decreasing cholesterol by 28%.

Being Neighborly Promotes a Healthy Heart

Eric S. Kim, a doctoral student in psychology, University of Michigan, Ann Arbor. His study was published in the *Journal of Epidemiology & Community Health.*

You may chalk up the "hearty" longevity of older neighbors to good Old World genes, but new research is saying it's something more. In fact, there may be something more to heart health for everyone beyond genes, diet and exercise. This heart-health booster is something we don't think about, and yet there it is, right in front of our noses—if we take steps to get it. And this newly proven secret to heart health and longevity is free and not hard to do—all you have to do is be neighborly.

That's right—just be neighborly to live longer! *Here's why...*

HOWDY, NEIGHBOR

We know that negative aspects of physical environments—noise, traffic and pollution—can harm our health. It's a no-brainer. Even so, scientists have conducted study after study to prove it. But recently, researchers from the University of Michigan took a different tack, looking at the impact of positive rather than the negative aspects of neighborhood living. The research team wanted to find out whether feeling part of a community, trusting neighbors and feeling safe had an impact on heart health. They called these feelings about community connections perceived neighborhood social cohesion.

Drawing data from the University of Michigan's ongoing Health and Retirement Study, the researchers identified 5,276 heart-healthy people and followed them for four years. The average age of these folks was 70. As for the Health and Retirement Study, it's a large, national program that collects information on health, health-care economics, aging and quality of life in adults older than 50. Information is collected through questionnaires that are sent every two years to the more than 22,000 participants in the program.

So, to measure neighborhood social cohesion, researchers asked the participants how they felt about the area within a 20-minute walk or one-mile radius of their homes. *These study participants rated how much they agreed with these four statements...*

- **I really feel part of this area.**
- **If you were in trouble, there are lots of people in this area who would help you.**
- **Most people in this area can be trusted.**
- **Most people in this area are friendly.**

Depending on how strongly a participant agreed with each statement, he or she was put into one of four groups—low social cohesion, low-to-moderate, moderate-to-high, or high social cohesion.

During the four-year study period, 148 of the participants had heart attacks. The researchers took this information and sliced and diced it with the data they had collected about neighborhood social cohesion and demographic factors (for example, age, sex, race, marital status, education level and income) of their study population.

THE REAL EFFECT OF SOCIAL CONNECTEDNESS

When the researchers adjusted data to compensate for the impact of demographic factors on heart attack risk, they found that, compared with people with low neighborhood social cohesion, people with low-to-moderate social cohesion were 34% less likely to have heart attacks and people with the moderate-to-high or high social cohesion were about 45% less likely to have heart attacks.

Those are stunning numbers—you can potentially reduce your risk of heart attack by half by just being neighborly and liking and being involved with where you live.

Although studies have shown that keeping a positive attitude is good for your health, this study is the first to examine how feeling positive about your neighborhood impacts your risk of heart attack. But the results aren't that surprising, are they? They emphasize the importance of being comfortable, safe and contented in light of what we know about stress and anxiety and heart health. The findings can perhaps be summed up by this proverb: "Better is a neighbor who is near than a brother who is far away." When family isn't close at hand or willing to be supportive, it is a comfort to know that neighbors—people in your community—can provide a safety net for social, emotional and physical needs. And that knowledge, over time, can be a powerful stress reducer.

If you don't already feel connected to your neighborhood, why not get more involved? If neighbors stroll along the street where you live, sit out in front of your house or apartment and chat with them as they pass. Or visit the local coffee shop, but don't bury your head in a newspaper, book or laptop. Instead, make a point to strike up conversations with other patrons. Attend an "open mike" at a local bar or restaurant where amateur singers and musicians entertain each other and welcome you to perform as well. It's a festive way to become part of a community. Join a community center, enroll in an adult-education class or become involved with a local charity or civic cause—and the more local, the better. If you make it a goal, you can definitely make more friends and acquaintances in your neighborhood and therefore feel more connected to it.

When you think about it, these are all just examples of being more open-hearted—and now there's proof that an open heart is a stronger heart.

An Apple a Day...

Study by researchers at University of Oxford, England, published in the *BMJ*.

A British study found that eating one apple a day could prevent 8,500 deaths a year from heart attacks and strokes in people over age 50 in the UK. Apples act like statins to reduce LDL "bad" cholesterol, a risk factor for heart attacks and stroke.

Six Ways to Liven Up Your Heart-Healthy Diet

Janet Bond Brill, PhD, RD, an expert in nutrition and cardiovascular disease prevention based in Valley Forge, Pennsylvania. She is director of nutrition for Fitness Together, a franchise company of almost 500 personal fitness-training studios, has served as a nutrition consultant for several corporations and is the author of *Prevent a Second Heart Attack.* DrJanet.com

Just about everyone knows that a Mediterranean-style diet can help prevent heart disease. Even if you've already had a heart attack, this style of eating—emphasizing such foods as fish and vegetables—can reduce the risk for a second heart attack by up to 70%.

Problem: About 80% of patients with heart disease quit following dietary advice within one year after their initial diagnosis. That's often because they want more choices but aren't sure which foods have been proven to work.

Solution: Whether you already have heart disease or want to prevent it, you can liven up your diet by trying foods that usually don't get much attention for their heart-protective benefits...

***SECRET 1:* Popcorn.** It's more than just a snack. It's a whole grain that's high in cholesterol-lowering fiber. Surprisingly, popcorn contains more fiber, per ounce, than whole-wheat bread or brown rice.

Scientific evidence: Data from the 1999–2002 National Health and Nutrition Examination Survey found that people who eat popcorn daily get 22% more fiber than those who don't eat it.

Important: Eat "natural" popcorn, preferably air-popped or microwaved in a brown paper bag, without added oil. The commercially prepared popcorn packets generally contain too much salt, butter and other additives. Three cups of popped popcorn, which contain almost 6 g of fiber and 90 calories, is considered a serving of whole grains. Studies have shown that at least three servings of whole grains a day (other choices include oatmeal and brown rice) may help reduce the risk for heart disease, high cholesterol and obesity.

***SECRET 2:* Chia seeds.** You're probably familiar with Chia pets —those terra-cotta figures that sprout thick layers of grassy "fur." The same seeds, native to Mexico and Guatemala, are increasingly available in health-food stores. I consider them a superfood because they have a nutrient profile that rivals heart-healthy flaxseed.

In fact, chia seeds contain more omega-3 fatty acids than flaxseed. Omega-3s increase the body's production of anti-inflammatory eicosanoids, hormonelike substances that help prevent "adhesion molecules" from causing plaque buildup and increasing atherosclerosis.

Scientific evidence: A study published in the *Journal of the American College of Cardiology,* which looked at nearly 40,000 participants, found that an omega-3 rich diet can prevent and even reverse existing cardiovascular disease.

Other benefits: One ounce of chia seeds has 10 g of fiber, 5 g of alpha-linolenic acid and 18% of the Recommended Dietary Allowance for calcium for adults ages 19 to 50.

Chia seeds look and taste something like poppy seeds. You can add them to baked goods, such as muffins, or sprinkle them on salads and oatmeal or other cereals.

SECRET 3: **Figs.** They're extraordinarily rich in antioxidants with an oxygen radical absorbance capacity (ORAC) score of 3,383. Scientists use this ORAC scale to determine the antioxidant capacity of various foods. An orange, by comparison, scores only about 1,819. Fresh figs are among the best sources of beta-carotene and other heart-healthy carotenoids.

Scientific evidence: In a study published in the *Journal of the American College of Nutrition*, two groups of participants were "challenged" with sugary soft drinks, which are known to increase arterial oxidation. Oxidation in the arteries triggers atherosclerosis, a main risk factor for heart disease. Those who were given only soda had a drop in healthful antioxidant activity in the blood... those who were given figs as well as soda had an increase in blood antioxidant levels.

Bonus: Ten dried figs contain 140 mg of calcium. Other compounds in figs, such as quercetin, reduce inflammation and dilate the arteries. Perhaps for these reasons, people who eat figs regularly have much less heart disease than those who don't eat them, according to studies. Most dried figs contain added sulfites, so it's best to buy organic, sulfite-free dried figs.

SECRET 4: **Soy protein.** Tofu, soy milk and other soy foods are "complete proteins"—that is, they supply all of the essential amino acids that your body needs but without the cholesterol and large amount of saturated fat found in meat.

Scientific evidence: People who replace dairy or meat protein with soy will have an average drop in LDL "bad" cholesterol of 2% to 7%, according to research from the American Heart Association. Every 1% drop in LDL lowers heart disease risk about 2%.

A one-half cup serving of tofu provides 10 g of protein. An eight-ounce glass of soy milk gives about 7 g. Edamame (steamed or boiled green soybeans) has about 9 g per half cup. Avoid processed soy products, such as hydrogenated soybean oil (a trans fat), soy isoflavone powders and soy products with excess added sodium.

SECRET 5: **Lentils.** I call these "longevity legumes" because studies have shown that they can literally extend your life.

Best choices: Brown or black lentils.

Scientific evidence: In one study, published in the *Asia Pacific Journal of Clinical Nutrition,* the eating habits of five groups of older adults were compared. For every 20 g (a little less than three-fourths of an ounce) increase in the daily intake of lentils and/or other legumes, there was an 8% reduction in the risk of dying within seven years.

Lentils contain large amounts of fiber, plant protein and antioxidants along with folate, iron and magnesium—all of which are important for cardiovascular health.

Similarly, a Harvard study found that people who ate one serving of cooked beans (one-third cup) a day were 38% less likely to have a heart attack than those who ate beans less than once a month.

Caution: Beans have been shown to cause gout flare-ups in some people.

Important: Lentils cook much faster than other beans. They don't need presoaking. When simmered in water, they're ready in 20 to 30 minutes. You need about one-half cup of cooked lentils, beans or peas each day for heart health.

SECRET 6: **Pinot Noir and Cabernet Sauvignon.** All types of alcohol seem to have some heart-protective properties, but red wine offers the most.

Scientific evidence: People who drink alcohol regularly in moderation (one five-ounce glass of wine daily for women, and no more than two for men) have a 30% to 50% lower risk of dying from a heart attack than those who don't drink, according to research published in *Archives of Internal Medicine.*

Best choices: Pinot Noir, Cabernet Sauvignon and Tannat wines (made from Tannat red grapes). These wines have the highest concentrations of flavonoids, antioxidants that reduce arterial inflammation and inhibit the oxidation of LDL cholesterol. Oxidation is the process that makes cholesterol more likely to accumulate within artery walls.

Bonus: Red wines also contain resveratrol, a type of polyphenol that is thought to increase the synthesis of proteins that slow aging. Red wine has 10 times more polyphenols than white varieties.

In a four-year study of nearly 7,700 men and women nondrinkers, those who began to drink a moderate amount of red wine cut their risk for heart attack by 38% compared with nondrinkers.

If you are a nondrinker or currently drink less than the amounts described above, talk to your doctor before changing your alcohol intake. If you cannot drink alcohol, pomegranate or purple grape juice is a good alternative.

A Top Cardiologist Reveals the Best Supplements for Your Heart

Patrick M. Fratellone, MD, is an integrative cardiologist and executive medical director of Fratellone Medical Associates, New York City. FratelloneMedical.com

---

Put your hand on your heart. How's it doing in there? For too many women, the answer is, "Not so good." Despite the fact that we try to eat right, exercise and watch our weight, heart disease is still the number-one killer of women in America.

What are we doing wrong? For one thing, we're not getting enough of the nutrients that our hearts need to stay healthy. "Much of our food is depleted of life-sustaining vitamins and minerals," explained integrative cardiologist Patrick M. Fratellone, MD. "That's why many people can benefit from specific supplements—whether their goal is to prevent heart disease or to minimize harm from the particular cardiovascular risk factors they already have."

Here's how the various heart-healthy supplements work...and the protocols Dr. Fratellone typically recommends based on patients' particular risk factors.

Important: Check with your doctor before beginning any supplement regimen. Some supplements can interact with other supplements or medications and/or cause side effects for people with certain medical conditions.

HOW THE HEART HELPERS WORK

- **Coenzyme Q10 (CoQ10),** the energy generator of all cells, enhances the heart's pumping ability.

Caution: CoQ10 may decrease the effectiveness of blood-thinning medication, such as warfarin.

- **Folic acid,** a B vitamin, helps prevent the formation of homocysteine, an amino acid that damages artery linings.

Caution: Avoid folic acid supplementation if you have a history of cancer.

- **Hawthorn,** an herb, may strengthen heart contractions and reduce blood pressure by relaxing blood vessels.

Caution: Don't use hawthorn if you have low blood pressure or take a beta-blocker or calcium channel blocker medication.

- **L-carnitine,** an amino acid, increases the heart's pumping action... and may facilitate weight loss by increasing metabolism.

Caution: Don't use L-carnitine if you have kidney disease.

- **L-taurine,** another amino acid, dilates blood vessels, improves blood flow and helps reduce blood pressure.

Caution: L-taurine may not be appropriate if you take diuretic medication or have stomach ulcers.

- **Magnesium** regulates blood pressure and heart rate.

Caution: Don't take magnesium if your blood pressure is already low.

- **Omega-3 fatty acids,** found in fish oil, increase HDL (good) cholesterol...decrease LDL (bad) cholesterol and triglycerides...slow plaque buildup in arteries...reduce the risk for arrhythmia (abnormal heartbeat)...and reduce blood pressure.

- **Vitamin B-12** inhibits harmful homocysteine formation. Use a methylated form of B-12, since

40% of patients have a methylation problem (MTHFR) and cannot absorb B-12 if it is not methylated.

- **Vitamin D-3** helps prevent inflammation...reduces heart attack and stroke risk in people with high blood pressure...and may protect against heart failure.

Next step: To make use of the information above, you need to know which specific nutrients are most beneficial for you—and that depends on your personal health status.

TO PREVENT HEART PROBLEMS...

Below is Dr. Fratellone's heart-protecting supplement protocol (to be taken daily, continuing indefinitely) for the typical perimenopausal or postmenopausal woman who has not been diagnosed with any condition that increases cardiovascular risk. Ask your doctor if you should take any or all of these five supplements. If you take a multivitamin, check which of the nutrients below your multi already provides.

Preventive protocol...

- **CoQ10**—100 mg daily.
- **Magnesium**—350 mg daily.
- **Omega-3s (in the form of fish oil)**—1,000 mg to 2,000 mg daily of combined EPA and DHA, the most beneficial components.
- **Vitamin B-12**—1,000 micrograms (mcg) daily.
- **Vitamin D-3**—1,000 international units (IU) daily.

IF YOU ARE ALREADY AT RISK...

You may benefit from additional protection if you have a condition that increases cardiovascular risk. Dr. Fratellone said that it is generally advisable to continue taking the five supplements above, though in some cases, a higher dosage is appropriate (as detailed below)...and to consider additional supplements (observing the aforementioned cautions), depending on an individual's particular health problem.

Ask your doctor about modifying your regimen as follows if you have...

ATRIAL FIBRILLATION OR OTHER ARRHYTHMIA

- **Hawthorn (extract ratio 1:2)**—20 drops mixed with water three times daily.
- **Magnesium**—increase to 500 mg daily.
- **Omega-3s**—increase to 1,000 mg three times daily.

CONGESTIVE HEART FAILURE

- **Hawthorn (extract ratio 1:2)**—20 drops mixed with water three times daily.
- **Vitamin D-3**—increase to 2,000 IU daily.

CORONARY ARTERY DISEASE

- **Folic acid**—1,000 mcg daily.
- **L-carnitine**—1,000 mg three times daily.
- **L-taurine**—500 mg three time daily.
- **Omega-3s**—increase to 1,000 mg three times daily.

DIABETES

- **CoQ10**—increase to 100 mg three times daily.
- **L-carnitine**—1,000 mg three times daily.
- **Magnesium**—increase to 500 mg daily.

EXCESS WEIGHT (BODY MASS INDEX OF 25 OR HIGHER)

- **L-carnitine**—1,000 mg three times daily.

HIGH BLOOD PRESSURE

- **L-taurine**—500 mg three times daily.
- **Magnesium**—increase to 500 mg daily.
- **Omega-3s**—increase to 1,000 mg three times daily.
- **Vitamin D-3**—increase to 2,000 IU daily.

HIGH CHOLESTEROL

- **CoQ10**—increase to 100 mg three times daily.
- **L-taurine**—500 mg three times daily.
- **Omega-3s**—increase to 1,000 mg three times daily.

HIGH HOMOCYSTEINE

- **Folic acid**—1,000 mcg daily.

HIGH TRIGLYCERIDES

- **CoQ10**—increase to 100 mg twice daily.
- **Omega-3s**—increase to 1,000 mg three times daily.

Is Salt Harmful for Everyone? Why You May Not Need to Cut Back

James J. DiNicolantonio, PharmD, a cardiovascular research scientist and doctor of pharmacy at Saint Luke's Mid America Heart Institute in Kansas City, Missouri. Dr. DiNicolantonio is also an associate editor of *BMJ Open Heart*, on the editorial advisory board of *Progress in Cardiovascular Diseases* and other journals and author of *The Salt Fix*. The SaltFix.com

We've all been told that a high-salt diet is a leading cause of high blood pressure (hypertension), heart attack, stroke and heart failure. What doctors don't tell patients—what many doctors don't know themselves—is that salt doesn't have the same effect on everyone's blood pressure.

A surprising fact: Many people do better when they consume more than the USDA's recommended daily sodium limit of 2,300 mg (roughly the amount in one teaspoon of salt). *Other common misconceptions regarding sodium...*

MYTH #1: **Salt raises blood pressure in everyone.** It's true that doctors have a right to worry about the salt consumption for some patients. Salt sensitivity—generally defined as an increase of 5% or more in blood pressure when sodium is consumed—is most common in older adults, black people and people of Chinese descent.

Important: If you're sensitive to salt, exceeding the recommended daily limit of 2,300 mg of sodium can cause sharp rises in blood pressure.

But what's harmful for this subset of the population is not harmful for everyone. Research shows that salt sensitivity affects about half of people with high blood pressure and about 20% of people who have normal blood pressure.

MYTH #2: **Salt always increases heart disease.** If a high-salt diet increased blood pressure, it would obviously increase the risk for cardiovascular disease—but, as discussed earlier, this occurs only in some people. When researchers study whether eating highly salted foods increases the rates of high blood pressure and heart disease, the findings are mixed. Meanwhile, the correlation between high-salt diets and improved health is compelling.

Example: People consume staggering amounts of sodium in Japan, France and South Korea. The average South Korean, for example, consumes more than 4,000 mg of sodium a day. In France and other Mediterranean countries, very salty foods, such as prepared sardines, anchovies and many aged cheeses, are eaten with most meals. Yet these countries are among those with the lowest death rates from coronary heart disease in the world, and Japan and South Korea boast among the highest longevity.

Most people don't realize that a low-salt diet can sometimes raise blood pressure by stimulating the body's "rescue" system (the renin-angiotensin aldosterone system) that's designed to help the body retain salt and water. When this occurs, low salt intake can increase heart rate, blood clotting and the constriction of blood vessels. It's also been linked to insulin resistance and diabetes.

MYTH #3: **No one needs more salt.** The ubiquitous advice to reduce sodium intake might be justified if it helped some people and didn't hurt the rest. But this isn't always the case.

To remain in homeostasis, the physiological state that puts the least stress on the body, most people who are not salt sensitive need about 3,000 mg to 5,000 mg of sodium a day.

What's more, many of our food choices (sugar and caffeinated beverages, for example) deplete salt from the body. So do commonly prescribed medications such as some antidepressants, diuretics and diabetes drugs. In addition, the average nonathletic adult sweats out 600 mg of sodium a day.

MYTH #4: **Healthy diets are naturally low in salt.** The diets that experts recommend for disease prevention, such as the Mediterranean diet, do exclude many of the processed foods that happen to be high in salt (and other unhealthful ingredients)—but they're not low-salt diets overall. If anything, as mentioned above with such countries as Japan and South Korea, they contain more salt than Americans typically eat. Think seafood (clams, lobster, crab), olives, kimchi, etc.

Why do these countries have less cardiovascular disease than the US? While there is no definitive research that a high-salt diet is the reason, it's been my observation that people who indulge their salt cravings tend to eat more heart-healthy vegetables (particularly the bitter ones, such as bitter greens)...nuts...and seeds—most likely because these healthy foods taste better with salt.

What's more, there is often a lot of potassium in naturally salty foods—for example, spinach, Swiss chard and artichokes. When it comes to improving blood pressure and heart health, more potassium is probably more important than less sodium.

MYTH #5: **Everyone should check the sodium content on food labels.** Unless you eat a lot of pretzels, chips and other super-salty foods, you are unlikely to eat more salt than your body can handle—unless you're salt-sensitive (see below).

I do advise people to avoid processed foods—mainly because these foods tend to be high in sugar, which can increase the risk for high blood pressure, diabetes and obesity. Most processed foods also lack fiber, and a lack of fiber can cause sugar spikes. It's much better to indulge your salt cravings with foods that are naturally salty—for example, sea vegetables (kelp, seaweed and algae), seafood, cheese and olives.

ARE YOU SALT-SENSITIVE?

There are no readily available tests to determine whether a person is salt-sensitive. So how do you know whether a low-salt diet would help you or hurt you?

Try this: With your doctor's OK, for two weeks, reduce your sodium intake to less than 2,300 mg of sodium per day. If your blood pressure drops by 5% or more, chances are you are salt-sensitive. If your blood pressure does drop, be alert for dizziness, fatigue, nausea, muscle spasms/cramps and blurred vision—signs that your blood pressure may be too low. In these cases, you may be better off listening to your body's salt cravings and eating the salt that it demands rather than adhering to a strict low-sodium diet.

Important: Discuss this with your doctor, and monitor your blood pressure closely.

The Best Ways to Cut Back on Salt

Michelle Hauser, MD, MPA, a primary care physician, certified Le Cordon Bleu chef and nutrition educator. Dr. Hauser is also a postdoctoral research fellow in cardiovascular disease prevention at Stanford University School of Medicine, California. ChefInResidency.com

Has your doctor told you that you need to cut back on salty foods? You may already know that having too much sodium can increase blood pressure. Now a 20-year study published in the *Journal of the American College of Cardiology* says that individuals with the lowest sodium intake seem to have the lowest risk of dying early.

The salt threat: People who have high blood pressure, diabetes or kidney disease or who are African-American or age 51 and older are often salt-sensitive. That means they have a sharp increase in blood pressure when they eat salty foods and are at greater risk for stroke, heart attack and other dangerous health problems. However, many people don't realize that even those who are not salt-sensitive could have an increase in blood pressure if they eat too much sodium.

Here's the good news: There are many simple ways to reduce your sodium intake without sacrificing flavor!

A DOCTOR/CHEF'S TIPS FOR REDUCING SODIUM

The average sodium intake per day in the US is a whopping 3,400 mg (that's about one-and-one-half teaspoons of table salt). However, the American Heart Association advises just 1,500 mg per day (two-thirds of a teaspoon) or less for optimal health. It may be no surprise that fast-food items and deli meats have a lot of salt. But restaurant meals and store-bought sauces, salad dressings, soups and even bread tend to be loaded with sodium as well.

Michelle Hauser, MD, MPA, a primary care doctor and certified Le Cordon Bleu chef, says the absolute best way to cut back on salt is to prepare more meals at home using fresh, unprocessed ingredients. This not only enables you to control the amount of salt added to meals but also maximizes the flavor of food so that a little salt goes a long way.

Some people prefer to wean themselves off salt slowly, while others find it easier to go "cold turkey."

Either way, here are Dr. Hauser's flavor-packed suggestions...

• **Add some acid.** A few drops of a sour ingredient, like citrus juice or vinegar, wakes up the flavor in foods and enhances any salt you do use, allowing you to get by with less.

What to do: Add a squeeze of lime to low-sodium black bean soup (it will make the soup taste saltier and give it a Latin flavor)...include a teaspoon of balsamic vinegar in your homemade tomato sauce...add a few drops of Tabasco sauce (made from red peppers and vinegar) to chili...and use an orange juice–based marinade to tenderize and flavor chicken. Other tasty sources of acid include the juice of Meyer lemons or grapefruits. Another option: Flavored vinegars—some are infused with herbs such as thyme or rosemary...others contain fruits like raspberries or figs.

• **Salt smart.** Do you have trouble knowing how much salt to add to your dishes? *Here's how to get maximum flavor without going overboard...*

What to do: To get the hang of this technique, try it with an unsalted sauce. Taste the sauce, taking note of the flavors. Sip some water, then add a few drops of an acidic ingredient to the sauce (see above) and stir. Taste again, noticing how much brighter and flavorful the dish is. Next, add a pinch or two of salt, stir and taste. If you taste the salt only on the tip of your tongue, the sauce is undersalted. Take a sip of water, and add another pinch or two of salt. The dish is perfectly salted when you taste the salt on the middle to the back of your tongue. The food is oversalted if the flavor hits the back of your throat.

• **Try these tasty all-natural salt substitutes.** Forget the potassium chloride salt-substitute sold in shakers at the grocery store—they can have a chemical or metallic taste. Fresh and dried herbs and spices add delicious flavors to your dishes and boost the impact of a small amount of salt.

What to do: You can buy fresh or dried rosemary, thyme and basil in grocery stores, but it's very easy to grow these herbs at home. Also, stock up on store-bought garlic and onion powders (not salts), cumin, coriander, Mexican oregano, smoked paprika and cayenne pepper.

Premade seasoning mixes—like Mrs. Dash Salt-Free Seasoning Blends, combinations of herbs, spices and dried vegetables—are available in grocery stores. But you may want to add some international flavor by using spice mixes from India, Asia, the Middle East or Africa. For example, Ras-El-Hanout is a Moroccan spice mix made of cumin, turmeric, allspice, coriander and pepper. You can buy this mix in gourmet cooking stores or online...or make it yourself (see the recipe at ChefInResidency.com).

• **Try roasting or grilling vegetables.** These high-temperature cooking methods cause a chemical reaction that releases hundreds of rich, savory flavor compounds (think of roasted or grilled mushrooms). With all this natural flavor, you'll never even miss the salt! The key is making sure that the surface of the food is as dry as possible before cooking (oils and seasonings are fine, but no added water).

Caution: Grilling and frying meats and fish can produce carcinogenic compounds, so avoid charring or overcooking these foods.

OTHER HELPFUL TIPS

• **Consider flaked kosher salt**—it has about half the sodium per teaspoon of granulated salt.

Note: Some people think sea salt is healthier than table salt.

The facts: There are small amounts of minerals and micronutrients in sea salt, but if you are getting the appropriate amount of sodium, these nutrients are not likely to affect your health. And sea salt contains just as much sodium as table salt by weight.

• **Get more potassium.** A high-potassium diet can blunt the effect of salt on blood pressure by increasing sodium excretion from the body. Eating a variety of fruits and vegetables is the best way to get the 4,700 mg per day of potassium suggested by the Institute of Medicine.

Good sources of potassium: Leafy greens, beans, potatoes, bananas, avocados, papaya, dried fruit, nuts and seeds, fish, chili peppers and powder, and even dark chocolate.

Caution: Check with your doctor before increasing your potassium intake if you have a chronic health condition (such as kidney disease)or take medication.

- **Add some interest to your plate by eating foods with a variety of colors, textures and flavors.** When you eat with all your senses, you will be less likely to need salt.

Hit the Sauna to Reduce Cardiovascular Risk

Study of 2,315 men by researchers at University of Eastern Finland, Kuopio, published in *JAMA Internal Medicine*.

Saunas are associated with lower death risk. Men in Finland who used a dry sauna two to three times a week over the long term (nearly 21 years) for at least 11 minutes each time had a 22% lower risk of dying from a sudden cardiovascular event than men who used a sauna only once a week. Men who used saunas four to seven times a week had a 63% lower risk of dying from a cardiovascular event.

Possible reason: Sauna use increases the heart rate to a level similar to that when doing low-to-moderate exercise and helps to lower blood pressure.

Yogurt Is Heart Medicine

Lynn L. Moore, DSc, MPH, is director of nutrition and metabolism at Boston University School of Medicine and coauthor of a study published in *American Journal of Hypertension.*

Eating yogurt may reduce heart disease risk in people with high blood pressure, reports Lynn L. Moore, DSc, MPH. Men with high blood pressure who ate at least two servings of yogurt each week had 21% lower risk for heart attack or stroke. Risk was cut by 17% for women. The reason is unknown, but probiotics from fermentation in yogurt production may play a role.

HEPA for Your Heart

Masako Morishita, PhD, is an environmental-exposure science researcher at Michigan State University, East Lansing, and first author of the research published in *JAMA Internal Medicine.*

Inexpensive HEPA air filter may reduce your risk for heart attack, reports Masako Morishita, PhD. When study subjects (average age 67) used commercially available, portable HEPA filtration units (costing less than $70 each) at home, they experienced a small but significant decrease in blood pressure—which, if maintained long term, could be enough to decrease cardiovascular events by 16%. HEPA filters remove fine-particulate-matter pollution from the air in the home.

Meditation Cuts Heart Attack Risk in Half

Robert Schneider, MD, director, the NIH-funded Institute for Natural Medicine and Prevention, professor of physiology and health, Maharishi University of Management (MUM.edu), Fairfield, Iowa. Dr. Schneider is author of *Total Heart Health.*

Meditation can bring about a state of deep relaxation in which your heart rate, blood pressure and respiration slow down, giving your cardiovascular system a much needed rest. TM is a particular brand of meditation that is simple and precise. It is practiced for 20 minutes twice a day while sitting comfortably with eyes closed and silently repeating a calming word to produce a natural state of restful alertness. The health benefits of regular TM potentially include not only lower heart rate and blood pressure, but also reduced total cholesterol and insulin resistance, less need for blood pressure medication and a slowing or reversal of the hardening of arteries that contributes to heart disease.

Building on the results of past meditation studies, researchers examined the specific effect of TM on heart disease patients. In a randomized controlled trial, they assigned 201 men and women (average age 59) with narrowing of cardiovascular arteries to either a TM group or a control group. For an average of five years, all participants received regular medical care, including medication as needed and lifestyle advice about risk factors such as diet and exercise. In addition, the TM group meditated for 20 minutes twice a day at home while the control group attended classes on cardiovascular health.

The participants who had meditated...

- **Experienced a 47% reduction in heart attacks, strokes and death, compared with those who did not.**
- **Reduced their blood pressure by an average of five points.**
- **Had significant reductions in psychological stress as measured by standard psychological tests.**

Sponsored by the NIH, the study was done collaboratively by researchers at the Medical College of Wisconsin and the Maharishi University. Findings were presented at an annual meeting of the American Heart Association in Orlando.

A POWERFUL LIFESTYLE CHOICE

The dramatic effect of TM on heart patients equals the discovery of a whole new class of drug therapy—one that taps into the body's own natural pharmacy of healing resources.

TM's heart benefits cannot automatically be generalized to other meditation techniques since they weren't studied. That said, you can learn more about other ways to meditate (and meditation in general) at websites such as Relaxationresponse.org and How-to-meditate.org. Additional options include guided imagery or visualization (in which you imagine specific images during meditation)...mindfulness meditation (an increased awareness of the present moment)... and techniques such as yoga, tai chi and qi gong that combine meditation, breathing exercises and movements or postures.

Exercise Better Than Medication

Huseyin Naci, doctoral candidate in pharmaceutical policy and economics at London School of Economics, fellow at Harvard Medical School, Boston, and leader of an analysis of 305 studies, published in *BMJ*.

Exercise may work better than medication after a heart attack or stroke to prevent early death. At least two-and-a-half hours a week of moderate-intensity aerobic activity, such as brisk walking, was as good as drugs for heart attack patients and more effective than medicine for stroke patients who were capable of exercising—although such patients may have been healthier to begin with. Doctors should discuss lifestyle changes as well as medication use with patients who have had strokes or heart attacks—a combination of medicine and exercise may be best for many people.

Omega-3 Supplements May Save Your Life After a Heart Attack

Study titled "Effect of Purified Omega-3 Fatty Acids on Reducing Left Ventricular Remodeling After Acute Myocardial Infarction (Omega-remodel Study): A Double-blind Randomized Clinical Trial" by researchers in the department of cardiovascular medicine, Harvard Medical School, and Brigham and Women's Hospital, both in Boston, presented at the American College of Cardiology's 64th Annual Scientific Session in San Diego.

You've survived a heart attack. But you're worried—could another one be waiting to happen? After all, it's a vulnerable time. As your surviving heart muscle works harder to compensate for damaged tissue, you can experience further scarring and inflammation that can weaken your heart even more. But there's a simple, safe, natural, food-based supplement that cardiologists now recommend that can greatly improve your odds of keeping your heart healthy. And while it's no surprise that omega-3s are linked with heart health, this is different—a particular kind and dose of omega-3 could literally keep you alive. *Here's how to save your heart in three seconds a day...*

OMEGA-3 FOR A BROKEN HEART

Omega-3 fatty acids, the kind primarily found in cold-water fish such as salmon, have had a heart-healthy reputation for a long time. It's good for your heart to eat fish twice a week or, if you don't eat fish, to add other omega-3-rich–foods to your diet. And omega-3 supplements have been shown to reduce the risk for irregular heartbeat (arrhythmia) and prevent related fatalities, as well as reduce high triglycerides and high blood pressure, although there isn't enough evidence to determine whether taking them helps healthy people prevent heart disease, according to NIH's National Center for Complementary and Integrative Health.

The latest research makes it clear that there is at least one group of people for whom the benefits of high doses of omega-3s are extraordinarily powerful—people who've had a heart attack.

EIGHT OUNCES OF SALMON IN A PILL

In this study, 358 patients who had had heart attacks were randomly assigned to take four grams of purified prescription-only omega-3 fatty acids (about the amount found in eight ounces of salmon) or a placebo (a capsule of corn oil) each day for six months. They started within one month of the heart attack. *The researchers wanted to know how omega-3 fatty acids affected...*

- **The left ventricle of the heart, which usually deteriorates after a heart attack**

- **The size of the area damaged by their heart attacks, which can enlarge after a heart attack**

- **Signs of inflammation.**

Results: Compared with placebo, the omega-3 fatty acids were a powerhouse of heart help. Patients taking omega-3 fatty acids were 39% less likely to show deterioration in heart function than those taking placebo. Their hearts also showed much less scarring—very important because the more scarred the heart tissue is, the less well it functions. The omega-3 fatty acids also had a powerful anti-inflammatory effect, with inflammatory enzymes being way down in patients in the omega-3 group compared with patients in the placebo group.

TAKE THESE RESULTS TO HEART

Four grams of omega-3 fatty acids is a high dose—for Americans. The study researchers noted that most Americans do not get the amount of omega-3 they need, in large part because we don't eat oily fish such as sardines, tuna, trout and salmon twice a week as recommended by the American College of Cardiology and the American Heart Association. In fact, in the study of heart attack survivors, omega-3 blood levels in patients in the high-dose omega-3 group increased quite a bit, but only up to the same levels generally seen among some populations in Japan whose diet is rich in fish—and who have lower risks for heart disease and sudden death from heart attack than Americans.

Nor did the researchers report any side effects, such as interference with blood clotting, which is a concern since omega-3s are natural anticoagulants. Still, check with your doctor before taking high-dose omega-3s, especially if you are on a blood thinner. These researchers used a prescription-only form of omega-3 supplement, Lovaza, which is FDA-approved for reducing high triglyceride levels. There are many good omega-3 supplements on the market, but you'll want to see what your insurance will cover.

All of us can safely benefit from improving our blood levels of omega-3s by eating fatty fish twice a week or by getting omega-3s from other foods. But if you've had a heart attack or know someone who has, a discussion with the cardiologist about taking four grams of omega-3s in a supplement might be a lifesaving conversation.

Better Care After Heart Attack

Donald Edmondson, PhD, assistant professor of behavioral medicine, Columbia University Medical Center, New York City.

Researchers examined data from 24 studies involving 2,384 people (average age 60) who had suffered a heart attack or other coronary event.

Result: One in eight patients suffered posttraumatic stress disorder (PTSD) after the event. In the general population, fewer than one in 25 develops PTSD related to any type of traumatic event. PTSD doubled risk for another cardiac event and for dying within one to three years. If you are experiencing anxiety following a coronary event: Talk to your doctor about therapies for PTSD.

How to Prevent This Deadly Vascular Emergency

Cam Patterson, MD, MBA, the Ernest and Hazel Craige Distinguished Professor of Cardiovascular Medicine, chief of the division of cardiology and associate chair for research in the department of medicine at the University of North Carolina at Chapel Hill. He also is physician in chief of the University of North Carolina Center for Heart & Vascular Care.

When 69-year-old US diplomat Richard C. Holbrooke suffered a catastrophic rupture of the aorta, the largest blood vessel in the body, he had only about a 10% chance of surviving. After 21 hours of heroic emergency surgery, and a second procedure the following day, Holbrooke died, becoming one of about 13,000 Americans who are killed by aortic ruptures each year.

Good news: The rate of survival from this condition increases dramatically when patients with a partial aortic dissection, which can lead to an aortic rupture, recognize the symptoms and get to an emergency room immediately. Often it's possible to prevent an aortic dissection altogether by getting a screening test to diagnose arterial weakness before there's an emergency.

What you need to know to save your life—or that of a loved one...

A RUPTURED ARTERY

Every drop of blood in the body passes through the aorta. About the diameter of a garden hose, the aorta originates in the left ventricle of the heart, rises into the chest and then descends into the abdomen.

Most aortic dissections occur in a damaged section of artery known as an aneurysm—this balloonlike bulge thins and weakens that area of the artery. Within this area, a small tear can form in the inner layer (tunica intima) of the blood vessel, creating a dissection.

What happens: Blood forces its way into the tear, widening it and eventually separating, or dissecting, the three layers of the blood vessel. The continued force of blood cuts through the arterial layers and creates a "false channel," or lumen. Patients can survive this initial dissection—in some cases, they won't even know that anything is wrong if the damage stops there. But often it doesn't.

Without treatment, 15% to 20% of patients with an aortic dissection will suffer (usually within minutes or days) an acute rupture, in which the aorta is completely torn. When this happens, liters of blood are lost within a minute, and many victims die within seconds. Many others with an untreated aortic dissection suffer a rupture at some later date.

TELLTALE SYMPTOMS

The symptoms of an aortic dissection can mimic those of a heart attack. Most patients with an aortic dissection experience sudden pain that's centered in the chest, but pain can also occur in the back or neck. They often describe the pain as a brief "ripping" sensation.

Other symptoms may include nausea, shortness of breath or heavy sweating. Victims may suffer a precipitous drop in blood pressure from inadequate circulation, causing light-headedness or fainting. Some people with aortic dissection experience only vague discomfort, similar to indigestion. In rare cases, an aortic dissection may cause no symptoms and be discovered during an imaging test for some other medical condition.

Typically, however, an aortic dissection is diagnosed after the patient complains of symptoms and receives a CT or MRI scan or a transesophageal echocardiogram, in which an ultrasound device is inserted into the throat to create an image of the heart's valves and chambers. An aortic dissection cannot be ruled out with a chest X-ray or an electrocardiogram, which records the heart's electrical activity and is often used to diagnose a heart attack.

EMERGENCY REPAIR IS CRITICAL

When an aortic dissection is detected, emergency surgery is always recommended, unless the patient is too frail to undergo an operation.

About 50% of dissections occur in the ascending aorta (in the chest) and these almost always require…

• **Open surgery,** which involves opening the chest and cutting out the damaged section of artery and replacing it with a synthetic tube. It's a complicated procedure, but more than 90% of patients will survive when it's done by an experienced doctor, assuming that the patients get to the operating room in time.

Most of the other dissections occur in the descending portion of the aorta (in the abdomen) and are usually treated with…

• **Endovascular stents that restore normal blood flow.** Rather than cutting out the damaged section of artery with an open procedure, a catheter is inserted through a blood vessel in the groin and threaded upward into the damaged area. Then a fabric tube reinforced with metal stents (also known as a scaffold) is used to restore the circulation pathway.

This procedure is preferred, in appropriate cases, because patients recover more quickly and have a lower risk for kidney damage and neurological complications than those who undergo open surgery.

Important finding: A three-year study that looked at the medical records of 28,000 patients found that the risk of dying in the hospital following an endovascular repair of a rupture in the descending aorta was 1.9%, compared with 5.2% following open surgery.

Patients who can't undergo surgery, often due to other medical problems, may be treated with analgesics and medications that lower blood pressure and reduce the risk that a dissection will worsen. Blood pressure should be routinely monitored and a CT or MRI scan performed every six to 12 months.

BEST APPROACH: PREVENTION

Because aortic dissections almost always occur within aneurysms, detecting the bulging artery is the first step in prevention. This can be tricky because aneurysms typically cause no symptoms until a dissection—or a complete rupture—occurs. *Important…*

• **Get screened.** I advise everyone to have an ultrasound starting at age 60—or, in some cases, an MRI or contrast CT scan—to screen for aortic aneurysms. Earlier screening is typically recommended if you have a family history of aneurysm or aortic dissection.

Screening is crucial for men with a history of smoking. Men are twice as likely as women to have an aortic dissection, and smoking doubles the risk once again. Screening is also important for women if they have smoked or have a history of heart disease, or a family history of aneurysm or aortic dissection.

Patients with no sign of disease usually don't require additional tests/screening. However, high-risk patients, such as those with a family history of aneurysm or aortic dissection, should get retested at least every five years—more often if they already have an aneurysm.

• **Earlier treatment.** Aortic aneurysms usually grow slowly, at the rate of about 1/100 of an inch in diameter annually. Because smaller aneurysms may never grow to a size that will cause a serious risk, we currently don't advise surgery or stenting until an aneurysm reaches about two inches in diameter.

However, having the procedure done at the time of diagnosis is the safest choice for those who are most likely to suffer an aortic rupture—people with uncontrolled hypertension...a family history of aortic dissection or aortic aneurysm...or a genetic condition called Marfan syndrome, which weakens the artery wall.

• **Blood pressure control.** Along with not smoking, controlling blood pressure is the best way to prevent aortic dissection, since most cases occur in patients with hypertension. Keep your blood pressure under 120/80.

• **Risk factor sometimes overlooked: High cholesterol.** Aortic aneurysms and dissections usually occur in people with atherosclerosis, the accumulation of fatty deposits that weaken the artery walls. Maintaining healthy cholesterol is among the best ways to prevent this.

Statins for Bypass Surgery

Islam Elgendy, MD, is a cardiology fellow at University of Florida College of Medicine, Gainesville.

Almost all heart-bypass patients would benefit from taking statins before and after the surgery, says Islam Elgendy, MD. The cholesterol-lowering drugs reduce the incidence of atrial fibrillation by 58%. One study suggested that statins might reduce the risk of dying in the hospital by 43%. Though more research is needed, starting statins at least two weeks before surgery may provide some protection.

Calcium Caution

Qian Xiao, PhD, a cancer prevention fellow at the National Cancer Institute, Bethesda, Maryland, and leader of a study published in *JAMA Internal Medicine*.

In a recent finding, men who took more than 1,000 milligrams a day of calcium were 19% more likely to die from heart disease than men who took no calcium. Excess calcium in blood vessels may narrow and harden coronary arteries. Previous research shows that women may be at risk as well.

Live a Long Life...Even with Cardiac Arrhythmia

Jennifer E. Cummings, MD, director of electrophysiology research and staff cardiologist, department of cardiovascular medicine, Section of Electrophysiology and Pacing, Cleveland Clinic, Cleveland, Ohio.

Does your heart occasionally flutter or skip a beat? Does it pound unusually fast or unusually slow? If so, you may have a cardiac arrhythmia, an irregular or abnormal heartbeat that indicates a malfunction in the heart's electrical system. An arrhythmia may be no big deal—causing no symptoms, sometimes, and presenting no underlying damage or disease—or it could be a very big deal indeed, possibly leading to stroke or sudden cardiac death.

This, in fact, is what happened to political commentator Tim Russert in 2008. His death is believed to be the result of an arrhythmia caused by the rupture of plaque in his arteries. Especially in that election year, Russert was such a familiar face in American homes that many felt his loss personally—and also worried that they, too, might be vulnerable to such a fate. And since cardiovascular disease is still the number-one killer in the US, it's good to review what to do about heart arrhythmias, including an exploration of natural options for controlling this common problem. We spoke to two experts—cardiologist Jennifer E. Cummings, MD, director of electrophysiology research at the Cleveland Clinic and Michael Traub, ND, a naturopathic physician in Hawaii and former president of the American Association of Naturopathic Physicians. Both emphasized that anyone who experiences a cardiac arrhythmia should call their doctor and schedule an evaluation.

AT THE HEART OF THE MATTER

The causes for arrhythmia can range from important to insignificant. Cardiac arrhythmia may be triggered by serious, underlying heart disease... more controllable factors such as stress...medications...caffeine...or it may simply be a normal variant that will cause no symptoms or health problems and requires no treatment or lifestyle adjustment.

The only way to find out is to work with your cardiologist and undergo medical tests.

Diagnostic tests for heart arrhythmia include a Holter monitor (where your heartbeat is measured over the course of the day as you go about your normal activities), an electrocardiogram (EKG), echocardiogram (heart ultrasound), stress test (a test that measures arrhythmias that are brought on by exercise or stress) or cardiac catheterization (threading a tube into the heart to visualize vessels). There are several distinct kinds of arrhythmia—all potentially dangerous:

• **Atrial fibrillaton,** a fast and irregular heartbeat that is associated with stroke and heart failure. This is the most common arrhythmia in people over 60.

• **Bradycardia,** an abnormally slow rhythm that can cause fainting spells and, though only rarely, death.

• **Tachycardia,** an abnormally fast heart rate that can also cause sudden death.

MAINSTREAM MEDICAL TREATMENTS

Mainstream medical treatments for arrhythmia include drugs, pacemakers and other interventions, surgical or non-surgical. According to Dr. Cummings, the treatment recommendation takes into consideration both the type of arrhythmia and the overall health of the patient. An electrophysiologist (a cardiologist who specializes in treating arrhythmia) can be helpful in exploring the pros and cons of the various treatment alternatives.

Here are some of the most common treatment options...

• **Antiarrhythmic drugs.** Pharmaceutical drugs may be prescribed to block electrical impulses causing the arrhythmia. These work well but the dosage must be carefully monitored and controlled, since paradoxically this class of drugs has also shown an association with an increased risk for a different type of arrhythmia.

• **Anticoagulant or anti-platelet therapy.** Blood-thinning drugs—primarily warfarin or aspirin—may be prescribed to prevent blood clots in people with atrial fibrillation or those at risk for stroke. But, notes Dr. Cummings, aspirin is not for everyone and these treatments are not interchangeable.

• **Calcium channel blockers and beta blockers.** These drugs are prescribed to treat certain abnormal heart rhythms.

• **Pacemaker and implantable cardioverter-defibrillator (ICD) devices.** If non-invasive treatment alternatives aren't effective or appropriate, your doctor may advise implantation of a pacemaker (to regulate the heart beat) and/or an ICD (to deliver a shock when the rhythm is disrupted, in the hope this will reset the heart to beat more regularly). Typically, slow heart rhythms are treated with pacemakers, while rapid, high-risk ventricular heart rhythms are treated with ICDs.

• **Radio frequency ablation.** A thin, flexible tube called an ablation catheter is threaded into the heart. Pulses of energy get sent through the catheter to the heart, locating and destroying small areas of tissue that are causing the arrhythmias. A similar treatment called cardiac catheter cryoablation accomplishes the same goal, using cold temperatures rather than heat.

THE NATURAL PATH TO CONTROLLING ARRHYTHMIA

Many people may be unaware of simpler tools like lifestyle change, dietary adjustments and natural supplements that may be effective for the treatment of arrhythmias. Dr. Traub said that in his experience, naturopathic medicine can often be practiced in tandem with conventional medicine to bring an abnormal heartbeat under control.

The first thing to consider is whether making lifestyle changes or successfully controlling underlying conditions can make a difference. *For example...*

• **If you smoke, stop...**but (especially if you are a long-timer) seek medical oversight, as your nicotine may need to be tapered.

• **Stimulants.** If caffeine triggers symptoms, cut back on or eliminate products such as coffee, caffeinated soft drinks, tea, chocolate and anything that contains caffeine. You may need to ease back rather than stop suddenly.

• **Over-the-counter cough medicines with pseudo-epinephrine should be avoided,** as this is a stimulant that can trigger arrhythmias.

• **Limit alcohol intake.**

• **If you notice that abnormal heart rhythms are associated with specific activities** (such as certain stressful family gatherings or particularly demanding exercises), avoid them…at least until you have figured out a way to tolerate such events without having an intense physiological reaction to them. Discuss this with your doctor.

• **If a medication appears to bring on symptoms,** ask your physician if it is possible to prescribe an alternate drug.

• **Take steps to effectively manage stress.** There are hundreds of ways to do this—yoga, meditation, exercise, getting a pet, changing jobs. Examine what is contributing stress to your life, and see what can help you better manage or even change it.

NATURAL SUPPLEMENTS FOR TREATING ARRHYTHMIA

Of course, lifestyle changes alone are not always sufficient to control arrhythmias. *In more serious cases, Dr. Traub prescribes…*

• **Fish oil.** This rich source of omega-3 fatty acids is step one of Dr. Traub's treatment protocol. Fish oil is a natural anticoagulant that reduces the risk of blood clots, which can be associated with arrhythmias.

Caution: Fish oil should be taken with caution—and only under your physician's careful supervision—particularly if you take blood-thinning drugs such as *warfarin* (Coumadin) or aspirin.

• **Nattokinase.** This extract of the Japanese fermented soybean product natto inhibits development of blood clots. Use with caution—and under a doctor's supervision—if you take other blood thinners.

• **Magnesium and potassium.** Magnesium and potassium deficiencies may lead to a higher risk of arrhythmias. If blood tests confirm a deficiency, your doctor may prescribe supplements to help restore normal blood levels and reduce arrhythmia risk or occurrence.

• **Other supplements.** Additional supplements that have shown promise but require further research include *Allium cepa* and *Allium sativum* (onion and garlic), *Atropa belladonna, Cinnamomum camphora, Cordyceps sinensis* and *Crataegus oxyacantha.* Dr. Traub also points out that acetyl-L-carnitine is used in Europe to treat cardiac arrhythmias.

Cardiac arrhythmia is common—but that doesn't mean it is safe to ignore it. If you experience even one episode of arrhythmia, call your doctor. You may find that it is nothing at all…or you may learn what you need to do to save your life.

People Who Have Had a Heart Attack Should Avoid Certain Common Painkillers

Anne-Marie Schjerning Olsen, MD, is a research fellow at Gentofte Hospital, University of Copenhagen, Denmark, and lead author of a study published in *Circulation.*

Nonsteroidal anti-inflammatory drugs (NSAIDs), such as *celecoxib* (Celebrex) and *ibuprofen* (Advil, Motrin), can increase the risk for another heart attack or dying from coronary artery disease. The elevated risk persists for at least five years.

Self-defense: *Naproxen* (Aleve) has the lowest cardiovascular risk of any NSAID. (Aspirin was not studied.) Or talk to your doctor about alternative painkillers.

10

Life Habits for Better Aging

Live with Purpose... Live Longer?

Marc E. Agronin, MD, a geriatric psychiatrist at Miami Jewish Health in Florida. He is author of *How We Age: A Doctor's Journey into the Heart of Growing Old* and *The End of Old Age: Living a Longer, More Purposeful Life*. MarcAgronin.com. Dr. Agronin recently recorded a series of podcasts for Bottom Line's Conversations with the Experts. BottomLineInc.com/podcast-playlist/marc-agronin

First, let's start with some good news on the human life span. Based on the latest statistics, the average life expectancy for a male or female born in the US is close to 79 years. That's more than 10 years longer than the predicted life expectancy in 1950.

Meanwhile, there's an ever-increasing group of people who are exceeding these expectations. Centenarians are now one of the fastest-growing age groups in the country. And the majority of these older adults have a good quality of life until quite near the very end. While advances in medical care are a key driver of these positive trends, there's no question that healthier lifestyles also make a difference.

So, with this backdrop, most people are now wondering: "What can I do to increase my own longevity?"

Even though there are lots of ways that people try to extend their life spans, my favorite approach is represented by research on places where the people actually live the longest. Highlighted in research by longevity expert Dan Buettner, author of *The Blue Zones*, these communities, which are scattered around the planet, have essential characteristics that are similar. For example, the longest-living people maintain physically active lifestyles...eat plant-based diets without excess calories (and include a daily glass of wine in some places)...have strong community and/or religious ties...and hold fast to an outlook on life that is accepting and purposeful.

That last point is worth focusing on, because a bevy of research findings from the Midlife in the United States (MIDUS) study have shown that having a strong sense of purpose is associated with fewer heart attacks and strokes—and longer life spans. The leader of this study, Carol Ryff, PhD, a psychology professor at the University of Wisconsin-Madison, has found that having purpose is, in fact, one of the pillars of overall well-being.

Takeaway: People who make a point to create meaning and purpose to their lives—whether it's organizing activities for an alumni group, volunteering at a nearby homeless shelter, taking up oil painting or becoming a master mahjong player—are more apt to maintain good health longer than those whose lives have no real purpose.

Add to this the important findings of Becca Levy, PhD, a professor of epidemiology and psychology at Yale University, and you'll see that there's another crucial component to living a long and purposeful life. According to Dr. Levy's research, individuals with positive self-perceptions toward aging had a median survival that was 7.5 years longer, on average, than those with more negative self-perceptions.

Takeaway: If you embrace aging as a meaningful and positive period of transformation rather than a slow slide into decrepitude, then you're more likely to gain a few extra years.

So, rest assured, that purpose and positivity are both protective. It's a combination that helps us to not only live longer, but also to live better!

Lessons for Living Longer From the People Who Live the Longest

Dan Buettner is founder of Blue Zones, an organization that studies the regions of the world where people commonly live active lives past the age of 100, and author of *The Blue Zones*. Bluezones.com

---

On the Japanese island of Okinawa, there are approximately 50 centenarians (those who reach 100 years or more) per 100,000 people. In the US, at most 20 per 100,000 people reach this impressive milestone.

A long life is not an accident. Writer and longevity expert Dan Buettner, in conjunction with the National Institute on Aging and the nation's top gerontologists, has studied what he calls the world's Blue Zones, areas where people live unexpectedly long and healthy lives. In addition to Okinawa, the Blue Zones include Sardinia, Italy... Loma Linda, California (home to many Seventh-day Adventists)...and the Nicoya Peninsula in Costa Rica.

Important finding: Only about 25% of longevity is determined by genetics. The other 75% is largely determined by the choices that we make every day. *The average American could live up to 14 more good years by putting the following habits to work...*

CHOOSE ACTIVITY, NOT "EXERCISE"

In Sardinia, where the rate of centenarians is 208 per 100,000, many men work as shepherds. They hike for miles every day. Similarly, people in Okinawa get hours of daily exercise in their gardens. California's Seventh-day Adventists, one of the longest-living groups in the US, take frequent nature walks.

What these groups have in common is regular, low-intensity physical exercise. They don't necessarily lift weights or run marathons. They merely stay active—and they do it every day throughout their lives.

Daily physical activity improves balance and reduces the risk for falls, a common cause of death among seniors. It lowers blood pressure and improves cardiovascular health. It increases the odds that people will be functionally independent in their later years.

Recommended: 30 to 60 minutes of moderate physical activity daily. This could include riding a bicycle or walking instead of driving.

EAT LESS

Okinawan elders intone this adage before eating—*hara hachi bu*—a reminder to stop eating when their stomachs are 80% full.

People who quit eating when they're no longer hungry (rather than eating until they feel full) find it easy to maintain a healthy weight, which reduces the risk for heart disease. This approach is more natural than conventional diets. *Helpful...*

- **Serve yourself at the kitchen counter, then put the food away.** People who do this tend to eat about 14% less than those who don't.

- **Use smaller plates and bowls.** Doing so makes servings look larger, which helps you eat less. In one study, people who ate from a 34-ounce bowl took in 31% more than those who used a 17-ounce bowl. Similarly, people drink at least 25% more when they use short, wide glasses instead of tall, narrow ones.

• **Buy small.** Most people consume about 150 more calories when they take food from large packages than when they take it from smaller ones.

LIMIT MEAT

In every Blue Zone, meat is consumed, at most, a few times a month. People in these communities live mainly on beans, whole grains, vegetables and other plant foods. These foods are high in fiber, antioxidants and anticancer compounds. Traditional Sardinians, Nicoyans and Okinawans eat what is produced in their gardens supplemented by staples—durum wheat (Sardinia), sweet potato (Okinawa) and maize (Nicoya). Strict Adventists avoid meat entirely.

Studies of Seventh-day Adventists show that a relatively high proportion eat nuts (any kind). Those who eat about two ounces of nuts five or more times a week have heart disease rates that are only half those who rarely eat nuts.

CONSIDER WINE

Studies of long-lived people suggest that drinking alcohol in moderation is a powerful factor in living longer. It is consumed in three of the Blue Zones (Okinawa, Sardinia and Costa Rica). In Sardinia, the shepherds drink about one-quarter bottle of red wine a day. Their wine has two to three times more flavonoids than other wines (because of the hot climate and the way the wine is made). Flavonoids reduce arterial inflammation. Inflammation has been linked to atherosclerosis, diabetes and Alzheimer's disease.

CULTIVATE A SENSE OF PURPOSE

A study funded by the National Institutes of Health (NIH) found that people who are excited by life and feel that they're making a difference tend to live longer (and healthier) lives than those who just "get by."

Okinawans call it *ikigai* and Nicoyans call it *plan de vida*, but in both cultures, the phrase essentially translates to why I wake up in the morning. Anything that gives you a sense of purpose—even something as simple as taking pleasure in watching your children or grandchildren grow up well—can add years to your life.

DE-STRESS

Many people don't realize that the 24/7 American lifestyle is literally toxic. It produces a chronic increase in stress hormones that triggers inflammation throughout the body.

Most of the world's longest-lived people incorporate some form of meaningful downtime into their daily lives. Nicoyans take a break every afternoon to socialize with friends. For Adventists, the Saturday Sabbath is a time to rest.

EMBRACE YOUR SPIRITUAL SIDE

Faith is a key element that most centenarians have in common. The Sardinians and Nicoyans are mostly Catholic. Okinawans have a blended religion that stresses ancestor worship. The Adventists form a strong religious community. People who attend religious services are about one-third less likely to die in a given period than those who don't. Even among people who don't go to church, those with spiritual beliefs have less depression, better immunity and lower rates of heart disease.

PUT FAMILY FIRST

In the Blue Zones, a great emphasis is placed on family—and people who live with or maintain close ties with their families get sick less often than those without these ties. They also are more likely to maintain better mental and social skills throughout their lives.

It's Tee Time for Better Health!

Andrew Murray, MBChB, sports medicine consultant, University of Edinburgh, Scotland, UK.

New meta-analysis: Hitting the links increases longevity (by up to five years, according to one of the studies included) and improves risk for heart disease. Golf also is linked to better mental health, perhaps due to the social interactions and opportunities to connect with nature.

For the most benefits: Aim for 150 or more minutes playing time per week—and skip the cart and walk, if possible. Be sure to warm up before each round to prevent injury, and wear sunscreen to protect against skin cancer. For more details, go to GolfandHealth.org.

You Can Have a Much Younger Body and Mind

Mike Moreno, MD, who practices family medicine in San Diego, where he is on the board of the San Diego Chapter of the American Academy of Family Physicians. He is also the author of *The 17 Day Plan to Stop Aging.*

What is it that allows some people to remain robust and healthy well into their 80s and 90s while others become frail or virtually incapacitated? It's not just luck. New studies indicate that aging is largely determined by controllable factors.

Case in point: Millions of people have chronic inflammation, which has been linked to practically every "age-related" disease, including arthritis, heart disease and dementia.

Inflammation can usually be controlled with stress management, a healthful diet, weight loss (if needed) and other lifestyle changes, but there are other, even simpler, steps that can strengthen your body and brain so that they perform at the levels of a much younger person.

To turn back your biological clock...

CHALLENGE YOUR LUNGS

You shouldn't be short of breath when you climb a flight of stairs or have sex, but many adults find that they have more trouble breathing as they age—even if they don't have asthma or other lung diseases.

Why: The lungs tend to lose elasticity over time, particularly if you smoke or live in an area with high air pollution. "Stiff" lungs cannot move air efficiently and cause breathing difficulty.

Simple thing you can do: Breathe slowly in and out through a drinking straw for two to three minutes, once or twice daily. Breathe only through your mouth, not your nose. This stretches the lungs, increases lung capacity and improves lung function.

Helpful: Start with an extra-wide straw, and go to a regular straw as you get used to breathing this way.

DRINK THYME TEA

When the lungs do not expand and contract normally (see above), or when the tissues are unusually dry, you're more likely to get colds or other infections, including pneumonia. The herb thyme contains thymol, an antioxidant that may help prevent colds, bronchitis and pneumonia and soothe chronic respiratory problems such as asthma, allergies and emphysema.

Simple thing you can do: Add a cup of thyme tea to your daily routine. If you have a chronic or acute respiratory illness, drink two cups of thyme tea daily—one in the morning and one at night.

To make thyme tea: Steep one tablespoon of dried thyme (or two tablespoons of fresh thyme) in two cups of hot water for five minutes, or use thyme tea bags (available at most health-food stores).

If you take a blood thinner: Talk to your doctor before using thyme—it can increase risk for bleeding. Also, if you're allergic to oregano, you're probably allergic to thyme.

Another simple step: Drink at least six to eight eight-ounce glasses of water every day. This helps loosen lung mucus and flushes out irritants, such as bacteria and viruses.

LOWER YOUR HEART RATE

Heart disease is the leading cause of death in the US. The average American would live at least a decade longer if his/her heart pumped blood more efficiently.

Elite athletes typically have a resting heart rate of about 40 beats a minute, which is about half as fast as the average adult's resting heart rate. This reduced heart rate translates into lower blood pressure, healthier arteries and a much lower rate of heart disease. But you don't have to be an athlete to lower your heart rate—you just have to get a reasonable amount of aerobic exercise.

Simple thing you can do: Aim for a resting heart rate of 50 to 70 beats a minute—a good range for most adults. To do this, get 30 minutes of aerobic exercise, five days a week. Good aerobic workouts include fast walking, bicycling and swimming. Even if you're not in great shape, regular workouts will lower your resting heart rate.

To check your pulse: Put your index and middle fingers on the carotid artery in your neck, and count the beats for 15 seconds, then multiply by four. Check your pulse before, during and after exercise.

WALK JUST A LITTLE FASTER

A study published in *The Journal of the American Medical Association* found that people who walked faster (at least 2.25 miles per hour) lived longer than those who walked more slowly.

Why: Faster walking not only lowers your heart rate and blood pressure but also improves cholesterol and inhibits blood clots, the cause of most heart attacks.

Simple thing you can do: You don't have to be a speed-walker, but every time you go for a walk, or even when you're walking during the normal course of your day, increase your speed and distance slightly.

Time yourself and measure your distance to monitor your progress, and create new goals every two weeks. Walk as fast as you can but at a speed that still allows you to talk without gasping, or if you're alone, you should be able to whistle. You'll notice improvements in stamina and overall energy within about two to three weeks.

TRY THIS FOR BETTER MEMORY

A study found that people who got even moderate amounts of exercise—either leisurely 30-minute workouts, five days a week, or more intense 20-minute workouts, three times a week—had better memories than those who exercised less.

Why: Physical activity increases oxygen to the brain and boosts levels of neurotransmitters that improve mood as well as memory.

Simple thing you can do: Try an aerobic dance class, such as Zumba or salsa, or power yoga. These activities provide the physical activity needed to boost memory...and learning and remembering complicated routines will activate brain circuits and promote the growth of new brain cells for further brain benefit.

Bottom line: Just keep moving—even housecleaning and yard work count. *More on boosting brain function below...*

SHAKE UP YOUR MENTAL ROUTINES

In a study of about 3,000 older adults, those who performed mentally challenging tasks, such as memorizing a shopping list or surfing the Internet to research a complex topic, were found to have cognitive skills that were the typical equivalent of someone 10 years younger. You'll get the same benefit from other activities that promote thinking and concentration.

Why: These tasks trigger the development of new neurons in the brain, which boost cognitive function.

Simple thing you can do: Try to change your mental routines daily.

Fun ideas: If you're right-handed, use your left hand to write a note. Study the license number of the car in front of you, and see if you can remember it five minutes later. Listen to a type of music that's new to you. Rearrange your kitchen cabinets so that you have to think about where to find things. Overall, don't let your brain get into the rut of performing the same tasks over and over.

FIGHT BRAIN INFLAMMATION

You've probably heard that good oral hygiene can reduce the risk for heart disease. A new study suggests that it also can promote brain health. Researchers found that men and women over age 60 who had the lowest levels of oral bacteria did better on cognitive tests involving memory and calculations than those who had more bacteria.

Why: Bacteria associated with gum disease also cause inflammation in the brain. This low-level inflammation can damage brain cells and affect cognitive function.

Simple thing you can do: Brush your teeth after every meal—and floss twice a day. I also recommend using an antiseptic mouthwash, which helps eliminate bacteria.

The Longevity Secret That Most Doctors Forget to Talk About

Victor Zeines, DDS, a holistic dentist with practices in New York City and Woodstock, New York. He is a founder of the Institute for Nutritional Dentistry in Woodstock, New York, and author of *Healthy Mouth, Healthy Body: The Natural Dental Program for Total Wellness.* NatDent.com

Would you believe that you can add years to your life just by taking care of your mouth? Many people can. That's because the disease processes that lead to heart problems, stroke and even lung disease often first present themselves in the gums, teeth and tongue.

What few people realize: To avoid gum disease and tooth decay, you need to do more than brush your teeth and floss. These practices may keep your mouth clean, but they do not address one of the underlying causes of oral health problems—nutritional deficiencies.

Good news: Easy, natural treatments, as well as a type of laser therapy that is becoming more popular, can treat severe gum disease and help ward off medical conditions that may shorten your life. These treatments can help not only people who want to prevent gum disease, but also those who already have it.

DEFEATING GUM DISEASE

Why is poor oral health so dangerous? Harmful bacteria from the mouth enter the bloodstream via blood vessels in the mouth and then travel throughout the body, wreaking havoc. Infected gums quadruple your heart attack risk and triple your stroke risk.

Frighteningly, about 75% of adults have some form of gum disease, including gingivitis, which occurs when a bacteria-laden film accumulates on and irritates the gums at the base of the teeth.

The more advanced form, periodontitis, occurs when infection and/or inflammation of gum tissues is accompanied by tissue destruction. Warning signs include persistent bad breath, gums that bleed while brushing and/or tender or receding gums. *Here are several natural treatments that can help...*

- **Coenzyme Q10 (CoQ10).** Found naturally in the body, though not always at a high enough level, CoQ10 is linked to reduced risk for heart disease. However, CoQ10 also strengthens gum tissue and promotes faster tissue repair and healing. It is available as a supplement.

Typical dose for oral health: 200 mg daily. If you take a blood-thinning drug, such as *warfarin* (Coumadin), consult a doctor before taking CoQ10—it can reduce the drug's blood-thinning effect.

- **Calcium.** This mineral helps rebuild bone, which can be destroyed by gum disease. Strive for 1,000 mg daily if you are age 19 to 50 and 1,200 mg daily if you are age 51 or older by eating calcium-rich foods, such as green leafy vegetables and canned sardines with their bones, and/or taking a calcium supplement. To enhance calcium absorption, look for a formula with vitamin D.
- **Goldenseal, myrrh and calendula.** These herbs work together to inhibit bacteria, stimulate immunity and reduce inflammation. Combine equal amounts of each herb in tincture form. After brushing your teeth, rinse your mouth with one teaspoon of the liquid and spit it out. Store the mixture in a brown bottle in a dark place.
- **Massage your gums.** To increase blood supply and bring more oxygen and nutrients to the area (as well as infection-fighting white blood cells), gently rub your gums a few times a day with clean fingers.
- **Laser therapy.** Lasers are used in dentistry to treat gum disease. This type of therapy targets the infected area to get rid of bacteria. Since gum disease can promote bone loss, the lasers also can stimulate the body to regrow bone. Laser treatment, which often is accompanied by nutritional therapy, can last for six months to a year, depending on severity. Check with your insurer to see if laser therapy is covered.

BATTLING TOOTH DECAY

Cavities are a consequence of acid and bacteria eroding the enamel or outer coating of the tooth. This creates openings and holes that can penetrate to the inner layers of the tooth and eventually kill the nerves. Cavities aren't just the result of poor brushing skills, but rather a signal that the body is overwhelmed by acid-producing bacteria (often from excess sweets, dairy and most fats).

Important: Many people are allergic to dairy, which, when consumed, can weaken their immune system and produce even more acid-producing bacteria. *Best remedies to prevent tooth decay...*

- **Natural toothpastes that contain herbs are just as effective as mainstream toothpastes at cleaning the teeth but are more gentle.** In fact, most mainstream toothpastes have a warning on the label telling users to seek medical attention if more than a pea-sized amount is swallowed.

Remember: The main purpose of using toothpaste is to keep your teeth and mouth clean.

Natural toothpastes to try: Nature's Gate, Homeodent and Vicco. In addition to regular flossing, brush after every meal. If you're at a restaurant and can't brush, simply rinse your mouth with water after eating.

- **Alfalfa, dandelion and horsetail.** These herbs have minerals that are absorbed by the teeth, making them stronger and more decay resistant.

To help strengthen enamel: Open 200-mg capsules of each herb and mix the contents with water, making a sludgy paste. Place a small amount of the paste at the gumline and rub it around your teeth. Repeat after brushing, twice daily. You can make a few days' supply and refrigerate.

All natural remedies in this article are available at health-food stores. Always talk with your doctor before using any herbs or supplements. For more advice on natural remedies for oral health, contact the International Academy of Biological Dentistry and Medicine (281-651-1745, IABDM.org) to find a holistic dentist near you.

The Mother of All Health Tips: You Need This to Live Long

Julianne Holt-Lunstad, PhD, professor of psychology and neuroscience at Brigham Young University, Provo, Utah. Her research focuses on the long-term health effects of social connections and includes a meta-analysis on the effects of loneliness and social isolation on mortality.

Other than air, water, sleep and food, what is it that human adults need so badly that doing without it is as harmful to health as being an alcoholic or smoking a pack of cigarettes a day?

Hint: It is so important to your health that not having it is worse for you than being sedentary and is considered twice as dangerous as obesity. It's not sex—though that may well be a part of it. It's social interaction, and believe it or not, having strong ties to other people is so vital that it actually improves the odds that you'll live for any given period of time by 50%! *Here's why other people make your life better...*

PEOPLE NEED PEOPLE

Compelling statistics spelling out the importance of human relationships were identified in research published in *PLoS Medicine,* which analyzed 148 studies involving the social habits of 300,000 people over an average of seven and a half years. Until then, the link between lack of relationships and risk for death hadn't been widely explored. The researchers learned that social support provides numerous emotional benefits that translate into good health and longevity, specifically...

- **Social connections help** people handle difficult and uncomfortable emotions, including anxiety and anger.
- **Friends and family act as helpful naggers—**they tend to encourage healthy lifestyles by urging people who aren't healthy to sleep more, lose weight, eat healthfully, see a doctor, exercise or quit smoking.
- **Social relationships provide meaning and purpose in life,** and people who have a purpose are more likely to take better care of themselves and avoid unnecessary health risks.

WHAT ARE THE BENEFITS?

Our relationships influence long-term health through emotional and/or psychological responses that affect physiological processes. The data show us that real or perceived availability of social resources is linked to lower blood pressure, better immune functioning and decreased inflammatory processes for a number of different diseases. In one study participants wore a device that measures blood pressure throughout a 24-hour period—it showed that people with social support tend to have lower blood pressure. However, despite the numerous studies showing that relationships are associated with healthfulness, the exact mechanisms by which they do so are not clear.

EPIDEMIC OF LONELINESS

Humans are naturally social, note the researchers, but many aspects of modern life lead to isolation. For instance, in our highly mobile society, people often live far from all or most of their family members. Many delay getting married and having children, and because more people of all ages are living alone, loneliness seems to be a growing problem. According to a Duke University study published in the *American Sociological Review*, over the past few decades, the number of Americans who say that they have no close confidants has doubled—to 25%. Increasingly popular technology that keeps us glued to a computer or cell phone inhibits development of close personal relationships. The Internet may make it easier to meet people, but online interactions cannot take the place of in-person engagement. For instance, studies have shown that physical touch from a loved one has measurable health benefits, including pain reduction and lowered blood pressure. Cancer patients who received loving touch from friends or family members reported less fatigue and nausea than those who did not.

QUALITY TIME

Relationship quality is absolutely important...scientific evidence does show that "negative relationships" can hurt our health. Rather than using that as a reason to be loners, however, this is evidence that we should work to improve existing relationships in addition to looking for more opportunities to develop new ones. In fact, the quality of relationships is more significant than the quantity. Having even one true confidant or someone you know you can turn to when you need a favor is important. You might have 50 people around you and still feel lonely—we need to go beyond thinking about numbers. Whatever the cause of loneliness—a negative perception of yourself or others, poor social skills, few social contacts or lack of a confidant—this is one "medical treatment" that can be quite pleasant. Start by calling a friend today!

Don't Let Loneliness Harm Your Health

Carla Perissinotto, MD, associate professor of geriatrics at the University of California at San Francisco. Dr. Perissinotto's research into the association between loneliness and health was published in *Archives of Internal Medicine*.

Loneliness is a miserable feeling...and generic advice such as joining a hiking club or a senior center may not help. The key to relieving your own loneliness is to understand it. Why are you lonely?

It's an important question to answer because loneliness has been linked to a variety of health problems, such as weakened immunity and hardening of the arteries. Research also suggests that the dangers associated with loneliness are on par with those related to obesity and cigarette smoking.

Latest development: Loneliness is now considered a risk factor for Alzheimer's disease according to a study published in the *Archives of General Psychiatry.* Although the exact link between loneliness and the brain is unknown, some experts hypothesize that loneliness provokes a chronic stress reaction that promotes inflammation, which accumulating evidence suggests may contribute to Alzheimer's disease, the most common cause of dementia.

How to fight loneliness and its associated health risks...

BEING ALONE VS. BEING LONELY

Many people choose to live by themselves and are perfectly content. Conversely, you can be lonely without being alone. Many lonely people are married, and some even have lots of friends.

So what is this thing called loneliness? It can include feeling that you lack companionship, feeling left out and feeling isolated. You can even be lonely without knowing it—you can have one of these feelings and not recognize it as loneliness, in the same way that some depressed people do not identify their negative moods and lethargy as depression.

WHAT CAUSES LONELINESS?

Some people may be more vulnerable to feeling lonely because of their personalities. But other times, people are in situations that promote loneliness. For example, maybe they need to stay home due to an illness and miss seeing others...or perhaps they are living in a rural area where it's difficult to connect with others and they crave more daily contact with people.

Loneliness also increases with age. In one study, 43% of seniors reported feeling lonely. *Two main reasons for this...*

- **Relationships frequently dwindle with age.** Upon retirement, your career-long social network may crumble...friends and family may move away...a beloved life partner may die.

- **Our ageist, youth-centered culture tends to ignore the wisdom and experience that aging provides.** The elderly are often stigmatized as a burden on society. It's easy to believe that your life no longer has a purpose when you feel unacknowledged by a world in which you once played a productive role.

EASING LONELINESS

There's no one-size-fits-all remedy for loneliness. But if you ask yourself the important question—Why am I lonely?—you may discover a solution that works for you. The following suggestions often help people pinpoint the cause of their loneliness and allow them to overcome it.

If you feel that you lack companionship...

- **Connect with more people.** Connecting with people who share your strong interest in something may help fill that void. Try joining a book group if you love to read...or an activist group if you are passionate about politics. Consider volunteering to tutor children or serve meals at a shelter. Beneficial connections can happen one-on-one or in groups. Some people find that getting a pet is helpful.

Unfortunately, the loneliness of social isolation may have deep roots. Even if you are lonely for companionship, you may find it difficult or unpleasant to connect with others—particularly if the problem is long-standing. Dig down to find out why.

Some people never developed the social skills that foster friendships, and some hold maladaptive beliefs about themselves (a sense of inferiority or superiority, for example) or about others (such as mistrust). If this is the case, self-reflection and therapy can help.

- **Put technology to work.** Computer, tablet or smartphone applications like Skype and FaceTime allow you to talk with—and see—friends and family who aren't nearby. The apps are free (once you own the device).

If you're uncomfortable with technology, consider taking a free class at a public library or senior center. Check SeniorNet (SeniorNet.org), a nonprofit company that offers in-person classes across the country specially designed for older adults.

Useful: The AARP-sponsored website Connect2 Affect.org offers valuable information and an interactive guide to local resources, such as job opportunities, volunteer programs and tax preparation services. Also, SeniorCenterWithoutWalls.org enables isolated seniors to participate in groups via phone or computer.

Important: Social media, such as Facebook, provides a measure of connectedness but shouldn't displace real-life contact.

If you feel left out...

- **Deepen your relationships.** Taking steps to deepen your friendships—by revealing more about yourself and listening and responding wholeheartedly to what your friends have to say—may bring the warmth of true connection into your life. Here, too, a therapist can help by giving you the tools you need to deepen your relationships.

Is it your relationship with your life partner that needs more intimacy? If your marriage leaves you lonely, you and your spouse may benefit from couples counseling.

If you feel physically isolated…

• **Overcome barriers.** Mundane difficulties can cut you off from others. Transportation is often an issue for older people who have mobility problems or don't drive. Local agencies for the aging can provide help, as can the website Connect2Affect.org (mentioned above).

Consider using a "task-sharing" service where people trade skills for what they need—for example, you help someone with balancing her checkbook and she gives you a ride to the supermarket.

Websites to try: SwapRight.com or Simbi.com. You could also take a taxi or use Uber if you cannot get a ride otherwise.

Maybe your diminished hearing or vision makes you reluctant to socialize. If that's the case, talk to your doctor about ways to improve your hearing or sight.

Easy Way to Get a People Fix

Crista Crittenden, PhD, assistant teaching professor in Penn State University's department of biobehavioral health.

Close social bonds are the time-honored cure for long-term loneliness and social isolation, which are linked to poor fitness, lack of self-care, depression, even cognitive decline. "Being a spouse, being a parent, having deep friendships—that's great," says Crista Crittenden, PhD, assistant teaching professor in Penn State University's department of biobehavioral health. "But a lot of people don't have that." Especially as we age, close social bonds can be hard to maintain as grown children move away and friends, sometimes, pass away.

The good news: Casual acquaintances protect quite well against health risks linked to loneliness.

Example: When Crittenden and colleagues examined the connection between social isolation and age-related decline in lung function—a major indicator of mortality risk—they discovered that what matters is not the depth of our relationships but the number of different people we interact with, even in a small way. That could be the clerk at the corner store or the neighbor we chat with on the sidewalk.

So let's honor casual interactions. "If you find yourself getting isolated," says Crittenden, "join a book club, or go to church or even just to the store." You know—the one where you always see that checkout person and have a great little talk.

How Reading a Book Makes You Healthier

Michael Roizen, MD, chief wellness officer, Cleveland Clinic, Ohio.

Remember that big stack of novels your high school English teacher wanted you to read? You might—or might not—have actually plowed through all those pages.

But either way, there's a new twist on reading that you should take note of as an adult.

In a nod to English teachers everywhere, we now know that joining a social group, such as a book club, can be good for your health!

Book club members live longer, according to research published in *BMJ Open*. Yes, really. It's not that readers are necessarily healthier than nonreaders…but getting together to talk about books appears to provide health-promoting effects that are comparable to those of regular exercise.

Surprising finding: When Australian researchers analyzed the habits of more than 400 adults who were transitioning into retirement, they found that those who attended two social groups—such as book clubs and church groups—had a 2% risk of dying over the six-year study period. When participants gave up one group, the risk rose to 5%…and to 12% if they gave up both groups.

Combining friendship with reading and other mental activities is a win-win because it lowers stress, increases serotonin (a "feel-good" brain chemical) and may even promote the growth of new brain cells.

"Companionship and intellectual stimulation—and thinking quickly during book club discussions—all of these things are very healthy," explains Michael Roizen, MD, chief wellness officer at Cleveland Clinic in Ohio.

So why not give it a try?

To find a book club in your area, check with your local library and/or websites such as MeetUp.com or ReadersCircle.org.

And for some excellent book titles to suggest to your new book club, go to https://bottomlineinc.com/life/books/best-book-club-books-that-you-havent-read-yet for 12 great options—everything from a Vietnam era page-turner about a teenage runaway to a US Supreme Court justice's autobiography about growing up in a housing project.

Happy reading!

Good Relationships, Surprisingly Good for Your Health

Alexa Elkington, MS, marriage and family therapist with a private practice in Las Vegas who leads communication workshops.

Here are the key points to help strengthen the quality of our interactions and close relationships—thus contributing to health and happiness...

- **Accept differences.** Instead of trying to change others, recognize and accept that they are who they are—full of strong points and weak points, lovable qualities and some that aren't so lovable...in other words, completely human.

- **Think positive.** You can decide to view other people's annoying small habits as big negatives...as neutral behavior...or even as charming quirks. For example, grown children visiting your home are apt to leave a dish or two in the sink, just as they did as kids. You can get fired up about it or smile at their consistency.

- **Appreciate.** Remember to say thank you even for small actions—including chores that the other person is "supposed" to do. Gratitude cheers the heart and increases warm feelings.

- **Be understanding.** Recognize and respect that your style of handling conflict may be different from the other person's. Those who easily speak up find it hard to understand someone who stays quiet, for instance. But it is important to accept the difference...and for "self-silencers" to protect their health by learning to speak up.

Divorce Dangers

Annals of Behavioral Medicine.

People who were divorced or separated were 46% more likely to die during the 14-year study period than those who were still married.

Possible reason: A stressful divorce can increase smoking and reduce physical activity.

The Gray Divorce Epidemic

Michele Weiner-Davis, LCSW, founder of The Divorce Busting Center in Boulder, Colorado, and DivorceBusting.com, which helps on-the-brink couples save their marriages. She is the best-selling author of eight books including *Healing from Infidelity*, *The Sex-Starved Marriage* and *Divorce Remedy*.

As a marriage therapist who helps couples avoid unnecessary divorce, I find it reassuring that the divorce rate in our country has stabilized.

But there's a notable exception: Divorce is on the rise among people age 50 and older who have been married for 20 to 30 years.

According to data from the National Center for Health Statistics and the US Census Bureau, the number of married couples in their 50s who call it quits has doubled since the 1990s. Among couples age 65 and older, divorces have tripled since 1990. This trend to divorce later in life even has a name—

the gray divorce. *Here's what you can do to save your marriage...*

WHY DIVORCE NOW?

There are many reasons why long-term marriages are breaking up...

• **Kids leaving home.** When children still are home, people who are unhappily married often choose to put aside their own unhappiness, fearing that divorce will negatively impact their children. They opt to make the best of the situation until the kids are launched. Divorces are common when the youngest child leaves home.

• **Feeling disconnected.** The early stages of marriage typically are characterized by feelings of strong physical attraction and infatuation. But over time, this mutual love affair wanes. Spouses start leading separate lives. They focus on their careers, children, extended family, friends, hobbies and other commitments...anything but each other. Eventually, loneliness and emotional disconnection set in.

• **Remarriage.** Older people often are in second or third marriages—which, overall, have significantly higher rates of divorce than first marriages. Stressors arising from complicated stepfamily dynamics, challenging ex-spouses and overwhelming financial responsibilities often are at the root of why these marriages end.

• **Increased life expectancy.** It's not uncommon for people in their 50s or 60s to live another 20 to 30 years. Many seniors are wondering whether they really want to spend what remains of their lives with their current partners—and finding that the answer is no.

• **In search of more energetic partners.** If two partners have decidedly different levels of energy or ability or interest in engaging in activities requiring vitality—such as sex, athletics or active hobbies—the more vibrant spouse might desire a more active partner.

• **Focusing on oneself.** Some people complain that during the course of their marriages, their own needs have taken a backseat to caretaking for others—spouses, children, parents and in-laws. Believing that "time is running out," there is a growing sense of urgency to nurture oneself instead. Divorce is viewed as an opportunity to redefine and refocus one's life.

REASONS NOT TO GET A GRAY DIVORCE

Although the idea of getting a new lease on life might be appealing, there are good reasons to be cautious about ending a marriage later in life.

In their quiet moments, many people who divorce later in life—even those who are happily divorced—express sadness about not being able to reminisce together about good times, share family holidays and other important events, or even rejoice in grandchildren together.

Furthermore, the idea that older children aren't affected by their parents' divorces simply isn't true. Research suggests that children of all ages—even adult children—often struggle tremendously when their parents divorce. They wonder, Isn't anything permanent in life? They worry about the viability of their own marriages.

Because mature adult children are believed to be emotionally equipped to deal with the challenges of divorce, parents often openly discuss details about their failing marriages, leaving their children feeling caught in the middle.

Although some gray divorcees yearn for the solitude that single life has to offer, others fantasize about finding new, more compatible partners with whom they can create healthier, more loving relationships. But "gray dating" isn't necessarily easy. Becoming single again after many years of marriage has its challenges.

Finally, because many gray divorcees are retired—or close to it—they may be living on fixed incomes that don't go nearly as far when split between two independent people as when shared by a couple. This can diminish the quality of life and create financial worries.

HOW TO PREVENT A GRAY DIVORCE

Some older couples think, We've made it this far...we don't need to do anything different now. But if your marriage still is strong and you don't want to wake up one morning thinking, We have nothing in common anymore, you have to make your marriage your number-one priority.

Your marriage should take precedence over kids, careers, hobbies, extended family and any other commitments. This means spending regular time together as a couple and checking in with each other daily. *Also...*

• **Break out of communication ruts.** Couples who have been together a long time can get stuck in ineffective ways of communicating. If you're upset about something in your relationship but avoid discussing it or find conversations about it to be nonproductive or hurtful, over time it will destroy your feelings of love for your partner.

Although all marriages have their ups and downs, when resentment, hurt and anger are ever-present, it is essential to address and resolve underlying issues. If communication problems are at the root of destructive interactions, it's easy to think that you're both so set in your ways after being married for so long that change isn't possible. But this simply isn't true. When motivated, people can make life-altering changes that profoundly improve the quality of relationships.

Learning new relationship skills is one way to achieve these fundamental changes. Marriage-education classes offered by mental health professionals, religious organizations and universities can be extremely helpful. Simply Google "marriage education" in your area to find a local class. Also, self-help books outlining how to have successful relationships can be useful.

• **Don't give up on compliments.** Science tells us that our brains have a negativity bias—that is, we're most likely to notice things that are problematic. Although this vigilance serves us in terms of survival, it's extremely detrimental in marriage. Constantly focusing on what your spouse does wrong creates resentment, anger and hurt, which in turn leads to emotional distance.

Instead, couples in healthy relationships focus most on what their spouses do right. They are diligent about expressing appreciation and gratitude. Older couples sometimes stop giving each other compliments in the mistaken belief that they're not necessary. But making a habit of complimenting your spouse a few times a day is a powerful way to build goodwill and friendship—an important foundation for a lasting marriage.

• **Keep it sexy.** Reaching midlife does not mean giving up on staying fit and having a satisfying sexual relationship. In fact, many couples in their 50s and 60s (and beyond) report having active sex lives. As people age, however, what they find sexually arousing changes. What "worked" in their 20s may be quite different from what "works" in their 50s or 60s. That's why ongoing open communication about sexual preferences is imperative.

Often one spouse is more interested in sex than the other. In itself, this is not a problem—as long as the couple finds a way to bridge this desire gap so that they both can be happy. When the lower-desire spouse consistently rejects his/her partner's sexual advances, it causes deep resentment, hurt and, eventually, anger. For the lower-desire spouse, anger is a big turnoff, making sex even less likely. For more on how to address this, read my article at BottomLineInc.com (search "When a Spouse Doesn't Want to Have Sex").

• **Break the routine.** Older couples can get stuck in routines. But happily married couples continually reinvent themselves. They are creative. They have a passion for breaking out of the mold. Novelty keeps relationships fresh...and that freshness keeps people interested.

What to do: Do some of the things your spouse loves to do even if you're not crazy about those things. Experiment with new hobbies that you can do together. Travel to new places. Try new kinds of recipes and restaurants. Even if you have two left feet, take a dance class together. Having more time available in later life makes engaging in new activities more feasible.

• **Get help.** If you've tried the steps in this article and still are thinking of getting a divorce, seek qualified professional help. Look for a therapist who specializes in marriage therapy and understands the issues you are facing as you age. The website of the American Association for Marriage and Family Therapy (AAMFT.org) offers a helpful "therapist locator" tool.

Have More Fun in Your Relationship

Judy Kuriansky, PhD, is a clinical psychologist and sex therapist on the adjunct faculty of Teachers College, Columbia University in New York City. She is the author of five books, including *The Complete Idiot's Guide to a Healthy Relationship*. DrJudy.com

Ever feel like you and your partner are stuck in an unfun rut of never-ending obligations, petty arguments or simmering tensions? There's a simple antidote to such strains that can add laughter to your lives every day—and remind you both of how fabulous it feels to be head-over-heels with each other. The secret is to invite the fun back into your relationship. *Here's how...*

• **Believe in the power of fun.** There's truth to the saying, "All work and no play makes Jack a dull boy"—and Jill a dull girl. Boredom can endanger a relationship, leading to emotional withdrawal...increasing partners' propensity for fantasizing about being with someone else...and even setting the stage for an affair or separation. But by renewing your commitment to sharing fun times, you can fortify your bond.

Evidence: Research from the University of Denver Center for Marital and Family Studies shows that fun and marital happiness go together...a study from Stony Brook University confirms that doing new and exciting activities together leads to better relationships.

• **Clear away stresses that interfere with fun.** If both of you are able to turn off your worries as easily as you hit delete on your computer, that's wonderful. But many people need to resolve whatever is weighing on their minds before they can let the fun energy flow. So try some instant decompression-for-two by doing deep-breathing exercises together. Set aside time to talk out whatever is bothering you. If you owe an apology, offer it without delay, thus clearing the air so you can enjoy each other's company again.

• **Sync your schedules.** Spontaneous frivolity is super...but when work and/or other commitments jam your agenda, you must work within that framework. Sit down together with your calendars and don't get up until you have carved out some togetherness time. Start small, for instance, with two hour-long blocks during the week plus a three-hour chunk on the weekend. Then keep those times inviolable—don't make excuses for letting other responsibilities intrude. Once you see how rewarding this is, you'll naturally make even more space for fun in your schedules.

• **Explore new definitions of fun.** It's great if you and your guy already agree that diversion means going to the movies, say, or cycling in the park. But not all couples enjoy the same activities, especially as their interests or physical abilities change over time. So have a frank discussion about what fun means to each of you now. Are the most appealing activities done indoors or outdoors? During the day or at night? As a twosome or in a group? Stay open-minded, and you may discover that the bridge games you used to find boring are just right for your nimble mind and aching knees today. Keep talking until you compose a list of at least three activities that are fun for you both...then add three more ideas each week. Plug those merry pursuits into the time slots you set aside on your calendars. It's fine to repeat your favorites, as long as those activities remain fun rather than becoming routine.

• **Recapture your childhood.** For additional inspiration, think back to what you enjoyed as youngsters. If your memories are vague, visit a park and watch how kids cavort—tossing balls, soaring skyward on swings, having a pretend tea party or just horsing around. Give yourselves permission to let go of your dignity and inhibitions and act silly.

Ideas: Have a pillow fight...build a snowman...buy some board games or puzzles...try bowling or badminton.

• **Be funny.** The word fun is imbedded in the word funny—so get a book of jokes and take turns reading it aloud to each other at breakfast or bedtime. Make a point of noticing whatever made you laugh during your day, then tell your partner so he can share the mirth. Such momentary bursts of fun, repeated often enough throughout each day, can add up to a lifetime of joy together.

A Top Longevity Expert Tells How to Have Good Sex at Any Age...Live Longer, Too

The late **Robert N. Butler, MD,** professor of geriatrics at Mount Sinai School of Medicine in New York City and former president and CEO of the International Longevity Center (ILC-Alliance.org). He was founding director of the National Institute on Aging and the coauthor of *The New Love and Sex After 60*.

Despite what Hollywood would have us believe, sex isn't limited to people under age 40. In fact, recent research shows that a sizable percentage of Americans are remaining sexually active into their 70s, 80s and beyond. But let's be honest—there are obstacles, both physical and psychological, to maintaining a healthy sex life as we age.

Very good news: After years of research and clinical practice as a specialist in longevity, I have found six key principles that, taken together, can help the vast majority of couples—no matter what age—have a good sex life. And when a couple has a satisfying sex life, their feelings of fondness and intimacy can grow stronger—and that improves every aspect of their lives. *For a great sex life at any age...*

1. Realize that sex and intimacy can literally add years to your life. Numerous studies have shown that close relationships are a key to maintaining good mental and physical health as we get older. Of course, emotional closeness can exist without sexual intimacy—but to the degree that sexuality helps enrich our closest relationships, it can be an important contributor to a long, healthy life.

Bottom line: If you give up on a good sex life, you may die sooner.

2. Ignore what society tells us about aging and sex. The idea of older people having sex is thought of as a rarity. This stereotype couldn't be further from the truth. A 2007 study of sexual activity among older Americans, published in the *New England Journal of Medicine*, showed that more than one-half of men and women between the ages of 65 and 74 and more than one-quarter of those between 75 and 85 had been sexually active within the previous 12 months. And among those who reported that they were in good or excellent health, these figures were considerably higher.

Bottom line: Don't let society's false stereotype keep you from one of the great joys of life.

3. Take care of your health. A healthy blood flow to the sexual organs is essential for sexual response. That's why maintaining good cardiovascular health—including managing cholesterol levels and blood pressure as well as exercising—is key to a good sex life. *Also vital...*

- **If you have diabetes, control it.** Diabetes is a killer of sexuality because it damages the cardiovascular system and the body's peripheral nerves.
- **Discuss with your doctor whether any medications you take might be affecting your sexual desire or response.**

Examples: Antidepressants can significantly reduce libido, while diuretics and beta-blockers used for high blood pressure can cause erectile dysfunction. Ask about alternative drugs and/or drugs that might counter the sexual side effects.

4. Steer clear of alcohol. A character in Macbeth famously said of alcohol, "It provokes the desire, but it takes away the performance." He was right. Alcohol can make us want sex more—and some women, in particular, say that their sexual pleasure is increased after drinking, most likely because alcohol reduces psychological inhibition. But even one drink can reduce a woman's vaginal blood flow and lubrication and intensity of orgasm. For men, intoxication can severely reduce the ability to achieve an erection and the intensity of orgasm—and regular alcohol consumption (even without intoxication) lowers testosterone levels, affecting quality of erection and orgasm.

Bottom line: A little alcohol might help—or at least not hurt—your sex life. But it's best to save any imbibing for after sex.

5. Take advantage of medications and sex-related personal-care products. For older people, the introduction of the oral medications *sildenafil citrate* (Viagra), *vardenafil* (Levitra) and *tadalafil* (Cialis), which help men maintain erections, has been an important development.

Reason: Erectile dysfunction is one of the most frequently cited reasons that older couples are no longer sexually active. While they are safe and effective for most men, talk with your doctor about potential side effects before trying any of these drugs.

What many couples don't realize: It is normal for an older man to need to have his penis physically stimulated to achieve an erection—just thinking about sex, or even kissing and other foreplay, often isn't enough. Ladies, this is not an indication of diminished desire. *As we all know, hormones play a great role in sex...*

- **For men.** If you are unhappy with your sexual response after following the advice throughout this article, see an endocrinologist for a check on your levels of testosterone and thyroid hormones. A low level of either can dampen sexual desire and ability. Hormone supplements can be prescribed.

- **For women.** Older women often experience vaginal dryness, which can make intercourse far less enjoyable or sometimes impossible. This problem can be solved by applying an over-the-counter, non-oil-based lubricant, such as K-Y Jelly, Astroglide, or Slip, just before sex...or, to allow for more spontaneity, by using a moisturizing insert such as Lubrin (which lasts several hours) or Replens gel, which lasts several days. (Avoid oil-based lubricants, such as petroleum jelly and baby oil, which tend to remain in the vagina and create a breeding ground for infections.)

Alternative: If a lubricant isn't enough to make sex comfortable, ask your doctor about a topical form of the hormone estrogen, which can be applied to the vagina to increase your body's ability to lubricate itself.

6. Keep all the flames burning. If you're in a long-term relationship and you want a satisfying sex life, it's important to purposely set aside time for nonsexual intimacy on a regular basis.

Perfect example: Years ago, I lived next door to a couple who had a weekly candlelight dinner in their backyard. This kind of intimate encounter may not always lead to sex—but it creates a psychological closeness that encourages physical intimacy.

MORE FROM ROBERT N.BUTLER, MD...

If You Are Single, Divorced, Widowed...

For older unmarried people, finding an appropriate sexual (and life) partner is a challenge. This is especially true for older women, whose longer life span means they outnumber older men by about two to one.

But remember: The loss of a sexual partner wouldn't stop a 30-year-old from seeking a new relationship, so why should it stop you at age 60, 70, 80 or older?

To find a wonderful partner: The key is to frequently participate in activities that will expose you to potential partners, especially activities in which you have a strong interest, such as dancing, politics or art. This will give you the best chance of meeting someone you're attracted to and who shares your interests, an ideal starting place for developing a more intimate bond.

The Truth About Drinking Past 45

Robert L. Doyle, MD, a clinical instructor at Harvard Medical School in Boston and assistant medical director in the Child and Adolescent Inpatient Unit at McLean Hospital in Belmont, Massachusetts. Dr. Doyle also has a private psychiatry practice in Cambridge, Massachusetts, and is coauthor, with Joseph Nowinski, PhD, of *Almost Alcoholic: Is My (or My Loved One's) Drinking a Problem?*

Once we reach middle age (roughly age 45) and beyond, we can simply look in the mirror to get ample evidence that our bodies are aging. What's not so evident is the cascade of hidden physiological changes taking place that drastically alter how our bodies process beer, wine and liquor, creating a host of health dangers.

Important: Even if you don't drink excessively—and imbibe no more than you ever have—there are still crucial, little-known facts everyone should have about alcohol's effect on the body as we age.

To learn more, we recently spoke with Robert L. Doyle, MD, one of the country's leading authorities on alcohol use.

WHAT HAPPENS WHEN WE DRINK

Research showing an association between moderate drinking—usually defined as no more than two drinks daily for men...and one for women—and lower rates of heart disease has gotten a lot of attention. But that's only part of the story.

Alcohol is metabolized primarily by the liver, which undergoes significant change with age. This "detoxifier" is very similar to a car's air filter—the longer it's used, the more clogged it becomes. That's the main reason a hangover hits us harder when we're middle aged or older than it might have in college—and, even more importantly, problem drinking increases our risk of developing cirrhosis and other liver diseases.

But other parts of the body also are significantly affected by alcohol...

- **Brain.** Excessive drinking is just one of many cumulative "insults"—such as banging our heads—that can affect the brain. Whether you drink too much over time or on a single occasion, alcohol's effect on your brain can lead to changes in your mood and behavior and make it more difficult to think clearly and move with coordination.

- **Muscle mass.** We lose muscle mass—at an average rate of 5% for each decade after age 35. On top of that, our bodies tend to become pudgier and fat shifts to other places, such as the midsection. Combine this with the fact that many older adults are chronically dehydrated—if you get less fluid, you won't be running to the bathroom so often!—and it sets the stage for more alcohol to build up in the bloodstream. That's because fat does not absorb alcohol as much as muscle does, and less water means alcohol's effects are stronger. Because women tend to have a higher fat-to-muscle ratio, they generally have higher blood-alcohol levels than men when they consume the same number of drinks.

- **Enzymes.** Beginning roughly at middle age, we produce declining amounts of alcohol dehydrogenase, an enzyme that breaks down alcohol. This means that you get a bigger buzz from a smaller number of drinks.

THE GOOD AND THE BAD

Even though alcohol's link to reduced heart disease risk has been widely publicized, there are negative effects that most people don't know about.

For example...

- **Heartburn.** If you have a stomach ulcer or chronic heartburn stemming from gastroesophageal reflux disease (GERD), alcohol wears away the mucous lining of the gastrointestinal tract, increasing the risk for internal bleeding. These gastrointestinal conditions (and the medications that are used to treat them) also can prevent good absorption of some nutrients from your food, increasing alcohol's punch.

- **Pain.** Using alcohol to ease a backache or any other chronic pain condition is a bad idea. It often leads to an increasing reliance on booze, which can quickly result in alcohol abuse.

- **Stroke.** When it comes to stroke, the research is mixed. One drink per day may lower stroke risk, but drinking more than one to two drinks a day may increase your chances of having a stroke.

- **Memory loss.** New research shows that middle-aged men who consumed more than 2.5 drinks each day showed reductions in memory and executive function (decision-making ability) between 1.5 and six years sooner than those who had fewer drinks daily. The research also suggested a faster cognitive decline in women who drank heavily, but the results weren't statistically significant.

- **Cancer.** Excessive drinking has been linked to several types of cancer, such as malignancies of the mouth, esophagus, liver and colon. Women who drink even moderate amounts (one drink daily) have a slightly higher risk for breast cancer than nondrinkers. In fact, there is a 10% to 12% higher risk for breast cancer associated with each drink per day.

ALCOHOL AND MEDICATION

It's no secret that people tend to take more over-the-counter and prescription medications as they age. Many of these drugs—and herbal remedies—are metabolized by the same liver enzymes needed to process alcohol.

Mixing alcohol with medications such as blood thinners can cause gastrointestinal bleeding. And heartburn medications, such as *cimetidine* (Tagamet) and *ranitidine* (Zantac), interfere with alcohol metabolism, allowing blood-alcohol levels to spike. Other drugs that interact with alcohol include cold and flu medications, pain relievers, antidepressants and sleep aids.

For a list of medications and herbs that interact with alcohol, go to the website of the National Institute on Alcohol Abuse and Alcoholism, NIAAA.NIH.gov and search "Harmful Interactions."

Takeaway: Because alcohol affects the body in such complex ways, it's always wise to talk to your doctor honestly about your drinking habits and how alcohol could affect the medications you take...any chronic health conditions you may have...and/or your risk factors for disease. In general, the older we get, the less alcohol we should drink.

How Drinking Can Weaken Your Muscles

Study titled "Associations Between High-Risk Alcohol Consumption and Sarcopenia Among Postmenopausal Women," by Hee-Taik Kang, MD, Chungbuk National University College of Medicine, Republic of Korea, and colleagues, published in *Menopause: The Journal of the North American Menopause Society.*

There's a very common habit you may have that is silently robbing your body of the muscle mass and strength you'll need as you get older. The habit is drinking alcohol.

Surprised? You knew that alcohol could hurt your liver—but shrink your muscles?

It's so. A new study finds, in fact, that drinking is strongly linked to worsening sarcopenia, the age-related loss of muscle mass and strength. Sarcopenia is increasingly recognized as an important contributor to falls and fractures as well as many chronic diseases.

How much you drink is the key. A little bit—not to worry. If you're still drinking like you did when you were younger, however, it's time to ask yourself, Is my drinking setting me up for a fall?

Background: The US Centers for Disease Control and Prevention recently recognized sarcopenia, a combination of low muscle mass and weakness in older adults, as a diagnosable medical condition. It can affect balance and walking and interfere with the ability to take care of the activities of daily living that allow for independence. Muscle mass is also key to metabolic and cognitive health—sarcopenia is linked with increased risk for heart disease, diabetes and cognitive impairment. In short, minimizing or preventing sarcopenia can help you remain healthy, functional and independent at older ages.

We naturally start losing muscle mass in our 40s. By the 50s, the average man or woman loses 1.5% a year. After age 60, that goes up to 3% a year. Sarcopenia, as opposed to just normal age-related muscle loss, is defined as a substantial loss of both muscle mass and strength—so much so that walking is affected. While statistics vary, it is estimated that as many as 15% of Americans age 60 and older and 50% of those age 80 and older have sarcopenia.

A healthy lifestyle that includes regular exercise and a good diet helps prevent sarcopenia. But too little has been known about the role of alcohol, which is what researchers set out to address in the latest study.

Study: Using data from a large national patient registry, South Korean researchers pulled medical records on about 2,400 postmenopausal women. (The issue affects men, too.) The records included measurements of lean body mass (aka, muscle). The women filled out questionnaires about their frequency and quantity of alcohol use, whether they drank alcohol in the morning (a sign of problem drinking), guilt or concern about drinking and known alcohol-related injuries. Based on their responses, they were classified as either at low, medium or high risk for alcohol problems. On average, the women were 62 years old. About 8% had sarcopenia.

Results: Women who were at risk for alcohol problems were at substantially increased risk for sarcopenia. Here are the percentages of women who had sarcopenia associated with their drinking habits...

- **Low risk**—7.6% had sarcopenia.
- **Medium risk**—11%.
- **High risk**—22.7%.

Heavy drinkers, of course, also tend to have otherwise less healthy lifestyles than light drinkers or teetotalers. But even after adjusting for age, weight, blood pressure, cholesterol levels, blood sugar, smoking and exercise habits, high-risk drinkers in this study were more than four times more likely than those in the low-risk group to have sarcopenia.

And what about men? While this study looked only at women, there are reasons to be concerned about men as well. Physiological research has shown that excess alcohol consumption can contribute to sarcopenia regardless of gender.

Bottom line: It's not exactly shocking to learn that something that we already knew was bad for us—drinking too much—causes additional harms. (According to Dietary Guidelines for Americans, moderate drinking for women is an average of no more than seven drinks a week and for men, no more than 14. According to the National Institute on Alcohol Abuse and Alcoholism, over age 65, "low-risk drinking" for men and women is the same—no more than seven drinks a week and no more than three drinks in a single day.) But this new research might be a wake-up call to look at your own habits. Unfortunately, drinking problems are increasing faster among people over 65 than in any other age group. Plus, over the age of about 45, alcohol can be harder on your body than when you were younger—even if you're still just drinking like you used to. And there's new evidence that even moderate drinking may not be so great for your brain.

Surefire Ways to Prevent Muscle Loss

Stuart M. Phillips, PhD, professor, department of kinesiology and Michael G. DeGroote School of Medicine, McMaster University, Ontario, Canada.

Starting in your 30s, your muscles began shrinking, making you imperceptibly but steadily weaker. And now, as each year ticks by, you keep weakening—losing muscle mass at a rate of 0.5% to 1% a year—so that the loss of strength is more obvious. At some point, if it hasn't happened already, you'll be in your kitchen wrestling with a jar of spaghetti sauce and thinking, Why do they make these lids so much tighter than they used to?

Loss of muscle mass and strength isn't just an inconvenience. It's one of the most accurate indicators—for seniors and the middle-aged and the young—that disease and death may be in your near future.

Scary findings: Study after study shows that people with less strength are more likely to be hospitalized or to die of any cause, including heart disease, stroke, cancer and pneumonia, within a given period. Scientists haven't figured out all the reasons that strength predicts health and well-being, but it's not only because unhealthy people get weaker—in fact, a reduction in strength is a better predictor of dying from cardiovascular disease than is high blood pressure.

If you've told your doctor that you're a bit weaker these days, and he/she said it's a "normal part of aging"—ignore him. You can and should preserve and build muscle mass and strength at any age—it's as important to health and longevity as keeping your arteries free of plaque and your cells free of cancer. And you can do it with a surprisingly simple three-pronged strategy—a routine of three simple strengthening exercises (no gym required)...the right diet...and three particular nutritional supplements that are proven muscle protectors. *Here's how to do it...*

BEST EXERCISES

Preserve and build the muscles in your arms, legs, hips and back that you need for everyday strength and activity by doing these three exercises two or three times a week at home or anywhere else…

• **Body-weight squat.** Stand directly in front of a stable, not-too-high chair with no armrest and with your back toward the chair seat and your feet shoulder-width apart. Slowly bend your legs, keeping your back straight and arms at your sides and knees over your toes, and lower yourself onto the chair. Then stand up slowly by reversing the motion. Do this 30 times. If you can't do 30 repetitions at first (and many people can't), start with what you can do, and over a period of days or weeks, work up to 30. (The same goes for the next two exercises.) If you can do even more, all the better—but 30 should be your minimum target.

• **Lunge.** While standing, keep your upper body straight and your shoulders back, and step forward with one leg, lowering your hips until both knees are bent at a 90-degree angle. Return to the standing position. Do 15 times on each side for a total of 30.

• **Push-up or modified push-up.** This oldie but goodie develops the upper back, shoulders, arms, chest and wrists. If you can't yet do "full" push-ups (with only your hands and toes on the ground), start with modified push-ups in which your toes and knees are on the ground…or even with easier "wall push-ups" where you stand facing a wall and place your hands on the wall at shoulder height. Your ultimate goal is at least 30 full push-ups.

Also important: Aerobic exercise to maintain fitness. You don't have to run miles and miles. A 25-minute jog or vigorous cycling just three times a week…or a 30-minute brisk walk five times a week will do the trick.

BEST FOODS

The ideal strategy for staying strong is like a three-level pyramid. The base of the pyramid—the essential factor—is exercise as described above, and the most important dietary component for your muscles is protein, the material out of which muscles are made. And believe it or not, despite the prevalence of meat in the typical Western diet, many Americans don't get enough protein for the best possible muscle strength.

The government's Recommended Dietary Allowance (RDA) for protein is 0.36 grams (g) of protein per pound of body weight per day. But that level is the minimum, not the optimum. For preserving and building muscle, we need at least 50% more—0.54 g of protein per pound of body weight per day. And some studies indicate that 0.73 g per pound of body weight is even better. (More than that doesn't build more muscle or strength.)

Problem: Most seniors get only two-thirds of the RDA, or about 0.24 g of protein per pound of body weight per day.

How much protein should you eat? Don't go by the government's RDA. Instead multiply your body weight in pounds by 0.54 to get the minimum number of grams per day…and multiply your body weight by 0.73 to get the maximum daily grams of protein likely to help your muscles. Then each day, aim to eat an amount in between those two results.

Example: A person who weighs 150 pounds would multiply 150 by 0.54 to get a minimum daily protein goal of 81 g…and multiply 150 by 0.73 to get a maximum useful daily protein amount of 109 g.

Equally important: Not only do you need enough protein—you need the kind that your muscles can easily use. The best muscle-building protein has two features. It is digestible—the amino acids that are the building blocks of protein are easily absorbed. Protein from meat, poultry, fish and other seafood, eggs and dairy is far more digestible than protein from plants. And the best protein for muscles has a high level of the amino acid leucine, which kick-starts muscle-building. The digestible sources of protein mentioned above also have the most leucine.

To optimize muscle-building, you also need to get protein at every meal, because unlike unused carbohydrates and unused fat, unused protein is not stored by the body for later use.

Best strategy: Eat a highly digestible form of leucine-rich protein, chosen from the above sources, at every meal.

Examples: For breakfast, eat two eggs (12 g protein) and one-half cup of yogurt (6 g). For lunch, cut up four ounces of chicken breast (35 g protein) into a salad. For dinner, eat a six-ounce serving of high-quality (preferably organic) meat or fish (around 40 g protein) along with vegetables and whole grains. For a bedtime snack, have one-half cup of cottage cheese (12 g protein).

Grand total: 105 g of protein, or just about the perfect amount to help preserve strength for our 150-pounder.

Note: Some medical conditions, for example kidney disease, can make it dangerous to consume even moderate amounts of protein—check first with your physician.

BEST SUPPLEMENTS

In a recent study by my colleagues and me at McMaster University, we added three nutritional supplements to the diets of older men who also were engaged in an exercise program—and the supplements increased strength and muscle mass more than exercise alone (of course, check with your physician to make sure that any new supplement is safe for you)...

- **Whey protein.** Milk has two main proteins—casein and whey. Whey is separated from casein during cheese-making, and whey protein powder is a supplement containing that by-product. It is unusually rich in leucine.

Suggested amount: If you are meeting your target range of daily protein from food as described above, you don't need a protein supplement. If you fall a bit short, mix enough protein powder into the drink of your choice (many people use milk) to reach the total daily range of protein for your body weight as described above. (Check the label of your whey product to determine how much powder provides that much protein.) Don't get more than 50 g of daily protein from whey powder—it is not a total substitute for protein-rich food. When buying whey powder, look for "NSF" on the label—NSF is a third-party organization that certifies products that have met rigorous manufacturing standards.

Best timing: Take whey protein soon after exercise, which maximizes muscle-building. If you can't consume whey because of an allergy or some other reason, consider a soy protein supplement instead.

- **Creatine.** This amino acid boosts the body's ability to produce energy and helps build muscle.

Recent finding: In a study published in *Nutrients*, just six days of creatine supplementation improved upper-body strength by nearly 3%.

Suggested amount: Two capsules per day, in divided doses, that together total 4 g to 5 g.

- **Fish oil.** The omega-3 fatty acids in fish oil (EPA and DHA) make your muscles more sensitive to protein, encouraging muscle-building.

Suggested amount: 750 milligrams (mg) of EPA and 500 mg of DHA per day.

Just Breathe...the Right Way

Rebecca Dennis, a breath coach and founder of BreathingTree.co.uk, a website that's dedicated to health-promoting breathing strategies. Based in London, she is author of *And Breathe: The Complete Guide to Conscious Breathing for Health and Happiness.*

It's the first and last thing we do in this world—take a breath. But somewhere in between, far too many of us lose touch with how to breathe naturally, fully...and correctly. Though we inhale and exhale about 20,000 times each day, most of the time we take short, shallow breaths that I call "stress breaths."

Why does our innate sense of how to breathe properly slip away from us? Whether we're fighting traffic or multitasking, our fast-paced lives often throw us into a stress-driven spiral that interferes with our ability to optimally fuel our bodies with life-sustaining oxygen. People who are suppressing feelings such as anger or emotional pain tend to hold their breath. *Fortunately, a few simple strategies can help us reclaim our breathing skills...*

MORE THAN "BELLY BREATHING"

We have all heard the term "belly breathing," but the real key to proper breathing is not so much your belly but your diaphragm. Deeply breathing from this dome-shaped sheet of muscle at the bottom of the rib cage is vital for respiratory function.

True diaphragmatic breathing uses the entire respiratory system—starting with the belly, then moving on to the midsection and into the chest.

Try it: Inhale through your nose, directing your breath into your stomach. Allow your diaphragm to drop downward and the rib cage to expand, thus creating space for the lungs to inflate. Pause for a moment, then exhale through your mouth and feel the rib cage contract. The motion of breath should go in and out like a wave. To adopt this healthier way of breathing, practice for a minute or two several times a day until it feels natural.

This form of breathing stimulates the parasympathetic nervous system (PNS), which slows your heart rate and breathing, lowers blood pressure and diverts blood toward the digestive system.

THE HEALING EFFECTS

Proper breathing offers a number of powerful health benefits, including…

- **Reduced anxiety and depression.** Deep breathing is believed to help elevate levels of serotonin and endorphins, naturally occurring "feel-good" chemicals. A study by Harvard Medical School psychiatrists showed that those who meditated daily for four years—a practice that relies heavily on conscious breathing—had longer telomeres, the protective "caps" on the ends of chromosomes that serve as biomarkers of longevity and slower aging.
- **Protection against viruses.** Our lymphatic system, which moves cleansing, vital fluids through our muscles and tissues, relies on breathing, movement and gravity to continue flowing. By promoting a healthy lymphatic system, deep breathing can play a crucial role in protecting the body from viruses, bacteria and other health threats.
- **Less constipation.** Deeper breathing (and the stress reduction that goes along with it) promotes intestinal action and stimulates overall digestion. This can improve conditions such as constipation and irritable bowel syndrome.
- **Improved sleep.** The relaxation that occurs with deep breathing is likely responsible for its positive effect on sleep quality.

BEST BREATHING FIXES

Targeted breathing exercises can help you deal more effectively with stress…and day-to-day health challenges such as indigestion, insomnia and fatigue. The best part is that you can do these exercises anywhere. Among my favorite quick breathing fixes—they can also help with respiratory conditions such as asthma and chronic obstructive pulmonary disease (COPD)…

- **Alternate nostril breathing.** This breathing exercise helps put you in a calm and centered state.

What to do: Breathe in deeply through your right nostril while pressing the left nostril closed with your right index finger…then exhale through the left nostril while pressing the right nostril closed with your right thumb. Next, inhale through the left nostril (right nostril still closed)…then close the left nostril and exhale through the right. The exhalations should take about twice as long as the inhalations. Repeat the cycle 10 times.

- **4-7-8 breathing.** If you are plagued by insomnia, this breathing exercise can put you to sleep within minutes.

What to do: Exhale completely through your mouth, making a "whoosh" sound. Close your mouth and inhale quietly through your nose to a count of four. Hold your breath for a count of seven. Exhale completely through your mouth, making a "whoosh" sound, to a count of eight. This is one breath.

Now inhale again and repeat the cycle three more times. Do this exercise when you need help going to sleep or if you awaken and want to get back to sleep.

Daytime Dozing Danger

Bernadette Boden-Albala, PhD, assistant professor, sociomedical sciences, Columbia College of Physicians and Surgeons, New York City.

People in their 70s who dozed a lot during the day had more than four times the risk of having a stroke than those who didn't doze. They also had a higher risk for heart attack and other cardiovascular problems. People in their 70s who dozed moderately had a 2.5-fold increased stroke risk.

Self-defense: If you're dozing a lot during the day, tell your doctor.

Live Like a Caveman and Live Much Longer

Philip J. Goscienski, MD, retired clinical professor of pediatrics, department of community and family medicine at University of California, San Diego, School of Medicine. He is author of *Health Secrets of the Stone Age*. StoneAgeDoc.com

---

Our bodies reached their current stage of development—in terms of genetics, chemistry and metabolism—during the Stone Age, tens of thousands of years ago. But our lifestyles, in particular our diets and exercise habits, have undergone changes that our bodies aren't equipped to handle.

In particular, the development of agriculture and domesticated livestock has led to a plentiful food supply. Humans don't have to work as hard to find a good meal, and those meals are served more frequently. Obesity, once rare, is now a leading health threat.

Yet in modern hunter-gatherer societies, people live much as they did in the Stone Age—that's how we can make conclusions about the health of our Stone Age ancestors. Obesity is virtually unheard of in these groups. Members rarely get diabetes, hypertension or heart disease. Cancer is rare. Even in the absence of medical care, they often are healthier than the rest of us.

Here's what worked for our Stone Age ancestors...

STONE AGE FRUIT

Our Stone Age ancestors gathered wild fruits, which were much smaller and less attractive than we are used to today. The fruits that we buy in supermarkets are bred for appearance, sweetness and size. They have less fiber and antioxidants and more sugars than fruits that grow in the wild without human intervention.

A USDA study published in *Journal of the American College of Nutrition* found that nutrient levels in produce have declined significantly in just the last 60 years. There have been drops in protein, calcium, vitamin A, riboflavin and thiamine.

Self-defense: Opt for smaller fruits (such as apricots, cherries and berries), which have a greater ratio of skin to flesh, relative to their size, than larger ones, such as peaches. This is important because the largest concentration of fiber and antioxidants is found in the skin and the layers just beneath.

Also, if possible, switch from standard supermarket produce (which tends to be larger) to organic, wild-grown or heirloom varieties. The produce that is available at farmers' markets usually hasn't been bred solely for appearance (or ease of shipping). It naturally will have a higher concentration of nutrients and fiber, thus making it a superior option.

GAME MEATS

Our ancestors ate plenty of meat, but they ate game meats (antelope, venison, bison), which have very little saturated fat. High intake of saturated fat leads to obesity, which is a leading cause of heart disease and cancer.

Most of the saturated fat in the American diet (apart from that found in processed and restaurant foods) comes from domestic animal meats. These animals are fed grains, which are not part of their natural diet. The meat of grain-fed animals is marbled with saturated fat, making it sweeter and more tender.

What we can learn: Avoid grain-fed beef and pork. Many specialty markets feature meats from grass-fed animals, which are superior to grain-fed.

Even better: Look for game meats, which are high in healthful mono-unsaturated fat and low in saturated fat. For example, a four-ounce serving of venison has 1.4 grams (g) of saturated fat, about one-third as much as the same amount of rib eye steak.

WATER, NOT SODA

During the Stone Age, people had only water to drink. Recent studies, including one that looked at the average diet of preschoolers in England, found that many children now drink no water. They get virtually all of their fluids from high-calorie, high-sugar soft drinks and juices.

The average American consumes about two-and-a-half sugary soft drinks daily. Many soft drinks contain about 150 calories per serving. Someone who drinks two nondiet soft drinks a day for a year is consuming the caloric equivalent of about 30 extra pounds.

Even diet soda has been linked to health problems. A recent study found that diet soda drinkers have a higher risk for stroke and heart attack.

What we can learn: Water is the healthiest liquid you can drink. Most adults need about 60 ounces a day—enough to make the urine clear or lightly colored, instead of dark. Opt for filtered water whenever possible. Stone Agers didn't have to worry about industrial chemicals.

FAR LESS SALT

Our ancient ancestors probably consumed about 700 milligrams (mg) of sodium daily, about the same amount as those who live in hunter-gatherer societies today. People in these societies have virtually no high blood pressure. The average American now consumes about four times this much salt, and high blood pressure raises the risk for heart disease and stroke, leading causes of death in the US.

What we can learn: No one needs extra sodium. Every natural food, including fruits and vegetables, contains enough sodium to keep us healthy. Anything "extra" is unnecessary—and often unhealthy.

Recommended: No more than 1,500 mg of sodium daily. Less is better. Relatively little of the sodium in the American diet comes from the salt shaker—most comes from processed foods. Read labels carefully, even when you think a food is "healthy." A glass of tomato juice, for example, has more than 800 mg of sodium. One tablespoon of soy sauce has 1,200 mg.

MINIROBICS

During the Stone Age, the average adult most likely expended between 3,500 and 5,000 calories a day. Back then, people didn't "do exercise," because their lives were exercise. They walked miles to gather food, chased down game and used only hand tools.

In modern hunter-gatherer societies, dieting is unheard of—and unnecessary. People are naturally lean. They stay strong even into old age, unlike the 25% of Americans over the age of 65 who need assistance getting out of bed or bathing. They have healthier hearts because they are always moving.

Today only about 10% of Americans regularly get intense physical exercise. On average, our level of daily activity is about 75% less than it was at the beginning of the 20th century.

What we can learn: Current guidelines call for about 30 minutes of moderately intense exercise daily. That's not enough. Our "caveman bodies" seem to function best when we get at least 60 minutes of moderately intense exercise daily. This means exercise that is intense enough to get you breathing hard. It could be working in the yard, doing housework, bicycling or lifting weights.

My advice: If you don't care for formal exercise, you still can get benefits from what I call "minirobics"—daily habits that keep you moving. These include things such as taking stairs instead of elevators...and using a push-type mower rather than one powered with gasoline.

The average person can burn an extra few hundred calories daily (and lose a pound or two a month) simply by moving more throughout the day. And you're never too old to start using your body more. Researchers in Boston conducted a study in which residents of a convalescent home were put on a strength-training program. Their average age was 90. In eight weeks, they had tripled their strength and increased their muscle mass by 10%.

The Definitive Antidote to Sitting All Day

Bernard Duvivier, MD, PhD, a postdoctoral researcher at Maastricht University Medical Center, the Netherlands, and lead researcher of the study titled "Reducing Sitting Time Versus Adding Exercise: Differential Effects on Biomarkers of Endothelial Dysfunction and Metabolic Risk" published in *Scientific Reports*.

Emily Banks, MBBS, PhD, is a professor of epidemiology at the National Center for Epidemiology and Population Health at the Australian National University in Canberra.

O*ne thing we know for sure:* Sitting for most of the day is terrible for your health, raising your risk for diabetes, obesity, high cholesterol and high blood pressure. But the remedy has been confusing. First, we thought that getting 30 minutes of cardio exercise every day was the answer because it benefits heart health and overall health. Then the "marching orders" were to get up from our desks every hour to stand, walk or stretch because incremental amounts of movement seemed to help undo the negative effects of sitting. There were even reports (widely misinterpreted) that sitting a lot wasn't bad for you after all. (It is.) So, which is it? What recent research out of the Netherlands shows is that exercise and light activities benefit your heart and metabolic health in different ways—and that you need to do both.

Exercise improves endothelial health by "training" blood vessels—increasing blood flow temporarily stresses them, and as a result, they become healthier, in much the same way that muscles become stronger and healthier from the stress of strength training. Exercise helps reduce blood pressure by increasing nitric oxide levels.

Light activity—standing, walking, stretching—improves what's called insulin signaling. Your cells become more sensitive to insulin, and glucose is more easily cleared from the blood. It's also possible that simply walking and standing throughout the day keeps insulin levels steady because the muscles you engage use blood glucose for fuel. Light activity might help improve cholesterol, in part due to an increase in an enzyme that boosts levels of HDL, the good cholesterol, and helps your body break down triglycerides (blood fats).

WAYS TO SIT LESS

More studies are needed to better pinpoint the ideal dose of light activities, but recent guidelines from countries including Australia and Belgium suggest that you get up every 30 minutes. *But you can build that rather robotic regime into activities that more naturally match your lifestyle, for example…*

- **Hold walking meetings** (get outside when the weather's nice) and walk to colleagues' desks instead of sending e-mails.
- **Walk around the field during your child's sports games** and practices rather than sitting in the bleachers.
- **When watching TV**, do chores during the commercials.
- **Drink more water**—besides keeping you hydrated, you'll have to get up to visit the bathroom more often (choose the farthest one you have access to).
- **Set an alarm on your phone** to remind you to move every half-hour.
- **Ditch the car.** Since you have no choice but to sit when you're in a car, instead walk, bike or take public transportation (and stand while using it) whenever possible. If you must drive, park farther away from your destination (whether it's your office or the entrance to the supermarket, movie theater or mall).
- **Change how you work.** Stand and/or walk around while you're on the phone. If your coworkers are game, you might even bring in a counter-height table and have everyone stand around that for meetings. If you work on a laptop, prop it up higher during at least part of the day so that you can stand while using it. While it can be expensive (usually about $300 to $600), if possible, switch to a standing desk (a.k.a., an "adjustable height workstation"), which you can find at OfficeMax, Office Depot and Amazon.com.
- **Avoid the couch.** You may find that simply standing while watching TV feels weird—maybe because you consider relaxing to be the main reason for watching TV. But interestingly, it doesn't feel nearly as weird if you do something while watching TV—such as walk on a treadmill or perform standing stretches or even iron your clothes. And if you play video games at home—stand. Why should the video characters' legs be the only ones getting used?
- **Cook more.** Instead of ordering food, make it yourself. Not only is the food likely to be healthier, but you'll be working in the kitchen, which usually entails standing, lifting and reaching. Then stand while you eat.

Like TV a Little Too Much? Do This and It Won't Hurt Your Health

Study titled "Associations of Discretionary Screen Time with Mortality, Cardiovascular Disease and Cancer Are Attenuated by Strength, Fitness and Physical Activity: Findings from the Uk Biobank Study," by researchers at University of Glasgow, Scotland, published in *BMC Medicine.*

The hours you log surfing the web and zoning out in front of the TV are a recipe for heart disease and other conditions and early death, right? After all, screen time, by definition, is sedentary behavior, a major health risk factor.

Maybe not.

A new study reveals that what you do in the hours that you're not watching a screen makes a big difference in whether those screen hours really are harming your health. The results might be enough to get you up off that couch or out of your chair—or at worst, make you feel less guilty about binge-watching *Game of Thrones*. But it's not quite a free pass for TV addicts.

HAZARDS OF SCREEN TIME

Over the past several years, the very act of doing a lot of sitting has come to be regarded as a harmful activity that degrades our health, and that was thought to be true even if we were active when we weren't sitting. But is it really true? Researchers at Glasgow University wondered, so they analyzed data compiled on 390,089 men and women, ages 40 to 69, who participated in the UK Biobank, an ongoing, population-based study in England, Scotland and Wales that tracks many health factors, including diet and fitness. Participants were followed for a median of five years. Their screen time ranged from an average of less than two hours per day to more than five hours per day and included any TV viewing plus computer use that wasn't related to work. Screen time with phones and tablets wasn't tracked.

The researchers' most significant finding wasn't surprising at all. As the amount of time devoted to channel- and web-surfing increased, so too did the risk for cardiovascular disease, cancer and cancer deaths, as well as death from all causes. But when the researchers filtered the data for fitness levels, everything changed.

The striking finding: Screen-time-related health risk applied only to the men and women who were inactive when not watching TV or web surfing, out of shape and not so strong. Their risk was almost double that of the participants who were fit, active and strong—for whom there was little or no hazard from increasing screen time. (There was a slight trend toward a very small increased risk in the fit, but it wasn't statistically significant.)

THE THREE FITNESS MEASURES THAT MATTERED

The researchers looked at three separate measures of fitness. Two are well-known—physical activity level and cardiovascular fitness. The third is less common—grip strength.

To measure physical activity, researchers totaled the time participants spent walking every week, along with any moderate or vigorous activity they engaged in such as sports or gym time. Cardiovascular fitness was calculated by measuring how intensely individuals could exercise and how much oxygen they metabolized while pedaling on a stationary bike.

To measure grip strength, the researchers used a device called a hand dynamometer, which, when squeezed, records the strength of a person's hand and forearm. It tends to also be a good indicator of the overall muscle strength in a person's arms and legs and is fast and simple.

After adjusting for lifestyle factors including smoking, diet, blood pressure and BMI (body-mass index), the results were dramatic. Those in the lowest third of grip strength were at high health risk for extra screen time—health outcomes got worse as their average screen hours rose. But those in the top third of grip strength had no increased risk from extra screen time.

In fact, it didn't matter which of the three measures were analyzed—scoring in the top third of any of them was protective. The researchers acknowledge that genes connected with fitness and strength could play a part in explaining their results, as could physical activity earlier in life.

Every study has limitations, of course—this one is observational, so it can't establish cause and effect. But if future research does show causation, the authors conclude, it would mean that people with low fitness would reap the biggest benefits from spending less time in front of screens—while people who are fit have a lot less to worry about.

To be sure, this study doesn't give you carte blanche to binge-watch hours of TV every night—even if you are fit. Nonetheless, if you regularly engage in walking, biking, jogging, swimming, dancing or another form of aerobic exercise—as well as an activity that increases your strength—spending a few hours each day devoted to TV or computer use may not be harmful after all.

Relax, enjoy—you've earned it.

The One Sleep Habit That Most Helps Your Health

Study titled "Smoking, Screen-Based Sedentary Behavior, and Diet Associated with Habitual Sleep Duration and Chronotype: Data from the UK Biobank" by Freda Patterson, PhD, assistant professor of biobehavioral health and nutrition at University of Delaware, Newark, and colleagues published in *Annals of Behavioral Medicine*.

If you're trying to live a healthier life and resist the temptation to gobble down that extra piece of chocolate cake tonight and then blow off your workout tomorrow morning...here's a tip from the world of behavioral health science—go to sleep...earlier.

While lifestyle change is never easy, there's growing evidence that becoming less of a night owl and more of a morning lark is a good place to start. Hitting the sack earlier may not only help you get more sleep—a healthy thing in itself—but also make it easier to achieve other healthy lifestyle changes.

You've heard of gateway drugs. But an earlier bedtime may be the opposite...a gateway to healthier behavior.

Yes, you can change. Here's why you should—and how.

BODY CLOCKS, WATCHING TV AND WHAT YOU ATE LAST NIGHT

It's already well known that getting too little sleep, on a chronic basis, is strongly associated with an increased risk for heart disease, stroke, diabetes and other disorders. What the new research found is that when you hit the hay is linked with three other behaviors that are major risk factors for disease.

The study, published in *Annals of Behavioral Medicine*, which analyzed data from 440,000 British adults, found that those who characterized themselves as "morning people" compared with "evening people" ate 25% more fruit and 13% more vegetables...and spent less time on sedentary activities such as watching TV (about 20 fewer minutes a day) and computer screens (about eight fewer minutes a day). "Morning people" also were 60% less likely to be smokers.

CAN BECOMING A LARK LEAD TO HEALTHIER HABITS?

While the study does not show cause and effect, the study's lead author, Freda Patterson, PhD, assistant professor of health promotion in the department of behavioral health and nutrition at University of Delaware, believes there are good reasons to think that poor sleep habits lead to poor lifestyle habits—not the other way around.

One reason is a body of research about how people use time. People who go to bed later, Dr. Patterson noted, tend to have expanded evening recreation time, which might involve eating less healthy foods late at night and staying on the computer late at night. (Ask yourself—are you more likely to be eating fruits and veggies during the day...or late at night in front of the TV? Are those extra hours at the end of the day likely to be the ones in which you're exercising?)

Physiology plays a role, too. If you've had too little sleep, you may feel sluggish and need an energy boost in the evening...and eating sugary foods may feel like just the ticket. Smokers might get a similar lift from nicotine. Inadequate sleep is also related to stress and anxiety, added Dr. Patterson, which people might "treat" with these bad habits.

A good goal may be to shift your bedtime a half-hour earlier in five- to 10-minute increments, said

Dr. Patterson. You'll likely spend less time watching screens and munching, and you may find you have more energy the next day to resist food temptations, eat healthier and be more physically active. "If we can get people to improve sleep, it may percolate to also improve these other risk behaviors," says Dr. Patterson. "Sleep may be the behavior that could facilitate improvements in cardiovascular and metabolic health."

Night Owls Have More Health Problems

Study of 1,620 people by researchers at Korea University College of Medicine, Ansan, published in *Journal of Clinical Endocrinology & Metabolism.*

Night owls have more health problems than early risers. People who stay up late are more likely to develop diabetes, metabolic syndrome and sarcopenia (loss of muscle mass), even if they get the same amount of sleep. Staying awake later at night often causes sleep loss, poor sleep and eating at inappropriate times.

Go Green, Live Long

Study titled "Exposure to Greenness and Mortality in a Nationwide Prospective Cohort Study of Women" by researchers at Harvard T.H. Chan School of Public Health, Brigham and Women's Hospital and Harvard Medical School, all in Boston, published in *Environmental Health Perspectives.*

The greenery that surrounds your home is more than eye candy. It also protects your lungs, helps ward off depression, protects you from cancer, improves your kidney health—and might even help you live longer.

So finds a study of more than 100,000 women living in nearly all US states. Researchers analyzed health records and compared them with geographic satellite data for "greenness"—a measure of chlorophyll, and a pretty good gauge of how much vegetation surrounded their homes.

Over an eight-year period, women who lived in the top fifth for greenery, compared with those in the bottom fifth, were 12% less likely to die. That was true regardless of age, race, socioeconomic status or whether the residents smoked. While this particular study was focused on women, similar health benefits for greenery have also been reported for men, the researchers note.

Why the green longevity bonus? Vegetation, the researchers note, helps protect against pollutants that can increase the risk for lung and kidney disease and cancer, improves mood and provides opportunities to be more active. Further analysis revealed that women surrounded by more greenery were less likely to have respiratory illness, kidney disease, cancer or depression. They also used fewer antidepressants. Living in green areas may allow for a healthier lifestyle—in fact, the researchers did find an increase in physical activity as well.

Nor was it just homes with big lawns that were healthier. While the relationship was strongest for the 250 meters surrounding the homes, it also held true (although to a slightly lesser degree) for an area of 1,250 meters—nearly a mile. So even if you don't have a big, green property, if you live near parks and other green spaces, you're in the pink.

Forests, we're told, are the lungs of the earth. But the lawns and fields and trees that surround our homes also help our lungs—and our spirits. They may even help us hang around longer to enjoy the scenery.

If you live near clean grass, try walking on it barefoot to energize your body...and don't forget greenery inside your house. Even when you're in an office, you can stay mentally sharp by gazing at a green scene.

Step Outside

John La Puma, MD, FACP, board-certified internist and certified California naturalist, who runs an organic teaching farm in Santa Barbara, California.

People who spend just 30 minutes in a green outdoor space at least once a week are 7%

less likely to develop high blood pressure, and 9% less likely to develop depression, than people who spend little or no time, according to a study published in *Scientific Reports*.

More Sun, Longer Life?

Study titled "Avoidance of Sun Exposure as a Risk Factor for Major Causes of Death: A Competing Risk Analysis of the Melanoma in Southern Sweden Cohort" by researchers at Karolinska University Hospital, Lund University, both in Sweden, published in *Journal of Internal Medicine*.

Michael F. Holick, PhD, MD, professor of medicine, physiology and biophysics, Boston University School of Medicine, and author of *The Vitamin D Solution*.

Let the sunshine in. It's good for the heart, according to a new study. It's no excuse to start sunbathing for hours without sunscreen, to be sure, but the new research suggests that avoiding the sun might shorten your life.

A HEALTHIER HEART

Back in the early 1990s, nearly 30,000 Swedish women filled out a questionnaire about how often they spent time in the sun in the summer or went to sunny climes for holiday in the winter. Over the next 20 years, researchers reported a few years ago, those who had the most sun exposure, compared with those with the least, were half as likely to die from all causes.

In the latest study, the researchers determined that the reason the sun seekers were less likely to die earlier was an decreased incidence of cardiovascular disease, which can cause death from heart attacks and stroke.

The sun seekers did have a greater prevalence of cancers, both skin cancers and internal cancers. But that's most likely because they lived longer. Age is one of the strongest risk factors for cancer. Interestingly, those who had nonmelanoma skin cancers, such as squamous or basal cell cancer, which are rarely fatal, tended to have been exposed to the most sun—and had the lowest rates of overall mortality.

How much longer did sun seekers live? Depending on other risk factors, such as smoking, sun seekers lived between six months and two years longer than sun avoiders, on average.

This is an observational study, so it doesn't prove cause-and-effect relationships, but noted it does fit in with other research—in both men and women.

HOW SUN PROTECTS THE HEART

Vitamin D, which the body produces in response to sun exposure, is of course a likely protective factor. In the famous Framingham Heart Study, men and women with blood levels of vitamin D below 15 ng/mL were 50% more likely to have a heart attack than those with higher levels. For reference, the Endocrine Society recommends blood levels at or above 30 ng/mL.

Vitamin D is heart-healthy in many ways—it helps regulate blood pressure (by tamping down production of the pressure-raising protein renin), improves the functioning of blood vessels (by reducing production of "foam" cells that can lead to atherosclerosis) and helps strengthen the heart muscle itself.

But the sun also stimulates the skin to produce nitric oxide, which is then released into the bloodstream. Nitric oxide allows our blood vessels to relax, and that can reduce blood pressure. Sun exposure also promotes production and release of feel-good beta endorphins—one reason that sunny days may be mood boosters—which reduces stress, protecting the heart.

JUST ENOUGH SUN...PLUS VITAMIN D SUPPLEMENTS

Before you head out unprotected into the sunshine, remember that Swedes (the subjects of the latest research) are much more likely to suffer a sun drought than most Americans. Stockholm, for example, gets only about 1,800 hours of sunshine a year—compared with 3,200 hours in, for example, Grand Junction, Colorado.

Most Americans can get enough vitamin D in the summer by receiving sensible sun exposure.

To ensure adequate vitamin D all year round, a supplement is recommended—for children, 600 IU to 1,000 IU daily...for most adults 2,000 IU daily...and for obese adults 4,000 IU to 6,000 IU daily. That's because anyone living north of Atlanta can't make enough vitamin D from sun alone between

October and April. For the record, vitamin D-2 is just as effective as vitamin D-3, so it doesn't matter which form of the supplement you take.

Shop More, Live Longer

Yu-Hung Chang, PhD, is a researcher at the Institute of Population Health Sciences in Taiwan and leader of a study published in the *Journal of Epidemiology & Community Health.*

According to recent research, shopping is good for a person's health. This study involved 1,841 seniors ages 65 and older who were asked how often they went shopping. Possible answers ranged from "daily" to "never."

Findings: Participants who reported shopping every day were 27% less likely to die during the study period than those who ventured out to stores less frequently.

Theory: Shopping involves various factors believed to extend longevity, including physical activity and increased social interaction.

Bottom line: Next time you feel the need for some retail therapy, don't feel guilty. You can even save your money—because window-shopping works, too.

Don't Waste Your Time Volunteering... When You Do It, Do It Right

Mark A. Stengler, NMD, naturopathic medical doctor in private practice, Encinitas, California...adjunct associate clinical professor at the National College of Natural Medicine, Portland, Oregon...author of *The Natural Physician's Healing Therapies.*

I recently asked one of my patients—Joe, a retiree in his 80s—what he had been up to and joked with him that whatever it was, it was keeping him healthy. He told me that his favorite activity is volunteering as a docent at the local art museum. He got to learn about each new exhibition and got to know it so well that he could lead tours. Volunteering is a kind of "medicine" for many of my patients. It keeps people like Joe active, mentally alert and engaged with other people, all of which contribute to his overall health. But volunteer experiences are not all alike. Based on current research, there seems to be a "right" way to volunteer—and when that happens, it can help you, too, no matter how old you are.

BEING NEEDED AND VALUED

As study after study has found, we get a lot when we give. In 2007, the federal government's Corporation for National and Community Service evaluated the health benefits of volunteering. Volunteering offers a variety of benefits to people of different age groups. For younger adults, it expands their skill set and introduces them to new situations and people that they might not otherwise encounter. While volunteering, people of all ages can experience what's known as a "helper's high," a feeling of euphoria, often followed by an ongoing feeling of well-being created through the act of giving.

Older adults who volunteer also reap distinct health benefits, even more so than their younger counterparts. The 2007 government report, which looked at 730 studies, found that adults over age 60 experienced improved mental and physical health, greater satisfaction with life and less depression. Older adults who volunteer live longer than adults who don't volunteer—they also have a greater sense of purpose and accomplishment, improved functional ability and tend to be less lonely and isolated than nonvolunteering adults.

Recent research bears this out. A 2011 study by Penn State College of Medicine researchers found that volunteering in a kindergarten class helped older adults with mild-to-moderate dementia by lowering their stress and enhancing their quality of life, relationships and self-esteem.

HOW TO BENEFIT FROM VOLUNTEERING

Research shows that for older adults to reap the psychological and physical health benefits of volunteering, certain criteria must be met...

- **Amount of time.** Health benefits from volunteering become evident for both younger and older adults after a certain "volunteering threshold," as researchers call it, has been met. Volunteers who help on a sporadic, irregular basis do not receive any benefit. Instead, people benefit most when they volunteer for two or more organizations...and perform between 40 and 100 hours or more of service annually, says the 2007 government report. (The study did not find that giving more hours provided more benefit.)

• **Level of engagement.** People who reap the benefits of volunteering are engaged with what they are doing—they aren't bored or just whiling away the time.

Lesson: Do something you enjoy.

• **Motivation.** Attitude makes a difference. In a 2011 study published in *Health Psychology*, University of Michigan researchers found that people who volunteered regularly without concern for their own interests had a lower risk for death four years later. People who volunteered for self-centered reasons (as an escape from their own troubles or because of other people's opinions) had the same mortality risk as nonvolunteers. If you are not sincere about your motivation to help others, you won't reap the benefits.

Interested in volunteering? Several websites provide lists of opportunities by region and interest, including Volunteer Match (VolunteerMatch.com) and the US government's United We Serve program (Serve.gov). To find out about opportunities if you don't have access to a computer, inquire at schools, churches and hospitals in your area.

Want to Live Longer? Take a Vacation

Study "Increased Mortality Despite Successful Multifactorial Cardiovascular Risk Reduction in Healthy Men. 40-Year Follow-Up of the Helsinki Businessmen Study Intervention Trial" published in *The Journal of Nutrition, Health & Aging*.

If you are one of those nose-to-the-grindstone people who think you are too busy to take a vacation, you'd be smart to rethink that. Your life may depend on it!

That's the finding of an important new study from the University of Helsinki in Finland that looked at 1,222 middle-aged businessmen who had at least one risk factor for cardiovascular disease (CVD), such as smoking, high blood pressure, elevated triglycerides, etc.

Here's how the research unfolded...

Vacation time was part of a new analysis that was tacked on to a previous shorter study that compared men who got health advice (on such things as aerobic exercise and healthy diet) to help manage their CVD risk factors with men who didn't get that advice. When the health coaching didn't improve the men's risk factors, medication was prescribed (such as blood pressure drugs and lipid-lowering medication). The coaching and medication initially reduced the rate of CVD compared with the control group, but at the end of the 15-year follow-up period, the men in the group that got health advice and/or medication were surprisingly more likely to have died.

When the researchers dug deeper into the data, that's when they discovered how work, sleep and vacation played a role.

How much vacation made a difference? Among the men who got health coaching and/or medication, those who vacationed for three weeks or less every year had a 37% greater risk of dying over a 30-year period than those who vacationed more often.

Not surprisingly, the men who didn't get as much downtime also spent more time at work and fewer hours sleeping. The stressful trifecta of fewer vacations, more work and less sleep is believed to have cancelled any benefits from the health advice and/or medication.

"Don't think having an otherwise healthy lifestyle will compensate for working too hard and not taking holidays," said Timo Strandberg, MD, PhD, professor of geriatrics at the University of Helsinki and the lead study author. "Vacations can be a good way to relieve stress."

What about women? Even though this research did not include women, the Framingham Heart Study (which did!) reported similar results—women who vacationed twice every year were eight times less likely to have a heart attack or develop heart disease than those who vacationed only once every six years.

Bottom line: Lots of exercise and kale salads won't necessarily help you live longer if you work too hard and skip vacations. You don't have to save for a fancy vacation to an exotic destination. The location of your vacation isn't important. But stress reduction is! One of the best ways to dial down the stress is to get away from your workplace for some stress-free downtime.

Buddy Up When You Exercise

James H. O'Keefe, MD, is a cardiologist at Saint Luke's Mid America Heart Institute, Kansas City, Missouri, and coauthor of a study published in *Mayo Clinic Proceedings*.

Exercising with a friend is linked to longevity. While people who regularly run on a treadmill or use a stationary bike at a gym live just 1.5 years longer than people who don't exercise, playing soccer adds nearly five years and playing tennis adds 10 years. It's socialization, not duration of activity, that seems to enhance the benefits of physical activity.

Get Organized... Live Longer

Julie Morgenstern, author of *Organizing from the Inside Out* and *SHED Your Stuff, Change Your Life*. JulieMorgenstern.com

Before heading to the runway for takeoff, pilots must complete a procedural checklist to assure the aircraft is ready for flight. Now many hospitals require surgeons to complete a similar checklist before doing even the most minor procedures—including, to the amusement of some, confirming which limb or organ is to be operated upon. While it seems silly, it's not—it's a way to be assured that every possible step is being taken to assure patient safety. Research is demonstrating that when hospitals adopt this practice, there is a measurable improvement in outcome. A recent study in the *New England Journal of Medicine* found a reduction in both deaths and complications when hospitals used a 19-item surgical safety checklist.

It makes sense that if individuals establish a structure with routine procedures for health-related matters, it would not only reduce stress, but also help lower the risk of at-home medication mistakes and other mishaps that can have serious consequences. Many people put themselves at risk because they are haphazard about letting important papers pile up or, equally problematic, throwing out things they should keep for future reference.

Organization expert Julie Morgenstern, author of several books, including *Organizing from the Inside Out* shared her best strategies for organizing your home for optimal health. "First and foremost," she says, "being organized is calming. It gives you a sense of assurance and of being in control and that reduces anxiety." No more heart-pounding panicked searches for lost items, which saves time as well. According to Morgenstern, people spend an average of a full hour a day looking for lost items. And organization eases financial anxiety by saving money—no more late charges as you routinely pay bills on time and no more duplicate purchases of stuff you need right now but can't find.

A PLACE FOR PAPER

Paper—bills, vaccination records, medical history, prescriptions, household information—represents the greatest organizational challenge. The vast majority of health information is still passed along on paper and it's critical to keep virtually all of it. She recommends streamlining how you handle health-related paperwork in order to minimize the chaos. *Her suggested strategies...*

- **Designate a "paperwork station"** where you will process and keep all printed and written information.
- **Have everything you need in one place**—a clean surface, a supply drawer, file folders, a telephone, possibly a computer, and at least one file drawer or box where you will keep printed material. It's fine to keep other records (financial, house-

hold) in the same place, but make sure all files are clearly labeled.

Always open your mail right away and near a trash can and a shredder. Deal with it, file it away or dispose.

MEDICATIONS AND SUPPLEMENTS

Other areas of health and medical materials require their own procedures. Drugs and supplements should be stored where you take them, preferably in the kitchen. Health organizations warn against storing meds in bathrooms due to heat and humidity. Always check whether drugs you take regularly need to be kept dry or cool, and if so, designate a special spot in the fridge or closet. Morgenstern suggests noting on prescription drug labels the date you take the first pill.

The reason: People often don't start a drug regimen for several days after purchase and the doctor may need to know how long you have been on the medication. This way you can respond with certainty. Note whether it is a new prescription or a generic or different brand, in case you have a reaction. Also, highlight expiration dates on all vials and bottles for easy reminders about discarding those that are out of date. Mark on your calendar when to call for renewals.

Remember that vitamins and other supplements should be used under a physician's prescription and treated with the same respect as drugs. If you use pill organizers, it is best to retain the original containers for first dose and expiration dates. This will also allow you to recall information about the manufacturer and lot number of the product if any issues arise.

Keep a chart of all prescriptions and supplements that you take. Include product name, prescriber, dosing and the reason that you're taking the product. A copy of this should be kept in a file folder and in your wallet in case of emergency.

MEDICAL RECORDS

Medical records are crucial. They are a part of your health history, they play a role in future medical treatment decisions, and in this era of specialization, your records are likely to be hither and yon in a variety of medical offices. If like many people you haven't kept a careful set at home, this is easy to remedy. You have a right to copies of your medical records—make it part of your routine to request copies from every doctor's office you visit, and call to request past records you don't have. Records you will need are those that concern all major illnesses and treatments, immunizations, test results, injuries and surgeries. If they are computerized, you can store them on a flash drive in addition to on your computer hard drive—and keep a hard copy in a safe place in your home.

A SUMMARY IS A GOOD IDEA

Now, to enter the land of the truly efficient—prepare a medical summary. This can be done on paper (even handwritten) or stored in the computer.

On the first sheet, at the top, list names, specialties and contact information for all your doctors.

Follow this with a bulleted list encapsulating your medical history—all your major illnesses, treatments, screening tests, surgeries and accidents. Include dates and names of treating doctors.

Also, write a brief family medical history that includes major illnesses of all first and second-generation relatives. (The US government offers a free online family health record tool at CDC.gov/genomics/famhistory.) Keep this record current, just as you do your financial records, and keep a paper copy in its special file, so it can be easily reached anytime you visit a new doctor or are asked about your medical history.

On another sheet list all routine health checkups with the doctors' names and numbers...review it monthly and schedule the appointments accordingly.

Online medical records and personal health tools from Google, Microsoft and others are an increasingly popular alternative.

Imposing order on any aspect of your life—especially anything related to health—brings a sense of calm and a significant reduction in stress, which translates into improved health in the long run.

10-Minute Ritual for All-Day Energy

Nancy Lonsdorf, MD, ABIHM (board certified by the American Board of Integrative Holistic Medicine), is an Ayurvedic doctor specializing in healthy longevity and women's issues. She is author of *The Ageless Woman: Natural Health and Beauty After Forty with Maharishi Ayurveda* and a coauthor of *A Woman's Best Medicine: Health, Happiness, and Long Life through Maharishi Ayurveda*. DrNancyLonsdorf.com

---

Do you often feel sluggish, fatigued, foggy-brained or blue? There's a potential solution that is simple, takes as little as 10 minutes per day and costs absolutely nothing.

The secret: Take a walk outdoors in the fresh air, for at least 10 minutes, within an hour or two of dawn.

The rising sun and morning air are invigorating because they are filled with what Ayurveda calls prana, or life force. This gives you energy and clears out any morning brain fog. It has a revitalizing effect on the emotions, too, creating a positive mood for the whole day. A dawn walk also enhances ojas, a subtle essence of the physical body that helps keep you fully immune and strengthened against disease. From the perspective of Western medicine, she added, an early morning walk gets your circulation and metabolism going after you have been asleep all night and also is good for digestion.

For best effect: Get up by 6 am (called vata time in the Ayurvedic tradition). Then walk toward the rising sun, letting its light fall on your face. And don't worry about the weather—no matter whether it's hot or cold, sunny or rainy or snowing outside, your dawn walk will be richly rewarding.

11

Look Marvelous

Simple Ways to Look Younger

Eudene Harry, MD, medical director of Oasis Wellness & Rejuvenation Center in Orlando, Florida. She is board-certified in both emergency and holistic medicine and serves as medical director for the Women's Wellness Society, a national group that focuses on women's health. She is the author of *Live Younger in 8 Simple Steps: A Practical Guide to Slowing Down the Aging Process from the Inside Out.* LivingHealthyLooking Younger.com

It's a fact of life that our skin becomes more wrinkled as we age. But you may be surprised to learn that our skin starts changing as early as age 30 for both women and men. Of course, you can "refresh" your appearance with Botox and skin fillers, but even "inexpensive" cosmetic procedures cost hundreds of dollars.

A better option: Healthful foods and effective skin-care products. Used properly, natural approaches can take years off your appearance.

STEP 1: TWEAK YOUR DIET

While you might think that skin-care products are the logical choice to smooth wrinkled skin, it's wise to first work from the "inside out" to give your skin the nutrients it needs to look its best. *Increasing laboratory evidence and positive reports from patients suggest that the following foods promote younger-looking skin...*

- **High-sulfur foods.** Sulfur is known to be one of the "building blocks" of collagen, a protein that strengthens skin and gives it elasticity. Fortunately, sulfur is found in a number of foods.

My advice: At least once a day, eat sulfur-rich foods.

Good choices: Eggs, chives, legumes (such as black, white or kidney beans) and fish that is high in omega-3 fatty acids (such as salmon and sardines).

- **Grape juice or red wine.** These contain flavonoids known as proanthocyanidins and proteins called tenascins—both help make the skin smoother and more elastic.

My advice: Enjoy a daily glass of grape juice—or red wine if your doctor says daily alcohol consumption is appropriate for you. Both are high in proanthocyanidins.

In addition, a grape seed extract supplement (typical dose 200 mg once a day) is beneficial, but check first with your doctor if you take medication, especially a blood thinner—the supplement may interact with certain drugs.

- **Soy foods.** Tofu, soy milk and other foods derived from soy can make skin appear significantly younger. This is mainly due to genistein, an antioxidant in soy that slows skin aging and increases collagen. Genistein and other compounds are linked to increased skin elasticity and plumpness. These compounds give the skin a "glow" that makes it appear younger.

My advice: Have one or more daily servings of soy foods.

Good choices: Edamame (steamed soy beans) and miso (a fermented paste used in cooking). Check first with your doctor if you have breast cancer or kidney disease or take any medication. Soy may be harmful for some breast cancer and kidney disease patients...it may also interact with certain drugs, including blood thinners and some antidepressants.

Also: To help keep skin hydrated, drink eight eight-ounce glasses of water each day.

STEP 2: USE THE RIGHT SKIN-CARE PRODUCTS

Skin-care products can help smooth wrinkles and provide other benefits, but there are so many on the market that most people are confused about which to use. *Best choices for younger-looking skin...*

- **Topical vitamin C.** About 80% of the dermis (the second layer of skin) consists of that all-important protein collagen. Because collagen production declines with age, it's a good idea to promote collagen production any way you can.

That's where vitamin C enters the picture. The body uses vitamin C to produce collagen, but whatever is consumed orally doesn't reach adequate concentrations in the skin to boost collagen. That's why you need to apply it topically.

My advice: Use skin-care products (such as lotions and sunscreens) that have ascorbic acid (vitamin C)—the best form of the vitamin for absorption as well as collagen production and sun protection. Studies show that topical vitamin C can reduce the appearance of fine lines and wrinkles in as little as three months.

To save money: Buy powdered vitamin C at a health-food store, and mix in a small pinch each time you use a moisturizer/sunscreen that does not contain the vitamin.

- **Retinoic acid.** This is a form of vitamin A that is added to hundreds of over-the-counter (OTC) skin-care products. It is also available by prescription. Retinoic acid increases cellular turnover, the rate at which cells divide. This makes the skin appear brighter, smoother and plumper.

My advice: Use OTC retinol cream once daily. Apply it at night because it temporarily increases the skin's sensitivity to sun. Most products have a concentration of 1% or less. Prescription-strength retinoic acid usually is not necessary.

- **Moisturizer.** Everyone should use this as they age. Adding moisture to skin cells makes them expand, which improves skin volume and texture. Moisturizers protect the skin from environmental factors (heat, dryness and pollution) that undermine skin health.

My advice: Use moisturizer with sunscreen at least twice a day. I advise a vitamin C–enhanced moisturizer that includes green-tea extract. Both ingredients improve the skin's ability to absorb the moisturizer. Compounds in green tea also reduce skin inflammation and sun-related skin damage. Soy moisturizers may provide similar benefits.

Also important: Exfoliation, an effective form of controlled trauma that stimulates the skin to produce more collagen. Every week or two, use a gentle facial scrub with fine grains and a soft facial brush. This practice also removes the dead skin cells that dull your complexion.

Sensitive skin sometimes cannot tolerate even a mild scrub. An ultrasonic brush, such as Clarisonic ($100 to $200 at department stores and online), with a hydrating cleanser is a good alternative.

A chemical peel once or twice a year is another good way to remove dead skin cells. OTC peels contain glycolic acid, lactic acid or salicylic acid, usually in a concentration of about 5% to 10%. Peels should also contain moisturizing ingredients to minimize irritation. If you're new to chemical peels, talk with your dermatologist before using one of these products, since they can irritate skin, especially sensitive skin.

Do-It-Yourself Face-Lift

Shellie Goldstein, LAc, a licensed acupuncturist, esthetician and certified Chinese herbologist who maintains a private practice in New York City and Amagansett, New York (HamptonsAcupuncture.com). One of the first acupuncturists to work in hospitals and health-care facilities in New York state, Goldstein is the author of *Your Best Face Now: Look Younger in 20 Days with the Do-It-Yourself Acupressure Facelift.*

If you've got facial wrinkles that you would like to reduce but you don't want to get Botox injections or a surgical face-lift, there's a do-it-yourself option that's far less invasive and far less expensive.

With a technique known as facial acupressure (similar to acupuncture but performed without needles), you can take up to five to 10 years off your appearance—and perhaps even improve your overall health in the process.

Sound far-fetched?

I have treated hundreds of patients who were contemplating face-lifts but found success with acupressure.

Bonus: Unlike Botox or surgery, acupressure won't give you a tight, frozen or pulled-back appearance. The results are softer and more natural.

WHY ACUPRESSURE?

Acupressure is based on a Chinese healing technique that involves pressing or kneading key points on the body to stimulate energy flow, known as Qi (pronounced chee), through invisible pathways called meridians. It can be used to relax or tone muscles, boost circulation and even improve digestion.

The conventional view: From the Western medical perspective, wrinkles are formed by changes in the skin's composition, thickness and elasticity as well as continuous muscle activity—for example, forehead wrinkles may appear after years of furrowing your eyebrows or squinting. As a result, the skin covering the muscle creases, eventually creating a wrinkle.

Chinese medicine has a different perspective. For example, specific meridians (that correspond to organ systems, such as those for the "Liver" and "Gallbladder") are believed to affect certain body parts, but they don't always seem to correlate. For instance, a meridian located at the junction between your thumb and index finger corresponds to the head—rubbing that area can reduce headaches and, yes, wrinkles.

DO-IT-YOURSELF ROUTINES

To help reduce wrinkles and puffiness, use the following routines each day until you are satisfied with the results and then as needed...

- **Forehead wrinkles.**

What to do: Begin at the top of your right foot, in the junction between your big and second toes. (This point is called "Liver 3.") Using medium to firm (but not painful) pressure, massage the point in a clockwise circle 10 times. (If you have arthritic fingers, use your knuckle instead.) Repeat on left foot.

Next, move to the back side of your right hand between your right thumb and index finger ("Large Intestine 4"). In a clockwise circular motion, massage this point for 10 rotations. Repeat on the left hand.

Then, move to the back of your neck. Place both thumbs where your spine meets the base of your skull and move them two inches to either side until they each land in an indentation ("Gallbladder 20"). Massage clockwise with firm pressure for 10 rotations.

Lastly, move to your face. Place the pad of each index finger a half inch above the center of each eyebrow ("Gallbladder 14"). Massage with medium pressure in 10 clockwise (right to left) circles.

Repeat the entire sequence three times in a single session each day. For deeper wrinkles, do the sequence several times throughout the day. You should notice a reduction in forehead wrinkles within 20 days.

- **Under-eye puffiness (due to age or allergies).**

What to do: Place your index finger two inches above the inside of your right ankle between the bone and muscle ("Spleen 6"). Do 10 clockwise rotations using medium to firm pressure. Repeat on left leg.

Next, move to the back of your right hand ("Large Intestine 4"), as described earlier, and perform 10 clockwise rotations. Repeat on the left hand.

Then, with your arm at your side, bend your left elbow to make a 90° angle. Pinpoint the area located at the outside edge of the elbow crease, between the bend and the bone ("Large Intestine 11"). Use your index finger to massage 10 times in a clockwise rotation using medium to firm pressure. Repeat on your right elbow.

Lastly, move to your face. Place your right index finger just to the side of your right nostril. Move the finger laterally to a spot directly underneath the center of your eye, in your sinus area ("Stomach 3"). Press in and slightly upward, performing 10 clockwise rotations. Repeat on the left side.

Do the entire sequence three times daily. You should notice a reduction in puffiness under your eyes after a few days.

Natural Anti-Aging Treatments for Your Skin

Jamison Starbuck, ND, a naturopathic physician in family practice and a lecturer at the University of Montana, both in Missoula. She is past president of the American Association of Naturopathic Physicians and a contributing editor to *The Alternative Advisor: The Complete Guide to Natural Therapies and Alternative Treatments.*

Worldwide, people now spend more than $1 billion on anti-aging products, and the number of cosmetic procedures such as Botox injections has grown 20% in recent years. But even as aging baby boomers try to beat back time, many are loathe to do anything so drastic as injecting chemicals into their faces... instead they are jumping on the "green wagon" and looking for a more natural approach.

We consulted Jamison Starbuck, ND, a naturopathic physician in family practice and a lecturer at the University of Montana, both in Missoula, who said expensive and possibly risky high-tech interventions are not necessary. Healthy, glowing skin at all ages comes from inside. If you take good care of your body, your skin will reflect your good health. We asked her to share her natural strategies for keeping skin youthful.

FROM THE INSIDE OUT

You are what you eat, mom used to say, and—as usual—she was right. For optimal skin health, Dr. Starbuck advises following an anti-inflammatory, anti-aging diet. Replace trans fats, saturated fats and processed foods with fresh fruits and vegetables and foods rich in healthy fats (e.g., omega-3 fatty acids), such as walnuts, flaxseed and cold-water fish (wild salmon, sardines, mackerel, etc.). Since an anti-inflammatory diet is believed to improve circulation, you may find that within days of starting to eat this way, the puffiness and dark circles under the eyes begin to diminish.

According to Dr. Starbuck, the more colorful the produce, the richer it is in antioxidants, which help slow the aging process and maintain elasticity in skin and underlying tissue. Keep your kitchen stocked with bright, colorful fruits and veggies like blueberries, strawberries, spinach, carrots and broccoli.

PROTECT AGAINST THE SUN

To shield your skin from the ravages of the sun's ultraviolet rays—which range from harmless age spots to deadly melanoma—steer clear of the midday sun. During the spring and summer, when you are outdoors a lot, make the application of sunscreen part of your daily skin care routine. If you live closer to the equator, do this more often. Choose a product that contains zinc oxide to block the sun, as well as the antioxidant vitamins C and E and selenium, since Dr. Starbuck says sunscreens that contain antioxidants are more helpful in preventing skin damage. Use products with a sun protection factor (SPF) of 15 or higher and that offer protection against both UVA and UVB rays. Avoid chemicals and fragrances.

Also, Dr. Starbuck notes that many people believe they can apply sunscreen first thing in the morning and safely bask in the sun for hours. It doesn't work that way. Don't overestimate a sunscreen's ability to protect you from the sun's ultraviolet rays. If you are spending the day at the beach or in the sun, reapply every hour or so.

KICK THE BAD HABITS

Young people can stay out late or work till the wee hours and still look and feel fresh the next day. Not so as you grow older, when every indiscretion seems to show. *Dr. Starbuck's advice...*

- **Don't smoke or overindulge in alcohol.**
- **Reduce your exposure to toxic substances such as air pollutants, herbicides and household chemicals including cleaning products.** Use common sense and be aware of the environment around you. For example, stay inside as much as possible on smog alert days...avoid all harsh chemical products that cause skin irritation...choose natural alternatives whenever possible.
- **Avoid exposing your skin to harsh detergent and antibacterial soaps,** instead choosing milder, fragrance-free, chemical-free, natural cleansers. Another thing you can do to reduce the toxic load on your skin is go green in your home. Avoid cleaning products made from toxic ingredients. Dr. Starbuck recommends the natural, green cleaning products made by Melaleuca.

MORE EXERCISE GIVES YOU FIRMER SKIN TONE

When you're fit, your circulatory system works optimally to deliver a better supply of blood and oxygen to tissue and skin. Exercise also promotes firm muscles, resulting in less cellulite. The President's Council on Physical Fitness and Sports recommends at least three 20-minute aerobic workouts a week (e.g., brisk walking, bicycling or swimming) and three 30-minute strength training sessions. Don't forget to drink lots of water when you exercise. Dehydrated skin sags...not a pretty picture. Even worse, it is more vulnerable to damage from irritants of all kinds.

USE NATURAL SKIN CARE PRODUCTS

The more antioxidants and the fewer chemicals, the better, Dr. Starbuck advises. She recommends simple, fragrance-free, dye-free products, such as good, old-fashioned Ivory soap and naturally based soaps and moisturizers made with cucumber or calendula. For the best effect, use moisturizing creams immediately after bathing, when your skin is better able to absorb them.

Also, she says there is no need to waste money on expensive face creams that make false promises to banish wrinkles. A *Consumer Reports* study found no difference between pricey products (which can cost literally hundreds of dollars per ounce) at upscale department stores, and down-to-earth, economical drugstore brands. Also, other research shows that skin responds well to topical antioxidants. Choose skin care products that contain antioxidants such as vitamins C, A and E.

DR. STARBUCK'S PERSONAL FAVORITE

Dr. Starbuck says one of her most relaxing, effective and detoxifying treats is hydrotherapy. She explains that alternating hot and cold tones the body and stimulates blood and oxygen flow. Dr. Starbuck says that intense heat eliminates toxins through the skin, after which a brief plunge in cold water tightens pores, stimulating and invigorating both your skin and your mood. (*Caution*: This is not recommended for pregnant women or people with vascular problems such as hypertension.) This effect can easily be created in your own home. Just follow up a hot bath or shower with a 30-second cold rinse. This closes pores and brings refreshment and blood flow to skin.

LOVE THE SKIN YOU'RE IN

If you follow a lifestyle that emphasizes fitness and wellness, it will be reflected in your good health overall, including clear, firm and radiant skin.

Eat Chicken Soup and Other Secrets to Healthier Skin

Andrew L. Rubman, ND, founder and medical director, Southbury Clinic for Traditional Medicines, Southbury, Connecticut.

You don't need to buy lotions and creams at the drugstore or department store to reduce wrinkles, prevent breakouts, add color and moisture to your skin and/or reduce the uncomfortable and unappealing effects of problems such as oily skin, eczema, psoriasis and rosacea.

Not only are lotions and creams usually pricey, but they often are laced with potentially toxic and harsh chemicals such as parabens and formaldehyde that have been associated with hormonal disruption and even cancer (see page 87).

Even if you feel attached to your favorite brand of skin lotion, it might be time to give it up, because there's a safer and cheaper alternative—and it doesn't involve anything external.

You can improve your skin naturally—from the inside out—by consuming certain foods and supplements. *There's a natural potion that you can stir up yourself in your kitchen...*

CHICKEN SOUP—THE WRINKLE POTION

Simmer a quartered chicken (skin, bones and all) with some onion, celery, carrots and a bay leaf for two hours in enough water to cover the contents—leave the pot uncovered for the full two hours, which will allow for evaporation and concentrate the liquid. The poultry and vegetables will give up their flavor and nutrients to the remaining water, and after you remove the solids, you'll be left with a broth rich in hyaluronic acid (HA)—the same substance that we make in our own bodies that provides skin with fullness, volume and plumpness. As we grow older, our bodies produce less HA, which causes our skin to wrinkle and sag, so consuming extra HA may help, said Dr. Rubman. Organic and free-range chickens tend to produce more HA than traditionally-raised chickens because their diets are healthier and they're allowed to exercise more. Make a big pot of this concentrated chicken broth, and then freeze half and refrigerate half upon cooling. Have a warmed cup every evening before dinner spiced with a pinch of sea salt and fresh ground pepper for extra flavor. Feel free to adjust the recipe with your own choice of herbs and spices, and you'll still get the benefit. Chicken broth that you buy in a supermarket is just not the same, Dr. Rubman explained, because valuable compounds in the chicken skin and bones don't make their way into store-bought broths and bouillon cubes. If you find that this soup isn't helping your skin enough, ask your doctor about taking extra HA in supplement form, Dr. Rubman advised.

ADD COLOR AND MOISTURE

For great skin, be sure to consume enough of vitamins A, D, and E and the mineral zinc. Many people don't meet the recommended daily requirements, said Dr. Rubman. And that's too bad, because they can help protect your skin from the aging and cancerous effects of the sun's UV rays and from damaging environmental irritants, such as exhaust fumes and smog that can make skin dry and dull, he said. Foods high in vitamin A include sweet potatoes, carrots and dark, leafy greens...foods high in vitamin D include salmon, mushrooms and fortified milk...foods high in vitamin E include sunflower seeds, almonds and peanuts...and foods high in zinc include oysters, low-fat roast beef and lentils. Also, colorful fruits and vegetables are filled with carotenoids, organic pigments that can add color to your skin, giving you a literally healthy glow. The amount of foods that you should consume depends on how deficient you are. Dr. Rubman said that if you eat lots of the foods mentioned above and don't notice any results within a few months, ask your doctor whether it's a good idea to take daily supplements containing vitamins A, D and E and zinc, as well as a supplement complex that contains mixed carotenes and other carotenoids including lutein, lycopene and zeaxanthin.

PREVENT BREAKOUTS

Plenty of adults get pimples.

The best natural defense: Nuts and seeds, which are packed with antioxidants and omega-3 fatty acids that calm systemic and facial inflammation and therefore reduce the frequency and severity of outbreaks, said Dr. Rubman.

Anti-pimple dose: A one-ounce serving per day of almonds, Brazil nuts, walnuts, pecans or sunflower seeds. Try the foods first, and if the effect isn't strong enough within a few months, talk to your doctor about taking both antioxidant and omega-3 supplements, which might amplify the effect, Dr. Rubman advised. Your health-care provider can help you figure out how much you need. If you have a peanut allergy, Dr. Rubman suggests trying algae-sourced omega-3s and food-grade coconut oil for antioxidants. Note that those with a severe preexisting allergy should consult their doctors before introducing any new substance.

RELIEF FOR OILY SKIN, ECZEMA, PSORIASIS & ROSACEA

The skin problems listed above are sometimes signs of poor digestive health, said Dr. Rubman. And one key to healthy digestion is making sure that there's enough "good" bacteria in your gut. As we grow older, the army of beneficial bacteria that normally crowds out the "bad" bacteria declines, so it doesn't hurt to "call for backup," so to speak, in the form of probiotic supplementation, he explained. Eat a healthful diet—whole foods, not processed—because that creates the best environment for healthful bacteria. But probiotics contained in foods, such as yogurts, don't build up as well as those found in supplements, said Dr. Rubman. He suggests asking your doctor about taking a supplement containing both Lactobacillus and Bifidobacteria, which may help restore a proper balance of bacteria in your intestine...and lead to healthier, better-feeling, better-looking skin.

---

14 Things That Make You Look Older

Kim Johnson Gross, cocreator of the *Chic Simple* book series and author of *What to Wear for the Rest of Your Life* and *Chic Simple Dress Smart: Men*. Based in New York City, she is a former Ford model and has been fashion editor at *Town & Country* and *Esquire* magazines and a columnist for *More* and *InStyle*. KimJohnsonGross.com

Lauren Rothman, style and trend expert who has appeared on *Entertainment Tonight, CNN, E! News* and *ABC News*, among other news outlets. She is a style consultant for individuals and corporations in the greater Washington, DC, area and author of *Style Bible: What to Wear to Work*. StyleAuteur.com

---

As you get older, wardrobe and style choices that worked when you were younger may no longer be serving you well. This goes for both men and women. Without knowing it, you may be looking older than you are. This could cause others to treat you as older and potentially hold you back from employment opportunities and advancements. This also can make you feel like you are not up to your game or comfortable in your skin. When you are not style confident, you are less body confident, which makes you feel less life confident.

Helpful: Seek out style mentors—people who look elegant and modern without chasing youth-oriented trends. Observe them carefully, and adapt elements of their style to your own. TV newscasters make good style mentors because they are required to look contemporary while also projecting dignity and authority.

Give yourself a good, hard look, and ask yourself whether you are looking older than your actual age with any of these common signals...

1. Sneakers for everyday wear. Your feet should be comfortable, but sneakers outside the gym just look sloppy and careless. Young people get away with it—but there are more stylish options when you're older. These include loafers or driving moccasins for men and low-heeled pumps with cushioned soles for women. Wedge-soled shoes are a comfortable alternative to high heels.

2. Baggy pants. Although young men may look trendy in high-waisted, loose-fitting jeans, this style screams old on anyone else. For women, the rear end tends to flatten with age, causing pants to fit loosely in the rear. And front-pleated pants for women generally are unflattering and unstylish.

Better: Spend the time to find pants that fit well—or figure a tailor into your wardrobe budget. Baggy is dowdy, but overly tight makes you look heavier. Well-fitting clothes make you look slimmer and younger.

3. Boring colors. Skin tone gets duller with age, so the colors you wear should bring light to your face. If you are a woman who has worn black for years, it may be too harsh for you now. Brown makes men fade into the woodwork.

Better: Stand in front of a mirror, and experiment with colors that you never thought you could wear—you may be surprised at what flatters you. Avoid neon brights, which make older skin look sallow, but be open to the rest of the color spectrum. Try contemporary patterns and prints. For neutrals, gray and navy are softer alternatives to black for women, and any shade of blue is a good bet for men.

4. Boring glasses and jewelry. Men and women should have some fun with glasses. It's a great way to update your look and make it more modern. Tell your optician what you're looking for, or bring a stylish friend with you.

As for jewelry for women, wearing a large piece of fab faux jewelry (earrings, necklace, ring) or multiple bracelets adds great style and youth to your look.

5. Turtlenecks. You may think a turtleneck hides a sagging neck and chin, but it is more likely to draw attention to jowls.

Better: A cowl neckline for women, or a loosely draped scarf. A scarf is the single best item to help a woman look thinner, taller, prettier and more chic. YouTube has several "How to Tie a Scarf" instructional videos (a favorite is by Nordstrom). For a man, an oblong scarf, looped, is a stylish European look that adds a welcome shot of color.

6. "Matchy" outfits. Carrying a handbag that matches one's shoes was once considered stylish. These days it is associated with older women—young women tend to prefer a more casual, unmatched look. If you own sweater sets, break them up.

7. Stiff or one-tone hair. An overly styled helmet of hair looks old-fashioned. Hair that's a solid block of color looks unnatural and harsh.

Better: Whether hair is short or shoulder-length, women need layers around the face for softness. As for color, opt for subtle highlights in front and a slightly darker tone toward the back.

Keep in mind that gray hair can be beautiful, modern and sexy. You need a plan to go gray, though, which means a flattering cut and using hair products that enhance the gray. Ask your stylist for recommendations. Also, if your hair is a dull gray, consider getting silver highlights around your face to bring light and "energy" to your hair.

Men who dye their hair should allow a bit of gray at the temples—it looks more natural than monochrome hair. But avoid a comb-over or a toupee. A man who attempts to hide a receding hairline isn't fooling anyone—he just looks insecure.

Better: Treat your thinning hair as a badge of honor. Either keep it neatly trimmed or shave your head.

8. Missing (or bushy) eyebrows. Women's eyebrows tend to disappear with age. Men's are more likely to grow wild.

Better: Women should use eyebrow pencil, powder or both to fill in fading brows. Visit a high-end cosmetics counter, and ask the stylist to show you how. You may need to try several products to find out what works best. Men, make sure that your barber or hair stylist trims your eyebrows regularly.

Also: Women tend not to notice increased facial hair (especially stray hairs) on the chin and upper lip—a result of hormonal change. Pluck!

9. Flabby arms. Toned arm muscles can help you look younger—but which muscles you should target varies by gender. Consider working with a trainer to learn the best exercises for you.

Women: Sagging biceps and triceps in the upper arm can make women look old. Exercising with dumbbells is the best way to tone these. Start with very light dumbbells if necessary—even two-pound weights can make a difference. Do bicep curls, hammer curls and tricep exercises several times a week.

Men: Broad shoulders help men continue to look young and powerful as they age. Bench presses and/or push-ups help here.

10. Deeply tanned skin. Baby boomers grew up actively developing suntans using baby oil and sun reflectors. Now pale is the norm. A dark tan not only dates you, it increases your risk for skin cancer and worsens wrinkling.

Better: Wear a hat and sunscreen to shield your skin from sun damage.

11. Less-than-white teeth. Yellowing teeth add decades to your appearance. Everyone's teeth get yellower with age, but with so many teeth-whitening products available, there is no excuse to live with off-color teeth.

Better: Ask your dentist which whitening technique he/she recommends based on the condition of your teeth—over-the-counter whitening strips, bleaching in the dentist's office or a custom bleaching kit you can use at home.

12. Women: Nude or beige hose. Nude stockings on women look hopelessly out-of-date. Bare legs are the norm now for young women, but they are not a good option for older women who have dark veins.

Better: In winter, wear dark stockings or opaque tights. In summer, use spray-on tanner for a light tan...or wear nude fishnet stockings or slacks or capris.

13. Poor-fitting bra. Get a bra that fits. Most women don't know that bra size changes as your body does. Giving your breasts a lift will make you look younger and trimmer.

14. Excess makeup. Thick foundation, heavy eyeliner, bright blusher and red lipstick all add years to your face.

Better: Use a moisturizing (not matte) foundation, and dab it only where needed to even out skin tone. To add color to cheeks, use a small amount of tinted moisturizer, bronzer or cream blush. Use liquid eyeliner in soft shades such as deep blue or brown, and blend it well. For lips, choose soft pinks and mauves, depending on your skin tone.

Bottom line: The idea is to have fun putting yourself together. That inner spark and personal style will show that you are getting better with age.

Omega-3s Keep Hair Healthy

Susan M. Lark, MD, former editor, *Women's Wellness Today.*

Hair follicles need nutrient-rich blood. This requires consuming enough essential fatty acids, especially the omega-3s found in flaxseeds and wild-caught, cold-water fish, such as salmon and trout.

Best: Ingest four to six tablespoons of ground flaxseeds per day, along with plenty of water. You can use flaxseed in yogurt, cereal, smoothies and salads. Eat fish at least three times a week.

Natural Remedies for Thinning Hair

David Hoffmann, BSc, founding member and past president of the American Herbalists Guild, an advisory board member of the American Botanical Council. He teaches at the California School of Herbal Studies in Forestville and is the author of 17 books, including *Herbal Prescriptions After 50.*

If you are concerned about thinning hair, first see your doctor to find out whether there's an underlying medical problem, such as a thyroid disorder, that needs treating.

But if no such problem is found, don't be too quick to turn to conventional hair-loss treatments—because these can be problematic.

For instance: Topical medications can cause itching and increased facial or body hair...there's limited evidence for the effectiveness of laser therapy—and if you're a woman, costly hair-replacement surgery isn't appropriate for diffuse thinning throughout the scalp, the type of hair loss women often experience.

Fortunately, there are other options. Natural therapies for hair loss have a long tradition of use. Safe and economical, they offer do-it-yourself alternatives to conventional hair-loss treatment. (All products mentioned below are sold at health-food stores and online.)

SCALP CIRCULATION BOOSTERS

For many people, the key to reversing hair loss is to increase blood flow in the scalp. Try any or all of the following for six weeks. If you notice improvement, continue indefinitely or for as long as needed.

- **Massage with rosemary oil.** Rosemary oil works by widening tiny blood vessels in the scalp, thus stimulating hair follicles and helping promote hair growth. Massaging the scalp with your fingertips also promotes improved circulation.

Directions: Dilute rosemary oil with an equal amount of almond oil. This is important—rosemary oil by itself may be too strong and can irritate skin. Every evening (or every other evening, if you prefer), use your fingertips to massage a few drops of oil into your scalp, particularly where hair is thinning. Leave on overnight...wash off in the morning.

•**Rinse hair with nettle tea.** Nettle promotes hair growth not only by improving circulation, but also by reducing inflammation.

To prepare: Mix one-half tablespoon of dried nettle with one cup of water. Bring to a boil, reduce heat, cover and simmer for 30 minutes. Remove from heat. Let sit, covered, for 15 minutes. Strain through cheesecloth. Cool before using. Apply to hair, massaging into scalp for several minutes. Leave on for 15 minutes, then shampoo.

Easier: Steep two nettle tea bags in very hot water for 10 minutes. Cool, then apply as described above.

Good brand: Traditional Medicinals Organic Nettle Leaf tea bags (800-543-4372, Traditional Medicinals.com/products/nettle-leaf).

•**Drink herbal tea.** Consuming certain herbal teas can improve sluggish circulation from the inside out, which can stimulate hair growth. Choose either or both of the following teas and drink a total of three cups per day. *Options...*

•Hawthorn. Steep a heaping teaspoon of dried hawthorn berries in one cup of very hot water for five to 10 minutes, then strain. If you prefer, take hawthorn in supplement form as an extract of either dried berries or flowers and leaves at a dosage of 300 mg twice daily.

•Ginger. Add several slices of fresh ginger to one cup of water and boil for five minutes, then remove the ginger.

HAIR-SAVING STRESS BUSTERS

Emotional ordeals can provoke numerous physical reactions, including hair loss. To help manage stress, Hoffman suggested, practice a daily relaxation technique (such as deep breathing)...and follow a whole-foods—based diet that emphasizes fruits and vegetables and minimizes red meat and alcohol. *Also...*

•**Supplement with B vitamins.** The various B vitamins are needed to convert food to energy and help cells grow—but physical or emotional stress can deplete these key nutrients. Take a daily supplement of a B-complex formulation. Follow the dosage guidelines on the label and continue indefinitely.

•**Try an herbal adaptogen.** Adaptogenic herbs have been used for thousands of years to increase the body's resistance to stress, trauma, anxiety and fatigue. Their mechanism is not well understood, but they are thought to work in part by balancing hormones, Hoffmann explained. *Choose one of the following...*

•Ashwagandha (also called withania).

•Rhodiola.

•Siberian ginseng (not regular ginseng, which is too strong).

Select a product labeled "standardized" (indicating that the brand uses consistent amounts of the active ingredient), and follow the dosage instructions on the label. If you experience headaches, discontinue use. Otherwise, continue daily for one month. If you notice improvement, stay with it for another month, then give your body a two-week break. If you do not notice improvement after one month, try one of the other adaptogens listed above.

It's Not Just About Wrinkles: Secrets to Younger-Looking Skin

Neal B. Schultz, MD, assistant clinical professor at Mount Sinai School of Medicine, assistant adjunct physician at Lenox Hill Hospital and owner of Park Avenue Skin Care, all in New York City. He is coauthor, with Laura Morton, of *It's Not Just About Wrinkles*.

When people complain about looking older, they usually talk about lines and wrinkles. However, most people who are dissatisfied with their appearance have color or texture problems as well that make them look older than they should.

Well-known treatments, such as Botox and collagen, are very effective for lines and wrinkles, but they don't affect color and texture issues. About three-quarters of patients will notice a dramatic improvement when they treat these two important factors, too.

COLOR

Color problems are among the easiest skin defects to correct. They basically fall into two categories—browns (such as age spots and freckles) and reds (usually due to engorged or broken capillaries).

• **Browns.** Brown spots go by many different names—sunspots, liver spots, age spots, etc. They're almost always caused by sun exposure, which triggers excessive activity in some of the skin's pigment-producing cells. Most brown spots appear on exposed areas of the skin, such as the face, arms and back of the hands.

On the other hand, blotchy brown areas that don't have a clear border are usually caused by an imbalance of female hormones, such as during pregnancy or in women taking birth control pills.

Virtually all brown defects can be removed with laser treatments, which cost $400 to $1,200 per treatment. A less expensive but more time-consuming approach is to lighten the brown areas with exfoliation.

Best home treatment: A product with 8% glycolic acid used daily. Glycolic acid is one of the alpha hydroxy acids (AHAs). It dissolves keratin, the uppermost layer of dead skin. Over-the-counter products, such as Aqua Glycolic Face Cream, Glytone Day Cream for Dry Skin and Kinerase Cream, lighten brown spots and stop the formation of new pigment cells.

Glycolic acid begins to work within two weeks—and will significantly reduce brownness in four to six weeks.

Important: Continue to apply a sunscreen whenever you are going outdoors. Repeated sun exposure will cause the brownness to return.

Also helpful: Twice-daily applications of over-the-counter topical vitamin C, such as Stallex C Complex Rescue Serum or SkinMedica Vitamin C Complex. Topical vitamin C lightens brown spots and blocks cell-damaging free radicals. It can be used in addition to glycolic acid.

Skin cancer warning: If there is a change in a brown spot's or a mole's size, shape or color (other than lightening from treatment) or if it bleeds, itches or becomes painful, contact your dermatologist immediately.

• **Reds.** Most people have one or more red spots or lines on their faces. They're often present on the cheeks or alongside the nose and usually are due to dilated or broken capillaries.

Common types: Telangiectasias, which appear as tiny straight or curved red lines...spider hemangiomas, which are raised red bumps with red lines emanating from the center...or cherry hemangiomas, flat or dome-shaped spots. Another type of redness is caused by rosacea—an acne-like condition that's characterized by red blotches (telangiectasias) that appear intermittently on the cheeks and nose.

Best home treatment: An over-the-counter topical sulfur preparation— such as Rezamid Acne Treatment Lotion or Sulforcin Acne Treatment Lotion. Sulfur shrinks blood vessels and helps reduce redness. This can work for rosacea, too, but test an area the size of a dime first to see how your skin reacts.

Because it's difficult to eliminate skin redness entirely, I usually advise patients to conceal it by using color-correcting makeup—a green-tinted foundation works best. Neutrogena makes a good one.

Diet: Certain foods have dilating effects on blood vessels, causing them to temporarily increase in diameter. The most common perpetrators are alcohol and spicy foods. Also, certain medications and vitamins (the most common of which is any form of niacin, one of the B vitamins) are known to cause dilation of facial blood vessels and thus to increase their conspicuousness.

TEXTURE

Young skin is smooth, with a noticeable "slip factor" when you run a finger across the face. Older "dull" skin feels rough, or there are "bumps" when the finger passes over enlarged pores.

Both of the main texture problems—enlarged pores and dull, flaky skin—are caused by the retention of dead skin cells. Skin cells are supposed to shed every 28 days—but not all cells do this. This results in an uneven accumulation of dead cells.

Best home treatment: Exfoliation with glycolic acid. People should start with a product that has 8% glycolic acid. The concentration can be increased to 10% or 15% if needed.

Bonus: Exfoliating can remove early precancerous cells along with the dead skin cells.

In-office exfoliation treatments: There are two types of in-office exfoliation—chemical, with a prescription glycolic acid treatment...and mechanical with microdermabrasion. The latter involves the use of a machine by a properly trained doctor, nurse or esthetician that bombards the skin with sterilized aluminum-oxide crystals. It immediately strips away dead cells and leaves the skin looking uniform and fresh.

In-office treatments cost $100 to $200 per treatment. You will need six to 10 treatments done at one- to two-week intervals.

CONTOUR

After about age 40, just about everyone notices an increase in lines, wrinkles and sagging skin. These and other contour problems usually are treated with products such as Botox and/or "filler" materials, such as collagen.

Botox can cost $400 to $1,600 per treatment, depending on the area done, and lasts about three months. Fillers are $600 to $2,000 per treatment and last three to nine months, depending on the area done and the filler used.

The main contour problems and the best treatments...

- **Frown lines** (the vertical lines between the eyes) and **forehead lines** (horizontal lines across the forehead) are known as dynamic lines because they're most visible when the underlying muscles move. Injections of Botox often can eliminate these types of lines, but when the injections wear off in about three months, they have to be repeated.
- **Marionette lines** run from the nose down to the corner of the mouth. They're caused mainly by the age-related loss of fat and skin elasticity. Botox can't be used for these lines because it can paralyze the entire cheek muscle and prevent smiling. A better approach is to inject collagen or another filler, such as Restylane. These products add volume to the skin and fill out the hollow contours.
- **Crow's feet,** the lines that radiate from the corners of the eyes, often can be improved or eliminated with Botox. In about 20% of cases, patients require a combination of Botox plus collagen.
- **Smoker's lines on the lips** (also called "lipstick lines" because lipstick can "bleed" into the tiny crevices) will disappear when injected with a very fine form of collagen. Most patients also are given injections of Botox to reduce muscle contractions that cause the lines.

The Silicon Secret to Better Health and Greater Beauty

Mark A. Stengler, NMD, a naturopathic medical doctor and leading authority on the practice of alternative and integrated medicine. Dr. Stengler is author of the *Health Revelations* newsletter, author of *The Natural Physician's Healing Therapies* (Bottom Line Books), founder and medical director of the Stengler Center for Integrative Medicine in Encinitas, California. MarkStengler.com

---

Patients often are surprised when I recommend silicon for their thinning hair or brittle nails. I believe that this mineral is a well-kept secret in the medical world. Note that silicon, the mineral, is different from silicone, the synthetic compound that (in gel form) is used in some medical applications and products, including breast implants.

Silicon is amazing—it's the second most common mineral in the Earth's crust and is found in sand on beaches. While it was once believed to be an inert contaminant, researchers discovered more than a century ago that silicon was concentrated in many of the body's tissues. What's more, silicon plays a role in keeping us healthy by strengthening bone and joint cartilage and maintaining the health of hair, skin and fingernails. *How silicon can help you...*

HEALTH BENEFITS OF SILICON

You may have heard silicon referred to as a "trace mineral," a mineral needed by the body in only very small amounts. But there is growing evidence that silicon could eventually be regarded as a macro mineral, which is required in amounts larger than that provided by food alone.

We have silicon in every cell of our bodies. Concentrations of silicon are highest in bone, connective tissues, skin, fingernails and hair, as well as the trachea, tendons and aorta—tissues that need strength and/or resilience. *Silicon's main role is to enhance the structural integrity of specific tissues, such as...*

- **Collagen.** Scientific evidence points to silicon being involved in the synthesis and "stability" of collagen, the body's chief protein. We need collagen to make most of our organs, bone and the fibrous tissues of the skin, tendons and ligaments. Without adequate collagen production, bones and ligaments weaken and skin tissue is compromised.

- **Joint cartilage.** Collagen and noncollagen proteins are needed to make joint cartilage, the role of which is to protect the joints and enable bones to move freely.

- **Bone.** Silicon is a major constituent of bone-making cells. Concentrations of the mineral are especially high in cells actively forming new bone. The mineral enhances the absorption of calcium, and a lack of silicon reduces the calcium content of bone. High intake of silicon is associated with better bone-mineral density and stronger bones.

Several studies have found that taking supplemental silicon increases the mineral density of bones.

Example: A study of postmenopausal women published in *BMC Musculoskeletal Disorders* found that adding a silicon supplement improved bone-mineral density above and beyond what was achieved with just calcium and vitamin D supplementation.

- **Skin, hair, fingernails.** Several small but promising studies have found that supplemental silicon often can restore a younger- and healthier-looking appearance. This is probably related to collagen and elastin production. Elastin is a protein that, as the name suggests, gives skin the ability to stretch. One study found that a commercial silicon oral supplement called RegeneMax reduced micro-wrinkle depth by 30%. It also improved the youthful look, or elasticity, of the skin. Other studies have found that silicon supplements can increase the thickness of hair strands and strengthen fingernails, making them more resistant to breaking.

GETTING SILICON INTO YOUR BODY

While silicon was once plentiful in herbs and grains, farming methods have depleted silicon from the ground, so many plant foods are not as rich in silicon as they could be. Because of this, most people have suboptimal levels of silicon. We need 5 grams (g) to 20 g daily of silicon—and the best way to get this amount is to take supplemental silicon.

For those people who have thinning hair or lackluster, aging skin and want a more youthful appearance, I recommend taking 5 mg daily of choline-stabilized orthosilicic acid, which is biologically active and much better absorbed than silicon derived from herbal sources. It is available in liquid and capsule form. If you have severe osteoporosis or osteoarthritis or brittle nails or hair, consider taking 10 mg daily. If your body takes in more silicon than it needs, you excrete the excess (so taking in more than you need at these doses is not a problem).

Brands to try: BioSil by Natural Factors (800-322-8704, NaturalFactors.com for a store locator)...JarroSil by Jarrow Formulas (310-204-6936, Jarrow.com)...and Xymogen's RegeneMax (800-647-6100, Xymogen.com, available through health-care professionals).

There are no side effects, and silicon is safe to take with other medications. Silicon supplements should be avoided by people with chronic kidney disease (excess silicon could result in further kidney damage) and women who are pregnant.

Wrinkles Be Gone!

American Chemical Society.

Maple syrup isn't the only valuable by-product of maple trees.

Recent lab discovery: Extracts from maple leaves were found to help block the wrinkle-causing process—much like Botox.

How to Eliminate Stress from Your Face

Ginger Hodulik Downey holds a BS in foods and nutrition, an MS degree in nutrition and a CNS (Certified Nutrition Specialist). She is currently the co-owner and vice president of R&D for DermaMed Solutions. In addition to her work at DermaMed, Ginger devotes time to working with patients in private clinical practice. As a contributor, Ginger hopes to continue to share her passion for holistic health and wellness.

We all know that stress is bad for our mental health and can increase our blood pressure, but did you know that it can make you look less beautiful? I recently acquired a new toy to help me with this exact aspect of my wellness—stress management.

Beauty is real motivation for many, especially people like me who work in the skin-care field. When I'm stressed I notice two things—an increase in breakouts and rashes on my face (and all over my body)...and also oilier skin.

On the science side of things, I know that when we are stressed, we release excess cortisol—a stress hormone. Cortisol is known to reduce collagen production, which leads to wrinkles and sagging skin. Cortisol also impacts oil production, which can cause more breakouts.

That's not good.

I felt it was time to get that stress in check before it did some real damage to my skin so I bought a Spire (SpireHealth.com). (*Note*: There are other products out there that you can try as well, such as the wellness trackers available at Bellabeat.com. This does not count as an endorsement of Spire and I did not get paid to write this review. I just chose this device as a way to manage my stress.)

Spire is a device that looks like a small stone on a metal clip that you attach to your bra or waistband. It communicates with your smartphone and helps you to be mindful of times when you are stressed. The science behind Spire is fairly simple. When stress triggers the brain's fight-or-flight response, heart rate elevates, breathing becomes shallow and muscles tense up. Spire picks up the body's information and sends this data to your phone, which in turn signals you when a stress response occurs. When you are tense for a few minutes, you get a little buzz from the device. (I missed this in the instructions and practically had a heart attack the first time my Spire zinged me with a warning that I was stressed.) Anyway, once you hear the buzz, you look at your phone, which tells you that you have been tense for some period of time and invites you to do a breathing exercise to calm down. It's absolutely amazing how quickly a few slow, deep breaths can settle you down to a calm state again. Breath is so powerful!

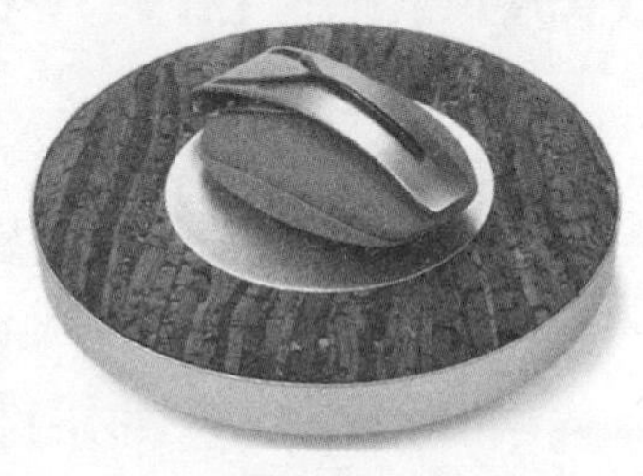

Overall, the idea behind the device is to create mindful moments where you notice the stress and do something constructive to counter it. I also found that wearing the device helped me to become aware of what triggers stress for ME personally. This is a powerful tool and, for me, brought some surprises.

I wore my Spire in all sorts of settings—on a business trip...during a regular work day...while just hanging with the kids. In my life, stressful times were tied to emotions more than to situations. I noticed that a long security line at the airport does not stress me, yet watching two people argue over their place in line in the airport restroom did. Simply thinking about an area of concern with my teenage son caused a tense moment and buzz, whereas face-to-face discussion with him about the same topic was not stress-provoking. I found that my internal thoughts are my stress triggers versus external events, which means that managing stress is totally within my control. (Of course!)

By creating a mindful moment, I am empowered to make a decision about how I will stop a stressful thought from settling into my body and doing harm. This is a must-have tool in my beauty toolkit, right alongside my favorite skin-care products!

12

Medical Care and Planning

Don't Let Dementia and Age-Related Diseases Catch You Off-Guard

Jullie Gray, MSW, LICSW, CMC, co-owner of Aging Wisdom, a life-care management firm in Seattle, president National Academy of Certified Care Managers, and past president, National Association of Professional Geriatric Care Managers.

Few situations could be more tragic for older adults than being treated as if they have Alzheimer's disease when they really have a treatable health issue, such as a drug side effect or depression. Equally disturbing is not knowing what is happening or where to turn if Alzheimer's or a movement disorder, such as Parkinson's disease, is setting in. This is especially true for older people who live alone and away from family. It happens every day to thousands of mature adults. They end up malnourished and living in squalor, forgotten in suboptimal nursing facilities—or on the street.

Help is available—help that can ensure you get the right diagnosis and treatment. And, just like estate planning, it can assist you in making arrangements in advance for health and physical needs if you have the beginnings of an incurable and progressive age-related disease.

WHEN DAILY LIVING BECOMES A CHALLENGE

The doorway to help is through a process called a geriatric assessment. Besides physical and psychological health, a geriatric assessment evaluates whether activities of daily living are becoming challenging. Activities include ordinary tasks such as eating, bathing and dressing as well as taking medications, keeping appointments, paying bills and getting around.

The first step is to make an appointment with your primary care physician for a geriatric assessment. The doctor will give you a physical exam and interview you to assess activities of daily living. If an age-related health issue is found, the doctor may act as the point person for a team of specialists who will take care of your health needs and help you plan for the future, whether that be making arrangements for physical therapy, optimizing your home to help you live there safely, getting transportation or a visiting nurse service or home-delivered meals, or arranging for nursing home care. Or the doctor may refer you to a geriatric specialist to assess your health and act as the point person for multispecialty care.

KNOW WHEN TO GO

A recent health alert by the division of geriatrics and palliative medicine at University at Buffalo, The State University of New York, gave guidance about when to arrange for a geriatric assessment of a parent, spouse or sibling by observing how that person manages the activities of daily living. It's easy to see when someone close to you is becoming frail and physically or mentally challenged—but what about when you have to make that decision about yourself? *A geriatric assessment may be wise if you answer yes to even one of these questions...*

- **Are you more forgetful, distracted and irritable than usual, and are you worried that your memory is failing?**
- **Do you feel not as steady on your feet, resulting in having a fall?**
- **Is taking care of your house, paying your bills and taking care of your health becoming more challenging?**
- **Do you have more than one chronic health problem?**
- **Are you worried about changes in your health and feel confused about what to do or who to turn to for help?**

PREPARING FOR AGING

Whether or not you decide to have a geriatric assessment, there are ways to ease age-related challenges that you can do on your own, such as optimizing your living space with better lighting, grab rails, easy-to-reach cabinets and drawers, elevated toilets and open showers. The key is to not delay.

Are You Just Getting Older or...Do You Need to See a Doctor?

Donnica Moore, MD, president of Sapphire Women's Health Group, a multimedia education and communications firm in Far Hills, New Jersey, and editor-in-chief of *Women's Health for Life*. She is a medical expert on ABC's *Good Morning America*. DrDonnica.com

You sigh with resignation when some annoying symptom appears or worsens, dismissing it as an inevitable sign of aging—but that can be a mistake.

Reasons: Often, simple self-help strategies correct the problem. In other cases, a visit to the doctor can prevent unnecessary suffering—or even save your life. *Symptoms to watch for...*

- **Seeing spots.** Gazing at a blank wall, you notice floaters—tiny dark specks or strings—in your field of vision.

Normal aging: The vitreous, a gel-like substance inside the eye, becomes more liquid, allowing microscopic fibers within to clump and cast shadows on the retina.

For self-help... Try nonprescription Dry Eye Relief Tear Stabilization Formula (CureFloaters.com). Its omega-3 fatty acids and other nutrients may reduce visual distortion from floaters by improving the cornea's film of tears.

See your doctor if... floaters are accompanied by gradual blurring or an overall yellowish or reddish hue to your visual field. You may have cataracts (clouding of the eyes' lenses), correctable with surgery.

Seek emergency care if... floaters suddenly increase significantly in number or are accompanied by flashing lights or hazy vision. You could have a retinal tear or detachment that requires immediate surgery to prevent vision loss.

- **Dizziness.** You stand up and your head spins.

Normal aging: The ear has fluid-filled structures that sense movement and balance. When tiny calcium crystals in the inner ear dislodge and float in this fluid, you may develop benign paroxysmal positional vertigo (BPPV). Other possibilities include orthostatic hypotension (postural low blood pressure), which occurs when blood pools in the legs, decreasing oxygen-rich blood flow to the brain...or hypoglycemia (low blood sugar).

Self-help... get up more slowly. In mild cases of BPPV or orthostatic hypotension, this prevents dizziness. BPPV also may be corrected with head movements called Epley or Semont maneuvers, which cause the crystals to lodge in a harmless area. For instructions online, see Dizziness-and-Balance.com (click on "Dizzy Patients"). To avoid blood sugar dips, each day eat three moderate meals and two healthful snacks that include some protein. Do not drive when dizzy!

See your doctor if...dizziness persists or is severe enough to create a risk of falling. A physician or physical therapist can guide your head through the Epley or Semont maneuvers. Low blood pressure can be corrected with diet, drugs and/or compression stockings. You also should be checked for medication side effects and underlying disorders (diabetes, anemia, ear or sinus infections) linked to dizziness.

Seek emergency care if...dizziness is accompanied by impaired vision, speech problems, and/or weakness or tingling on one side of the body. These may indicate a stroke.

- **Indigestion.** You feel a burning sensation beneath your breastbone.

Normal aging: When the sphincter between the esophagus and stomach weakens, digestive acids can move upward and irritate the esophagus.

Self-help...limit foods and beverages likely to trigger discomfort—citrus, onions, tomatoes, mint, spicy or high-fat foods, coffee, alcohol. Do not eat within three hours of bedtime. Lose excess weight. Wear clothing that is loose at the waist. Do not smoke. Use blocks to raise the head of your bed by about six inches.

See your doctor if...symptoms occur more than twice per week—chronic heartburn may warrant medication or surgery. If you also experience swallowing difficulties, vomiting, tarry stools or unintended weight loss, get screened for gastrointestinal ulcers and cancer.

Seek emergency care if...upper abdominal pain occurs along with unusual fatigue, shortness of breath, nausea and/or back pain. These can be signs of a heart attack.

- **Leaking urine.** You sneeze or are hurrying to the bathroom and—whoops! Some urine escapes.

Normal aging: Pelvic muscles that control urination weaken over time...and declining estrogen thins the walls of the urethra, creating a wider and weaker channel for urine to leave the bladder.

Self-help...six times each day, do "fast-and-slow" Kegel exercises.

How: Contract the muscles around your vagina and anus, lifting them upward and inward...hold for 10 seconds, then relax for 10 seconds...repeat 10 times. Next, contract for one second, then relax for one second...repeat 10 times. Avoid caffeine and carbonated beverages—they can irritate the bladder.

See your doctor if...you often leak urine or use the toilet more than eight times per day or more than twice at night.

Treatments: A probe inserted into the vagina emits a current that may stimulate and strengthen pelvic muscles over time. Collagen injected into the bladder outlet may improve closure...Botox injected into the bladder lining can reduce spasms. Surgical options include inserting a sling to support the urethra...or implanting a nerve-stimulating device that calms spasms in an overactive bladder.

Seek emergency care if...there is blood in your urine. You must be checked for kidney stones, pyelonephritis (a kidney infection), severe urinary tract infection and/or urinary tract cancer.

- **Poor memory.** You made plans to see a friend but cannot remember where to meet.

Normal aging: As the body produces lower levels of chemicals that brain cells need to function optimally, memory worsens.

Self-help...try daily crossword or Sudoku puzzles or games that challenge brain speed (see GamesForTheBrain.com). Get regular aerobic exercise to increase cerebral blood flow and promote neuron regeneration. Aim for seven to nine hours of sleep per night. Do not smoke or consume more than one alcoholic drink daily—people with these bad habits develop Alzheimer's disease an average of 2.3 to 4.8 years earlier, respectively, than nonsmokers and nondrinkers.

See your doctor if...forgetfulness interferes with day-to-day tasks or if loved ones say that they notice behavioral changes. High blood pressure and diabetes increase dementia risk, so work with your doctor to control these conditions. Ask your doctor if memory problems may be linked to medication or an underlying problem, such as a vitamin B-12 deficiency, sleep disorder, anemia, low thyroid or depression.

Seek emergency care if... a memory lapse occurs suddenly and is accompanied by changes in vision, speech and/or balance—this could signal a stroke. Also get immediate help if memory problems occur after a head injury, even a seemingly minor one. This can signal bleeding within or around the brain. Emergency surgery can be lifesaving.

Hey Doc, Treat Me... Not My Age!

Mark Lachs, MD, MPH, professor of medicine and co-chief of the division of geriatrics and gerontology at Weill Cornell Medical College in New York City. He is director of Cornell's Center for Aging Research and Clinical Care and director of geriatrics for the New York-Presbyterian Health System. He is author of *Treat Me, Not My Age*.

It's not surprising that older adults have more health problems than young people. What is surprising is how poorly this older population is served by our health-care system.

This is partly due to medical ageism, a subtle type of age discrimination that makes it harder to navigate the health-care system as you get older. In a Duke University survey, nearly 80% of respondents older than 60 had been told at least once by their doctors that their ailments were due to age—the implication being that the ailment is simply a result of getting older, so the doctor isn't going to treat it.

Many of the conditions that get more common with age, such as pain, hearing loss and depression, are never fully investigated. Similarly, a doctor might feel that a little knee pain or the leakage of urine is "normal" in older adults. This attitude means that underlying problems might never be diagnosed.

Undertreatment is one consequence of medical ageism...overtreatment is another. Doctors who practice what is known as "cookbook medicine" tend to recommend the same tests and procedures for everyone.

Your doctor should treat you, not your age. *Here's what to watch out for—and what to do to make sure that medical ageism doesn't hurt you or a loved one...*

UNDERTREATMENT

Rationing health care is among the most common forms of medical ageism. A doctor looks at the patient's medical record, notes the birth date and then makes certain assumptions.

Example: A patient who complained that he hurt his knee during a tennis match might be advised to take up a less physically demanding sport, such as golf. Or he might simply be told to "take it easy."

I know plenty of 70- and 80-year-olds who are in great shape and play a tough game of tennis, and a few 40-year-olds who are frail. The doctor's job is to address the problem, not to ignore the problem with age-based assumptions.

Self-protection: Don't let your doctor brush off any health issue with a reference to age. Be wary if he/she performs a perfunctory exam or rushes through your history. You should be asked detailed questions such as, "When did the pain start?"..."How many days are there when it doesn't hurt?"..."How's your range of motion?" etc.

It's possible that there won't be an easy solution, or any solution, for your problem. If that's the case, make sure that your doctor tells you why. "You're just getting older" is not an acceptable answer.

OUTDATED EXAM

The traditional office exam is not effective for older adults. It was created more than 100 years ago, when people didn't live as long. Information about blood pressure, reflexes, heart sounds, etc., is helpful, but it tells little about how well you function in daily life.

Example: A patient who appears perfectly healthy based on the standard medical exam might be falling every day at home.

Self-protection: Don't wait for your doctor to discover things. Make a list before you go, which might include balance problems, declines in muscle strength, poor hearing or even social isolation, which can lead to depression. These and other functional issues often are more important for long-term health than what is revealed by an exam.

Ideally, your doctor also will perform tests to see how you actually function. He might speak at different volumes to check your "real-life" hearing.

You might be asked to walk or to stand up and then sit down. You might be given a list of words and numbers and asked to repeat them.

Helpful: Ask friends and family members if they've noticed things that you haven't. Maybe you keep turning up the volume on the television or asking people to repeat themselves. You might be getting tired more easily or forgetting names more often.

ARE YOU DEPRESSED?

Depression is common in the elderly, but doctors often fail to diagnosis it. This is partly because it takes time to perform a mental health evaluation, so most doctors don't routinely do it. It's also because older adults often experience different symptoms of depression than those who are younger.

Self-protection: Tell your doctor if you've been feeling more irritable lately...have been losing weight...or are eating less regularly. These are common signs of depression in older adults.

Important: If you're suffering from depression, ask for a referral to a gerontologist (an internist who specializes in treating older patients) or a geriatric psychiatrist. Medicines can be helpful, especially when used in conjunction with supportive psychotherapy, but older people respond differently to antidepressants. They may require different doses and/or durations of treatment than younger adults.

OVERCARE

Too much medical care is just as dangerous as too little, particularly for those who are taking multiple medications, have underlying health problems and generally are frail.

Example: The mother of a friend of mine has Alzheimer's disease and dementia, as well as diabetes. The doctors and nurses who care for her always are tracking her blood sugar. This requires multiple daily blood sticks...which she thinks is a sign that they're trying to kill her, making her agitated and unhappy. For a patient like this, treating the diabetes this aggressively doesn't make a lot of sense.

Similarly, I would hesitate to subject an 82-year-old woman to the inconvenience and stress of a mammogram, particularly if she has had many negative mammograms in the past, no history of breast problems and no family history of breast cancer.

Self-protection: Don't agree to any test or procedure without asking your doctor if the results will change or improve your outcome. You also should ask questions such as, "What will happen if I do nothing?"..."Will the results of this test lead to more tests?"..."What are the side effects of testing?"

A patient might reasonably decide that he wants every possible test and treatment—it's just as reasonable to do the opposite in some cases.

AVOID THE ER

According to 2007 data from the National Center for Health Statistics (the most recent data available), about 25% of Americans older than 75 went to the emergency room at least once that year. That's the last place that you want to be except in a real emergency.

In the ER, there's too much care—and too little. Examinations are rushed. There's often a lack of communication among doctors. Patients may be given tests that they don't really need. It's an extremely stressful environment.

My advice: Ask your doctor how you can contact him, or an assistant, at any hour. Certainly don't delay in getting to the ER if you have serious symptoms, such as those of a stroke or heart attack, but other conditions might wait until the next day if you can get the over-the-phone OK from your doctor.

"You're just getting older" is not an acceptable response from a doctor.

Don't Let Your Doctor Get It Wrong

Helen Haskell, MA, president of Mothers Against Medical Error, a nonprofit patient-safety organization.

Fifteen years ago, my teenage son Lewis went to the hospital for an elective surgical procedure. After the operation, his doctors failed to notice that he was suffering from an undetected infection and blood loss from an ulcer caused by pain medication. They believed his symptoms were an indication of constipation from other pain medications he was taking. This mistake cost my son his life—he died four days after entering the hospital.

Now: I teach patients skills that can help them avoid a similar tragedy.

A "BLIND SPOT" IN MEDICINE

A groundbreaking new report from the prestigious Institute of Medicine (IOM) concluded that most Americans will experience at least one diagnostic error—that is, an inaccurate, missed or delayed diagnosis, as determined by later definitive testing—at some point in their lives.

The IOM report called diagnostic errors a "blind spot" in the delivery of quality health care. Each year, about one in 20 patients who seek outpatient care will suffer from a wrong or delayed diagnosis. According to autopsy studies, diagnostic mistakes contribute to about 10% of patient deaths. Unfortunately, diagnostic errors haven't gotten as much attention as treatment and surgical errors—for example, operating on the wrong body part—partially because the latter are easier and quicker to identify. Now patient-safety experts are taking steps to better understand why diagnostic errors occur. *Key reasons...*

- **Tests help—and hurt.** Patients may be given a staggering number of tests—X-rays, blood tests, biopsies and more. The process of ordering, conducting and conveying the results of a test, however, can be complex and poorly organized.

- **Poor communication.** Can you count on the internist to talk to the nurse? Will the radiologist convey all of the pertinent information to the surgeon? Don't count on it. Patients also play a role. They should tell their doctors about all the symptoms they're having and whether they're getting better or worse after starting a new treatment.

- **Snap judgments.** Doctors often develop a working diagnosis within the first few minutes of hearing the patient's reported symptoms. The danger is that doctors can develop a so-called anchoring bias that leads them to cling to their initial diagnosis and prevents them from fully considering new information or looking for other possibilities.

HOW TO MAKE SURE YOUR DOCTOR GETS IT RIGHT

Major medical groups, including the Society to Improve Diagnosis in Medicine, have identified a number of institutional factors—such as stronger teamwork—to reduce errors. But no one has more at stake in these situations than the patients themselves. *Four steps you can take to avoid a misdiagnosis...*

***STEP 1:* Organize your thoughts.** Most of the time, doctors have only 15 minutes with each patient, so you need to make the most of your time together.

Plan ahead: Your medical history—including a description of symptoms and when the problem started—is the most important part of an exam. Describe the nature and context of your symptoms in as much detail as you can. When do you feel them? What makes them worse or better? Why are you worried? Keep it concise and on topic, but include your own thoughts so the doctor can address the issues that concern you.

My advice: If possible, before you see the doctor, use the Internet to investigate your symptoms and the likely causes. Your findings should not be used to challenge your doctor, but rather as a way to have a more informed conversation. If you don't have confidence in your own abilities to do research, take advantage of a service like Expert HealthSearch (ImproveDiagnosis.org/?page=ExpertHealthSearch), a free service that puts you in touch with a medical librarian who can search the literature for you.

***STEP 2:* Don't be afraid to question test results.** They are more prone to error than most people imagine. In one study, experts who reviewed biopsies of more than 6,000 cancer patients concluded that 86 had been given a wrong diagnosis. Samples can be too small or even contaminated...technicians can make mistakes...and there can be false-negatives or false-positives. Results can be misinterpreted, or even more often, they can go unreported to the patient.

My advice: If a test result seems to fly in the face of the symptoms you are experiencing, consider asking to repeat the test or have a second doctor review it. And never assume that no news is good news. Follow up to be sure that your test results have been received and reviewed and that you know what they are.

STEP 3: **Ask about alternatives.** Many common symptoms—such as fatigue, muscle aches and abdominal pain—are known as nonspecific symptoms. They can be caused by dozens of conditions.

My advice: To help understand your doctor's thinking, ask him/her this question: Could you please explain your differential diagnoses? This is a list of possible diagnoses ranked in order of likelihood. It's a thought process that helps a diagnostician avoid overlooking any likely possibilities. The most serious conditions on the list should be ruled out before settling on a less serious diagnosis, and the doctor should be looking for causes and not just treating symptoms.

What to ask: If there is any question about a diagnosis, patients can help assess the "fit" by asking three important questions: Does this diagnosis match all my symptoms? What else could it be? Could there be more than one thing going on?

STEP 4: **Don't skip the second opinion.** I cannot stress this enough. In the study of cancer patients cited earlier, Johns Hopkins University researchers found that one to two of every 100 who got a second opinion with definitive testing after a tumor biopsy had gotten a wrong diagnosis the first time.

My advice: It's not always possible to get a second opinion—sometimes in medicine you have to move fast. But if you can, a second (or even a third) opinion is smart when symptoms seem severe...if your doctor is recommending surgery...or if you are told that you have a rare or fatal condition. Check first, but usually insurance will pay for a second opinion. Outside of emergencies, most of the time a brief delay in treatment while you get a second opinion will not affect your outcome.

Don't Forget Your Doctor's Words

Charles B. Inlander is a consumer advocate and health-care consultant based in Fogelsville, Pennsylvania. He was the founding president of the nonprofit People's Medical Society, a consumer advocacy organization credited with key improvements in the quality of US health care, and is the author or coauthor of more than 20 consumer-health books.

A friend of mine recently called me about an hour after his doctor had told him that he had prostate cancer and asked if I could help him decide on the best way to proceed. Of course, I was happy to help. But when I asked exactly what his doctor had said, my friend didn't know! All he remembered hearing were two words—"prostate cancer."

Not remembering what your doctor tells you is extremely common—especially if it's a scary diagnosis or a complicated explanation laden with medical terms. In fact, a classic study conducted by researchers at Allegheny College found that 40% to 80% of the information told to patients by health-care providers is forgotten immediately! The greater the amount of information shared, the greater the percentage that was forgotten. *What helps—you can do any or all of the following, depending on your needs...*

- **Get it in writing and in a picture.** It's long been known that we retain information best when we receive it both verbally and visually. Research backs this up. A study found that when patients were given only verbal medical instructions, just 14% of the information was retained compared with 85% when a visual and text were provided. That means you should always ask your doctor to write down—or give you preprinted information—about your diagnosis. You probably already bring your own pad and pen to take notes at your appointment. But that may not be enough. Ask your doctor to also show you a picture or diagram of what is wrong with you—he/she could use an X-ray, a plastic anatomical model or textbook drawing of the problem area. You can take a photo of the visual with your phone.

Also important: Ask your doctor to give you written instructions about follow-up care and/or how to use prescribed medications, even if you expect to get similar information from your pharmacy. Your doctor may suggest taking the drug less frequently at first or have some other reason for adjusting its typical use.

• **Don't go alone.** We all know that it's smart to bring a family member or friend to important medical appointments so you'll have a second set of ears to remember what the doctor has said. You have a right to have someone with you in the examining room to ask questions or seek clarification. When I recently had surgery, I made sure my wife came with me to every pre- and postoperative appointment. She asked questions I had not thought of and described things that happened during my recovery that I had forgotten.

• **Make a recording.** One of the best ways to not forget what your doctor tells you is to make a brief voice and/or video recording of your medical appointment. Your smartphone should have an app that enables it to function as a mini tape recorder. If not, you can download one of these apps from your phone's app store. Either hold the phone or put it on a nearby table. Make sure you know how to record beforehand. You can also use your phone's camera to make a video recording (with sound) of your doctor appointment. If you don't have a smartphone, it's worth purchasing a battery-operated handheld digital recorder. You can get one for less than $50. Whatever method you use, just be sure to ask your doctor if it's OK to record the conversation.

Germy Stethoscopes

Ronald Collman, MD, professor of medicine and microbiology, University of Pennsylvania Perelman School of Medicine, Philadelphia.

In a recent study, all 40 stethoscopes used in a hospital intensive care unit (ICU) were significantly contaminated with bacteria.

Best: Ask your doctor if a stethoscope can be kept by your bedside and used only for you.

Your Doctor Might Not Be Your Advocate

Eva Kahana, PhD, humanities professor, Case Western Reserve University, Cleveland, and coauthor of a study published in *Clinical Interventions in Aging*.

Older adults view doctors as their advocates. This is the old medical model, in which doctors had more personal relationships and continuity with their patients. But the more people age 65 and older trust their doctors, the less likely those patients are to be advocates for their own health concerns—for instance, by requesting referrals to specialists or requesting specific prescriptions. But this can mean that some older adults are receiving poorer health care now, because in current medicine, doctors have less time to spend with patients or get to know them, and patients are increasingly expected to take the initiative regarding their own care.

Get In to See Your Busy Doctor

Charles B. Inlander, a consumer advocate and healthcare consultant based in Fogelsville, Pennsylvania. He was founding president of the nonprofit People's Medical Society, a consumer advocacy organization credited with key improvements in the quality of US health care, and is author or coauthor of more than 20 consumer-health books.

Not too long ago, I was concerned about what I thought was a suspicious lesion on my back, so I called my dermatologist's office for an appointment. The receptionist told me that the earliest available appointment was two months away. Before I hung up, though, I got scheduled for an appointment just two days away! Below, I'll tell you how I did it.

But first, let me explain what's happening all over the country. Over the past few years, more and more patients have been complaining about how long it takes to get appointments with their doctors—even doctors they have been seeing for years. While the problem tends to occur more often with specialists, who are harder to come by than primary care doctors in some locales, the declining number of primary care doctors is creating a backlog for some practices, too. But with the help of the following secrets, you'll greatly increase your chances of getting a medical appointment sooner. *What works best...*

• **Talk to the right person.** The receptionist answering the phone at a medical practice usually has little discretion over scheduling. She'll book you into an opening on the calendar, often weeks or months away. If you need a quicker appointment, ask to speak to the nurse who works with your doctor. That's what I did to get my appointment with the dermatologist so much quicker. Even if you have never been to the practice before, this usually works.

Insider secret: Don't cry wolf. When you talk to the nurse, give a legitimate medical reason (such as a recurrence of a previously treated condition) for the expedited appointment.

• **Do not ask about a "waiting list."** If you can't get through to the nurse, you'll probably assume that you should ask to be put on a waiting list (so you'll be called if there's a cancellation).

Don't do that! Insider secret: Instead of mentioning a waiting list, ask the receptionist if you can be put on the "quick call" list. This is the term that most medical practices use when referring to the list for people who get priority appointments when a cancellation or opening occurs. Asking for the quick call list tells the receptionist that you are something of an insider, which will help you get priority status.

• **Consider an urgent-care center.** If you are having a nonemergency problem (such as flulike symptoms or pain due to a minor injury) but cannot get a timely appointment with your primary care doctor or a specialist, head to your nearest hospital-affiliated or freestanding urgent-care center or even one at your local drugstore or supermarket. These walk-in practices can quickly determine if you need to see a specialist (or need hospital care)...and, if needed, usually can get you a quick appointment with an affiliated specialist (sometimes on the same day). If you're trying to see a specialist for an initial appointment, a call from your primary care doctor may help you get in sooner.

Important: For serious problems, such as chest pains, high fever, breathing difficulties or burns, go to an emergency room!

• **Get a new doctor.** If one of your current doctors regularly makes you wait several weeks or longer for an appointment, don't hesitate to find a new doctor. While he/she may be busy, your time is valuable too, and it's reasonable to expect to be seen within a month for a routine appointment or within a few days for a special need.

Is Doctor Burnout Putting You at Risk?

Tait Shanafelt, MD, chief wellness officer at Stanford Medicine and associate dean at Stanford School of Medicine, California. Dr. Shanafelt, a hematologist/oncologist, is a leading researcher in the field of physician wellness.

Patients aren't the only ones who are stressed these days about our health-care system.

Shocking research: A surprisingly large number (42%) of physicians described themselves as "burned out," according to the *Medscape National Physician Burnout & Depression Report 2018.*

Other research has found that at least half of physicians are experiencing professional burnout.

What's causing all this discontent? The unhappy and stressed-out doctors most often blamed bureaucracy—all the record-keeping and other tasks that take time away from patient care.

Many also cited long hours and lack of respect from administrators, colleagues and even patients. Even more troubling, research shows that when physicians are burned out, their patients suffer, too.

To find out what medical consumers need to know about this increasingly common problem and how to get what they need from their doctors, we spoke with Tait Shanafelt, MD, a leading physician and researcher who has extensively studied physician burnout.

Are some doctors more at risk than others?

Yes. Doctors on the front lines of patient care, including internists, family doctors and emergency physicians, appear to be at the highest risk—perhaps, in part, because they bear such a heavy administrative/clerical burden in coordinating care and communicating via the electronic portal, refilling prescriptions, etc.

Women in medicine are more likely than men to report burnout—perhaps because of their need to juggle more responsibilities at home than their male colleagues. And while burnout can show up as early as medical school, it peaks in the middle-career years.

How does this affect patients?

When physicians are burned out, it may impact their personal relationships first—but patients eventually will be affected as well. Studies have linked physician burnout to poorer quality care, reduced safety and reduced patient satisfaction.

Burned-out physicians also report more medical errors. Studies have suggested that when doctors are burned out or dissatisfied, their patients are less likely to follow instructions—perhaps due to a lack of trust and/or a lack of compassion demonstrated by the physician.

Patients treated by burned-out doctors even recover from surgery more slowly than the patients of more engaged doctors, though the reasons for this are not fully understood.

Burned-out physicians also are more likely to cut back and work part-time…or even retire early—decisions that can contribute not only to physician shortages in some communities but also to a lack of continuity in patient care.

What might a burned-out physician look like in the eyes of a patient?

Most patients will not notice anything—at least not at first. That's because most physicians want to serve their patients and will try to hold things together professionally, even when they are struggling on the inside.

Eventually, however, some physicians may become noticeably less patient and empathetic and more distracted. They may come across as callous or cynical. They may be less responsive to questions during doctor appointments, phone calls and electronic messages.

New patients may believe that the doctor has always been that way—and unfortunately, the profession certainly includes some doctors who fit that mold.

But a patient who has a long-standing relationship with a caring and skilled physician may well notice the change. In fact, physicians who start out as the most empathetic and committed caregivers sometimes have the hardest time setting healthy limits around work.

As a result, these often-beloved physicians may have higher risks of eventually burning out because they are more likely to take extra time with patients, which means that they then must update charts after hours or on weekends.

If I think my doctor might be burned out or headed for burnout—and I want to continue the relationship—is there anything I can do?

It's easy to primarily view doctors through the professional lens and forget that they are human, too. They like to hear that their hard work and effort on behalf of their patients are making a difference. So if you feel grateful for your doctor's care, write a note or just say a few words of thanks at the end of your visit.

If you have a close relationship with your doctor and you do notice signs of burnout, it is also OK to say something such as, "I'm worried about you. You seem tired. Are you taking care of yourself?" If you initiate such a conversation, communicate kindness. That kind of concern from a patient could be a wake-up call for a physician who does not realize that his/her work has started to suffer.

What can I do to steer clear of burned-out physicians in the first place?

Look for medical practices, hospitals and other institutions that are well run and adequately staffed.

How can you know if this is the case?

For one thing, if you are having a good experience—in everything from scheduling your appointments to getting your follow-up phone calls returned—there is a good chance that the doctors working there are having good experiences, too. That's because they are backed by a supportive team and an efficient system.

In a well-run medical practice, you should get prompt attention from staff as you check in and go to an exam room. If the doctor does not see you right away, another member of the team should come in to check your vital signs and ask some questions.

When the doctor comes in, he/she may be accompanied by a scribe who will take notes or a nurse who will help you with follow-up instructions—research shows that this extra support in note-taking increases physician satisfaction.

If a practice does not have that level of support staffing, then appointment times should be generous enough for the physician to give you adequate attention and to attend to electronic record-keeping and other logistics.

If you leave a medical appointment feeling rushed and harried, your physician may feel this way, too—and both of you could suffer.

WHAT EXACTLY IS PHYSICIAN BURNOUT?

Burnout, in any profession, has three components—emotional exhaustion, cynicism and a diminishing sense of effectiveness.

Burned-out doctors have...

- **Lost enthusiasm for their work.**
- **Lost their sense of human connection with colleagues and patients.**
- **Have started to feel that nothing they do really matters.** They no longer believe that they can make a difference—even if that's the reason they became doctors in the first place.

Doctor's Gender May Matter

Ashish Jha, MD, MPH, professor of health policy, Harvard T.H. Chan School of Public Health, Boston.

Among more than one million patients age 65 and older who were treated for sepsis, pneumonia or other conditions, those with female internists were 4% less likely to die prematurely and 5% less likely to be readmitted to the hospital within 30 days than those with male doctors.

Possible reason: Previous studies have suggested that women internists may be more likely to have better communication with patients and to follow established recommendations for care.

Video Consultations Help Rural Patients Live Longer

Study titled "Virtual Consultations Through the Veterans Administration SCAN-ECHO Project Improves Survival for Veterans with Liver Disease," led by researchers at University of Michigan, Ann Arbor, was published in *Hepatology*. In the study, researchers reviewed the records for 513 patients with liver disease whose primary care doctors took advantage of videoconferencing with liver specialists and compared them with similar patients who did not consult with a specialist.

Living in the country, far from crowded cities, may be peaceful and quiet. But what if you're sick and need treatment by a specialist who doesn't have an office nearby?

For a person with hepatitis C or some other form of serious liver disease, this question is crucial because these conditions are traditionally treated by liver specialists or specialists in infectious disease. If you live far from the cities where such specialists tend to settle, doctor visits are challenging—especially when you have liver disease, which often requires repeat visits for treatment.

For a University of Michigan gastroenterologist, Grace L. Su, MD, finding a solution was a personal quest. After a patient of hers died because he couldn't make it to a follow-up visit, she was determined to research how technology could solve the problem. She knew that videoconferencing, which connected primary care doctors in remote areas with highly trained specialists in other parts of the country, had been shown to help patients with hepatitis C.

But Dr. Su, who is also chief of gastroenterology at the VA Ann Arbor Healthcare System, wanted to study whether this form of telemedicine would work for patients with other liver diseases, including cirrhosis (scarring of the liver) and other forms of hepatitis.

Study results: Patients with primary care doctors who used videoconferencing were more likely to receive screening for liver cancer and other serious complications of liver disease...and these patients were 46% less likely to die than patients who did not have a specialist visit during the nearly four-year follow-up period.

Bottom line: While this study focused on patients with liver disease, long-distance consultation with other medical specialists is widely available and could also be potentially lifesaving.

How to Tell Your Doctor to Wash His Hands

David J. Shulkin, MD, internist and immediate past president and chief executive officer of Beth Israel Medical Center in New York City. He is professor of medicine at Albert Einstein College of Medicine and editor of the journal *Hospital Physician*.

As the chief executive of a major medical center, I have reviewed dozens of cases in which patients knew something was wrong with their care but were too polite, too uncomfortable or too intimidated to speak up.

Example: One woman didn't say anything when she was called by the wrong name. She just went along—and wound up having extensive tests that were intended for another patient.

No serious harm was done in this case, but others aren't so lucky. I've seen people needlessly suffer severe pain because they didn't want to question their doctor's judgment...or risk a serious infection because they felt that it was rude to tell someone to wash his/her hands.

It's normal to feel intimidated in the authoritarian environment of a doctor's office or a medical center—but it's better to be tough. Studies show that so-called difficult patients, ones who demand the highest level of care, recover more quickly and with fewer complications than those who are passive.

Some common "sticky" situations—and how to respond...

UNWASHED HANDS

You might feel rude telling someone to wash his hands. Do it anyway. Every year, nearly two million infections are spread in hospitals. The Centers for Disease Control and Prevention (CDC) estimates that this number could be reduced by as much as 70% if health-care workers would consistently wash their hands before and after treating each patient.

Reducing infection, particularly from potentially deadly organisms such as methicillin-resistant Staphylococcus aureus (MRSA), is more important than not saying anything because you're embarrassed. *Don't let anyone in the hospital touch you until...*

- **You've seen him wash his hands, either in a sink or with an alcohol-based gel sanitizer.** You can say something like, "I'm sorry, but I'm really afraid of infections. Would you mind washing your hands before we start?"
- **You've seen him wash before he puts on gloves.** The gloves won't protect you if they're contaminated from unwashed hands.
- **He has wiped and sanitized instruments that will touch you, including blood pressure cuffs and stethoscopes.** Hospital staff use alcohol pads or cleaning cloths with disinfectants, such as ammonia, to clean equipment.

STOPPING A PROCEDURE

You are never required to continue a treatment or procedure that's going badly.

Examples: A nurse might fail to properly insert an intravenous (IV) needle after multiple attempts... or a resident might have a hard time doing a spinal tap.

When someone has a needle in your back, it might not feel like the best time to complain, but it's your right to do so...to ask someone else to take over...or even to stop the procedure.

At teaching hospitals, many procedures are done by residents. If a procedure or treatment is taking too long or causing too much pain, ask for a more experienced attending physician to take over. You could say something like, "This seems to be taking too long. I would appreciate having someone with more experience try." If the staff argues—or, worse, ignores you—ask to speak to a nursing supervisor.

Helpful: Ask a friend or family member to be present during procedures. Patients understandably are reluctant to challenge their health-care team. An advocate, however, is more dispassionate and can watch out for your best interests. He/she might say something like, "I think she's had enough. We need to take a break for a moment."

YOU SUSPECT A WRONG DIAGNOSIS

Suppose that you've been having headaches. Your doctor might make the diagnosis of migraines and prescribe a strong prescription drug. That might be the correct decision—but what if later you wonder if the headaches are linked to something in your diet and that the medication might not be necessary?

Don't be silent. The average patient knows more about his symptoms than the doctor. Most doctors welcome additional information, even when that information changes the original hypothesis. In this case, reporting a food sensitivity could be an important part of your treatment because migraines often are linked to dietary factors.

Important: If your doctor seems threatened by your questions or dismisses your ideas out of hand, find another doctor.

ASKING FOR MORE DRUGS

It's common for patients to needlessly suffer postsurgical pain because they don't want to seem like complainers or because they're afraid that their doctors will suspect they're drug abusers, but adequate pain control is critical. Patients who experience little or no pain are more ambulatory, less likely to get pneumonia, have a lower risk for blood clots and leave the hospital, on average, one to two days sooner than those whose pain is managed poorly.

There are no tests that can accurately gauge a patient's pain, so self-reports are critical. Addiction is rare when drugs are used for temporary pain relief—and doctors know this. *What to do…*

- **Never assume that your level of pain is normal.** If you think the pain is intolerable, it needs to be treated. Make sure that your pain is taken seriously.

- **Request a pain assessment.** Pain is considered a vital sign, along with factors such as blood pressure, pulse and temperature. As soon as you notice pain, ask for a formal assessment. You'll probably be asked to rate your pain on a numeric scale, with zero indicating no pain and 10 indicating the worst pain imaginable. Most patients can attain levels of two or below with the right medication.

If you need a higher dose, or more frequent dosing, say so. Your doctor will understand if you say that the pain treatment isn't working. Everyone responds to painkillers differently.

Recommended: Patient-controlled analgesia (PCA). These devices deliver small regular doses of medication, usually intravenously, when you push a button. They now are the preferred method for controlling postsurgical pain.

DOORWAY VISITS

A hospital doctor sometimes will poke his head in your doorway, ask how you're doing and then rush off before you have a chance to discuss concerns.

Doorway visits are always inappropriate. If you're nervous about confronting the doctor directly—or he never sticks around long enough for you to say anything—you might keep a notebook by your bedside. Write down your questions and concerns. Then, when the doctor makes his rounds, hold up the notebook and say something like, "I'm glad you're here. I have just a few issues that I've written down. I'd like to go through them with you."

NEGOTIATING FEES

Don't be embarrassed to discuss financial issues with your doctor or the hospital, particularly if you don't have insurance. Negotiating fees and payment schedules is routine.

Example: Suppose that you have recently lost your job and health insurance. Bring it up the next time you see your doctor. Say something like, "I want to make sure that I get the best care, but I don't have health insurance right now. Cost is important, so I would be grateful if we could discuss it."

Doctors often reduce fees for patients who don't have insurance. They also can reduce costs in other ways, such as prescribing generic rather than brand-name drugs, ordering only essential tests and scheduling telephone follow-ups rather than office visits.

Exception: Health-care fees established by government insurance plans may not be negotiable. It's illegal, for example, for your doctor to waive Medicare copayments or deductibles.

Postmenopausal? What Your Doctor Should Know About Your Pregnancies

George Saade, MD, is a professor and chief of obstetrics and maternal-fetal medicine at the University of Texas Medical Branch in Galveston. He also is the president of the Society for Maternal-Fetal Medicine.

Unless you have been with the same primary care physician since before all of your babies were born, your current doctor may not know about any pregnancy complications you experienced.

Why this could be hazardous to your health: Problems during pregnancy, even if they occurred long ago, provide important clues about your current and future risk for potentially serious disorders—clues your doctor must be aware of in order to offer you optimal care.

Pregnancy complications are equally as important risk factors as whether you smoke or have a family history of chronic health conditions like heart disease or diabetes—it's alarming that many doctors neglect to ask patients about their pregnancy history.

Pregnancy complications of concern include…

- **Gestational hypertension** (high blood pressure that develops during pregnancy) or preeclampsia (high blood pressure and excess protein in the urine after the twentieth week of pregnancy).
- **Gestational diabetes** (diabetes that develops during pregnancy).
- **Delivering a baby with a low birth weight** (below five pounds, eight ounces).
- **Delivering a premature baby** (before 37 weeks' gestation).
- **Stillbirth.**

A history of such complications may increase your risk for…

- **Cardiovascular problems.** A recent study in *Obstetrics & Gynecology* looked at 15,065 Norwegian women who gave birth to their first child between 1967 and 1995, examining various aspects of their health an average of 16.5 years after their pregnancies. Compared with participants who had normal blood pressure during pregnancy, those who had had hypertension while pregnant had higher blood pressure and unfavorable levels of total cholesterol, LDL "bad" cholesterol and triglycerides (a type of blood fat). These factors increase a person's risk for heart attack and stroke.

That's not all. Other studies found that women with a history of preeclampsia had approximately double the risk for coronary heart disease, stroke and blood clots…that women who had delivered a preterm infant had nearly triple the risk for cardiovascular disease…and that women who delivered a low-birth-weight baby had seven to 11 times the usual risk of dying from cardiovascular causes.

- **Diabetes.** Even if their blood glucose levels return to normal in the postpartum period, women who had gestational diabetes are at significantly increased risk for developing type 2 diabetes later in life. Women with a history of preterm delivery also are more likely to develop diabetes later on. And according to a Danish study, women who had had blood pressure problems during pregnancy had a more than threefold increased risk for subsequent diabetes.
- **Kidney disease.** Studies link preeclampsia, preterm delivery and/or having a low-birth-weight baby with later development of kidney problems. Also, Israeli researchers found that women who had delivered stillborn babies had a 4.7-fold increased risk of dying from kidney-related causes.

Though researchers don't yet fully understand why pregnancy complications increase certain health risks later in life, it is likely that pregnancy unmasks a predisposition to these chronic diseases or conditions. If you are already predisposed to hypertension, for example, it may first show up when you're pregnant because of the additional demands that pregnancy puts on your body.

To protect yourself...

• **Describe any pregnancy complications to your primary care doctor in as much detail as you can recall...** if possible, get a copy of your medical records from your obstetrician. If you experienced problems during more than one pregnancy, emphasize that fact—studies show that repeated pregnancy complications put you at even greater risk.

• **With your doctor, discuss getting extra screening tests for cardiovascular, metabolic and kidney disorders, as appropriate.**

• **Prevention is the best medicine**—so it is especially important that you commit to a healthy lifestyle. Eating nutritious foods, exercising regularly, controlling your weight and not smoking can go a long way toward offsetting the future health risks that accompanied the pregnancy complications of your past.

Is That Medical Test Really Necessary?

Dennis Gottfried, MD, an associate professor of medicine at University of Connecticut School of Medicine, Farmington, and a general internist with a private practice in Torrington, Connecticut. He is author of *Too Much Medicine: A Doctor's Prescription for Better and More Affordable Health Care.*

Getting all the health screening tests possible sounds like a great idea. After all, frequent screening tests help detect diseases early and help you live longer, right? *Not always...*

DO YOU NEED THAT TEST?

People who are sick obviously need medical attention and appropriate tests. So do those at high risk for certain diseases. If you have a family history of melanoma, for example, I believe an annual skin check is wise. But many tests administered to millions of healthy people every year have no clear benefits. So why, then, do doctors order unnecessary tests? According to a 2014 physician survey, more than half admitted that they do it to protect themselves from malpractice lawsuits...36% said they recommend these tests "just to be safe"...and 28% said they do it because patients insist.

My advice: Before getting any medical test, ask your doctor why he/she is recommending it and what he will do with the information. Will the test reveal a problem that needs to be fixed? Is it likely that you will live longer if your doctor confirms a tiny thyroid nodule? If the answer is no, the test might be unnecessary—and needlessly risky.

Common tests you may not need...

LATE-LIFE COLONOSCOPY

Most people are advised to have a colonoscopy every 10 years, starting at age 50. The benefits seem obvious. Colonoscopy allows doctors to detect early-stage cancers and remove precancerous growths. Overall, the test has reduced the risk for death from colorectal cancer by about 40%.

Exception: For those who are age 75 or older, the risks of colonoscopies usually outweigh their benefits. A Harvard study looked at data from more than 1.3 million Medicare patients between the ages of 70 and 79. The researchers found that while colonoscopy slightly reduced cancer death rates in those who were under age 75, the test made little to no difference in those who were older.

Why: Between 30% and 50% of Americans will eventually develop polyps in the colon, but the vast majority of polyps will never turn into cancer. This is particularly true in the elderly because cancers take a long time to develop. Someone who's age 75 or older probably won't live long enough for the polyps to become cancerous.

Routine colonoscopies are generally safe but not totally risk-free. Bleeding and perforations can occur, and in rare cases, there have been deaths as a result of complications of colonoscopy. Plus, the test is expensive, and the "bowel prep" can be very unpleasant.

My advice: Get a colonoscopy every 10 years starting at age 50 (or as directed by your doctor), but if nothing serious is ever found, you can skip the test after age 75.

SKIN EXAMS

Millions of Americans ask their dermatologists to perform an annual head-to-toe skin exam. The early detection and removal of melanoma skin cancers is critical. More than 80,000 cases are diagnosed annually, and almost 10,000 people will die from melanoma. But only about 1% of all skin cancers are melanomas. The vast majority of skin cancers are basal and squamous cell carcinomas, which are slow-growing and present little health risk.

The US Preventive Services Task Force (USPSTF), an independent group of national experts that makes evidence-based recommendations about tests and other medical services, concludes that the evidence is insufficient to recommend for or against annual dermatological screening for melanomas. According to the group, the downsides of screening include overdiagnosis (the detection of diseases that are unlikely to ever be a threat) and the possibility of disfigurement caused by needless biopsies. There is also the expense of procedures and visits to the dermatologist. The USPSTF consciously did not address screening for basal and squamous cell carcinomas because of their relative medical insignificance.

My advice: An annual skin screening by a dermatologist doesn't make sense for everyone—particularly individuals who don't have a personal or family history of melanoma or those who are not severely immune impaired, such as people who have HIV. However, do be sure to see a dermatologist if you notice a mole, growth or "spot" that meets the ABCDE criteria—Asymmetrical...Border irregularity...Color that is not uniform (often with shades of black, brown or tan)...Diameter greater than 6 mm (which is about the size of a pencil eraser)...and Evolving size, shape or color, or new symptoms such as bleeding or itching. These are the changes that are most likely to signal melanoma.

PROSTATE-SPECIFIC ANTIGEN (PSA) TEST

Before this blood test was developed, about 70,000 men in the US were diagnosed with prostate cancer every year. With the advent of PSA testing in the 1990s, that number has increased to about 161,000 per year, and at the same time, the number of men dying from prostate cancer has decreased slightly. Is this due to early diagnosis using PSA testing? Many experts believe that the decline in prostate cancer death is from improved treatment of advanced prostate cancer, not early detection.

The vast majority of cancers that are discovered by routine PSA tests are indolent, meaning that they grow so slowly that they're unlikely to ever threaten a man's health. In fact, prostate cancer is typical in aging men. By age 80, about 60% of men have cancer in the prostate gland, but most never know it and go on to die from something else. Finding these cancers early is of no value and even may cause harm.

PSA test findings can lead to treatments that are not risk-free. For example, men who have elevated PSA levels will often be advised to undergo biopsies, which carry risks, such as bleeding and infection. Others will have radiation therapy, which can cause fatigue and frequent urination...or surgery, which can cause incontinence, impotence and, in rare cases, death. Plus many men will have to live with the scary knowledge that they have cancer, even though most of the cancers pose no risk at all.

The USPSTF recommends that men ages 55 to 69 discuss the benefits and harms of PSA screening with their doctors in order to make the best decisions for themselves based on their values and preferences. But for men age 70 and older, the group has concluded that the risks of routine testing outweigh the likely benefit and that PSA testing should not be done.

The USPSTF does not address PSA screening in men under age 55, but the American Cancer Society recommends that men at average risk for prostate cancer discuss screening with their doctors beginning at age 50 and that men at high risk consider screening at age 45. The American Urological Association recommends that men discuss PSA screening with their doctors before age 55 if they are at high risk for prostate cancer...between the ages of 55 and 69 if they are at average risk...and at age 70 or older if they have a greater than 10-year life expectancy.

Bottom line: Men should be sure to discuss the pros and cons of PSA testing with their doctors.

THYROID SCREENING

Ultrasound technology has made it easier to find and evaluate growths in the thyroid gland. As a result, there has been a threefold increase in the diagnosis of thyroid cancers, but there hasn't been any change in the thyroid cancer death rate.

A study from the Department of Veterans Affairs Medical Center and Dartmouth Geisel School of Medicine concluded that the apparent increase in thyroid cancer was mainly due to improved detection. About 87% of the cancers measured were just 2 cm or smaller and were unlikely to ever pose a threat. Yet patients were treated surgically with the risk for bleeding, vocal cord paralysis and disfigurement. They also had to deal with the psychological trauma of being told they had cancer. Radiation is also standard treatment for thyroid cancer and can cause side effects. Additionally, radiation exposure presents a cumulative lifetime risk of developing cancer.

My advice: Don't get routinely screened for thyroid cancer. However, if you have a neck mass or lump...you notice changes in your voice...or have a family history of medullary thyroid cancer, an ultrasound of your thyroid may be advised.

Remember: At the proper age and appropriate intervals, screening tests, such as colonoscopy, mammograms and Pap smears, are necessary. Also be sure to get a cholesterol test every five years and blood pressure checks annually...and regular dental and eye exams.

Thyroid Treatment Risk

Jeffrey L. Anderson, MD, distinguished clinical and research physician, Intermountain Medical Center Heart Institute, Murray, Utah.

Overtreating thyroid disease may raise stroke risk. Among 170,000 people tested for blood levels of the hormone free thyroxine (FT4)—low levels indicate an underactive thyroid—those with the highest levels, but within what is still considered the normal range, had a 40% greater risk of developing atrial fibrillation (AFib) than those with the lowest levels. AFib, a common heart-rhythm disorder, increases risk for stroke.

When to Think Twice About Medical Advice

H. Gilbert Welch, MD, MPH, an internist at White River Junction VA Medical Center, Vermont, and a professor of medicine at The Dartmouth Institute for Health Policy & Clinical Practice, where he specializes in the effects of medical testing. He is author of *Less Medicine, More Health: 7 Assumptions That Drive Too Much Medical Care.*

It's natural to assume that more health care is better than less—that checkups, tests and treatments make people healthier. But that isn't always the case.

Obviously, people who are sick need to see doctors and get the necessary tests. Those who are healthy may benefit from preventive medicine. But many of the assumed benefits of medicine don't always pan out.

Here are four common but false assumptions about medical care...

FALSE: **It never hurts to get more information.** It would seem that getting as much medical information as possible would be a good thing. Not necessarily.

Example: A colleague's father was 85 years old and in good health when his doctor noticed an abdominal bulge during a checkup. He ordered an ultrasound, which showed that the bulge wasn't a problem—but the test did reveal a possible problem with the pancreas. To check it out, the doctor ordered a CT scan. The pancreas was normal, but the test showed a possible nodule on the liver. A biopsy showed that the liver was healthy, but the biopsy caused serious bleeding and other complications, necessitating a week in the hospital.

More data can produce more problems, which require more tests, which can create problems of their own. And all this can cost you real money—yet not improve your health.

More data also can distract your doctor. Minor laboratory abnormalities identified during a routine visit—such as slightly elevated cholesterol or slightly depressed thyroid function—often draw physicians away from the problems you want to talk about.

My advice: Expect more and more opportunities to get tested for a variety of conditions. Know that while all these tests may serve the financial interests of their manufacturers, they may not serve your interests. Before agreeing to any test, ask your doctor what he/she is looking for. Is there a specific problem you are likely to have? Or is it a fishing expedition? Avoid the latter—it's too easy to catch trash fish (meaningless abnormalities). Also, ask your doctor whether more information will change what you should do. If not, don't seek more information.

FALSE: **It's always better to fix the problem.**

All medical treatments are a bit of a gamble. You might improve when a problem is "fixed." Or things could go wrong and you could get worse. It's often better to manage a problem than to bring out the big guns.

Consider coronary artery disease. It's potentially life-threatening, so it needs to be treated. Many doctors recommend balloon angioplasty, a procedure to expand the arterial opening and restore normal blood flow. It can eliminate symptoms almost immediately, but it also carries significant risks to the patient.

With medical management, on the other hand, your doctor will treat the problem with medications and advice for a healthier lifestyle. You'll still have the underlying problem, but you'll learn to live with it.

How do the approaches compare? One large study found that patients with stable angina who had balloon angioplasty were no less likely to die or have a heart attack than those who depended on lower-risk medical management.

My advice: When you're faced with a medical decision—scheduling a test, having surgery, starting medications—tell your doctor that you want to take a stepwise approach. Start with the easiest, safest treatments first. You can always add more aggressive treatments later.

Think about upper-respiratory infections. Sure, you could get pneumonia, and you might eventually need antibiotics. But most people can just wait it out. Don't get tests or treatments unless your doctor convinces you, with good evidence, that you need them.

FALSE: **It's always better to find it sooner.**

The argument for cancer screening seems obvious. If you had cancer, wouldn't you want to know as soon as possible? Screening (looking for disease in large populations) does turn up a lot of cancers. Does this save lives? Less often than you might think.

Take mammography. It's been used for widespread screening for 30 years, yet the number of women who are diagnosed with metastatic breast cancer is about the same now as it was before. For every 1,000 women who get the screenings, at most three (likely closer to less than one) will avoid dying from breast cancer as a result. The numbers are roughly the same for men who are screened for prostate cancer.

The benefits are huge if you happen to be in one of these small groups, but what about the rest? They're faced with the cost and inconvenience of the initial test. Many will be advised to get biopsies or other follow-up tests. Some will have surgery or radiation for cancers that probably would have done nothing.

I'm not saying that screening tests are all bad—just that they aren't all good.

My advice: Ask your doctor if he/she is confident that you, as an individual, will benefit from screening tests.

***FALSE:* Newer treatments are always better.**

There's a saying in medicine, "When you have a new hammer, everything looks like a nail." When doctors discover a new treatment, such as a drug or a particular surgery, they tend to want to use it again and again.

Some new drugs really are superior to old ones—but not that often. Vioxx is a good example. It's an aspirin-like arthritis drug that got a lot of attention because it was somewhat less likely than similar drugs to cause stomach bleeding. But a few years after it was approved by the FDA, it was removed from the market because it was found to increase the risk for heart attack and stroke.

New drugs are tested in relatively small numbers of people. It can take many years before their benefits and risks become fully apparent.

My advice: Unless you have to take a new, breakthrough drug, tell your doctor that you would prefer something tried and true—preferably a drug that's been on the market for seven years or more.

Don't Let Your Doctor Become Your Drug Dealer!

Anna Lembke, MD, a psychiatrist, assistant professor and chief of addiction medicine at Stanford University School of Medicine in California. She is the author of *Drug Dealer, MD: How Doctors Were Duped, Patients Got Hooked, and Why It's So Hard to Stop.*

With all the alarming headlines warning us against the full-blown opioid epidemic that is gripping the US, you'd think that patients and doctors would be on high alert for possible misuse of these drugs. *Yet the problem continues...*

Shocking statistics: More than 91 Americans die every day from an opioid overdose, according to the Centers for Disease Control and Prevention (CDC).

Surprisingly, only 7% of people who misuse or are addicted to these powerful painkillers get them from strangers or dealers—the vast majority are obtained with legitimate prescriptions or from friends or relatives who presumably obtained them from their doctors.

Why do doctors continue to prescribe drugs that are known to cause addiction—and why do so many patients demand drugs that are not effective for long-term pain?

To learn more, we spoke with Anna Lembke, MD, a psychiatrist and addiction specialist who has extensively studied the misuse of prescription drugs.

Which drugs are most likely to cause addiction?

The opioid painkillers—morphine, *hydrocodone*, *oxycodone* (OxyContin, Percocet), *fentanyl* (Sublimaze, Duragesic), etc.—are the main offenders. They're classified by the FDA as Schedule II drugs, meaning they carry a high risk for addiction.

Some stimulant drugs, including *methylphenidate* (Ritalin) and other medications used to treat attention deficit hyperactivity disorder, can also be addictive, particularly when they're used by patients who are also taking opioid painkillers or other mood-altering drugs.

Are prescription medications more addictive than street drugs?

They may not be inherently more addictive (this would depend on the different chemical properties), but they're more readily available—and that's a big part of addiction. In the 1960s, 80% of heroin (an illicit opioid) users started out with heroin. Today, most heroin users begin with prescription opioid painkillers before moving on to heroin.

Opioids are routinely prescribed by pain specialists, surgeons and family doctors. Patients acquire the drugs from emergency rooms, walk-in clinics and online pharmacies. They're everywhere.

Who is most likely to get addicted?

Patients with a previous history of addiction—to alcohol and/or drugs—have the highest risk. Addiction is also common in those with a family history of addiction or a personal history of depression or other psychiatric disorders. Before prescribing opioids, doctors should ask if a patient has any history of addiction or mental illness as well as if there is any family history of addiction. If a doctor does not ask about this (many don't), a patient should be sure to alert his/her doctor regarding these issues.

However, we've also found that patients with no history of addiction/drug use are also at risk. Studies have shown that about 25% of patients who use these drugs for legitimate medical reasons for three months or more will begin to misuse these medications—meaning they take more than prescribed or don't take the medication as prescribed (for example, they binge or hoard medication). This is a first step on the road to addiction.

Why do doctors keep prescribing opioids?

Many believe, mistakenly, that patients who take these drugs for pain—as opposed to using them recreationally—are unlikely to become addicted. There's an old (and flawed) statistic that pain patients have less than a 1% chance of becoming addicted. We now know that this is not true.

Other factors: Doctors want to ease pain... pleasing patients is part of their DNA. Prescribing a powerful painkiller can feel like a better alternative than possibly letting someone suffer.

How do patients get more medication than they need?

Many of them "doctor shop"—they exaggerate their symptoms while collecting prescriptions from many different doctors. Some patients claim to have lost or misplaced their prescriptions before the refill date. Others create so much disruption in doctors' offices—begging for drugs, threatening lawsuits, intimidating the staff, etc.—that they're given prescriptions just to be rid of them.

Note: Some insurance companies are now closely monitoring claims and alerting prescribers about suspicious activity, so some patients pay out of pocket to avoid getting caught.

Don't patients know that they're becoming addicted?

Surprisingly, they don't. Addictive drugs work on the brain's reward pathways. Patients feel so good when they take the drugs that they lose insight into all the negative consequences—lost jobs, damaged relationships, etc.

Who should take these drugs?

Opioids are very effective painkillers. Anyone who's suffered a severe, acute injury—a broken leg, for example—will clearly benefit in the short term. Those who have had major surgery almost always need them. They're also a good choice for those with acute pain related to cancer, such as metastatic cancer lesions on the bone. And opioids are an essential tool in the last few hours of life to help ease the passage to death.

But for chronic pain, opioids should be the very last choice. Nonmedication alternatives, such as psychotherapy, physical therapy, acupuncture, massage, meditation, etc., should be tried first, followed by nonopioid medications, such as *ibuprofen* (Motrin) or *acetaminophen* (Tylenol). These approaches can also be tried in combination.

For people who don't respond to the approaches above, opioids may be required, but doctors need to proceed with caution. I advise intermittent dosing—say, using the drugs three days a week, without using them in between. This will still reduce pain but with less risk for addiction. Patients don't take the drug regularly enough to build up a tolerance and dependence, so they shouldn't have withdrawal symptoms.

Can anything else be done to help?

Doctors who prescribe these drugs should take advantage of prescription drug monitoring programs. These state-by-state databases (available in every state except Missouri) allow doctors to see every prescription (for opioids and other scheduled drugs) that a patient has received within a certain time. They'll know how many prescriptions a patient has received...how many doctors they're getting them from...the doses they're taking, etc. This information goes into the database when a patient picks up the prescription at the pharmacy.

Are Your Medications Making Your Life Worse?

Barbara Farrell, PharmD, assistant professor in the department of family medicine and an adjunct assistant professor in the School of Pharmacy, both at University of Waterloo, Canada. She was named Pharmacist of the Year by the Canadian Pharmacist Association in 2011 and is cofounder of the Canadian Deprescribing Network. Follow her research team on Twitter (@deprescribing). Deprescribing.org

It happens for the best of reasons. Your cardiologist, say, prescribes one medication, then you see your endocrinologist and get another, and your rheumatologist gives you another—and the doctors don't talk to one another. Each is trying to help you—but collectively, they could be hurting you...possibly badly.

Polypharmacy—taking a combination of medications that does more harm than good—is a national epidemic, and it's getting worse. The truth is, our medical system is a lot better at prescribing medications than at stopping ones that are no longer needed—deprescribing. Yet doing so, carefully and under medical supervision, reduces the adverse side effects and often improves health. Would it help you to deprescribe?

A SNEAKY MULTIPLICATION

Polypharmacy can happen before you know it.

Case in point: Many medications, regardless of the conditions they're prescribed for, can have depression as a side effect. They include certain blood pressure drugs...heart drugs...drugs for heartburn (proton pump inhibitors)...even painkillers. The more of these drugs you take, the higher your statistical risk of developing depression.

Polypharmacy also is associated with a host of other adverse effects including an increased risk for falls and cognitive impairment that can lead to emergency room visits and hospitalization. The problem often gets worse as you get older—you're not only likely to need more medications, but your body's ability to process those medications declines. A drug or dosage that was appropriate when initially prescribed might no longer be safe or appropriate. However, polypharmacy can happen at any age.

A "MIRACULOUS" RECOVERY

You now understand polypharmacy. *For an idea of how deprescribing can work, consider this case study...*

The woman sat slumped over in her chair—and then slid out onto the floor when she tried to stand. She had been diagnosed with dementia and was on the waiting list for a long-term-care facility, where she seemed likely to live out her remaining days. Instead, 10 weeks later, she was walking and living an active life. Her long-term-care stay had been canceled—her doctors realized that she did not even have dementia!

What changed? A medical team reviewed this woman's case and discovered that she was taking 32 prescription medications each day—and together, the medications that had been prescribed to help this woman instead were ruining her life. The review team gradually eliminated 15 of those drugs and reduced the dosages of several others.

For most, polypharmacy's effects are subtler. And to determine whether it's happening to you, you probably will need to press your doctor or doctors. Most physicians are far more likely to write prescriptions than to review and eliminate them. That's slowly changing, but for now it's up to you to take the lead. *Here's how...*

- **Make a medications list.** It's a good idea to put all your prescription drugs, over-the-counter medications, vitamins and other supplements in a bag and bring them to your doctor and ask for a review. But also bring a list of each of these, including dosages, to help your doctor review them accurately and quickly. Group drugs together on the list by their purpose—heart drugs, pain drugs, etc.

- **Call your doctor's attention to medications that are likely to be problematic.** *Certain kinds of prescription drugs, if used long term, are particularly likely to cause problems...*

  - Sleeping pills
  - Blood sugar drugs (especially sulfonylurea drugs)
  - Blood pressure drugs (especially if they lead to low-pressure episodes)
  - Narcotic pain drugs
  - Heartburn/GERD drugs (proton pump inhibitors)

•**Ask your doctor—or doctors—to review all your medications.** You might start a conversation this way—"I read an article about the dangers of polypharmacy, and I want to take a serious look at all of the medications I am taking..." For any particular medication, you might ask, "Is this prescription and dosage a problem to take for as long as I've been on it? Is it appropriate for my age? Could I be on a lower dose?" If you see several specialists, have this conversation with each one.

• **If you are prescribed medications after a hospital stay, follow up with your own doctor.** According to a study of elderly patients discharged from 11 Veterans Affairs medical centers, 44% were prescribed one or more unnecessary drugs.

And even if the medications are appropriate for you at discharge, ask your doctor—or the hospital pharmacist—which ones you can stop taking a few weeks or a month later.

AVOID FUTURE UNNECESSARY PRESCRIPTIONS

To reduce your odds of being given unnecessary prescriptions in the first place...

•**If you develop a new health problem, raise the possibility that drugs are causing it.** Ask, "Could this be a side effect of any of the drugs I'm currently taking or the combination of drugs?" It might not be, but you'll ensure that your doctor considers that possibility.

•**Ask the following questions about any new medication**—how long should you take it...how will you know whether it's working...and what side effects should you watch for.

•**Explore lifestyle changes that can reduce the need for certain prescriptions.**

Example: Consider relaxation techniques before resorting to sleeping pills. Jot down your questions before you see your doctor.

•**Talk to your pharmacist.** With any new prescription, raise the question of polypharmacy with your pharmacist. If he/she has a concern that your doctor did not bring up, ask him to call your doctor's office to resolve the situation.

Helpful: Use the same pharmacy for all your prescriptions. That increases the odds that the pharmacist will spot potentially problematic drug interactions even before you ask about them.

•**Be aware of the risks of stopping certain medications too quickly.** Discontinuing certain prescription drugs can cause side effects—and some can be dangerous. This is especially true for certain classes of medications including antidepressants, blood pressure drugs called beta-blockers and sleeping pills. But there are others, too. So don't reduce or stop any drug without guidance from your doctor...and if a doctor does recommend ending a drug, ask whether it needs to be tapered and, if so, ask for detailed instructions on how to do that properly.

Surprisingly Dangerous Medicines

Robert Steven Gold, RPh, hospital pharmacist and affiliate instructor of clinical pharmacy at Purdue University, West Lafayette, Indiana. He is author of *Are Your Meds Making You Sick? A Pharmacist's Guide to Avoiding Dangerous Drug Interactions, Reactions and Side Effects.*

Some medicines are obviously risky. Most people know that codeine and driving don't mix...and that you might bleed too much when taking a blood thinner such as warfarin.

What people don't realize is that every drug, including over-the-counter medications, potentially can cause serious side effects. A study in *The Journal of the American Medical Association* reported that adverse drug reactions were responsible for 700,000 emergency room visits in just one year.

Here, medicines that seem safe but have unexpected risks...

•**Mineral oil**

It's been used for generations for treating constipation. It's inexpensive, effective and available in supermarkets and pharmacies.

The danger: Lipoid pneumonia, a type of lung inflammation caused by inhaling an oil-based substance.

It's common to inhale (aspirate) substances into the lungs. This often happens when we eat or drink. The natural response is to cough—but mineral oil soothes the throat and calms the cough reflex.

Result: Particles of oil stay in the lungs and cause irritation that can lead to pneumonia. The symptoms include a persistent cough or difficulty breathing...and the irritation can increase your risk for a bacterial infection in addition to pneumonia.

To be safe: Don't exceed the recommended dose of one to three tablespoons daily. The more you take, the more you increase your risk for aspirating some of the oil.

Also important: Don't swallow mineral oil when you're lying down—it's more likely to get into the lungs. Consuming mineral oil after you've been drinking alcohol also is risky because alcohol impairs the body's ability to swallow normally.

I advise patients who need a laxative to use newer, safer products, such as Metamucil or Colace.

• **Calcium carbonate antacids** (Rolaids, Tums)

People don't believe me when I tell them that antacids can be risky. Believe it. Up to 10% of patients who frequently use calcium-based antacids to relieve heartburn or increase calcium intake experience side effects.

The danger: High doses of calcium carbonate can lead to hypercalcemia, elevated blood calcium, which can cause heart problems.

Warning signs: Nausea, abdominal and/or lower back pain, increased urination and/or impaired thinking.

To be safe: Follow the dosing instructions on the label, and don't take the tablets for more than two weeks without a doctor's supervision.

Also, ask yourself if you really need an antacid. People who frequently use aspirin or *naproxen* (Aleve), for example, may experience gastrointestinal (GI) irritation that feels like heartburn. *Acetaminophen* (Tylenol) may be less likely to cause GI problems.

Alternative: For relief from heartburn, you occasionally can substitute other, noncalcium types of antacids, such as Maalox or Alka-Seltzer.

• **The diuretic *Furosemide* (Lasix)**

It's among the most frequently prescribed diuretics—"water pills" that remove excess fluid from patients with cardiovascular problems such as hypertension and heart failure.

The danger: Hearing loss. Drugs in this class, known as loop diuretics (others include bumetanide and ethacrynic acid), affect the concentration of potassium and other electrolytes in the inner ear. When given at high doses, usually in intravenous treatment, they're estimated to cause hearing loss in up to 100,000 patients a year.

To be safe: Talk to your doctor if you notice hearing loss in both ears soon after starting the medication. You might need to take a lower dose...or your doctor might switch you to a different medication that doesn't affect hearing.

Hearing usually returns once the dose and/or medication is changed—but the risk for permanent damage increases the longer you take the medication.

• **The diuretic *Spironolactone* (Aldactone)**

This drug is used to reduce edema (fluid retention) in patients with heart, liver or kidney disease. It also can be used to treat hypertension.

The danger: It sometimes causes a dangerous increase in blood potassium, a condition known as hyperkalemia, which can cause an irregular heartbeat that is potentially deadly.

To be safe: Patients who take this drug must undergo frequent testing for blood potassium. When you are first prescribed it, you will need to have an electrolyte panel two to four weeks later... a follow-up test after three months...and regular tests about every six months.

If your potassium is elevated, your doctor might advise you to stop taking the drug. This will allow potassium levels to drop back to normal.

Also helpful: Don't combine this medication with supplements—such as energy drinks or multinutrients—that contain potassium.

• **Metformin** (such as Glucophage) for diabetes.

One of the main drugs for type 2 diabetes, metformin improves the body's sensitivity to insulin and decreases production of glucose (blood sugar) in the liver.

The danger: It can cause lactic acidosis, a rare but potentially deadly complication that occurs when a metabolic by-product, known as lactate, accumulates in the body. Only about five in 100,000 patients who take metformin will develop lactic acidosis, but it's fatal in up to 50% of cases.

To be safe: Know the signs. The onset of lactic acidosis often is subtle and accompanied by symptoms such as fatigue, muscle pain and respiratory distress.

Patients with kidney or liver disease usually are advised not to take metformin—or, if they do take it, to undergo frequent (every three to six months) blood and urine tests.

Also don't combine metformin with *cimetidine* (Tagamet), a medication used for heartburn and ulcers. It can increase the amount of metformin in the body by up to 40%. Other GI-protecting drugs, such as *famotidine* (Pepcid), don't have this effect.

• **Serotonin for depression.**

Millions of Americans take selective serotonin reuptake inhibitors (SSRIs), the most frequently used medications for depression. SSRIs such as *escitalopram* (Lexapro) and *paroxetine* (Paxil) increase brain levels of serotonin, a neurotransmitter that affects mood.

The danger: Some people retain too much serotonin, a condition known as medication-induced serotonin syndrome. It can cause muscle twitches, loss of coordination, agitation, heavy sweating and other symptoms, including shivering or diarrhea. It is fatal in rare cases.

To be safe: Ask your doctor to review all your medications before starting treatment with an SSRI antidepressant. The risk for serotonin syndrome increases when SSRIs are combined with other medications, including dextromethorphan (an ingredient in cough medications), the antibiotics *linezolid* (Zyvox) and *ritonavir* (Norvir), and narcotic painkillers such as codeine.

Important: Don't take the herbal supplement St. John's wort if you're also taking an SSRI. St. John's wort increases serotonin.

Medication Mistakes We All Make—Some Can Be Deadly

Matthew Grissinger, RPh, director of Error Reporting Programs at the Institute for Safe Medication Practices. ConsumerMedSafety.org

Nearly two million Americans are hurt every year by the medication mistakes of others, such as being given the wrong drug or the wrong dose. But this total includes only the errors that are caused by doctors or in hospitals. It doesn't include the mistakes that many of us make on our own, such as forgetting to take a pill or accidentally double dosing.

Thankfully, most of these errors are not fatal, but they can be. *Common mistakes—and how to avoid them…*

MISTAKE: **Taking two different products with the same ingredient.** Suppose that you normally take acetaminophen several times a day to reduce pain from arthritis. Each dose contains 325 milligrams (mg). Then you get a cold. So you take an over-the-counter cold remedy such as NyQuil. Many cold medications contain about 650 mg of acetaminophen per dose.

You could wind up getting 2,500 mg of acetaminophen from several doses of the cold remedy… in addition to the acetaminophen that you're taking for arthritis. You could exceed the maximum safe dose of 4,000 mg a day without even knowing it.

Self-protection: Always read labels. Don't take any medication without knowing what it contains. Many have more than one active ingredient. If a new medication contains an ingredient that you're already taking, ask your doctor or pharmacist if the combined dose is safe.

Also, drugs can have similar actions even if the active ingredients are different. Some antidepressants, for example, lower blood pressure as a side effect. Your pressure could drop too low if you're also taking medication for hypertension. Again, never take any combination of drugs without consulting your doctor first.

MISTAKE: **Assuming two doses are better than one.** Many people think that more is better. For example, if one dose of a painkiller gives some relief, they tell themselves that a double dose will be even more effective.

Not true. For example, you'll get the same relief from 400 mg of ibuprofen (the usual adult dose for mild-to-moderate pain), taken every four to six hours, as you would from one dose of 800 mg—with less risk for side effects.

Most of the common painkillers, such as aspirin and ibuprofen, take time to work. You might not notice much improvement in the first hour or two. After that, the medication gets more effective as it changes your body's chemistry. Be patient.

Self-protection: Take the recommended dose for at least a few days. If your problem still isn't under control, ask your doctor if you should take a higher dose—or if another painkiller might be more effective.

MISTAKE: **Missing a dose.** Everyone forgets to take medication sometimes. It rarely matters, particularly if a drug is used for treating a long-term condition such as hypertension or high cholesterol. Just take your next scheduled dose.

Exception: Medication that you need for an acute problem, such as an infection. If you're taking an antibiotic four times daily and you miss the morning dose, you usually can take a double dose at lunchtime, then return to the normal schedule.

But check with your doctor or pharmacist because doubling up is dangerous with some medications.

Examples: Patients taking Coumadin, a blood thinner, could experience excessive bleeding if they take a double dose. With blood pressure drugs, you could suffer from hypotension, pressure that falls too low.

Self-protection: When you get a new prescription, ask your doctor or pharmacist what to do if you miss a dose. The rules are different depending on the medication.

MISTAKE: **Using a regular spoon to measure medications.** People routinely use kitchen spoons to measure their liquid medications. Don't do it. A study in *Annals of Internal Medicine* found that participants who used kitchen spoons to measure medications wound up taking either too much or too little.

Self-protection: Some liquid or powder medications are packaged with a measuring device, such as a graduated cap. These devices are far more accurate than a kitchen spoon. Or you can buy dosing syringes or other appropriate measuring devices at pharmacies.

MISTAKE: **Unsafe splitting.** In an effort to save money, many patients ask their doctors to prescribe a higher-strength pill, which they split in two to get the correct dose.

This isn't necessarily a bad idea. The cost of a 5-mg dose usually is about the same as you would pay for 10 mg. You'll probably get the right dose if the pill is scored for easy cutting. But if it is not scored for cutting and you cut it anyway, you could get uneven doses.

Self-protection: To split tablets that are hard, very small or have an unusual shape, use a pill splitter, available at pharmacies. They have sharp blades and are designed to hold pills in the correct position when cut.

Never split or separate capsules—and don't split medications that have a time-release mechanism. Breaking the coating could cause the medication to be absorbed too quickly—or even, in some cases, not absorbed at all.

MISTAKE: **Buying or taking the wrong drug.** This happens more often than you might think. Name confusion is among the most common types of drug errors. The US Pharmacopeia, an organization that sets drug standards, estimates that more than 1,400 commonly used medications have names that are so similar that people often confuse them.

Examples: It would be easy to confuse the osteoporosis medication Fosamax with Flomax (used to treat an enlarged prostate gland). Are you supposed to take Lamictal to prevent seizures or Lamisil to treat a fungal infection? Even names that don't sound alike, such as Avandia and Coumadin, may look similar on handwritten prescriptions.

Self-protection: Know the correct name of every drug that you're taking and why you're taking it. Never take pills in a dark room.

Helpful: When your doctor is writing a prescription, ask him/her to jot a note on the prescription saying what the drug is for. If the prescription is for Coumadin, for example, the note might read "to thin the blood." The pharmacist will be less likely to make a mistake. Also, confirm with the pharmacist what the drug is for when you pick up your prescription.

Heartburn Drugs Can Be Dangerous to Your Kidneys

Ziyad Al-Aly, MD, assistant professor of medicine, Washington University School of Medicine, St. Louis.

Long-term use (over two weeks) of proton pump inhibitors (PPIs), such as *omeprazole* (Prilosec) and *esomeprazole* (Nexium), is known to increase risk for acute kidney problems, such as fluid retention and fatigue.

New research: PPIs can cause serious long-term kidney problems (even renal failure) without initially causing symptoms.

If you use a PPI: Follow label directions unless your doctor advises otherwise. If you're using PPIs for longer than 14 days, make sure your doctor is monitoring your kidney function.

How to Choose the Right Hospital for You

Steven Z. Kussin, MD, gastroenterologist and founder of the Shared Decision Center of Central New York. He has taught at Albert Einstein College of Medicine and Columbia College of Physicians and Surgeons, both in New York City. He is author of *Doctor, Your Patient Will See You Now: Gaining the Upper Hand in Your Medical Care*. He appears on WKTV in Utica, New York, as *The Medical Advocate*.

Sooner or later, nearly everyone winds up in a hospital. It might be for testing...an ER visit ...or treatment for serious illness.

If you get hit by a bus, the best hospital is the closest one. Fortunately, most health problems aren't that pressing. It makes sense to choose a hospital with the best record for treating patients with your particular condition.

How can you tell which hospital? It may not be easy. You can't trust the billboards that appear in metropolitan areas. (Hospitals and other healthcare facilities spend billions on advertising every year.) Recommendations from friends and family members generally are based on limited anecdotes and are not authoritative. Even your doctor might not have the best advice. *Here's how to find the right hospital for you...*

DIFFERENCES MATTER

People spend more time shopping for flat-screen TVs than choosing hospitals. They just assume that all hospitals provide more-or-less equal care.

They don't. One study found that heart attack patients who went to higher-quality hospitals had a 1% increase in survival. That is significant in itself, and for patients who need procedures for certain conditions such as some cancers or abdominal aortic aneurysms, the differences are starker. There might be a three- or four-fold difference in survival and complication rates between great and so-so hospitals.

CHOOSE THE BEST

Everyone wants to use a hospital that's close to home. Your local hospital may be superb, but you can't count on it.

To find the best, investigate the following...

- **Web-based lookups.** *There are many resources to choose from including...*
  - Medicare's Hospital Compare (Medicare.gov/hospitalcompare)
  - Why Not the Best (WhyNotTheBest.org)
  - The Leapfrog Group (LeapfrogGroup.org).

These and other websites use publically available data to rate hospitals on various measures of performance—death rates from serious conditions (such as heart failure and pneumonia)...frequency of hospital-acquired infections...patient satisfaction...etc.

On these websites, you plug in your zip code to find hospitals in your area. You then can check to see how well (or poorly) each hospital manages patients with various conditions.

These web-based services are useful even when they don't discuss your particular condition. Some hospitals cultivate a culture of excellence. If they rate highly in one area, they're more likely to do well in others.

• **Hospitals farther away.** When patients are given a choice, they almost always choose the hospital that's closest to home. It might be the best hospital in your area—but a better one might be just a little farther away.

Surgical death rates tend to be higher at small, local hospitals than at regional medical centers. Hospitals that treat large numbers of select patients do better than those that treat fewer. If you're seriously ill and need a risky procedure, you should be willing to drive the extra miles to get the best possible care.

In one interesting study, patients were given a hypothetical scenario. They were asked to imagine that they had pancreatic cancer and needed surgery...and they could choose among different hospitals. All of the patients preferred having surgery locally if the risk of dying was the same as at a regional hospital. But when they were told that the risk of dying was twice as high at a local hospital, 45% still chose to stay close to home!

Don't use a second-rate hospital just because you're reluctant to travel. For routine procedures, it probably doesn't matter—the risks will be negligible wherever you go. But for serious illnesses or higher-risk procedures, a large, regional medical center probably will be the safer choice.

• **Number of patients.** Suppose that you need a back operation or a bypass procedure. Do you want to go to a hospital that does a handful of procedures a year? Or should you choose one that packs them in by the hundreds?

An analysis by *US News & World Report* found that the risk for death for patients with congestive heart failure and chronic obstructive pulmonary disease was 20% higher at facilities that saw the fewest patients.

My advice: Choose a hospital that treats a lot of patients with your particular condition—ask a hospital administrator or patient-care supervisor how many of your procedures are done each year. If you can't get this information, ask the surgeon how many he/she does. One study found that endocrine surgeons who did 100 or more operations a year accounted for 5% of total complications, while those who did three or fewer a year accounted for 32%.

• **Doctor qualifications.** Your doctor's experience is just as important as your hospital's. As mentioned above, doctors who see a lot of patients with similar conditions tend to have better track records. Those who work at top medical centers usually are better than those at smaller facilities—but not always.

ProPublica (a nonprofit investigative news service) looked at data from more than 2.3 million Medicare patients. The analysis revealed that a small number of surgeons accounted for about 25% of all surgical complications. Some had complication rates that were two or three times the national average, and some of them worked at the nation's most prestigious medical centers.

It's difficult to assess a doctor's competence. One thing you can do is ask other doctors, including your own, about a particular doctor's expertise. In addition, you can check out his/her education on the Web. It might sound snobbish, but other things being equal, I'd prefer to see a doctor who went to a great college, medical school and training program rather than lower-tier institutions.

You also can ask a prospective surgeon about his/her success and failure rate and rates of complications. Some surgeons won't discuss these matters. The good ones probably will be proud to do so.

Helpful resource: Healthgrades.com allows you to enter medical conditions and procedures into a search window and then provides the doctors who treat them and their Healthgrades ratings.

• **Patient satisfaction.** Patient satisfaction isn't a perfect proxy for quality, but you might glean some useful information. Check the patient-satisfaction measures on hospital-comparison websites.

How long did it take for nurses to answer calls? Were the doctors warm or brusque? Was the food delicious or dreadful? These might seem like minor considerations, but research has shown that patient satisfaction and good health care often go together.

7 Ways to Make Outpatient Surgery Safer

David Sherer, MD, an anesthesiologist and former physician-director of risk management for a major HMO in the metropolitan Washington, DC, area. He is author, with Maryann Karinch, of *Dr. David Sherer's Hospital Survival Guide* and *The House of Black and White*, a memoir of growing up in a medical family. DrDavidSherer.com

Ever since Joan Rivers died after a routine surgical procedure at an outpatient center in Manhattan, people have been wondering if they're better off having surgery in a hospital.

The reality is that the vast majority of outpatient procedures go off without a hitch. But you can reduce your risk by getting involved before the procedure. *Important steps...*

CHECK YOUR PHYSICAL STATUS

Ask your doctor about your "physical status classification." The American Society of Anesthesiologists uses a numerical scale to assess a patient's surgical risks. Patients with higher physical status (PS) scores (four or five) because of health problems should have procedures done in hospitals because their risk for complications is higher.

Example: A patient who needs a knee replacement also might have poorly controlled diabetes, kidney insufficiency and nerve damage. His/her PS might be rated as four—too high to safely have a major procedure at an outpatient center.

In general, patients with PS scores of one through three—with one being generally healthy and three indicating that they have serious diseases that aren't life-threatening—are good candidates for outpatient procedures.

PICK YOUR SURGEON CAREFULLY

Don't assume that every surgeon in an outpatient center has the same experience—or the same credentials.

Suppose that you're planning to get Botox or Restylane injections. These are not as simple as most people think. For the best results—and the lowest risk for complications—you should have the procedure done by a physician who is board-certified in plastic and reconstructive surgery.

Caution: In many states, many procedures can be done by any physician who has undergone minimal training in these procedures, such as a weekend course or three-day seminar. These doctors might be board-certified in something but not necessarily in the field that concerns you.

Also important: The amount of experience. Studies have clearly shown that doctors who do a lot of procedures have better results, with fewer complications, than those who do them less often.

Example: If I were planning to have LASIK eye surgery, I wouldn't feel comfortable seeing a surgeon who had done the procedure 50 times. I would want someone whose total cases numbered in the hundreds or even thousands.

INSIST ON PAIN CONTROL

Most people assume that their surgeons will do everything possible to minimize postoperative pain. Not true. Some doctors are reluctant to order strong painkillers on an ongoing basis because they worry that the patient will become addicted. Or they mainly use narcotics (opioids, such as codeine and morphine) that dull pain but can cause unpleasant and sometimes dangerous side effects, including impaired breathing, constipation, itching, nausea and vomiting.

Poorly controlled pain is among the most serious postoperative complications. It impairs immunity and increases the risk for infection...slows healing times...and can increase the risk for blood clots when patients hurt too much to move normally.

My advice: Tell your surgeon that you're terrified of pain. Ask what he/she plans to use to relieve your pain—and emphasize that you would like to avoid narcotics if at all possible.

Also, ask about *bupivacaine* (Exparel), a non-narcotic anesthetic that was recently approved by the FDA. The active ingredient is encapsulated in liposomal (fat-based) particles and slowly released over 72 hours. When injected into the surgical area, it relieves pain as effectively as narcotics with fewer side effects.

BEWARE OF SUPPLEMENTS

Tell your doctor about everything that you're taking. Surgeons and anesthesiologists routinely ask patients about medications that they're using. They don't always think to ask about supplements.

This is a dangerous oversight because many supplements—along with garden-variety over-the-counter medications such as aspirin—can interact with the drugs that are used during and after surgery.

Examples: Garlic supplements increase the risk for excessive bleeding, particularly when they're combined with aspirin. The herbs ephedra and kava can interfere with anesthetics.

Patients who are taking natural remedies—including vitamin E, echinacea, ginseng, valerian and St. John's wort—should ask their doctors if they need to quit taking them. You may need to stop two weeks or more before the procedure. Aspirin should be discontinued two to three days before.

PLAN FOR THE WORST

Even routine procedures sometimes go south. Most outpatient surgical centers are equipped with crash carts (used for cardiac emergencies) and other equipment and drugs for handling serious complications—but some don't have these on hand.

Ask the surgeon if a crash cart will be available. *Also ask...*

- **Is there *dantrolene* (Dantrium)?** It can reverse a rare but deadly complication from anesthesia known as malignant hyperthermia. The drug is always stocked in hospitals, but an outpatient center might not have it.

- **Is there *succinylcholine* (Anectine, Quelicin)?** It's a fast-acting paralytic agent that assists doctors in quickly intubating patients who can't breathe—one of the most dangerous complications of anesthesia. It has been reported that Joan Rivers might have lived if this drug had been available.

DON'T PUT UP WITH NAUSEA

It is estimated that 30% of all postsurgical patients will experience nausea, retching or vomiting. These are among the most common surgical complications.

My advice: Tell your anesthesiologist/surgeon if you've suffered from surgery-related nausea in the past. He/she can administer *granisetron* or *ondansetron* (Zofran), which helps prevent nausea in most patients.

GET MOVING

Try to get moving as soon as you can. Surgeons used to recommend lengthy bed rest for postsurgical patients. They now know that it's better to move around as soon as possible to prevent constipation, urinary retention and muscle weakness, among other common complications.

As soon as you're able, get up and walk (with your doctor's permission, of course). If you can't stand right away, at least move in bed. Stretch your legs. Move your arms. Roll over, sit up, etc. Any kind of physical movement increases blood flow and improves recovery times. It also improves the movement of your lungs, which can help prevent postsurgical pneumonia.

When "Simple" Surgeries Turn Deadly

Frank Overdyk, MD, a patient-safety advocate and anesthesiologist in Charleston, South Carolina. Dr. Overdyk is a member of the board of advisors of the Physician-Patient Alliance for Health & Safety, PPAHS.org. He received the 2018 AAMI (Association for the Advancement of Medical Instrumentation) & Becton Dickinson Patient Safety Award.

Some surgeries and procedures are considered "minor" when compared with lengthy, invasive operations such as heart or brain surgery...or a hip or knee replacement.

The so-called simple procedures—performed about 40 million times each year in the US—often take place in ambulatory surgery centers (ASCs), where you're sent home in a few hours. But what happens when simple surgeries go wrong—or even turn deadly?

NOT SO SIMPLE AFTER ALL

Since their introduction in the US in the 1970s, ASCs have been a valuable resource, helping patients avoid hospital-acquired infections and speeding recovery at home in more comfortable surroundings.

However, the risks are real. Deaths resulting from treatment at ASCs are not officially tracked, but according to a recent investigative report published by *USA Today Network* and *Kaiser Health News*, more than 260 ASC patients died from surgical complications (such as internal bleeding and cardiac arrest) over the last five years. *Some key risks—and how to protect yourself...*

- **Cosmetic surgery (such as a face-lift).**

What can go wrong: Particularly during any type of cosmetic surgery, in which a surgeon is operating near the mouth, nose, vocal cords or neck, general anesthesia (the use of a drug to make the patient unresponsive and unconscious) or "deep sedation" (similar to general anesthesia but often does not involve a breathing tube) can interfere with a patient's ability to breathe.

To protect yourself: If your surgeon plans to use deep sedation, ask whether a dedicated sedation provider will be involved (by law, general anesthesia requires an anesthesiologist, nurse-anesthetist and/or anesthesiologist assistant). Or ask whether the surgeon can use local anesthesia or a nerve block instead. With a nerve block, local anesthetic is injected near nerves and specific body parts that will be affected by the surgery. Nerve blocks have different risks from general anesthesia and deep sedation but usually don't impede your ability to breathe or your level of consciousness.

- **Tonsillectomy.** Nearly 300,000 tonsil-removal surgeries are performed each year in adults—often prompted by frequent sore throats. But chronically swollen tonsils also contribute to sleep apnea, which raises risks for serious conditions, such as heart attack and stroke.

What can go wrong: Tonsillectomy involves the airway and blood vessels. Persistent bleeding in the airway after tonsillectomy is an infrequent but serious complication that requires immediate attention and can arise hours after the procedure... long after the ASC closes.

To protect yourself: Ask to be the first case of the day. This is the best time to schedule any procedure—but especially this one. Scheduling early in the day gives the most time for any complication to be addressed on-site.

- **Bunionectomy.**

What can go wrong: Recovery from bunion removal can be very painful, and opioid pain relievers often are prescribed for the immediate post-op period and beyond. This can be dangerous, especially for patients with sleep apnea, obesity or advanced age. In addition to depressed breathing, opioids can trigger a variety of side effects, including nausea/vomiting and urinary dysfunction.

To protect yourself: Before your procedure, discuss the plan for post-op pain management. Ask your doctor how you can limit opioid use by instead relying on alternatives, including nonsteroidal anti-inflammatory drugs (NSAIDs) and the COX-2 inhibitor *celecoxib* (Celebrex). These drugs target enzymes responsible for inflammation and pain without such a high risk for side effects.

- **Endoscopy.**

What can go wrong: With endoscopy, which involves the use of deep sedation, both the doctor performing the procedure and the anesthesia provider are working inside your airway. This means that contents from your stomach could get into your lungs (aspiration).

To protect yourself: Make sure you are a suitable candidate and without an acute illness (see below).

ARE YOU AN ASC CANDIDATE?

If you're elderly and/or have chronic health problems that increase your risk for complications during or after your surgery—such as moderate-to-severe sleep apnea, morbid obesity or chronic obstructive pulmonary disease (COPD), discuss with your primary care doctor and the doctor performing the procedure whether you're a suitable candidate for outpatient surgery at an ASC.

Also, if you have a cold, the flu or a fever, call to notify your outpatient facility—you may be asked to reschedule the procedure to a time when you are well. Similarly, if your blood sugar or blood pressure is high or unstable...or you have shortness of breath from asthma or heart failure, notify the doctor performing the procedure and get advice on the best plan of action.

OTHER SAFEGUARDS YOU NEED

Before undergoing treatment at an ASC, also make sure that...

- **The facility only rarely needs to transfer a patient to a hospital for more advanced care.** The hospital also should be relatively close.
- **There will be electronic monitors and "crash carts" on-site.**
- **A dedicated anesthesiologist, nurse-anesthetist or anesthesiologist assistant will be on hand during the procedure.** This is crucial if you will be receiving general anesthesia or deep sedation. Deep sedation carries greater risks than "conscious sedation," during which the patient is able to respond to verbal prompts and commands.

Note: If you are comfortable with taking oral medication for anxiety and prefer not to take the additional risks associated with deep sedation, ask for conscious sedation, and make sure your consent form indicates this.

- **Your oxygen saturation and exhaled carbon dioxide ("capnography") will be continuously monitored by the dedicated provider mentioned above during all procedures requiring deep sedation or general anesthesia.** Oxygen saturation also should be monitored continuously during recovery from deep sedation or general anesthesia. The recovery area should be staffed by a qualified professional trained in basic and advanced cardio life support.
- **The doctor performing the procedure has board certification** by a board that is a member of the American Board of Medical Specialties, ABMS.org. This credential is highly recommended and offers an added layer of safety.

How to Take Charge in the ER

Steven Z. Kussin, MD, previously a gastroenterologist and founder of The Shared Decision Center in Utica, New York. He has taught at Albert Einstein College of Medicine of Yeshiva University and Columbia University College of Physicians and Surgeons, both in New York City. Dr. Kussin is author of *Doctor, Your Patient Will See You Now: Gaining the Upper Hand in Your Medical Care.*

Emergency rooms are crowded, chaotic and confusing places. Americans now make about 130 million ER visits each year. It's estimated that about half of all hospital admissions now come from ER referrals.

Problem: Patients who are seen in ERs (or "emergency departments") and/or admitted to the hospital may be subjected to disjointed care, medication errors, misdiagnoses and poor outcomes and huge costs.

Solution: To protect yourself or a loved one, it's more important than ever to be both assertive and savvy about managing your own care in the ER and/or hospital.

IN THE ER

People have been known to die in ER waiting rooms. It's not uncommon to wait three hours or longer. But if you're really sick and getting sicker, you need to get attention now. *Here's how...*

- **Go to the head of the line.** ER nurses assess each new arrival (this is called triage), and the sickest or most badly hurt patients see doctors first. When you're asked why you're there, don't waffle or give a long-winded reason. Keep to the point. Say something like "chest pain" or "excruciating headache."
- **Stick to your worst symptoms.** Pain and other symptoms tend to cycle from bad to bearable. Don't downplay discomfort. If your pain was severe two hours earlier, focus on that. This is not the time to be stoic. Get their attention.
- **Go over their heads.** If you're not getting triaged or end up sitting for hours after you're put in an examining room, you (or a family member) should check in every 20 minutes or so with the triage nurse. If this doesn't help, ask to see a caseworker. They're responsible for coordinating medi-

cal care and making sure that patients get what they need—including a nurse's or doctor's attention.

Important: If your condition is worsening, notify the ER staff immediately.

• **Get your test results.** When you leave the ER, get copies of the results of any tests you received. It might take extra time, but it's worth the wait. Even though you'd assume that the ER would forward this to the proper hospital floor if you're admitted (and to your personal doctor), it's safer to have these test results with you. This ensures that hospital physicians have the information they need to treat you.

IN THE HOSPITAL

First make sure you are admitted. If you are a Medicare patient and are admitted "under observation," you are not an in-patient. You may be billed an amount of money that will sicken you more than the reason for the initial visit. There is no appeal. And if you subsequently need nursing home care, you will not receive Medicare coverage for it. Patients can be hospitalized for days undergoing exams, tests and receiving drugs—without officially being admitted to the hospital. This is an expensive mistake. Always insist on admission, and ask for an appear before the fact.

If you are admitted to a hospital for any reason, be sure to bring your relevant medical records and the prescription bottles for any medications you're taking. If you aren't able to do this, send a relative to your primary care physician's office to get copies of your records from at least the last year and to your home to get your pill bottles.

Poor communication causes about 40% of all medication errors—one-quarter of which occur when doctors don't get a complete medical history or fail to review your prior medical records. Fortunately, many hospitals now have electronic medical records, which allow doctors to easily access most records. *What to do...*

• **Get your doctor on board.** Most hospital care is now managed by hospitalists, doctors who are trained in acute and inpatient care. But a hospitalist will not know you.

Why it matters: Your regular doctor knows your health background, which can affect treatment. The hospitalist will not. If you are the patient, you are likely to be very sick and unable to communicate clearly on your own behalf. If this is the case, try to have a family member—one who isn't afraid to speak up—with you at all times.

Important: Find out which hospitalist is assigned to your case, and let your regular doctor know who it is. Ask your doctor if he/she will drop by every other day to check on things...talk to the hospitalist...and review your test results. Also let the hospitalist know the name and phone number of your primary care doctor and insist that they communicate.

• **Wait for test results.** Hospitals discharge patients much more quickly than they used to—sometimes you are on the street even before test results are in. One study found that 40% of lab and x-ray outcomes were still pending when patients left hospitals—and some results could have affected treatment options or even the diagnosis.

My advice: When you check into a hospital, ask to meet with the hospitalist and the discharge planner. Tell them that you'd like to have your entire hospital record—including all test results—on the day you're discharged. If the hospital staff says that only a discharge summary can be made available, ask your primary care doctor to follow up within 48 hours for your full hospital record.

• **See your doctor soon after you leave the hospital.** Don't wait more than two weeks—sooner is better. Research has shown that patients who don't schedule follow-up visits with their doctors are up to 10 times more likely to be readmitted to the hospital within 30 days.

GO TO THE RIGHT ER FOR SEVERE INJURIES

Choosing the right ER before an emergency can greatly improve your quality of care...and could save your life. If you've suffered a severe injury (for example, in a serious car accident or a bad fall) and are able to express your preference regarding the hospital you go to, ask to be taken to a Level I trauma center, or if that's not possible, a Level II trauma center. Both types of ERs are always staffed with surgeons, anesthesiologists and other specialists. To find a trauma center near you, go to FACS.org/trauma/verified.html.

Important: I don't recommend urgent-care centers or nonhospital-affiliated emergency facilities for serious emergencies. Use urgent care only for problems that you already know aren't too serious. An urgent-care center might be an option for familiar symptoms you've had in the past and that have been previously evaluated. A cough, cold, slight fever, bruise or the like are neither new nor worrisome to most of us.

If your symptoms are sudden, new, debilitating to any degree and/or scare you, that's enough to make the ER visit a wise choice. It is not the place for routine care.

The Secrets to Getting the Best Hospital Care

Iris Atkins, RN, works in the radiation oncology department at a large medical center in Chula Vista, California. She has 50 years of experience and has been a nurse supervisor and worked in the hospital's intensive care direct observation unit and cardiology department.

Want to make sure that you get the best care possible during your hospital stay? Get on your nurse's good side.

A recent study from researchers at the University of Pennsylvania in Philadelphia found that if a nurse perceives his or her hospital's care to be "excellent," that is usually correct—a nurse's perception usually matches the hospital's data on patient outcomes and other measures of quality of care. And if a nurse can easily recognize what good care looks like, chances are she knows how patients can get it, too!

We sought out advice from Iris Atkins, RN, a nurse with 50 years of experience who works in the radiation oncology department at a large medical center in Chula Vista, California.

When it comes to interacting with a nurse at a hospital, she revealed a few key tips that patients should remember. They'll help keep your nurse happy, which is bound to help keep you happy and healthy in return!

HOW TO GET ON YOUR NURSE'S GOOD SIDE

First of all, it's worth noting that Atkins herself didn't make any crazy confessions during our conversation. For example, she said that she has never treated any patients rudely or poorly—even ones who were difficult.

Is this true for all healthcare workers? Probably not. Nurses are professionals, sure, but they're also human beings. And when you treat them with respect and ask the right kinds of questions, you're likely to get a greater amount of attention, friendliness and helpfulness in return. *Here's what Atkins advised...*

- **Ask about your nurse's personal life.** This might sound intrusive, but showing that you care about your nurse as a person (not as a servant) can make him or her feel more valued. Plus, you may find that you have something in common—whether it's an overprotective older brother, growing up in a small town, a passion for running or a love for cheesecake—and that will create a bond between you.

- **Make her smile.** Joke about yourself...tell your nurse your favorite one-liner...or even ask a family member or friend to bake a batch of brownies for her. And don't worry about being seen as a kiss-up. Nurses have intense, stressful jobs, so anything that you can do to put her in a good mood might encourage her to come visit your room more often.

- **Be polite.** You'd be surprised to learn how often patients ignore their nurses when nurses enter the room...and then speak in a condescending tone or bark out orders when they do say something. Granted, there's a good chance you aren't feeling well when you are in the hospital—but you can say "hello," "good-bye," "please" and "thank you," right?

- **Speak up—but not too often.** You're familiar with the phrase "the squeaky wheel gets the grease." That definitely applies in a hospital! If there's something that you need, don't expect your nurse to read your mind—ask her about it. Of course, you don't want to buzz her into your room again and again for nonemergency requests, so consolidate these requests—whether for a room-temperature change, a pillow adjustment, a drink or even something larger like a room change—and then tell her that you've saved up requests to save her some trips.

Keep these tips in mind the next time you're in a hospital. Your nurse can be your greatest advocate—and you can help make her exactly that.

The Flu Can Be Missed...and Become Deadly

Leslie Kernisan, MD, MPH, a geriatrician and founder of the aging health podcast and website, BetterHealth WhileAging.net. Study titled "Underdiagnosis of Influenza Virus Infection in Hospitalized Older Adults" by researchers at Vanderbilt University School of Medicine in Nashville, Tennessee, published in *Journal of the American Geriatrics Society.*

Did you know that you can have the flu without having flu symptoms? It's particularly true for people over age 65—and it can be really dangerous. People over 65 are more vulnerable than younger people to flu-related serious illness (such as pneumonia), hospitalization and death.

Here's the shocker: A recent study found that older people going to hospitals with respiratory illnesses—during flu season—were less likely than younger people to be tested for the flu! *Here's what the study found—and how to protect yourself...*

UNDERCOVER OPERATION

Researchers analyzed how often flu tests were ordered for 1,422 patients who were admitted to four Tennessee hospitals during several of the past flu seasons. Many, but not all, had symptoms that can signal the flu, including cough or fever. The researchers looked at the rates of testing for the flu according to doctors' orders. They also independently—and surreptitiously—tested each patient for the flu themselves.

Results: Doctors flu-tested only 28% of patients, and were only about half as likely to order flu testing for patients 65 or older than they were for patients who were younger.

Important finding: More than one-quarter of the older people with confirmed influenza infection in this study did not have classic influenza-like signs such as cough and fever.

Here's why: Older people often don't develop the cardinal signs of infection from the flu—their immune systems do not respond as vigorously as younger people's. For example, they're less likely to develop a fever, which is one of nature's defenses against many viruses and bacteria. Plus, older people may have lower normal temperatures, so the typical definition of fever (above 100.4°F) may not be the right guide.

As a result, in older people with the flu, it might initially seem like a worsening of symptoms of chronic conditions they already have, such as asthma, congestive heart failure or chronic obstructive pulmonary disease (COPD). Or they might just feel fatigued and under the weather. But doctors should know better—especially during flu season—because these patients are actually in grave danger.

WHY PROMPT DIAGNOSIS MATTERS

Knowing that you have the flu is critically important. Even though early symptoms of the flu may appear less worrisome in older people than in younger people, the flu can—and often does—ultimately come roaring forth in these older people and turn very serious very quickly. Research suggests that in people who are "high risk"—and everyone age 65 or older is considered high risk—early use of antiviral medications can significantly reduce the risk for serious complications of the flu, including bronchitis, pneumonia and death.

Important: The 15-minute rapid-flu test often used in doctors' offices and hospitals frequently results in "false negatives," meaning you may have the flu but the test doesn't detect it. So if your rapid test is negative, ask your doctor to also give you a follow-up test, which can take a few hours.

If you've already had the flu shot and you feel ill during flu season, ask to be tested for the flu anyway. It is quite possible to get the flu even though you've been vaccinated.

INSIST ON GETTING TESTED

If you are over 65 and you don't feel well, get tested for the flu even if you do not have a fever or cough. Don't wait to see what happens or until you get much sicker—anti-influenza medication works best the sooner you start it and can help you avoid hospitalization. It's possible that doctors and hospitals may be more attuned to flu testing during a bad-flu year, but if it is not offered, ask to have the test.

More ways to protect yourself...

- **Make sure to get the flu shot.** It's not 100% effective, but it's better than not getting it at all.
- **Ask your doctor about getting vaccinated against pneumococcal disease** to protect you against pneumonia and other illnesses that can make the flu particularly deadly. The onetime-only vaccination series (usually two shots administered one year apart) is recommended for all people age 65 and older.

Beware These Surprising Hospital Dangers

Elizabeth Eckstrom, MD, MPH, professor and chief of geriatrics in the division of general internal medicine & geriatrics at Oregon Health & Science University in Portland. Dr. Eckstrom is coauthor, with Marcy Cottrell Houle, MS, of *The Gift of Caring: Saving Our Parents from the Perils of Modern Healthcare.*

No one loves hospitals. But we need them. If you are over age 70, however, there is a one in three chance that you will leave the hospital in worse overall shape than before you got sick or injured. The phenomenon has become so pervasive that health professionals have dubbed such a problem a "hospitalization-associated disability"—caused not by your illness or injury but by your hospitalization.

But it doesn't have to be that way. *Here are eight secrets that can protect you or a loved one from a downward spiral in the hospital...*

SECRET #1: **Start out strong.** As we age, we lose muscle mass and our hearts and lungs work less efficiently. But we are not helpless. A regular exercise routine—including moves to get your heart pumping, increase strength and improve balance—can help stave off frailty. That will put you in better fighting shape should you ever require hospitalization. So will a nutritious diet. A Mediterranean-style diet, which is rich in fruits, vegetables, nuts, fish and healthy oils, is an ideal choice.

If you know that you are going to have surgery or go into a hospital for some other reason, ask your health-care providers about prehabilitation (also known as "prehab")—an exercise-and-nutrition program designed to prepare you for the rigors ahead. Specific therapies are available that will help reduce your chances of functional decline from surgery, cancer treatments or other health issues. Depending on your insurance plan, therapy and counseling prescribed by your doctors related to prehab may be covered.

SECRET #2: **Document your baseline.** Every older adult should (with assistance, if needed) fill out and routinely update a health history sheet, listing health-care providers, medications, major medical problems and, crucially, details about how independently the person handles "activities of daily living," such as walking, dressing, bathing, housework and navigating the community. This is each individual's "baseline"—and you want to make sure that all the doctors seeing you or your loved one in a crisis know what it is. Otherwise, they might not realize when you have suffered a setback.

SECRET #3: **Stay oriented.** When hospitalized, many otherwise sharp older adults can develop delirium, an acute state of confusion brought on by an acute medical illness, in just a few days. If you have dementia or memory problems, you are even more likely to develop delirium in the hospital. So it's important to do everything you can to keep yourself or a loved one oriented to reality.

Wear your hearing aids and glasses. If the hospital asks to send either of these home for safety, a family member or friend should try to bring these items in for at least several hours per day to ensure that the older adult can participate in conversations, health planning and therapy sessions. Stick to as many daily routines as possible, including getting up to dress, wash up and use the toilet, if possible.

Also: Brush and floss your teeth at least twice a day. This will help you feel more like yourself, and some research suggests that it may even help stave off pneumonia by reducing the amount of oral bacteria that can migrate into the lungs.

SECRET #4: **Mind the meds.** Ask the medical staff about the risks and side effects of any new medications prescribed. Watch out especially for any that are on the American Geriatrics Society's Beers Criteria of drugs that are potentially inappropriate for adults over age 65 (known as the Beers list).* Some of these medications can cause confusion and other side effects that raise the risk for hospital-associated declines.

If you or your loved one is prescribed one of these drugs, ask to speak with the physician and/or pharmacist about safer alternatives or lower doses.

SECRET #5: **Get moving.** Within the first week of being in bed, some older adults lose the ability to walk independently. Unused muscles quickly become stiffer and smaller. Lung function declines.

Anyone who can get out of bed should do it—even if it just means shuffling to a nearby chair or the bathroom a few times a day. And don't depend on flimsy hospital slippers. Walking shoes with good tread and a closed heel are best to prevent falls. Some walking-shoe companies (such as ASICS) make a slip-on walking shoe that is easier to get on and off in the hospital.

If a patient must be in bed, a physical therapist should be called in on day one to prescribe bed exercises and make a plan to get the patient up and moving as soon as possible. Nurses should turn immobile patients in bed every two to four hours to prevent bedsores.

SECRET #6: **Speak up for sleep.** Despite widespread calls for change, some hospitals still disturb sleeping patients—at all hours of the night—to check vital signs and perform other care. If that's happening, ask if it's necessary and if you or your loved one might be left to sleep from 10 pm to 6 am. If there is no medical reason to interrupt your sleep during the night, ask the doctor to write an order to not disturb you between those hours.

Also helpful: Open the window blinds during the day, and turn off the lights at night to keep your sleep-wake cycle on track...and stick to mealtimes and other day and night routines. Earplugs can decrease the inevitable hospital noises.

SECRET #7: **Pay attention to fluids.** Dehydration can lead to delirium, urinary infections and constipation, all of which can be major contributors to hospital-associated declines. So make sure that you or your loved one drinks plenty of water (at least 48 ounces daily).

SECRET #8: **Don't go it alone.** It's always a good idea to have a loved one with you at the hospital to watch out for signs of trouble and communicate with the medical staff. Having someone stay overnight is ideal.

Also: Some hospitals have units, known as Acute Care of the Elderly (ACE) units, staffed by teams of geriatric specialists. Such units have been shown to reduce the risks for functional decline and increase the chances that patients will be discharged back to their homes instead of to nursing homes or other care facilities.

Ask if any hospital near you has an ACE unit. If not, then ask if there's a geriatrician on the hospital staff who could see the patient if needed.

*For a copy of the list, go to AmericanGeriatrics.org and search "Beers Criteria." Then click on "Updated AGS Beers Criteria."

Beware These RX Mistakes

Frank Moriarty, PhD, senior research fellow, HRB Centre for Primary Care Research, Royal College of Surgeons in Ireland, Dublin.

In a review of 38,229 primary care patients age 65 and older, about half were prescribed potentially inappropriate medications, and the percentage was even higher among those who were hospitalized.

Examples of inappropriate prescribing practices: Receiving a higher dose of a current medication...and failure to stop or reduce a drug dosage after hospital discharge.

Self-defense: Carry a list of the medications you are currently taking (with dosages and reasons for use) whenever you see your primary care doctor or are admitted to the hospital—and review any changes with your doctor.

Hiring an In-Home Caregiver —What You Must Know

Jullie Gray, LICSW, CMC, principal of Aging Wisdom, a geriatric-care-management company based in Bellevue, Washington. She is a certified care manager and licensed independent clinical social worker with three decades of experience working with older adults. AgingWisdom.com

The vast majority of Americans would rather remain in their homes than move to an assisted-living facility, according to surveys by AARP. Hiring an in-home caregiver could make it possible to remain at home even after you no longer can live fully independently—but it's a trade-off in challenges compared with a nursing home–type facility. The experience can be pretty horrible, in fact, if you don't take the right steps.

Here's how to select and manage an in-home caregiver...

ASSESSING YOUR NEEDS

As a first step, it is very worthwhile to have a professional geriatric care manager (often called "aging life care expert") assess the senior's needs. For example, does the senior mainly need companionship during the day? Housekeeping? Meals prepared and served? Medication doled out? Does he/she need help with activities of daily living, such as toileting, bathing and dressing? Are there health issues that require trained assistance, such as giving injections to a person with diabetes or assistance with physical therapy exercises? Do you need an aide who can drive—on outings, errands and to doctor appointments...and will you provide a car or will you require the use of the aide's car? (The care manager also can recommend caregiver agencies and/or caregivers.)

This assessment usually takes about two hours at $100 to $150 an hour. Aging Life Care Association (formally National Association of Geriatric Care Managers*) can help you find a care manager in your area (visit AgingLifeCare.org). Or ask local senior centers, Area Agency on Aging offices or the senior's doctor if he/she can recommend agencies or care providers.

HIRE THROUGH AN AGENCY

In-home caregivers can be hired directly or through an agency, but agencies are the safer and simpler option.

Hiring in-home help directly might save you a few dollars an hour, but in general, the savings are significant only for people who hire an undocumented immigrant and/or don't pay the required taxes. Doing either of these things could lead to legal problems for both of you. (If you hire someone directly, that person will be your employee, creating insurance and tax obligations—you are required to pay payroll taxes, obtain the worker's liability insurance and file employer tax forms with the state and federal governments.)

Hiring directly also means that you will have to conduct a background check on this person yourself and find a replacement on short notice if he/she is sick, needs time off, quits or is fired. Hiring an undocumented immigrant also makes it virtually impossible to run a full background check on the caregiver. That's a big risk when you consider that this person essentially will be unsupervised in the senior's home.

A reputable agency should handle all of these issues for you.

When you speak with an agency, ask the following...

- **Are you licensed by the state?** Some, though not all, states require licensing—your local Area Agency on Aging office should know if yours does.
- **Are you a member of the American Association for Homecare?** Belonging to this professional

*Jullie Gray is past-president of this organization.

association suggests a commitment to professionalism (AAHomeCare.org).

Also ask about the process for requesting a new caregiver if the first one assigned doesn't work out or is sick. You should be able to do this relatively quickly and easily.

Make sure the senior meets any potential caregivers during the interview process so that he will be more welcoming when you actually make a hire.

MAKING THE CAREGIVING RELATIONSHIP WORK

• **Be very clear with the caregiver about your expectations.** Explain precisely what you want him/her to do. Are there specific household or personal tasks that should be prioritized? Is social interaction for the senior a priority?

Lack of communication about needs and expectations is a common cause of problems. If you want something done, ask. If you don't like how something is being done, give instructive feedback.

• **Lock up all valuables, or move the valuables to the home of a trusted relative before allowing a caregiver to work in the home.** Secure any checkbooks, credit cards and documents containing Social Security numbers or other personal data, too, and keep a close eye on accounts and credit reports for any signs of identity theft. These measures are important even if you eventually come to know and trust a caregiver.

• **Plan ahead for backup.** It is best to hire multiple caregivers on a rotating schedule—possibly one for weekdays and one for weekends—if your caregiving needs are truly full-time. Even if you hire a live-in, no one can work 24/7. And even if the caregiver tells you that he wants to work every day to make more money, everyone needs days off for vacation, sick days and doctor visits. It will be easiest on your senior, both physically and emotionally, if his care is consistently provided by caregivers he knows and who are adequately trained in his needs.

• **Visit randomly.** Close friends and relatives of the senior should drop in without warning occasionally when the caregiver is working to make sure that he is doing his job and that the senior is happy and safe in his care.

WHAT WILL THIS COST?

Extensive in-home support is expensive. In-home care costs an average of $18 an hour—around $19 if "personal care" such as help bathing, dressing and/or using the bathroom is required. These hourly rates vary by region and can easily reach $25 or more per hour in high cost-of-living areas. Agencies typically have four-hour minimums per day. Round-the-clock live-in assistance averages around $350 a day, nearly three times the price of the typical assisted-living facility. There might be additional one-time costs associated with remaining in the home as well, such as modifying the house to allow wheelchair access, installing an easy-access bathtub and grab bars throughout the home or adding a bedroom for a live-in caregiver.

How to Choose the Right Medical Advocate

Charles B. Inlander, a consumer advocate and health-care consultant based in Fogelsville, Pennsylvania. He was the founding president of the nonprofit People's Medical Society, a consumer advocacy organization credited with key improvements in the quality of US health care, and author or coauthor of more than 20 consumer-health books.

Chances are you have a living will. This document (also known as an advance directive) spells out exactly what you wish to have done—or not done—when end-of-life medical decisions must be made. (*Note*: If you don't have a living will, the website CaringInfo.org has free downloadable advance directives with instructions for each state. You can also go to DoYourOwnWill.com).

But there are many other times when you may be unable or unwilling to make an important medical decision. You may be hospitalized for major surgery, a stroke or some other serious condition, and due to the powerful medications and/or treatments you're receiving, you can easily become confused—or even delusional. Or you may be home but too weak because of a chronic, debilitating condition to be fully aware of your medical options. In these cases, unless you have a spouse or have legally designated another family member or friend as your advocate, medical personnel can (and usually do) make the decisions.

That's why it's so important to choose an advocate while you are still in full control of your faculties. *Points to consider when choosing an advocate...*

- **Look for someone who will doggedly represent you.** It should be a person you know well and trust completely. It may be a family member or a close friend. If possible, the person should live near you so that he/she can be there when needed. Be sure to tell that person the key facts about your health, such as chronic conditions, medication allergies, etc. (It's most helpful to give this information in writing.)

Insider tip: Be sure your advocate understands your philosophy about life. For example, would you want to extend your life for a certain period...even if the quality was significantly limited? Do you have religious beliefs, such as not having blood transfusions, that might be counter to what doctors may advise?

- **Make sure it's legal.** To avoid any confusion when decisions must be made, it's best to make your choice of an advocate legally binding. If you are married, under the law, your spouse automatically becomes your legal health-care advocate, and no paperwork is needed. However, if you do not want your husband or wife as your advocate or your spouse is unable to perform the duties, you can create a legal document known as a Durable Power of Attorney (POA) for Health/Medical Care (different states have slightly different names for this form, such as Medical Power of Attorney) to indicate the person you have selected to have that power.

Note: Most states do not require this to be drawn up by a lawyer, but you should be very specific about what your preferences are in the document itself and have it notarized if the state requires it. There are websites with free power of attorney forms that are tailored to your state's laws. I like PowerOfAttorney.com because it has samples of the various types of power of attorney forms you might consider, such as a separate POA that grants someone else control over your finances. POAs for health care go into effect when a doctor says that you are unable to make your own decisions.

Insider tip: Power of attorney forms do not supersede a living will. Because living wills apply only to end-of-life care, you should have both. Make sure your advocate has a copy of your living will so that he can present both documents in any medical circumstance where they may be needed.

Beware the Hospital-Nursing Home Shuttle

Robert Martensen, MD, PhD, is director of the Office of History at the National Institutes of Health in Bethesda, Maryland. He has cared for thousands of critically ill patients and taught bioethics and medical history at Harvard Medical School in Boston and at Tulane University in New Orleans. He is the author of *A Life Worth Living: A Doctor's Reflections on Illness in a High-Tech Era.*

Many Americans with serious chronic illnesses spend their last months or years being shuttled from a nursing home to the hospital and back to the nursing home—again and again. During each hospital stay, they may be subjected to painful, invasive and expensive procedures that neither ease discomfort nor extend life.

It's a chilling scenario, but all too common—particularly for women. Robert Martensen, MD, PhD, author of *A Life Worth Living: A Doctor's Reflections on Illness in a High-Tech Era*, explained, "Many more older women than men are single because women live longer, on average. If a patient cannot speak for herself regarding her preferences on end-of-life care—and no family member speaks for her—she is at the mercy of the 'default behavior' of medical institutions. Typically, this means that the nursing home automatically sends the patient to the hospital if her health becomes unstable...and that the hospital aggressively treats her until she is stable enough to be discharged back to the nursing home—even if treatment does not increase comfort or restore any physical function that improves quality of life. It goes around and around this way until the patient's body no longer responds to treatment."

Do you have a loved one in, or headed for, a nursing home? Don't let this happen to her. And you don't want this to happen to you.

If the patient can participate in decisions about her own care...

Clarify your (or your loved one's) preferences. Dr. Martensen said, "When a person with serious chronic illnesses starts to lose significant function (recurrent hospitalizations are an indicator of that) or says that she 'doesn't expect to live much longer,' it's time to talk." Discuss how intensively she wants to be treated when it's likely that no aggressive treatments will restore function and comfort.

Help her prepare an advance directive. This legal document, which the patient can revise at any time, outlines her preferences regarding future medical care. A lawyer can handle this...or you can do it yourself by getting advance directive forms from the hospital admissions department or the Internet (do a search for the patient's state plus "advance directive"). Copies should go to the patient's doctor, hospital, nursing home and closest relatives.

State laws vary, but basically there are two types of advance directives—and it's wise to have both. A living will specifies the type of treatment a person wants or does not want under various circumstances. A durable power of attorney for health care appoints a particular person to make health-care decisions in the event that the patient can no longer do so. Dr. Martensen explained, "Since it is hard to predict how a final illness will play out, a living will checklist may not cover all contingencies. For example, administering intravenous antibiotics may make sense in some situations and not in others—so it helps to have someone who can assert the patient's preferences in terms of a specific therapy." [*Editor's note*: While you're at it, it's prudent to prepare an advance directive for yourself, too, especially if you live alone.]

If your loved one cannot speak for herself...

• **Ask questions if aggressive treatments are proposed.** "Advanced interventions, such as mechanical ventilation or artificial nutrition, were designed as bridges from a medical catastrophe to reasonably good health," Dr. Martensen said. "When crossing the bridge is not going to lead to reasonably good health, we must look at what really matters to the patient."

Example: Using a ventilator may make sense if it helps a pneumonia patient recover... but may not make sense as a semipermanent mode of living to a person with advanced chronic lung and heart disease whose lungs will no longer function on their own.

So: Ask the doctor, "What is the goal of the proposed treatment? How will it affect the patient's comfort, function and longevity? How long would treatment be continued?" If the answer is basically "I don't know," you may want to agree to a trial period of a few days or a week and then reevaluate.

• **Request a palliative consultation.** Palliative approaches, including hospice, aim to find a balance between a treatment's potential benefits and its harms (such as pain and being utterly dependent on machines and other people). Once a palliative care plan is in place, your loved one can get off the hospital-nursing home shuttle...and live out her days in greater peace.

Easing the Way Through Debilitating Disease

Diane E. Meier, MD, director, Center to Advance Palliative Care (CAPC.org), director, Lilian and Benjamin Hertzberg Palliative Care Institute, both at Mount Sinai Medical Center, New York City.

No one wants to think about seeing a specialist in palliative care... it sounds like the end of a long, sad road. But actually, palliative care, by definition, is about improving life's quality—and it is not just for the dying. It's about relieving pain and making life better for any patient suffering from a chronic and/or long-term illness by using a variety of tools, including medication, support and other methods to improve comfort and quality of life. Palliative care has been shown to make life worth living—and to prolong it.

If you mistakenly thought palliative care described only end-of-life comfort measures, you're in good company. Many people confuse it with hospice care, which is for patients at the end of their lives who can no longer benefit from curative treatment. This misunderstanding about palliative care is even shared by many doctors. The unhappy result is that people who would benefit from palliative care suffer needlessly.

LIFE GETS BETTER

According to Diane E. Meier, MD, director of the Center to Advance Palliative Care (CAPC.org) and the Lilian and Benjamin Hertzberg Palliative Care Institute at Mount Sinai Medical Center in New York City, palliative care is appropriate from the point of diagnosis with a serious or chronic illness. That includes cancer, heart disease, diabetes, respiratory ailments, kidney failure, Alzheimer's, multiple sclerosis, ALS, etc. Since the goal is to ease suffering and offer the best quality of life for as long as possible—and since a better quality of life helps people live longer—why wait?

There is new research demonstrating that palliative-care programs actually do help people live longer. Published in the *New England Journal of Medicine*, the Massachusetts General Hospital study randomly assigned 151 patients with lung cancer to receive either traditional lung cancer treatment or the same treatment along with palliative care. The patients receiving palliative care lived nearly three months longer than the others, on average. They also had fewer symptoms of depression and a markedly better quality of life.

You may be surprised to learn that this type of care is not available at all hospitals, though dramatic progress has been made. The US now has 1,800 hospitals with palliative-care programs, which means that more than 80% of US patients who are hospitalized for serious illness have access to this service.

Certain types of hospitals are more likely than others to offer such care. In a recent survey, 98% of National Cancer Institute (NCI)-designated cancer centers reported having palliative-care programs, versus 78% of non-NCI cancer centers. Dr. Meier adds that teaching and nonprofit hospitals offer more palliative-care programs than nonteaching and for-profit facilities. In areas where this kind of care is not easily available, some palliative-care programs now extend their reach into the community—for instance, by training visiting nurses to deliver palliative care to patients at home.

DON'T SUFFER IN SILENCE

"Suffering is not noble," Dr. Meier said. "Pain is extremely debilitating, and living with it increases the risk for other illnesses and death." If you experience symptoms such as pain and/or fatigue that do not respond to standard treatment, whether they occur as a result of your illness or as a side effect of treatment, ask your doctor for a referral to a palliative-care team. Who is on such teams varies from hospital to hospital, but generally there is a physician, nurse, nurse practitioner and social worker, all specializing in pain and symptom management and providing practical and psychological support to patients and their family caregivers. Also, depending on availability and your own needs, you may see a psychiatrist or psychologist, physical therapist, occupational therapist, nutritionist, massage therapist or yoga therapist.

Here's what Dr. Meier says you can expect from palliative care...

- **Pain and symptom management.** Since patients are typically first referred for pain relief, appropriate analgesic medications (even morphine derivatives, if that's what it takes) are used to get pain under control. Additional treatments (including medications) are used to relieve other symptoms as needed—physical ones such as nausea, fatigue, constipation, loss of appetite, shortness of breath and difficulty sleeping, as well as psychological symptoms like sadness, depression and anxiety and general stress.

- **Nondrug treatments to relieve pain and discomfort.** Techniques such as massage, acupuncture and music and art therapy may be used to help patients and family members feel better.

- **Support for patients and family.** Palliative-care specialists provide support and information as you sort through complex treatment decisions to arrive at the treatment plan that best fits your personal needs. They also offer counseling to help patients and family members cope with emotional issues.

- **Coordination of transitions.** Palliative-care teams can help patients with the transition from hospital to home by offering practical advice and emotional support...information about where to get part-time or full-time help with nursing or practical chores at home...and someone to call if something goes wrong at 3:00 in the afternoon or 3:00 in the morning.

Most insurance plans cover palliative care that you receive in the hospital. Coverage of home care is spottier, however, so it is important to be sure you understand what your policy will and will not pay for. To find a palliative-care program in your area, visit GetPalliativeCare.org/providers.

And remember, this really is a call you should make sooner, not later.

13

Natural Ways to Live Longer

6 Herbs That Slow Aging

Donald R. Yance, CN, MH, RH (AHG), clinical master herbalist and certified nutritionist. He is author of *Adaptogens in Medical Herbalism* and *Herbal Medicine, Healing & Cancer*. DonnieYance.com

You can't escape aging. But many Americans are aging prematurely. *Surprising fact:* The US ranks 42nd out of 191 countries in life expectancy, according to the Census Bureau and the National Center for Health Statistics.

The leading cause of this rapid, premature aging is chronic stress. Stress is any factor, positive or negative, that requires the body to make a response or change to adapt. It can be psychological stress, including the modern addiction to nonstop stimulation and speed. Or it can be physiological stress—such as eating a highly processed diet…sitting for hours every day…absorbing toxins from food, water and air…and spending time in artificial light.

Chronic stress overwhelms the body's homeostasis, its inborn ability to adapt to stress and stay balanced, strong and healthy. The result?

Your hormonal and immune systems are weakened. Inflammation flares up, damaging cells. Daily energy decreases, fatigue increases, and you can't manage life as effectively. You suffer from one or more illnesses, take several medications and find yourself in a downward spiral of worsening health. Even though you might live to be 75 or older, you're surviving, not thriving.

We can reduce stress by making lifestyle changes such as eating better and exercising. You also can help beat stress and slow aging with adaptogens. These powerful herbs balance and strengthen the hormonal and immune systems…give you more energy…and repair cellular damage—thereby boosting your body's ability to adapt to chronic stress.

Important: Adaptogens are generally safe, but always talk with your doctor before taking any supplement.

Here are six of the most powerful adaptogens (based on Ayurveda and Traditional Chinese medicine)…

- **Ashwagandha.** This adaptogen from Ayurveda (the ancient system of natural healing from India) can help with a wide range of conditions.

Main actions: It is energizing and improves sleep, and it can help with arthritis, anxiety, depression, dementia and respiratory disorders, such as asthma, bronchitis and emphysema.

Important benefit: It is uniquely useful for cancer—it can reduce the toxicity of chemotherapy (and prevent resistance to chemotherapeutic drugs)...relieve cancer-caused fatigue...and possibly prevent recurrence.

• **Eleuthero.** This is the most well-researched adaptogen (with more than 3,000 published studies). It often is called the "king" of adaptogens. (It was introduced in the US as "Siberian ginseng," but it is not a ginseng.)

Main actions: Along with providing energy and vitality, eleuthero protects the body against the ill effects of any kind of stress, such as extremes of heat or cold, excessive exercise and radiation. More than any other adaptogen, it helps normalize any type of physiological abnormality—including high or low blood pressure...and high or low blood sugar.

Important benefit: Eleuthero is a superb "ergogenic" (performance-enhancing) aid that can help anyone involved in sports improve strength and endurance and recover from injury.

• **Ginseng.** Used as a traditional medicine in Asia for more than 5,000 years and the subject of more than 500 scientific papers, ginseng has two primary species—Panax ginseng (Korean or Asian ginseng) and Panax quinquefolius (American ginseng).

Main actions: Ginseng is antifatigue and antiaging. It increases muscle strength and endurance and improves reaction times. It also strengthens the immune system and the heart and helps regulate blood sugar.

Important benefits: American ginseng can be beneficial for recovering from the common cold, pneumonia or bronchitis (particularly with a dry cough)...and chronic stress accompanied by depression or anxiety.

Korean or Asian ginseng is helpful for increasing physical performance, especially endurance and energy. It is effective for restoring adrenal function and neurological health such as learning and memory.

• **Rhaponticum.** This herb contains more anabolic (strengthening and muscle-building) compounds than any other plant. It is my number-one favorite herb for increasing stamina and strength.

Main actions: It normalizes the central nervous and cardiovascular systems...improves sleep, appetite and mood...and increases the ability to work and function under stressful conditions.

Important benefit: This herb is wonderful for anyone recovering from injury, trauma or surgery.

• **Rhodiola.** Rhodiola has gained popularity over the past few years as studies show that it rivals eleuthero and ginseng as an adaptogen. It is widely used by Russian athletes to increase energy.

Main actions: Rhodiola increases blood supply to the muscles and the brain, enhancing physical and mental performance, including memory. It normalizes the cardiovascular system and protects the heart from stress. It also strengthens immunity.

Red flag: Don't use rhodiola alone—it is extremely astringent and drying. It is best used along with other adaptogens in a formula.

• **Schisandra.** This herb has a long history of use as an adaptogen in China, Russia, Japan, Korea and Tibet. The fruit is commonly used, but the seed is more powerful.

Main actions: Schisandra can treat stress-induced fatigue...protect and detoxify the liver... treat insomnia, depression and vision problems... and enhance athletic performance.

Important benefit: This adaptogen may help night vision—one study showed it improved adaptation to darkness by 90%.

COMBINATIONS ARE BEST

Any one herb has limitations in its healing power. But a combination or formula of adaptogenic herbs overcomes those limitations—because the adaptogens act in concert, making them more powerful.

This concept of synergy—multiple herbs acting together are more effective than one herb acting alone—is key to the effectiveness of the herbal formulas of traditional Chinese medicine (TCM) and Ayurveda. Both these ancient forms of medicine often employ a dozen or more herbs in their formulas.

But it's not only the combination of herbs that makes them effective—it's also the quality of the herbs. There are many more poor-quality adaptogens on the market than high-quality (or even mediocre-quality).

My advice: Look for an herbalist or herbal company that knows all about the source and content of the herbs it uses.

Example: Herbalist & Alchemist, a company that grows most of the herbs used in its products.

Or find a product sold to health practitioners, who then sell it to their patients—this type of product is more likely to be high-quality.

Example: MediHerb, from Standard Process.

Herbal formulas from my company, Natura Health Products, also meet these criteria for high quality.

Our Experts Agree: Nearly Everyone Should Take These 5 Vitamins

Hyla Cass, MD, integrative physician in private practice in Los Angeles, natural supplement formulator and consultant, and coauthor of several books including *8 Weeks to Vibrant Health*. CassMD.com

Joshua Levitt, ND, naturopathic physician in private practice in Hamden, Connecticut, a clinical preceptor for Yale School of Medicine and author of *The Honey Phenomenon: How This Liquid Gold Heals Your Ailing Body*. WholeHealthCT.com

Michael Murray, ND, author or coauthor of more than 30 books featuring natural approaches to health, including *The Encyclopedia of Nutritional Supplements* and *Bottom Line's Encyclopedia of Healing Foods*. He is based near Scottsdale, Arizona. DoctorMurray.com

Andrew Rubman, ND, director of Southbury Clinic for Traditional Medicines in Southbury, Connecticut, and author of the blog "Nature Doc's Patient Diary" at BottomLineInc.com. SouthburyClinic.com

Jacob Teitelbaum, MD, holistic fibromyalgia and pain specialist in private practice in Kailua Kona, Hawaii, and coauthor of *Real Cause, Real Cure*. EndFatigue.com

Are there nutritional supplements that everyone should consider taking? We posed that question to five nutrition-savvy doctors who have served as experts for Bottom Line Inc. for years. Surprisingly, they not only all said "yes," but they all generally agreed on what these nutritional supplements are.

That consensus is even more surprising given the negative attention that multivitamin/mineral supplements have gotten lately. Some studies have failed to find that they protect against heart disease, for example. But that's not why most people even take multis—or should, our experts say.

Better reason: To ensure that you are getting adequate amounts of essential nutrients to function at your best day to day.

Many Americans don't get enough. According to the latest Dietary Guidelines report, common nutritional shortfalls include the B vitamin folate, vitamin D and magnesium. And deficiencies become more common for certain nutrients after age 50, when nutrient absorption often declines.

Important: Our experts agreed that in addition to the specific recommendations below, everyone should take a multivitamin/mineral supplement that supplies 100% of the Recommended Daily Intake (RDI) for most vitamins, minerals and trace elements (especially selenium, chromium and iodine).

Exception: Iron deficiency is rare in people over age 50, so iron should be part of your multi only if a doctor-ordered test shows that you are iron-deficient. Why? Too much acts as an unhealthy oxidant.

A healthy diet always comes first, our experts agree.

Example: Fruits, vegetables and beans provide fiber and potassium that supplements generally don't provide.

Does everyone need all these supplements? No. If you eat fatty seafood at least twice a week, for example, you could safely skip omega-3 supplements. But most of us would benefit from taking all of these supplements.

What follows are the amounts that our experts agree are safe and beneficial for everyone. They often prescribe higher amounts for certain patients.

Important: Share your supplementation plan with your health-care provider, who can offer individual guidance.

A good multi is just the beginning, our experts told us. *Here are four additional daily supplements that benefit nearly everyone…*

- **Magnesium.** Magnesium strengthens muscles, builds bone, energizes the brain, regulates the heart, reduces high blood pressure, balances blood sugar, aids sleep, eases pain, improves digestion, helps your body utilize calcium and more. Before processed food dominated the diet, Americans consumed 600 milligrams (mg) of magnesium a day on average. Today, that number is about 275 mg—well below the RDI of 420 mg for men and 320 mg for women.

Recommended daily dose: Our experts most often prescribe 200 mg twice a day—once in the morning, once in the evening—for a daily total of 400 mg.

Avoid: Magnesium oxide, which can sometimes cause loose stools.

Best: Magnesium glycinate.

• **B vitamins.** B vitamins play important roles in the health of your brain and nerves, blood, digestive tract, muscles, skin and eyes. They help power every cell in the body. Our experts put a special emphasis on folate, B-6 and B-12.

Recommended daily dose: Take a "B-50-complex" supplement either once a day or in divided doses twice a day. This formulation, sold under a number of different brands, includes all the Bs. The name refers to the fact that the daily dosage is 50 mg or 50 micrograms (mcg) for many of the Bs. Those levels exceed the RDI in most cases but are safe to take daily.

Additional recommendation: If you are a vegetarian or a vegan or are over age 50, also take a separate B-12 supplement. While a B-50-complex supplement will have a small amount of B-12 (typically 50 mcg), taking an additional B-12 supplement is important because B-12 deficiency is particularly common as we age, in part because we produce less of the stomach acid needed to absorb it from food.

Tip: Look for a sublingual (under-the-tongue) product providing the most active form—methylcobalamin—at a daily dose of 1,000 mcg.

• **Vitamin D.** Vitamin-D deficiency is disturbingly common in the US. Indeed, most Americans have blood levels below a minimally healthy level of 30 nanograms per milliliter (ng/mL). Our experts agreed that blood levels above 50 ng/mL (but not higher than 80 ng/mL) are best for peak functioning of muscles, bones, digestion, immunity, hormones and circulation. Vitamin D also may help prevent breast and colon cancers.

Recommended daily dose: 2,000 international units (IU) of D-3, the form that's best absorbed. That supports a blood level of 50 ng/mL for most people and is safe to take daily long-term.

Important: Get your vitamin-D level tested. If it's very low, your doctor may prescribe higher doses, up to 10,000 IU daily.

• **Fish oil.** Fatty fish such as salmon and sardines are rich in the omega-3 fatty acids EPA (eicosapentaenoic acid) and DHA (docosahexaenoic acid). If you don't eat fatty fish at least twice a week, consider a daily omega-3 supplement.

It's true that recent studies have failed to find that these supplements prevent heart disease in healthy people. But omega-3s are key nutrients for every cell in the body, and most Americans don't get enough. And there is evidence that they are key to lifelong health.

Example: In a study from Harvard Medical School and several other leading institutions, researchers looked at 15 years of health data on more than 6,500 postmenopausal women and found that those with the highest levels of EPA and DHA were 11% less likely to die from any cause during the study than those with the lowest levels. Another recent study conducted at Tufts University on men and women found that higher blood levels of omega-3s were linked to healthier aging.

Reason: Omega-3 fatty acids make all cell membranes more flexible and youthful—and every part of the body benefits. They can ease arthritis, improve mood and ward off depression, protect against dementia, reduce high triglycerides (blood fats) and even slow skin aging.

Recommended daily dose: A supplement that supplies 1,000 mg of EPA and DHA combined. Higher doses may be prescribed to reduce high triglycerides.

Caution: Omega-3 supplements act as anticoagulants, so talk to your doctor before taking one if you already are taking a prescription anticoagulant.

Omega-3s for Longer Life

Study of 2,692 people, average age 74, by researchers at Harvard School of Public Health, Boston, published in *Annals of Internal Medicine.*

In a recent finding, people over age 65 with the highest blood levels of omega-3 fatty acids were 27% less likely to die of any cause during the study period...40% less likely to die of coronary heart disease...and 45% less likely to die of an arrhythmia than people with the lowest levels of omega-3s. Overall, those with the highest omega-3 levels lived an average of 2.2 years longer than those with the lowest levels.

How to Choose the Perfect Omega-3 Supplement

C. Leigh Broadhurst, PhD, a physical chemist with a major government agricultural research laboratory in Beltsville, Maryland. Dr. Broadhurst has conducted peer-reviewed research on omega-3 fatty acids for nearly 20 years.

Millions of Americans now pop omega-3 supplements as routinely as they shower and brush their teeth. And with good reason. Omega-3s help fight everything from arthritis and depression to macular degeneration and high triglycerides.

But with so many of these supplements on the market, how do you know which is best for you? For answers, *Bottom Line/Health* turned to C. Leigh Broadhurst, PhD, a chemist and leading expert on omega-3 supplements.*

DO YOU NEED MORE?

Omega-3s are essential fatty acids. As such, these nutrients cannot be manufactured by the body, so they need to be obtained from foods or supplements.

As with most nutrients, it's preferable to get your omega-3s from food, which also provides a slew of beneficial vitamins and minerals. For example, the richest omega-3 food sources, including oily fish such as salmon, sardines and trout, are also high in immune-supporting vitamin D and selenium.

What you may not know: Getting enough omega-3s from one's diet is tough. In fact, the US Dietary Guidelines Advisory Committee has estimated that about 70% of Americans are deficient in this crucial nutrient.

Unless your daily diet includes marine sources of omega-3s, such as oily fish, you should consider taking omega-3 supplements. Walnuts, flaxseed and other plant sources have the omega-3 alpha-linolenic acid, which the body does not convert very efficiently to *eicosapentaenoic acid* (EPA) and *docosahexaenoic acid* (DHA)—the two main types of omega-3s. Therefore, plant foods don't provide nearly as much of these crucial omega-3s as do the fish listed earlier.

WHICH IS RIGHT FOR YOU?

Several omega-3 sources are available in supplement form, including fish oil, krill oil and algae (see descriptions of each below). To ensure that you're getting an adequate dose of EPA and DHA, look for an omega-3 supplement that is labeled "concentrated."

My advice: Take two 1,000-mg capsules of fish oil daily (at least 400 mg of EPA...and 200 mg of DHA in each capsule).**

Good product for general health: Jarrow Formulas' EPA-DHA Balance, $11.57 for 120 capsules, Amazon.com. This is a highly concentrated, purified fish oil (made with anchovies and sardines), produced by a reputable manufacturer.

When larger doses of omega-3s may be needed: Individuals who suffer from severe rheumatoid arthritis or who have heart disease should eat seafood at least twice a week. In addition, the National Institutes of Health recommends that rheumatoid arthritis sufferers get 3.8 g of EPA and 2 g of DHA daily via supplements...those with heart disease should get up to 6 g of EPA and up to 3.7 g of DHA daily.

Caution: Taking 3 g or more daily of omega-3s may cause excessive bleeding in some people, so

*Dr. Broadhurst has been a consultant in the natural products industry but has no financial interest in any of the products mentioned in this article.

**Consult your doctor before starting an omega-3 regimen.

this much fish oil should be taken only when recommended by a physician for a specific purpose.

To avoid taking multiple capsules, consider trying a pourable variety of omega-3s—a single teaspoon contains about 2 g of omega-3s, which is the equivalent of two 1,000-mg capsules. Liquids are generally more cost-effective, too.

If you're worried about the taste of an omega-3 liquid: Try a flavored fish oil (such as lemon, orange or mint) or mix your omega-3 dose in orange juice or pineapple juice. Good liquid omega-3 products are available from Twinlab and Nordic Naturals.

If you're allergic to fish or you are a vegetarian: Many algae-based omega-3 products are available. DSM Nutritional Products makes life'sDHA, which is a highly purified and concentrated source of DHA (available at lifesDHA.com).

What about krill oil? This omega-3 product is derived from krill—tiny, shrimplike crustaceans that are normally eaten by whales, penguins and seals. Some people find that krill oil helps relieve joint pain faster than fish oil does.

Good krill oil supplements are available from Twinlab, Jarrow, Nature's Way and Natrol.

MAKE SURE IT'S PURE

A final point to consider in choosing an omega-3 supplement is the quality of the manufacturing process. To ensure that the company is complying with high manufacturing standards, choose omega-3 products that are labeled with the Good Manufacturing Practices (GMP) certification. This certification, granted by the Natural Products Association, shows that the company's manufacturing facility has been inspected every two years by an independent third-party auditor who checks production processes and that the product meets specifications in such areas as purity and strength. For a list of GMP-certified companies, go to the website of the Natural Products Association, NPAnational.org.

An alternative to look for: Certification from NSF International, an independent testing organization, NSF.org, indicates that an independent accredited lab has confirmed that the product contains what is on the label and on-site inspections have been made at the manufacturing facility.

MORE FROM DR. BROADHURST

Fatty Acid Face-Off: EPA vs. DHA

There are two main types of omega-3 fatty acids—eicosapentaenoic acid (EPA) and docosahexaenoic acid (DHA). Each of these fatty acids plays a different role in keeping our bodies healthy. EPA inhibits a key enzyme that fuels the production of inflammatory hormones. As a result, it is slightly more effective than DHA against certain types of inflammatory conditions, such as arthritis and joint and tendon problems. DHA, on the other hand, will boost the health of your brain's neurotransmitters.

For the greatest benefit: It's wise to choose an omega-3 supplement that contains both EPA and DHA. Just as calcium and vitamin D work synergistically, so do EPA and DHA.

Turmeric vs. Curcumin—Which Is Better for Your Health?

Andrew L. Rubman, ND, naturopathic doctor, founder and medical director, Southbury Clinic for Traditional Medicines, Southbury, Connecticut. He is author of the *Bottom Line* blog "Nature Doc's Patient Diary." SouthburyClinic.com

Which is better, curcumin or turmeric? Aren't they basically the same thing? The answer is that curcumin and turmeric have some of the same benefits...as well as their own unique ones. What's common to both are antioxidant and anti-inflammatory properties.

Turmeric is a bright yellow spice commonly used for flavoring, especially in curries and Middle Eastern dishes. Sometimes called "Indian saffron," turmeric comes from the root of the Curcuma longa plant, a relative of the ginger family. Turmeric also is used as a traditional treatment in Indian and Chinese Traditional Medicine for a range of conditions, including arthritis, laryngitis, bronchitis and diabetes.

Curcumin is the primary active ingredient in turmeric. It is one of the family of antioxidants called curcuminoids and is the component of turmeric that has been most extensively studied. In fact, research finds that curcumin can reduce ulcerative colitis flare-ups and postsurgery pain...help with anxiety and depression...help prevent type 2 diabetes...and may be a preventive for several types of cancer, including cancers of the prostate, breast, skin and colon.

Turmeric has been less well-studied. Nevertheless, research finds that it prevents heart attacks after bypass surgery...reduces skin irritation after radiation treatments...helps control cholesterol...helps reduce obesity...fights fungal infection...and reduces gall bladder disease. Other research finds that turmeric (and curcumin) reduce the joint pain, swelling and inflammation of arthritis.

So to answer which you should take—turmeric or curcumin—to get the most benefit, you should take both.

WHAT TO LOOK FOR

Choose a turmeric supplement fortified with extra curcumin—ideally, one that is 95% curcuminoids. A typical dose is 400 milligrams (mg) to 600 mg taken two or three times a day (a total of 1,200 mg to 1,800 mg/day). Also, since neither turmeric nor curcumin is well absorbed in the digestive tract, look for a supplement that includes piperine, a pepper extract that aids absorption.

Note: You also can boost turmeric's health benefits when eating curry by adding pepper—but you'll need to eat a lot of curry to get benefits equal to taking supplements.)

And you can apply turmeric directly to skin for arthritis pain relief...

Turmeric paste for pain relief: Mix one tablespoon of turmeric spice with enough coconut oil to make a paste. Apply to affected body part and let sit for three hours...then wash off with warm water. Repeat two to three times a week. (Note: Your skin may take on a slight golden hue, but that will fade with time.)

Turmeric is considered safe at doses mentioned above. But it's always best to talk to your doctor before taking this or any other supplement. The most common side effect of larger doses is upset stomach. Piperine can interfere with some prescription drugs, including *phenytoin* (Dilantin), *propranolol* (Inderal), *theophylline* and some chemotherapy drugs for breast cancer.

Magnesium for Healthier Bones, Muscles, Blood Sugar, Blood Pressure—and More

Mark Stengler, NMD, a naturopathic medical doctor and leading authority on the practice of alternative and integrated medicine. Dr. Stengler is author of the *Health Revelations* newsletter, author of *The Natural Physician's Healing Therapies*, founder and medical director of the Stengler Center for Integrative Medicine in Encinitas, California, and adjunct associate clinical professor at the National College of Natural Medicine in Portland, Oregon. MarkStengler.com

One patient had muscle cramps. Another had headaches. And a third had an irregular heartbeat. These were vastly different medical conditions, and yet the solution that I recommended for each patient was the same—magnesium. It helped each of these patients—and did so quickly.

Few nutrients possess the remarkable and diverse benefits of magnesium. It is the fourth most abundant mineral in cells after calcium, phosphorus and potassium. Magnesium is found in our bones...muscles...blood...and other tissues. It is needed by the body for energy production...fat and protein synthesis...muscle relaxation...nervous system function...and calcium metabolism.

According to US Department of Agriculture data, two out of every three Americans don't meet average daily intake requirements for magnesium, which are 300 milligrams (mg) to 420 mg daily for adults. In addition, many people have a magnesium deficiency due to stress...genetics...or a medication, such as a diuretic (usually taken to control blood pressure). As a consequence, these people face an increased risk for health problems. Maintaining adequate levels of magnesium can help reduce muscle cramps, stabilize blood sugar, lower the risk for heart disease, ease migraine headaches, strengthen bones and slow the aging process.

Consider one of my patients, Robert, who limped into my clinic. He was suffering from painful leg-muscle spasms that woke him at night and plagued him during the day. Muscle spasms often are related to low magnesium. Since magnesium relaxes muscles, I started Robert on an intravenous (IV) drip of magnesium sulfate. Within an hour, the pain in his leg eased. I had Robert begin taking a daily magnesium supplement, which helped to reduce subsequent leg-muscle spasms.

Magnesium is so important that it is sometimes hyped as a miracle cure.

Truth: Boosting magnesium levels can lead to recoveries that seem almost miraculous. Here's how magnesium could help you...

- **Muscle strength.** In addition to cramp relief, magnesium has many other muscle-related benefits. The reason that people often say that they feel an increase in energy after starting to take magnesium supplements is that the mineral is involved in the body's production of energy, most of which occurs in muscle cells. In a study conducted at the University of Palermo, Italy, researchers found that seniors with the highest levels of magnesium had the greatest muscle strength, including better grip strength, lower-leg muscle power, knee-extension torque and ankle strength. People with low magnesium levels had poor muscle function and strength.

- **Bone health.** Almost two-thirds of the body's magnesium is found in bone, where it works with calcium to provide structural support. Researchers at Yale University gave girls ages eight to 14 either magnesium or a placebo twice daily for one year.

Result: The girls who took magnesium developed much stronger bones compared with girls who took a placebo.

- **Stress buster.** Many people manifest stress physically by tensing the muscles of their back and shoulders, leading to tightness. Because magnesium is such a good muscle relaxant, it often can help ease muscle tension. Magnesium also stimulates the body's production of the calming brain chemical gamma amino butyric acid (GABA), so it also helps people to mentally relax.

- **Heart benefits.** Magnesium helps relax blood vessel walls, which reduces blood pressure. Magnesium sulfate is sometimes administered via IV in the hospital to reduce the risk for arrhythmia (irregular heartbeat). It also eases heart palpitations. Magnesium can help other heart problems, such as cardiomyopathy, a condition in which the heart fails to pump blood adequately.

There's more: Doctors at Harvard Medical School report that high levels of magnesium were associated with a significantly lower risk for sudden cardiac death, which causes about half of all deaths from coronary artery disease. The study found that people with the highest blood levels of magnesium were 77% less likely to suffer sudden death from cardiac arrest.

- **Diabetes.** Magnesium deficiency is common among people with type 2 diabetes. Earlier this year, German researchers conducted a study in which they gave magnesium supplements to overweight, prediabetic men and women. Those taking magnesium had a significant reduction in fasting blood sugar, better insulin resistance and lower blood pressure compared with those given a placebo.

- **Neuropathic pain.** Soaking in a bath with Epsom salts, which are granules of magnesium sulfate, is a well-known way to ease aches and pains. But I believe that magnesium's role in relieving severe pain has been barely tapped. In one study, British doctors used IV magnesium to treat people with postherpetic neuralgia, intense pain after a shingles (herpes zoster) outbreak. Pain was significantly reduced after just 30 minutes of receiving magnesium. Another study found that a one-time IV dose of 500 mg to 1,000 mg of magnesium sulfate eliminated nerve pain related to metastases in cancer patients.

In my own practice, I find that a combination of IV and oral magnesium eases nerve pain.

• **Asthma.** Magnesium can block the bronchial reactivity common in asthma attacks. In one study, doctors from Brazil reported that supplements of magnesium glycinate decreased bronchial reactivity by 30%. When taken in supplement form, magnesium glycinate is a well-absorbed and well-tolerated type of magnesium. In the study, subjects became more resistant to common asthmatic triggers (such as cold air and allergens) and were able to reduce their asthma medication by almost 40%. I have found similar results with my patients.

• **Headaches.** Several studies have shown that supplementing with magnesium can reduce the frequency of migraine headaches. IV magnesium sulfate also has been found to relieve the pain of cluster headaches in people with low blood levels of magnesium. Research has found that magnesium levels affect serotonin receptors and other brain chemicals that affect headache.

• **Anti-aging.** Magnesium also might help keep you younger. Studies show that magnesium is required to maintain telomeres, the protective tips of chromosomes (which contain your genes). Researchers have found that magnesium-deficient cells have an abnormal shortening of their telomeres, which is strongly associated with rapid aging.

MY ADVICE

Many foods contain magnesium, although most people don't get enough magnesium from their diet. Foods rich in magnesium include green vegetables, such as spinach and dark-leaf lettuce. The green color of vegetables comes from chlorophyll, which contains magnesium. Other excellent sources of magnesium are halibut, almonds, cashews, whole grains, pumpkin seeds and lentils.

I recommend that my patients have their magnesium levels checked. This can be done with a red blood cell magnesium test, which is not part of a regular blood test so you will have to ask for it.

Based on the results of this test, I find that most patients do need to supplement with magnesium. I usually recommend that these adults (both men and women) eat foods high in magnesium and take 200 mg of magnesium glycinate two or three times a day. Most multivitamins don't contain that amount, but many calcium-magnesium formulas do.

Magnesium of any kind can have a laxative effect if you take too much. If you have kidney problems, speak with your doctor before taking magnesium because the mineral could exacerbate kidney disease.

Magnesium Supplements

Mark A. Stengler, NMD, naturopathic medical doctor in private practice, Encinitas, California...adjunct associate clinical professor at the National College of Natural Medicine, Portland, Oregon...author of *The Natural Physician's Healing Therapies*.

Most magnesium supplements have magnesium oxide as the main ingredient, not magnesium glycinate. *What is the difference?*

Both forms of magnesium are commonly available as over-the-counter nutritional supplements—and both are effective. However, I prefer that patients use the glycinate form, especially when taking doses above 400 mg. This is because magnesium glycinate is less likely to cause loose stool than the oxide form. But if you can't find the glycinate form, it's OK to use the oxide version as long as it doesn't give you loose stool.

How a Quick Massage Can Help You Live Longer

Mark Tarnopolsky, MD, PhD, professor in the departments of pediatrics and medicine, McMaster University, Ontario, Canada.

No one wants to be overweight, have diabetes or grow old prematurely. Tough to overcome it all, right? Maybe not. A recent study shows that there's a simple strategy that may help prevent all three that is actually quite fun and relaxing.

A massage might do the trick!

And we're not talking about an expensive, hour-long massage, either—research shows that an inexpensive massage lasting just 10 minutes can be beneficial.

MASSAGING YOUR MUSCLES TO FIGHT DISEASE

Researchers were interested in studying massage immediately after exercise for two reasons. For one thing, practically speaking, that's a common time for people to get a massage, since many people say that massage helps reduce muscle soreness from exercise. Another reason is that, biologically, it's easier to measure differences in the effect of massage on cells after exercise, because exercise puts the body into a state of temporary stress.

Volunteers in the study included 11 healthy, active men in their 20s who provided a bit of muscle tissue from one thigh for a baseline biopsy. Then researchers had the volunteers do 70 minutes of fast-paced cycling on a stationary bike. The volunteers rested for 10 minutes and then had a 10-minute massage on one thigh only. Immediately after the massage, researchers took second muscle biopsies, but this time from both thighs in order to compare massaged tissue versus nonmassaged tissue. Two and a half hours after the second biopsies, the volunteers underwent a third set of biopsies on both thighs to capture any changes that might have occurred a bit later after their massages.

To learn about the findings, we called Mark Tarnopolsky, MD, PhD, a professor of medicine and head of neuromuscular and neurometabolic disease at McMaster University in Canada, who was a coauthor of the study published in *Science Translational Medicine*.

STOP THE DAMAGE!

Dr. Tarnopolsky said that the researchers found two very interesting differences in the muscles that had been massaged...

A gene pathway that causes muscle inflammation was "dialed down" in these muscles both immediately after the massage and 2.5 hours after the massage. (Specific genes can be present in our tissues but not always active.) Dr. Tarnopolsky said that this is helpful knowledge because muscle inflammation is a contributor to delayed-onset muscle soreness, so it confirms biologically what we've always believed through anecdotal observation—a post-exercise massage can help relieve muscle soreness.

Conversely, another sort of gene was "turned on" by the massage—this is a gene that increases the activity of mitochondria in muscle cells. You probably know that mitochondria are considered the "power packs" of our muscles for their role in creating usable energy. Now, it's true that better mitochondrial functioning has been shown by other studies to help decrease insulin resistance (a key risk factor for type 2 diabetes) and obesity and even to slow aging. Is it a stretch to link post-exercise massage to these benefits? Dr. Tarnopolsky said that it's not unreasonable—there is a potential connection, and future research will need to be done to confirm it.

TREAT YOURSELF TO MASSAGE

The massage type that Dr. Tarnopolsky and his colleagues used was a standard combination of three techniques that are commonly used for post-exercise massage—effleurage (light stroking)...petrissage (firm compression and release)...and stripping (repeated longitudinal strokes). It's easy to find massage therapists in spas, salons, fitness centers and private practices who use these techniques. Or you could ask your spouse or a friend to try some of these moves on you (even if his or her technique isn't perfect) because there's a chance that it could provide the benefits, said Dr. Tarnopolsky—he just can't say for sure, since that wasn't studied.

Dr. Tarnopolsky studied massage only after exercise, so that's when he would recommend getting one, but it's possible that massaging any muscles at any time may have similar benefits—more research will need to be done to find out.

Remember, you don't have to break the bank on a prolonged 60-minute massage—a simple 10- or 20-minute rubdown (which usually cost $10 to $40) can do the trick.

PRP Magic: Look Younger, Feel Younger with Platelet- Rich Plasma

Laurie Steelsmith, ND, LAc, licensed naturopathic physician and acupuncturist in private practice in Honolulu. She writes Bottom Line's "Natural Healing Secrets for Women" blog and is coauthor of three books—the best-selling *Natural Choices for Women's Health*, the critically acclaimed *Great Sex, Naturally* and her latest, *Growing Younger Every Day.* DrSteelsmith.com

Blood may not be the sexiest topic but your own blood may be the secret to health and vitality.

Sound bizarre? Think again. Here in the realm of naturopathic medicine, we live by the tenet that our bodies are built to heal themselves. Proof of this emerges in myriad ways, from scabs that eventually form fresh skin to an (albeit exasperating) itch—a sure sign that blood is moving towards a wound in the name of healing. Overall, the human body is a miraculous creation, designed for curing itself and tremendous resilience.

And we can harness this power even more by using platelet-rich plasma. The therapy, widely known as PRP, utilizes injections of a patient's own blood to jumpstart the healing process and rejuvenate specific areas of concern. First discovered in the 1970s in the field of hematology, PRP began to be used a decade later, initially in maxillofacial surgery before moving into a variety of medical procedures, including cardiac surgery, gynecology, oral surgery and ophthalmology.

But what, exactly, is PRP—and how does it work?

In PRP, a small amount of blood (30 to 60 milligrams, or two to four tablespoons) is drawn from the patient and placed into a centrifuge. As the blood spins at a very fast rate, red blood cells are separated from plasma (the clear liquid that transports blood throughout the body) and platelets. The removal of red blood cells leaves us with platelet-rich plasma—plasma so rich in platelets, in fact, that it contains 10 times as much as whole blood. In PRP therapy, the platelet-rich plasma is either injected into the region of the patient's body that requires treatment, applied topically or administered through microneedling—a minimally invasive procedure in which ultra-fine needles are inserted into the skin.

So what does this platelet-rich plasma do? Plenty. Platelets play a variety of roles in your body, from encouraging blood to clot to encouraging wounds to heal—or, as the National Institutes of Health frames it, they're on "continual 'call of duty' because inside of them lies one of the most powerful reservoirs of factors responsible for tissue repair." This is thanks to the fact that they're jam-packed with properties that aid in regeneration, including platelet-derived growth factor, transforming-growth factor B, fibroblast activation, insulin-like growth factor, epidermal growth factor and cytokines—cell-signaling proteins that impact immunity and inflammation (among other functions). Ultimately, platelets affect the stem cells in our tissues and stimulate them to produce whatever they're programmed to make—whether it's cartilage, connective tissue, elastin or hair.

As expected, the applications of PRP are broad and exciting, offering the potential of tissue regeneration in everything from sexual wellness to orthopedics. Here's a closer look at how PRP has helped others—and how it might one day help you.

ORTHOPEDICS

Kari, a 68-year-old woman, arrived at my office suffering from chronic ankle and knee pain, which had been plaguing her since a motor vehicle accident 18 years earlier. I treated her joints with PRP three times, with each session one month apart.

By the end of our time together, she reported an increased range of motion and radically reduced pain. The science is there, too. Therapeutic PRP injections for joints, ligaments and tendons have been studied extensively, and show particular promise in the arena of cartilage repair.

Indeed, PRP can be an absolute windfall for those suffering from osteoarthritis, a form of arthritis that affects 27 million Americans. It can be due to wear and tear of the joint or, as in the case of Kari, from trauma. When cartilage breaks down inside a joint—whether it's from a car accident, heredity, obesity or another cause—it can cause pain, swelling, inflammation and a limited range of motion. PRP has the capacity to aid in this by fueling new cartilage production. It can also help repair chronically inflamed tendons and partially torn ligaments. In some cases—including Kari's—patients can forgo surgery after receiving PRP injections.

OPHTHALMOLOGY

My esteemed associate, naturopath and acupuncturist Dr. Kristen Coles, has treated a few patients with severe dry eye disease. Otherwise known as dry eye syndrome, the malady is marked by a chronic lack of sufficient lubrication and moisture, the results of which manifest as constant irritation, inflammation and even scarring.

For example, for Bree—who had severe dry eye disease secondary to Graves' ophthalmopathy—Dr. Coles recommended one PRP drop per eye, once a day, for eight weeks. Bree began to experience relief nearly immediately—as in, within the first two weeks of treatment. At the end of her regimen, her ophthalmologist noted that she had increased moisture in her eyes.

Dr. Coles' patients, of course, aren't alone. A 2017 study published in *Ophthalmology Therapy* evaluated the topical use of PRP in 368 patients with dry eye syndrome. The results were startling. After six weeks of treatment, symptoms improved in 322 cases. The authors stated that PRP is an "effective treatment to improve signs and symptoms in patients suffering from moderate-to-severe chronic dry eye syndrome." Another 2017 study, this one published in the *Journal of Ophthalmology*, demonstrated that PRP can mend dry eye syndrome post-LASIK surgery. In short, PRP may be a godsend for anyone suffering from the debilitating side effects of severe dry eye disease.

SEXUAL WELLNESS AND GYNECOLOGY

Menopause often arrives with a series of symptoms that can dramatically affect a woman's sex life. Such was the case with Stella, who, at 57, was suffering not only from vaginal dryness but also incontinence and "reduced" sexual sensation. Following a PRP treatment—affectionately known as an O-Shot® (as developed by Charles Runels, MD)—her libido was revived and her orgasms were "better than ever."

Hers was far from an isolated case. One of PRP's biggest claims to fame is the impact it can have on one's sexual health. During these sessions, PRP is injected into the intimate areas of women and men (in which case, they're called "P" shots.) In men, PRP is injected into the shaft of the penis to support girth and enhance sexual sensation, and in women it is injected into the vulva and the area around the urethra to decrease urinary incontinence and to also enrich sexual pleasure.

Sound painful? Don't despair! A patient is prepped with a numbing cream and given a nerve block that prevents pain. Indeed, the most "painful" part is the idea of having any kind of injection "down there." But I can assure you, if it's done right, it doesn't hurt—and the results can be nothing short of rejuvenating.

I have been doing PRP injections for sexual wellness primarily on women and every woman I have treated—from postmenopausal women to a 30-year-old who wanted to boost her sexual enjoyment—has reported positive effects, from increased sensation to greater vaginal lubrication.

This is thanks, again, to PRP's rich concentration of important growth factors, which can help invigorate the nerves, muscles, connective tissues and blood vessels of the lower pelvic floor (including the clitoris, urethra, vulva, and vaginal wall). Because of the structural support that PRP provides, many women also report resolution of their stress and urge incontinence after a PRP treatment. What's more, given that the treatment is derived from a woman's own body, authors of a 2017 study argued that there is no risk of a reaction to foreign bodies. (To which we women say, hallelujah!)

AESTHETICS

Aside from the distinction PRP has earned in the world of sports medicine—Tiger Woods, Kobe Bryant and Reggie Jackson are just a few of its fans—PRP's utmost renown may be in the field of aesthetics. The technique for a PRP facial utilizes either the relatively pain-free (and aforementioned) microneedling or it can be injected. In some cases, the PRP is applied simultaneously with a facial filler, applied directly to the problem with a syringe, or smeared on following microdermabrasion or a laser treatment. The end results, meanwhile, can be downright dramatic.

As Mona Gohara, MD, puts it, "PRP theoretically acts as a matrix that promotes collagen production, parlaying into softer wrinkles, firmer skin, more hair and, in some endorsements, lifted breasts." Numerous studies published in the *Journal of Cosmetic Dermatology* confirm this. The data also demonstrates that PRP can significantly reduce the appearance of brown spots, diminish wrinkles, increase skin firmness and, overall, have a "significant, reproducible, positive impact on biological facial rejuvenation." PRP can also be used to offer volume to cheekbones and nasolabial folds.

Following a PRP procedure, your cells will continue to regenerate for three to six months, with the effects lasting up to a year. It's a swell side effect (and deal), considering that my 65-year-old patient Shauna claimed a series of facial PRP treatments took 10 years off of her face—and she was just one of many patients who saw a major transformation.

Once-a-year treatments are recommended to maintain healthy collagen production. If a woman is older, she may choose to do a series of six treatments one month apart. It is about creating and maintaining healthy, vibrant-looking skin, and supporting collagen, which, as we age, tends to break down.

PRP is also making waves—literally—in the domain of hair regrowth. Again, this comes down to the growth factors it boasts, which, when inserted into the scalp, can activate hair follicles and foster hair regrowth. According to Neil Sadick, MD—a dermatologist in New York City and the director of the Sadick Research Group, studying and treating hair loss (an issue that affects 1 in 5 Americans, and can take a huge emotional toll on both men and women)—the use of PRP is "a great treatment option for hair loss because it has a number of scientifically based articles showing its efficacy in increasing hair count, hair thickness and the growth phase of the hair cycle."

WHAT ABOUT COST?

You may be wondering about insurance coverage for PRP procedures. My practice does not take insurance and so I never considered the question, but I doubt that it currently is. And PRP procedures can be expensive. For example, treating one joint in my office using a 30-mL kit costs $550...a 60-mL kit costs around $650. The facial PRP cost is about $650 per treatment. Cost for the O shot is $1,200. But prices vary depending on where you live (most doctors on the mainland charge more than we do).

Yet these costs may not sound so high when you consider the magical results that PRP treatments can yield.

Live Longer By Meditating

Robert H. Schneider, MD, director, Institute for Natural Medicine and Prevention, Maharashi University of Management, Maharashi Vedic City, Iowa.

Background: Transcendental meditation (TM), a technique that produces a state of "restful alertness," has been shown to reduce stress levels and lower blood pressure.

People with hypertension (average age 72) who regularly practiced TM for 20 minutes twice daily were 30% less likely to die from heart disease over an 18-year period than those who did not practice TM.

Theory: TM lowers levels of adrenaline and cortisol, stress-related hormones, in the body.

Helpful: Practice TM for 20 minutes twice daily.

Meditation for People Who Don't Like to Meditate

Sharon Salzberg, cofounder of the Insight Meditation Society meditation center in Barre, Massachusetts. She has taught meditation since 1974 and written numerous books, including *Real Happiness: The Power of Meditation* and *Real Love: The Art of Mindful Connection.*

Despite all its virtues, meditation can be seemingly impossible for many people to do. Fortunately, there are simple solutions for virtually all of the reasons that people cite for not being able to meditate.

DO IT YOUR WAY

The most familiar form of meditation involves sitting or lying down for about 30 minutes and focusing on your breathing—how it feels as air enters and leaves your nose or as your chest or abdomen rises and falls. For most people, it takes about 30 minutes to calm their stress-based thinking—I forgot to call so-and-so, etc.—and reach a deeper level of concentration.

It's simple but not easy. It is common to become frustrated with your mind's constant chatter, or you may feel so restless, bored or distracted that you give up.

My solutions for the most common reasons that people don't try meditation—or give it up…

Problem: Feeling too restless to meditate. Some people find it impossible to sit still for an extended period of time.

Solution: Try walking meditation. Find a quiet, unobstructed, flat area where you can take at least 20 steps before turning around. As you walk slowly, let your attention rest on your feet and legs. Be aware of the sensations in each foot as it lifts off the ground, moves through the air, then settles down.

Feel the contact of the ground in your toes and the soles of your feet. Notice how the muscles of each leg tighten and then relax as you walk. Observe the sensations in the foot (and the leg) that is not bearing weight.

Note: Walking meditation is also ideal for people who tend to fall asleep while meditating in a chair or lying down.

Problem: Getting distracted by noise. It's not always easy to find a quiet place to meditate, and some people are very sensitive to noise.

Solution: Make sound the object of your meditation. The distinction between sound and noise is important. "Sound" is a purely physical phenomenon, while "noise" is sound plus a negative judgment. The idea is simply to notice sounds as they arise—beep, rumble, clang, hiss—without speculating about where they come from.

When you become aware that you're reacting to a sound, observe the thoughts you have about the sound. What does the anger or irritation feel like? Then go back to just hearing it.

Problem: The "mind chatter" won't stop. You may hope that meditation will clear your mind of thoughts, but invariably the thoughts keep on coming—a conversation you had last week…what you want to eat for dinner. Your mind just won't shut down.

Solution: Don't fight the thoughts. Just observe them as they pass through your mind.

It's like sitting on the bank of a river and watching the water float by, noticing leaves, twigs, fish, flashes of sunlight and shadow—without being swept up by the current.

If the thoughts persist, gently bring your attention back to the sensations of breathing…or the feeling of your feet on the floor. When more thoughts arise, repeat the process.

Problem: There's no time to meditate. When your schedule is busy, it may not be possible to devote a half hour (or even 20 minutes) to meditation every day.

Solution: Start with 10 minutes. For many people, it's easier to find three 10-minute periods in the course of the day than to arrange a time for a lengthier break. If 10 minutes seem too long, you can even start with five.

How can five or 10 minutes of meditation be enough to benefit you? The reason is that the dailiness of meditation—making it a regular part of your routine—is more important than the amount of time you meditate. And many people find that after several weeks of five-minute meditation periods, it seems natural—and possible—to meditate longer.

14

Save Your Senses

Cataract Surgery: Better Vision and Perhaps a Longer Life

David F. Chang, MD, clinical professor of ophthalmology at University of California, San Francisco, and past president of the American Society of Cataract and Refractive Surgery. He is an international authority on cataract surgery who frequently lectures surgeons about advanced cataract techniques and the newest lens implants. He is coauthor of *Cataracts: A Patient's Guide to Treatment*.

No one wants to have surgery—any surgery. But once you have had cataract surgery, you'll probably wonder why you waited so long.

Recent developments: Cataract surgery now takes about 20 minutes for most people. You'll go home soon after the procedure...serious, vision-threatening complications, such as infection, are extremely rare...and it's successful in about 99% of cases, making it one of the most effective of all surgeries.

The benefits are undeniable. Within days, you'll see better—with sharper vision, better nighttime eyesight and fewer bright-light "halos." But that's not all.

The procedure, which usually is done on one eye at a time, is performed while you're awake and while your eye is numbed with eye-drop anesthesia, so it's not even painful. Most health insurance plans pick up the tab.

To learn more about the latest advances in cataract surgery, *Bottom Line Health* spoke with David F. Chang, MD, a noted authority on cataract techniques.

IS IT YOUR TIME?

Most people are familiar with the telltale signs of cataracts—the normally clear lens within your eye becomes cloudy and/or discolored. Because the lens focuses incoming visual images and transmits them to the retina, these changes, though generally gradual (occurring over a period of years), can cause significant vision loss if untreated.

Important: The lens sits behind the iris and pupil, so you can't self-diagnose cataracts by looking in a mirror. Only an eye doctor using a special microscope can actually see cataracts.

That's why it's important to see an eye doctor (in addition to having routine eye exams) if you're experiencing vision problems, including blurred vision, difficulty seeing details (such as small print or road signs) and glare or poor night-driving vision.

Age is the main risk factor for cataracts. When you're young, the proteins that form the lenses of your eyes are arranged in a way that makes the structures crystal-clear. Over time, these proteins eventually start to clump together and reduce the amount of light that passes through.

By your 60s and 70s, these changes will have gradually begun to occur. Most people, if they live long enough, will develop cataracts that are advanced enough for them to consider surgery.

Earlier-onset of cataracts has been associated with such risk factors as smoking, diabetes, prior retinal surgery, severe nearsightedness, excessive sun exposure and prolonged use of certain medications such as steroids.

WHAT ARE YOU WAITING FOR?

Cataracts can affect one or both eyes, either simultaneously or at different times. In the past, doctors advised patients to delay surgery until a cataract was "ripe"—meaning that it was so advanced that the benefits justified the lengthy recovery and the potential for complications due to the large incision that was used at that time. Unfortunately, many people are still operating under this misconception.

Newer thinking: You don't need to wait so long. If the cataract is impairing your daily activities, such as reading and/or driving, it makes sense to have cataract surgery sooner rather than later because of the procedure's exceptionally high success rate.

Now the lens is broken up into many small pieces using ultrasonic vibrations within the eye, then suctioned out. The incisions are so small that stitches aren't required—and cataracts can be safely removed at an earlier stage. The replacement artificial lens lasts a lifetime and is folded so that it can pass through the tiny (about one-eighth inch) incision.

The timing is important because cataracts can get so bad that they increase a person's risk for falls and auto/pedestrian accidents, as well as contribute to depression.

These factors may have something to do with the recent research regarding cataract surgery that was published online in the journal *JAMA Ophthalmology.*

Key findings: This study of more than 74,000 women ages 65 and older found that those who had undergone cataract surgery had a 60% lower risk of dying over the 20-year study period than those who did not get treated.

BETTER VISION WITHOUT GLASSES

You'll obviously see better once a cataract is removed. What some people don't realize is that they might see better than they ever did.

The surgeon will remove the cloudy lens and replace it with a clear, artificial lens that comes in more than 50 different powers.

Suppose that you have always worn glasses to see well in the distance. When you have cataract surgery, a replacement lens can be chosen to correct your particular type/degree of optical error. For example, some lenses correct for astigmatism (blurred vision that is caused by incorrect corneal curvature). Certain artificial lenses function like bifocals and reduce how frequently people must rely on reading glasses.

In most cases, cataract surgery won't completely eliminate the need for glasses. Most people will have excellent distance vision without glasses following cataract surgery. However, most will need reading glasses—but can perhaps use them less often and/or get by with a lower-power prescription.

WHAT ELSE CAN YOU DO?

Surgery is the only treatment for cataracts, and it is a permanent solution—the new lens will remain transparent forever. Unfortunately, there is no medication that can halt or reverse cataract formation. What can one do to prevent cataracts?

- **Wear sunglasses outdoors.** The UV radiation in sunlight damages eye proteins and can lead to cloudiness. A large study that reviewed data from more than a half million people found a strong association between cataracts and skin cancer—more evidence that UV exposure is a major risk factor.

What to do: Wear sunglasses with UV protection whenever you plan to spend prolonged periods of time outdoors. Virtually all sunglasses today are UV-protected.

- **Wear a broad-brimmed hat to block UV radiation.** It will reduce your risk for eyelid skin cancer as well as cataracts.

• **Eat a nutritious diet.** Many studies have found an association between a healthy diet and fewer cataracts—but that's not the same as proof.

For example, several studies have suggested that particular nutrients—alone or in combination—can help prevent cataracts. The large Age-Related Eye Disease Study (AREDS) reported that people with cataracts who got the most lutein and zeaxanthin (antioxidants that are found in leafy greens and other fruits/vegetables) were 32% less likely to need cataract surgery.

Other research has looked at the effects of fish oil supplements (or regular meals including fatty fish)...vitamin C...vitamin E...and other nutrients.

It's common sense to eat a nutritious diet. If you want to take one of the AREDS formulations, check with your doctor first if you are a current or former smoker. Certain versions of these supplements (with lutein and zeaxanthin) also contain beta-carotene, which has been linked to increased risk for lung cancer in current and former smokers.

How to Protect Your Eyesight!

Mrinali Patel Gupta, MD, a retina specialist and assistant professor of ophthalmology at Weill Cornell Medicine in New York City. Her research has been published in many professional journals, and she was a recipient of the Howard Hughes Medical Institute-National Institutes of Health Research Fellowship for her work on AMD at the National Eye Institute.

How would you feel if you lost your eyesight? When asked this question, nearly half of Americans recently surveyed by researchers at Johns Hopkins University said that it would be the worst possible thing that could happen to their health. Ironically, half of the respondents in the same survey were completely unaware of age-related macular degeneration (AMD), a leading cause of blindness in the US.

THE BASICS OF AMD

The word "age" in AMD doesn't mean that the condition affects only the elderly. Rather, it means that the incidence of AMD rises with age. The exact causes of AMD are unknown, but some risk factors are well established—such as age, gender (women get it more often than men) and race (whites face a higher risk than other races).

Other risk factors: Having blue eyes...obesity...and high blood pressure. A healthy lifestyle that includes not smoking and a nutritious diet are the best ways to help reduce the risk for AMD.

DRY AND WET AMD

AMD affects and damages the macula of the retina—the region of the retina responsible for central vision (seeing what's right in front of us) and fine acuity vision (seeing fine details).

There are two forms of AMD—dry and wet. The dry form accounts for 90% of people with AMD. In the early stages, dry AMD may cause no visual symptoms, which is why routine eye exams are important for diagnosis. As dry AMD progresses, patients may start to notice subtle changes or distortions in central vision such as straight lines that appear wavy or written words that seem to be missing letters. In the late stages of dry AMD, patients may have severe vision loss. In general, however, the progression of dry AMD is slow and occurs over many years, and some patients may never have vision loss.

Wet AMD is characterized by abnormal blood vessels that grow under and into the retina. The blood vessels can leak blood and fluid that reduce vision and damage the retina. Wet AMD causes the majority of cases of AMD-related blindness and can progress rapidly.

The dry form of AMD can progress to the wet form—risk of conversion from dry to wet AMD is approximately 14% to 20% over five years. There may be no symptoms early in the conversion of dry to wet AMD. Subsequently, patients may notice subtle vision changes such as those described above. Severe vision loss, such as dramatic reduction in overall vision or a large dark area in central vision, can develop, especially if wet AMD goes untreated.

DIAGNOSIS OF AMD

Because most people with dry AMD may have no symptoms, regular eye exams are important to identify the early signs of the disease. AMD can be diagnosed during a routine dilated eye exam done by an ophthalmologist or optometrist. The American Academy of Ophthalmology advises a baseline eye exam at age 40 (earlier if you have eye disease or are at risk for developing eye disease) and an exam every year or two at age 65 and older. However, your doctor may advise more frequent exams based on your specific situation.

If you experience any slowly progressive (over weeks or months) vision changes, get promptly evaluated by an ophthalmologist. And if you have severe and sudden vision loss, see an eye doctor immediately, preferably on the same day, for an evaluation to determine if you need emergency treatment.

TREATMENT FOR DRY AMD

If you have dry AMD, there are currently no medical treatments, but it can be effectively managed to prevent progression. *What to do...*

• **Maintain a healthy lifestyle**—don't smoke and eat a nutritious diet.

• **Get an eye exam once or twice yearly,** including an optical coherence tomography scan to check for progression from dry to wet AMD. This noninvasive imaging test allows doctors to examine the retina to detect the abnormal blood vessels of wet AMD at very early stages. Your doctor may repeat the test at every visit. The test is also used to monitor wet AMD.

• **Self-monitor.** Use the Amsler grid—with horizontal and vertical lines—at least a few times a week to check for subtle vision changes in each eye. If there's any change in the grid when looking at it, such as straight lines that appear crooked/wavy or parts of the grid are missing, you should contact your eye doctor. A downloadable Amsler grid is available at AmslerGrid.org, and grids are also available as a smartphone app.

Also: For some patients, getting the right nutrients may prevent dry AMD from worsening. An eye doctor can tell you if your situation warrants vitamins for your eyes.

What the research shows: A large clinical trial led by the National Institutes of Health found that patients with intermediate or advanced AMD in only one eye who took an antioxidant mix—500 mg of vitamin C...400 international units (IU) of vitamin E...15 mg of beta-carotene...80 mg of zinc...and 2 mg of copper (known as the AREDS formula)—were less likely to have progression of AMD.

Note: Current or former smokers should use the newer AREDS2 formula, which has lutein and zeaxanthin instead of beta-carotene—beta-carotene is associated with increased risk for lung cancer in smokers.

These mixes are available over-the-counter in pharmacies.

BREAKTHROUGH INJECTIONS

Previously, the average patient with wet AMD quickly lost significant vision (two to three lines on the vision chart in the first two years alone). But with the advent of anti-vascular endothelial growth factor (VEGF) therapy, vision can be stabilized or improved in roughly half of patients.

Multiple large clinical trials have demonstrated that intravitreal injection (into the eye) of medications that block VEGF, such as *bevacizumab* (Avastin) and *aflibercept* (Eylea), dramatically reduce vision loss in wet AMD.

The procedure is done with local anesthesia in the ophthalmologist's office. It's quick and usually painless. The injections are often given monthly...or on a less frequent basis, depending on how the patient is doing. Some people need long-term therapy, while others can over time reduce or discontinue it but are monitored closely as many patients subsequently need additional treatments (when the wet AMD becomes active again). The treatment controls wet AMD but is not a cure. The risk associated with injections is very low but includes cataracts, retinal detachment, bleeding or infection/inflammation in the eye.

An Orange a Day Keeps Macular Degeneration Away

Bamini Gopinath, PhD, is principal research fellow at Westmead Institute for Medical Research, Westmead, Australia, and lead author of a study published in *The American Journal of Clinical Nutrition.*

An orange a day may keep macular degeneration away, reports Bamini Gopinath, PhD. People who consumed at least one orange daily were 60% less likely to have age-related macular degeneration 15 years later than people who did not eat oranges. The protective effect may be due to the flavonoids in oranges—but no benefit was found from consuming other flavonoid-rich foods, such as apples, or from flavonoid supplements.

How to See Better in the Dark

Marc Grossman, OD, LAc, is a holistic developmental/behavioral optometrist, licensed acupuncturist and medical director of Natural Eye Care, New Paltz, New York. He is coauthor of *Greater Vision* and *Natural Eye Care*. NaturalEyeCare.com

Aging often brings a reduction in the ability to see well in low light.

Reasons: Night vision has two elements. First, the pupils must dilate to let in as much light as possible. Normally this happens within seconds of entering a darkened environment—but as we age, the muscles that control pupil dilation weaken, slowing down and/or limiting dilation. Second, chemical changes must occur in the light-sensitive photoreceptors (called rods and cones) of the retina at the back of the eyeball. Some of these changes take several minutes and some take longer, so normally full night vision is not achieved for about 20 minutes. Even brief exposure to bright light (such as oncoming headlights) reverses these chemical changes, so the processes must start over. With age, these chemical changes occur more slowly... and some of our photoreceptors may be lost.

While we cannot restore the eyes' full youthful function, we can take steps to preserve and even improve our ability to see in low light. *Here's how...*

- **First, see your eye doctor to investigate possible underlying medical problems.** Various eye disorders can cause or contribute to reduced night vision, including cataracts (clouding of the eye's lens), retinitis pigmentosa (a disease that damages the retina's rods and cones) and macular degeneration (in which objects in the center of the field of vision cannot be seen). Night vision also can be compromised by liver cirrhosis or the digestive disorder celiac disease, which can lead to deficiencies of eye-protecting nutrients...or diabetes, which can damage eye nerves and blood vessels. Diagnosing any underlying disorder is vital because the sooner it is treated, the better the outcome is likely to be.

- **Adopt an eye-healthy diet.** Eat foods rich in the vision-supporting nutrients below...and ask your doctor whether supplementation is right for you. *Especially important...*

  - Lutein, a yellow pigment and antioxidant found in corn, dark green leafy vegetables, egg yolks, kiwi fruit, oranges and yellow squash.

    Typical supplement dosage: 6 milligrams (mg) daily.

  - Vitamin A, found in carrots, Chinese cabbage, dark green leafy vegetables, pumpkin, sweet potatoes and winter squash.

    Typical supplement dosage: 10,000 international units (IU) daily.

  - Zeaxanthin, a yellow pigment and antioxidant found in corn, egg yolks, kiwi fruit, orange peppers and oranges.

    Typical supplement dosage: 300 micrograms daily.

  - Zinc, found in beans, beef, crab, duck, lamb, oat bran, oysters, ricotta cheese, turkey and yogurt.

    Typical supplement dosage: 20 mg daily.

- **Update prescription lenses.** Many people just keep wearing the same old glasses even though vision tends to change over time—so new glasses with the correct prescription often can improve night vision.

- **Keep eyeglasses and contacts clean.** Smudges bend rays of light and distort what you see.

- **Wear sunglasses outdoors on sunny days,** especially between noon and 3 pm. This is particularly important for people with light-colored eyes, which are more vulnerable to the sun's damaging ultraviolet rays. Excessive sun exposure is a leading cause of eye disorders (such as cataracts) that can impair eyesight, including night vision. Amber or gray lenses are best for sunglasses because they absorb light frequencies most evenly.

• **Do not use yellow-tinted lenses at night.** These often are marketed as "night driving" glasses, implying that they sharpen contrast and reduce glare in low light. However, Dr. Grossman cautioned that any tint only further impairs night vision.

Safest: If you wear prescription glasses, stick to untinted, clear lenses—but do ask your optometrist about adding an antireflective or antiglare coating.

• **Exercise your night vision.** This won't speed up the eyes' process of adjusting to the dark but may encourage a mental focus that helps the brain and eyes work better together—thus improving your ability to perceive objects in a darkened environment.

What to do: For 20 minutes four times per week, go into a familiar room at night and turn off the lights. As your eyes are adjusting, look directly toward a specific object that you know is there...focus on it, trying to make out its shape and details and to distinguish it from surrounding shadows. With practice, your visual perception should improve. For an additional challenge, do the exercise outdoors at night... while looking at unfamiliar objects in a dark room...or while using peripheral vision rather than looking directly at an object.

When driving at night, avoid looking directly at oncoming headlights. Shifting your gaze slightly to the right of center minimizes the eye changes that would temporarily impair your night vision, yet still allows you to see traffic.

Also: Use the night setting on rearview mirrors to reduce reflected glare.

• **Clean car windows and lights.** When was the last time you used glass cleaner on the inside of your windshield...or on rear and side windows... or on headlights and taillights? For the clearest possible view and minimal distortion from smudges, keep all windows and lights squeaky clean.

Can We Say Good-Bye to Reading Glasses?

Marc Grossman, OD, LAc, is a holistic developmental/behavioral optometrist, licensed acupuncturist and medical director of Natural Eye Care in New Paltz, New York. He is the coauthor of *Greater Vision* and *Natural Eye Care*. NaturalEyeCare.com

When it comes to signs of aging, different people have different pet peeves. Some of us really don't like those gray hairs... others sigh over a lost silhouette...still others hate needing reading glasses to see what's on the menu.

Since exercise improves the strength, flexibility and function of our bodies, it makes sense that eye exercises could improve our ability to see close up. Yet this is a controversial topic. Though various studies have found no clear benefit from eye exercises, many holistic practitioners and their patients say that vision can indeed be improved.

The challenge with aging eyes: Many people first become farsighted—meaning that nearby objects look blurry even though more distant objects are clear—starting in their 40s. This is due to presbyopia, a condition in which the aging lens of the eye becomes too stiff to focus clearly up close.

Detractors of eye exercise say that it won't restore lens elasticity. But supporters say that's not the point. Marc Grossman, OD, LAc, a holistic developmental/behavioral optometrist in New Paltz, New York, and coauthor of *Greater Vision*, explained, "Eye exercises can improve the strength, flexibility and adaptability of muscles that control eye movement and encourage a mental focus that helps the brain and eyes work better together. This can slow the progression of farsightedness and possibly improve vision."

So the answer to the question, "Can eye exercises help us say good riddance to reading glasses?" seems to be yes for some people—and it certainly can't hurt to try.

Dr. Grossman recommended four exercises for improving close-up vision. "While you do the exercises, remember to keep breathing and keep blinking. And smile! Smiling reduces tension, which helps your muscles work optimally and your brain focus on what's around you," he said.

Try to do the exercises while not wearing any reading glasses—or if your close-up vision is not good enough for that, wear weaker reading glasses than you normally do. If you usually wear glasses or contacts for distance vision, it is OK to wear those while doing the exercises.

How long to practice: Do each exercise for three to four minutes, for a total practice time of about 15 minutes per session, at least three times weekly. If you get headaches while exercising your eyes, reduce the time spent on each exercise—and see your eye doctor if the problem persists.

• **Letter reading**—for better scanning accuracy and conscious eye control when reading or using a computer.

Preparation: Type up a chart with four rows of random letters, just large enough that you can read them while holding the page at a typical reading distance (type size will vary depending on an individual's vision). Leave space between each row. In row one, type all capitals, one space in between each letter...row two, all lowercase, one space in between each letter...row three, all lowercase, no spaces...row four, wordlike groups of random letters arranged as if in a sentence.

Exercise: Hold the chart with both hands. Looking at row one, read each letter aloud left to right, then right to left. Then read every second letter...then every third letter. If your mind wanders, start over.

Over time: When you master row one, try the same techniques with row two...then row three... then row four. If you find that you have memorized parts of the chart, make a new one using different letters.

• **Near and far**—for improved focus and focusing speed when switching your gaze from close objects to distant objects (such as when checking gauges on a car as you drive).

Preparation: Type a chart with six to eight rows of random capital letters, each letter about one-half inch tall (or as tall as necessary for you to read them from 10 feet away). Tack the chart to a wall and stand back 10 feet.

Exercise: Hold a pencil horizontally, with its embossed letters facing you, about six inches from your nose (or as close as possible without it looking blurry). Read any letter on the pencil, then read any letter on the chart. Keep doing this, switching back and forth as fast as you can without letting the letters blur.

Over time: Do this with one eye covered, then the other.

• **Pencil pushups**—to promote eye teamwork. All you need is a pencil.

Exercise: Hold a pencil horizontally at eye level 12 inches from your face (or as far as necessary to see the pencil clearly). With both eyes, look at one particular letter on the pencil...keep looking while bringing the pencil closer to your face. If the letter blurs or doubles, it means that one eye is no longer accurately on target—so move the pencil back until the letter is clear once more...then try again to slowly bring the pencil closer while keeping the letter in focus.

• **The "hot dog"**—for improved flexibility of the muscles within the eye that allow the lens to change shape. No props are needed.

Exercise: With your hands at chest height about eight inches in front of you, point your index fingers and touch the tips together, so that your index fingers are horizontal. Gaze at any target in the distance and, without changing your focus, raise your fingers into your line of sight. Notice that a "mini hot dog" has appeared between the tips of your fingers. Still gazing at the distant object, pull your fingertips apart slightly—and observe that the hot dog is now floating in the air. Keep the hot dog there for two breaths...then look directly at your fingers for two breaths, noticing that the hot dog disappears. Look again at the distant object and find the hot dog once again. Continue switching your gaze back and forth every two breaths.

As your close-up vision improves, you may find that you need less-powerful reading glasses—or none at all—for your day-to-day activities.

Secrets to Choosing the Best Glasses for You . . .

Melvin Schrier, OD, FAAO, an optometry consultant based in Rancho Palos Verdes, California. A fellow of the American Academy of Optometry and past president of the New York Academy of Optometry, he operated a private optometry practice in New York City for more than 40 years and has written numerous journal articles and book chapters on eye health.

With all the lenses that are available today—from sophisticated progressives to drugstore readers—and an array of contacts and fashionable frames to choose from, you might think that selecting your eyewear has never been easier.

The truth is, there now are so many choices out there—each with its own quirks and pitfalls—that you really need to know what you're doing to avoid making costly, potentially eye-damaging mistakes.

How to guard against the most common mistakes…

MISTAKE #1: **Assuming that progressives are always the best choice.** Those nifty lenses known as "progressives," which offer a continuum of clear vision from near to far (close-up, midrange and distance) within a single pair of glasses or contacts, may seem like the ideal solution for aging eyes. Unlike bifocals and trifocals, progressives have no line separating the different viewing zones.

But for many people, progressives are not all they're cracked up to be. Stationary objects may sometimes appear to be moving because the edges of the optical zones are somewhat blurred by design. This also can make driving tricky—for example, you must move your head to the right or left rather than glancing to the sides, where the edges will be blurred.

On top of that, progressives are more expensive than traditional bifocals and trifocals—about $400 and up versus about $200 to $300 for bifocals or trifocals, which have separate viewing zones separated by lines.

If your eye doctor agrees that progressives are a good choice for you, ask about lenses from manufacturers that are pulling out all the stops to try to address some of the common pitfalls.

Two progressive lenses you may want to discuss with your doctor…

- **Varilux X Series.** To help do away with blurry peripheral vision, these new lenses use a patented design that is intended to even out the magnification across the lens. For more information, go to EssilorUSA.com/products/varilux.
- **Shamir Golf glasses.** These progressive lenses are designed to provide sharp focus for the distances that are most important to golfers—for the scorecard in their hands…the ball at their feet when putting or teeing off…and the green in the distance. For more details, go to ShamirLens.com.

MISTAKE #2: **Expecting one set of eyewear to do the trick.** Even if you can get by with a pair of progressives, you may want to have more than one set of eyewear to get the best possible vision correction for different tasks.

For example, if you spend long hours in front of a desktop or laptop computer, you may need a prescription for single-vision glasses designed specifically for the distance between you and the screen. These glasses will help reduce eyestrain and fatigue, dry eyes and blurred vision.

Very helpful: Measure the distance from the bridge of your nose to your computer screen (laptop or desktop), and take this measurement to your eye exam. The American Optometric Association recommends that the computer screen be placed 20 to 28 inches from the user's eyes.

So-called "computer glasses" can even be made with lenses that selectively filter out harmful blue light, also known as high-energy visible (HEV) light. In the blue and violet part of the light spectrum, HEV is a particularly intense light wave that is emitted from electronic devices, including computers, tablets and smartphones. (Certain bands of blue light, such as blue-turquoise, are found in the sun's UV rays and are beneficial, aiding in color perception and vision sharpness.)

Studies published in the *Archives of Ophthalmology* show that chronic exposure to harmful blue light may damage the retina, the light-sensitive tissue of the eye, and may increase risk for eye disorders such as age-related macular degeneration and cataracts.

Single-vision eyeglasses designed specifically for computer work usually offer the best correction for heavy computer users. If you're over age 40, however, you may want to consider using bifocal computer glasses. This allows you to see the computer screen clearly and read written material on your desk.

For eyeglasses that are designed to block out harmful blue light and glare, you may want to talk to your eye doctor about the following high-quality lenses: Crizal Prevencia No-Glare blue-light lenses, CrizalUSA.com.

If you are a computer user and prefer progressives, ask your doctor about these well-crafted lenses: Zeiss Office lens, Zeiss.com (search "Office lens")...and Seiko PCWide, SeikoEyewear.com.

MISTAKE #3: **Opting for fashion over function.** Lots of people accept less than excellent vision in exchange for chic eyewear, but this can set you up for trouble.

Examples: If the frames are too big for you, your eyes will not be optimally centered, which could cause visual distortion...if you favor the look of small frames, there may not be enough room for the bifocal or progressive lenses you need.

Either way, you are increasing your risk for blurry vision, headaches and neck pain.

MISTAKE #4: **Not getting the right fit.** No matter what your prescription and frames, your eyes should sit precisely in the center of the eyeglass (this may not be the center of the frame) to see clearly.

Progressive lenses have the least room for error. If they're off by even a millimeter, you may have trouble seeing at all three distances.

Important: A precise fit is something online retailers can't offer. Sure, purchasing glasses online may save you money, but this could also prevent you from having clear and comfortable vision.

Better approach: Get your exam from an eye-care professional (optometrist or ophthalmologist), and purchase your glasses there for easy follow-up in case there are any problems.

Also: There is no reason to accept thick, "Coke-bottle" type lenses these days. The technology now is available for even very strong prescriptions to be made in relatively thin lenses.

MISTAKE #5: **Not getting double-checked.** Many people never revisit their eye-care specialists even if they suspect there's a problem.

Good rule of thumb: It may take up to three days to get used to a new prescription and frames—but if you're uncomfortable after that time, go back to the eye-care doctor who gave you the prescription.

Sometimes all it takes is a simple adjustment to your frames. In many people, for example, one ear sits slightly higher than the other, so such an adjustment is needed.

MISTAKE #6: **Getting hooked on drugstore readers.** You can't beat the price! And these simple reading glasses do offer various levels of magnification.

However, because these readers provide identical magnification in both lenses, they're a viable option only for people who need the same level of vision correction in both eyes—something that rarely occurs.

Many adults have a condition known as anisometropia, in which the eyes require significantly different prescriptions. In fact, a new study has found that nearly one-third of people over age 75 have the condition.

If you have anisometropia and try to get by with drugstore readers, your vision will not be as clear as it would be if you wore prescription readers—not to mention the ill effect it will have on your ability to complete your weekly crossword puzzle!

Surprising Eye Protector

American Academy of Ophthalmology annual meeting.

People with diabetes who took the diabetes drug *metformin* were only half as likely to develop age-related macular degeneration (AMD) as those not taking the medication.

Theory: The drug's inflammation-fighting properties may also help guard against AMD.

If I Have Glaucoma, Can I Get Cataract Surgery?

David F. Chang, MD, clinical professor of ophthalmology at University of California San Francisco and past president of the American Society of Cataract and Refractive Surgery. He is an international authority on cataract surgery who frequently lectures surgeons about advanced cataract techniques and the newest lens implants. He is coauthor of *Cataracts: A Patient's Guide to Treatment*.

Most patients who do not have significant vision loss from glaucoma—a condition in which the internal pressure of the eye is so high that it damages the optic nerve—can expect good results from cataract surgery. In fact, eye pressure frequently decreases in glaucoma patients after cataract surgery, which gives them a bonus benefit along with improved eyesight. (It's important to realize that any vision loss due to advanced glaucoma is permanent, and that portion of vision impairment can't be restored with cataract surgery.) If you have glaucoma and cataracts and want to treat the cataracts, it's important to get the timing right.

WHY TIMING IS IMPORTANT

Cataract surgery is recommended when blurry vision from the cataracts starts to interfere with daily tasks such as driving. However, because cataracts are the normal aging of the natural lens, delaying surgery won't actually damage the eye. On the other hand, glaucoma, if it isn't controlled, damages the optic nerve, causing permanent vision loss—so getting your glaucoma under control must never be delayed and takes priority over cataract surgery.

Once your glaucoma is under control, cataract surgery can frequently be done without any special precautions. Most people will continue using their pressure-reducing glaucoma drops immediately before and after cataract surgery. (Your doctor will let you know the specifics.)

If your doctor believes that it would be safer to reduce your eye pressure even further, he/she may suggest combining cataract surgery with a new type of glaucoma surgery to reduce your eye pressure.

Called minimally invasive glaucoma surgeries (MIGS), these procedures (there are several variations) are safe and usually don't lengthen the recovery time from the cataract operation. Studies have shown that when combined with cataract surgery, MIGS devices reduce the eye pressure more than cataract surgery alone would have. Traditional "filtering" glaucoma surgeries reduce eye pressure the most, but these are more invasive than MIGS. They carry more risk, require a longer recuperation and are reserved for patients with more advanced glaucoma.

A MIGS procedure involves implanting a tiny drainage device, or stent, in the eye. Typical stents reduce eye pressure by increasing the fluid outflow through the eyeball's natural drainage system. Although they will not "cure" your glaucoma, a stent might reduce the number of glaucoma medications you need.

Cataract surgery is the ideal time for MIGS because the stent can be inserted through the same incision made for cataract removal.

Many glaucoma patients also wonder whether having glaucoma reduces their chances for successful cataract surgery. In general, the answer is that unless you already have significant vision loss from the glaucoma, you can expect good results from cataract surgery.

Exercise Fights Glaucoma

Victoria Tseng, MD, PhD, ophthalmologist, UCLA Jules Stein Eye Institute, California.

The most physically active people (those who exercised moderately to vigorously 30 minutes a day, five days a week) were 73% less likely to develop glaucoma than the least physically active, according to a study that tracked 5,000 adults over several decades.

Theory: Exercise may change the blood flow to the optic nerve or affect intraocular pressure. More study is needed.

Study Shows That Hearing Loss Is Linked to Dementia

Frank R. Lin, MD, PhD, assistant professor, division of otology, neurotology and skull base surgery, Johns Hopkins School of Medicine, core faculty, Center on Aging and Health, Johns Hopkins Medical Institutions, Baltimore.

How many times have you heard someone say, "I'd love to live to 100 or more—if I had my wits about me!" Fear of dementia is something that worries most everyone at some time or another because there seems so little to do to treat or avoid it. But now researchers have discovered a fascinating link between dementia and hearing loss—and that link may offer helpful strategies for all of us concerned about our wits...

GREATER HEARING LOSS = GREATER RISK OF DEMENTIA

First let's look at the study, which took place in Baltimore at the National Institute on Aging. Johns Hopkins assistant professor of otology Frank R. Lin, MD, PhD, and his colleagues followed more than 600 adults between the ages of 36 and 90 for approximately 12 years. None of these people had had dementia, but about 25% had some level of hearing loss at the beginning of the study. Over time, 9% developed dementia—with two-thirds of these having Alzheimer's.

In analyzing their data, Dr. Lin and his colleagues discovered that participants who had hearing loss at the beginning of the study were significantly more likely than the others to develop dementia. Specifically, they found that the risk for dementia increased even in those with only mild hearing loss (25 decibels) and rose further as hearing worsened. In fact, for each 10 decibels of hearing loss, there was a 20% jump in dementia risk!

So does hearing loss cause dementia? Dr. Lin explained his findings: "There are three different pathways through which hearing loss may contribute to dementia," he said. *These are...*

- **A common brain pathology.** To some extent, basic neuronal aging in the brain may lie at the root of both hearing loss and dementia—in which case, there is little we can do to improve the symptoms that a patient is struggling with. But as you'll see in the instances below, there are indeed chances for significant improvement.

- **Hearing loss itself.** Dr. Lin and his research team speculate that for people with hearing loss, the strain of decoding ill-heard messages over the years puts a load on the brain that may lead to cognitive decline. Your brain might be compelled to reallocate vital resources to help with hearing at the expense of cognition, exhausting your cognitive reserve, Dr. Lin said. "That may explain in part why straining to hear conversations over background noise in a loud restaurant can be mentally exhausting for anyone, hard of hearing or not," he added.

- **Social isolation.** Hearing loss often triggers social inactivity, which is itself strongly associated with dementia. In an unrelated 2011 study at Rush University Medical Center in Chicago, investigators found that older adults (average age 80) who enjoyed the highest level of social interaction had only one-quarter the level of cognitive decline experienced by the least social individuals.

When we address the problems of hearing loss and social isolation, we could possibly affect the second two pathways and potentially delay the onset of dementia, Dr. Lin observed. These findings were published in the February 2011 issue of *Archives of Neurology*.

REDUCE YOUR RISK FOR DEMENTIA

Interventions that slow dementia even by just one year could lead to a 10% drop in its prevalence over the coming decades, say researchers. *While further study is necessary to identify which interventions are most effective, many are dictated by common sense...*

- **Get a hearing aid.** If you have difficulty hearing, the Johns Hopkins study gives you a powerful new reason not to ignore it out of stubbornness or vanity, as many people do. Today's digital hearing aids not only offer much better sound quality than previous technology, they also can be quite small and discreet.

- **Learn to use your hearing aid properly.** At the audiologist's office, practice putting in and taking out your hearing aid...cleaning it...replacing batteries…and adjusting volume. Continue to work with your audiologist until you feel comfortable and satisfied. Your audiologist will also help you tune your hearing aid for your specific needs.

• **Take advantage of other hearing assistance.** Use the hearing-assistance systems now available in many concert halls, theaters, museums and places of worship…and choose telephones (home, cell and office) with built-in amplifiers. There are many models available now.

• **Socialize your way to a sharper brain.** Visit friends and family, attend parties, join a book or bridge club, volunteer and/or attend religious services. The latest research suggests that socializing is just as important—and maybe even more important—in keeping your mind sharp than solitary brainteasers like crossword puzzles.

"A lot of people ignore hearing loss because it's a slow and insidious process as we age," Lin said. But even if it creeps up on you, chances are that deep down you know that your hearing isn't what it should be. If that describes you, let your doctor know, and take care of your hearing to take care of your brain!

Your "Memory Problems" May Actually Be Due to Hearing Loss

The study "Considering Age-Related Hearing Loss in Neuropsychological Practice: Findings from a Feasibility Study" was conducted by a neuropsychology and cognitive health research team at Baycrest, a geriatric care program affiliated with University of Toronto, and published in *Canadian Journal on Aging*.

Forgetfulness can be frustrating…and frightening, causing you to worry that you have early symptoms of Alzheimer's disease if you can't remember what your spouse told you to pick up at the grocery store, for example, or the name of the restaurant where your friend said to meet.

But don't be too quick to panic.

A Canadian team of researchers recently took a closer look at 20 older adults who were undergoing cognitive evaluations and discovered that "forgetfulness" may have more to do with a person's hearing than an actual memory problem.

When clinical neuropsychologists analyzed the cognitive evaluations of the study participants, along with assessments of their hearing, 56% of those being tested because they were concerned about memory/thinking problems and possible brain disorders had some degree of hearing loss, ranging from mild to severe, with only about 20% of them wearing hearing aids. Interestingly, 25% of the individuals who were worried about potential memory problems had no signs that a brain disorder was causing their forgetfulness.

Because none of us can remember what we never heard, this research suggests that hearing difficulties can masquerade as forgetfulness. Even when a person's brain is otherwise healthy, hearing loss can cause communication problems, social isolation and loneliness—all of which are associated with an increased risk for dementia. Getting treatment for hearing loss can help preserve your physical and mental well-being.

Takeaway: If you're concerned about your memory, ask your primary care doctor to perform a hearing examination in addition to cognitive testing. On the basis of your results, your doctor may give you tips on how to communicate better…suggest an over-the-counter sound amplifier…or recommend that you see an audiologist for a full workup. These hearing professionals can determine the best way to improve your hearing…and if that includes the use of a hearing aid, they can explain how to correctly operate and maintain it. To find an audiologist near you, visit the American Academy of Audiology's website (Audiology.org) for a searchable list.

Important: Today's hearing aids are not the big, ugly, screechy appliances that your grandparents used. They are much more sophisticated now, and some are barely noticeable. They can be expensive, though—typical costs, which usually aren't covered by insurance, range from $800 to $4,000 per ear—so be sure to work with a professional who can help you find what's right for you.

Prevent Hearing Loss

Murray Grossan, MD, an otolaryngologist and head and neck surgeon with the Tower Ear, Nose and Throat Clinic at Cedars-Sinai Medical Center in Los Angeles. He is coauthor of *The Sinus Cure: 7 Simple Steps to Relieve Sinusitis and Other Ear, Nose, and Throat Conditions.*

Normal aging can undoubtedly impair hearing, but millions of Americans suffer unnecessarily from hearing and other ear problems that can largely be avoided. *Most common preventable causes of hearing loss—and my advice...*

NOISE

Loud noise is one of the primary causes of hearing loss. The vibrations from loud noise damage the sensory structures (hair cells) of the inner ear. This damage permanently impedes the hair cells' ability to transmit the electrical signals to the brain that allow us to hear.

Exposure to loud noises before about age 15, when the ear is most vulnerable, is usually the most damaging, but sounds that we hear every day, such as sirens, also can reach the threshold for ear damage in people of any age.

Rule of thumb: If people must speak louder than usual to be heard, the setting is noisy enough to warrant taking precautions to avoid hearing problems.

Best prevention strategies...

- **Stick your fingers in your ears to block the sound of passing sirens.** A siren on an emergency vehicle can produce up to 140 decibels—loud enough to cause permanent damage after a single exposure.

Important: If you suffer hearing loss and/or ringing in the ears (tinnitus) after exposure to loud sounds—from a siren or gunshots, for example—see a doctor if these symptoms have not subsided within 24 hours. Your doctor can prescribe medication that may help restore hearing.

- **Wear ear protection in the yard and/or garage.** Earmuffs that have a rubber seal and completely cover the outer ear (available online for $14 to $40) are more effective than earplugs at blocking the noise from power tools, drills, saws, vacuums, chain saws and lawn mowers. Airplane mechanics use this kind of earmuff.

- **Get a set of customized earplugs** (available from most hearing-aid dealers for about $25) if you go to car racetracks, work at a construction site, attend loud concerts or spend time in other noisy environments. Customized earplugs are designed to exactly fit an individual's ear canals.

- **Consider buying noise-canceling headphones** (available at most electronics stores and online for about $130 to $300) if you listen to digital music players (such as iPods with earbuds or earphones) in noisy environments.

These headphones block external sounds—from jet engines and crowds, for example—so you don't have to turn up the volume so high on your digital music player, which increases the risk for ear damage. Digital music players are safe when used at a normal volume in a quiet room.

EARWAX

Earwax (cerumen) lines the ear canal and keeps bacteria-promoting dirt and debris from reaching the eardrum. Old wax normally moves out of the ear canal as new wax is secreted, usually every three months. But some people have a genetic tendency to produce excessive wax, which can fill the ear canal and cause hearing loss, a feeling of "fullness" in the ears and/or ringing in the ears.

The only way to know if earwax is causing hearing loss is for a doctor to examine the ear canal. If you know you've had problems with earwax in the past, you may want to try to remove it at home. *My advice...*

- **Apply several drops of a wax-dissolving medication** (such as Debrox or Murine Ear Drops) that contains carbamide peroxide twice daily for up to four days. After the wax is softened, use a bulb syringe to gently flush the ear with body-temperature water. Do not insert the syringe beyond the entrance to the ear canal—if you block the canal, injury may result. If symptoms, such as hearing loss, don't improve within four days, your doctor may need to remove the wax with irrigation and suction.

Caution: Avoid cotton swabs. People who attempt to remove wax from the ear canal with a cotton swab are more likely to compress it than remove it, making it harder to remove and leading to painful pressure on the eardrum.

EAR INFECTIONS

Ear infections are very common in children, but adults get them, too. The infection usually occurs in the middle ear—often following a cold or another viral infection—and can be intensely painful. Ear infections can lead to permanent hearing loss. *My advice...*

- **Blow your nose gently.** Blowing too vigorously can force mucus and bacteria from the nose into the eustachian tube, which connects the middle ear to the back of the nose. When blowing your nose, do it slowly and gently—and do not press on one nostril while blowing out the other.

AIRPLANE EAR

The rapid changes in air pressure that occur when flying—particularly during takeoff and landing—can cause the eardrum to bulge outward or pull inward.

Result: A condition called barotrauma, which causes pain, discomfort and/or fluid buildup in the middle ear, can lead to temporary hearing loss. *My advice...*

- **Don't sleep during takeoffs or landings.** You need to be awake to yawn, chew gum or open your mouth—all of which open the eustachian tube. Opening the tube allows air to flow in and stabilize the pressure.
- **Use enzyme lozenges.** Pineapple and papaya enzymes (available at health-food stores) reduce swelling of the eustachian tube and relieve congestion. Don't chew the enzyme lozenges—acids in the stomach will neutralize the enzymes. Let them melt between the cheek and gums.

Recommended dosage: One lozenge three times on the day before the flight and again on the day of flight.

- **Drink hot tea.** Both black and green teas contain chemicals that stimulate the nasal cilia (tiny hairs that protect the respiratory tract from dust and other pollutants), which helps open the eustachian tube. Drink a cup or two of hot tea before and during the flight.

Important: If you have a cold or allergies, use a decongestant nasal inhaler, such as *propylhexedrine* (Benzedrex), or a decongestant, such as *pseudoephedrine* (Sudafed)—now sold "behind the counter"—before the plane takes off. Reducing congestion makes it easier for the eustachian tube to open.

Losing Your Sense of Smell?

Richard L. Doty, PhD, FAAN, director of the Smell and Taste Center and professor of psychology in otorhinolaryngology: head and neck surgery at the Perelman School of Medicine, University of Pennsylvania, Philadelphia. He is an internationally recognized expert on taste and smell dysfunction and author or editor of 11 books, including *The Great Pheromone Myth* and *Smell and Taste Disorders.*

If you've noticed that your sense of smell (aka olfaction) isn't what it used to be, you're not alone. For some 20 million Americans, the ability to detect everyday smells, from baking bread to burning wood, is slipping away...or even gone.

Why this matters: Even though primary care physicians rarely ask patients about loss of smell, it can be an early red flag for certain chronic medical conditions.

A MULTITASKING SENSE

Few people appreciate the multitude of daily functions tied to their sense of smell. *This all-too-often neglected sense serves as...*

- **A key to appetite.** Smell is responsible for most of our sense of taste. People with a diminished sense of smell often have a poor appetite, remarking that food is tasteless or just doesn't taste the same. While taste buds can distinguish basic levels of sweet, sour, bitter, salty and umami (a savory, earthy taste), smell also plays an important but often underappreciated role in our ability to taste foods.
- **A harbinger of serious disorders.** A diminished sense of smell is often an early symptom of Parkinson's disease and Alzheimer's disease. In fact, smell dysfunction is the most common early symptom reported by Parkinson's patients even be-

fore they suffer motor-related symptoms, such as tremors or walking difficulties.

A HARD-TO-SPOT DEFICIENCY

Because few primary care physicians test for smell problems, you need to be alert for any suspected loss of this sense.

This can be challenging because the loss of smell that tends to occur with aging happens gradually, and most people with health problems don't recognize that they have lost their sense of smell. For example, loss of smell is present in about 90% of people with Parkinson's disease, but most don't recognize that they have a problem.

Self-defense: Even if you only suspect a change, you should report this to your doctor. If there is no obvious reason for the loss of smell, such as a cold, allergies or nasal congestion, then smell testing is recommended.

SMELL TESTING

A number of tests are available to assess one's ability to smell. These range from simple three-item scratch-and-sniff screening tests...the 16-item Sniffin' Sticks odor identification test that uses felt-tip pens to dispense odors...to longer tests, such as the 40-item University of Pennsylvania Smell Identification Test (UPSIT).* With the 15-minute UPSIT, you are asked to smell a series of odors (such as rose, pizza, cinnamon and mint) and identify each odor from a list of choices.

The UPSIT, which can be ordered by physicians online for a nominal cost, helps doctors to determine both the absolute and relative (to one's age and sex) degrees of smell loss.

TREATMENT OPTIONS

The first step in treatment is to identify the cause of the smell loss. Olfactory problems related to Parkinson's disease or brain damage are generally believed to be irreversible, but early detection is helpful in planning medical treatment.

There is strong evidence in a 2013 paper published in *JAMA Otolaryngology–Head & Neck Surgery* that regular exercise can help to maintain the ability to smell in later life, much like it can help to avert or delay the onset of dementia. However, it is not known whether exercise can reverse such impairment once it is present.

If the loss is due to simple inflammation, including that caused by chronic sinusitis, then treatment with powerful anti-inflammatories (such as corticosteroids) may bring back some sense of smell. Oral steroids typically restore smell function within about a week. Continued topical therapy with steroid sprays or washes can, in some cases, maintain the restored function. If nasal polyps are to blame, surgical removal can be helpful.

Promising therapy: Some evidence shows that the antioxidant alpha-lipoic acid may help one regain the sense of smell in certain cases, such as long-lasting dysfunction due to upper respiratory infections. The suggested dosage is 400 mg to 600 mg daily.

Important: Before trying alpha-lipoic acid, talk to your doctor. This supplement has been shown to lower blood sugar, so people with diabetes need to use caution. It could also interact with some medications, including antibiotics, anti-inflammatories, tranquilizers, heart medications and chemotherapy drugs.

Another option: Small amounts of smell-restoring alpha-lipoic acid can be found in foods.

Good sources: Organ meats (such as kidneys and liver)...spinach...and broccoli.

Are you at risk?

There are dozens of possible causes for smell loss. *Among the most common...*

- **Aging.** With age, the nerves that are involved in smell weaken, and odor-detecting membranes lining the nose become thin and dry.
- **Smoking.** Because it irritates nasal passages, smoking impairs one's sense of smell. The good news is that normal smelling function can return in less than a year after quitting in light smokers and over the course of several years in heavy smokers—providing another reason to quit.
- **Air pollution.** Research published in 2016 in *Environmental Health Perspectives* noted that the tiny particulates in polluted air enter the nose, cross

*Dr. Doty is president of Sensonics International, the manufacturer and distributor of the UPSIT.

through the olfactory bulb and actually enter the brain. There the stray microparticles, commonly found in diesel exhaust and air pollutants, can induce an inflammatory response that can lead to brain tissue damage, the development of Alzheimer's-like pathology and a loss of smell.

- **Certain medications.** More than 70 medications can affect one's sense of smell. The list includes heart drugs, such as the cholesterol-lowering medication *atorvastatin* (Lipitor) and blood pressure drugs such as *amlodipine* (Norvasc) and *enalapril* (Vasotec), and some decongestant nasal sprays. Unfortunately, there is not much data indicating whether stopping such drugs will reverse smell loss.

- **Head injury.** Even a relatively minor head injury, as might occur when one hits the back of the head on the pavement after slipping on ice, can permanently damage the delicate nerve connections to the brain that control your sense of smell.

Coping with Taste or Smell Disorders

Ronald DeVere, MD, a board-certified neurologist and medical director of the Taste & Smell Disorders Clinic in Austin, Texas. Dr. DeVere is coauthor of *Navigating Smell and Taste Disorders*.

Smell and taste disorders can severely affect a person's quality of life, especially social interactions. Since meals are no longer enjoyable, dining with family and friends loses much of its attraction.

With dysosmia (distorted sense of smell) and dysgeusia (distorted sense of taste), eating becomes so unpleasant that it can lead to dangerous weight loss and, in severe cases, malnourishment. Depression is also common among these patients.

The inability to taste or smell properly also can be dangerous, as sufferers may inadvertently eat, say, spoiled meat or not detect the smell of leaking gas.

HOW TO COPE

Because the majority of smell and taste disorders are due to age-related damage of the smell or taste receptors in the nose and/or mouth and the nerve pathways, there is no specific treatment for these types of problems with smelling.

However, if your smell loss is due to a vitamin B-12 or zinc deficiency or low thyroid levels, treating these conditions should help. If you are suffering from a loss or distortion of smell or taste, it's wise to consult an ear, nose and throat doctor or a neurologist.

If smell loss is due to an ailment such as a cold, improvement usually occurs over time—anywhere from six months to three to four years.

Interesting finding: When the University of Pennsylvania did a 20-year follow-up study of individuals with various types of smell impairment, many of them continued to improve over 10 to 20 years.

If your smell or taste disorder is caused by medication, simply switching to a different prescription may be the answer.

For people who have dysosmia (a distorted sense of smell that's often unpleasant), it often helps to use one to one and one-half teaspoons (three to four times daily) of normal saline and squirt it into each nostril with a small syringe. Do this while in the head-down position so that the saline forms a film of fluid over the nerve cells that identify odors and different flavors. This helps prevent outside odors from getting to the injured smell system. This approach works for about half of all sufferers.

Also helpful: Off-label use of medications such as the antiseizure medication *gabapentin* (Neurontin) can block abnormal electrical impulses that occur in dysosmia. Such medication helps decrease or stop dysosmia in about 60% of patients with the disorder.

Removal of the olfactory bulb is often a last-ditch effort to remove the bad smells and is very successful. Partial loss of smell will result, but loss of taste does not usually worsen after surgery.

The bad tastes of dysgeusia can be helped by trying Cepacol anesthetic lozenges, Xylocaine gel or lidocaine mouthwash and/or the medication gabapentin.

COOKING TRICKS

Because smell and taste disorders inhibit one's ability to fully savor and enjoy food, many of my patients with partial smell or taste loss have learned to change the way they prepare meals, emphasizing texture, temperature, tartness and spiciness.

Even if you have a taste impairment due to smell loss, you can still appreciate some basic tastes, textures and temperatures. *For example, it helps to...*

- **Add spicy salsa to a baked potato** (instead of sour cream, which has no flavor in the smell impaired). Try other spicy condiments, such as horseradish or mustard.
- **Marinate meats with sweet fruit juices, sweet wine or sweet-and-sour sauce.**
- **Eat tart foods,** such as grapefruit and oranges.

Trouble Swallowing?

JoAnne Robbins, PhD, a leading specialist in swallowing disorders and professor in the department of medicine at the University of Wisconsin School of Medicine and Public Health in Madison. She is coauthor of *Easy-to-Swallow, Easy-to-Chew Cookbook*.

Eating and drinking are among life's greatest pleasures, yet about 15 million Americans have difficulty swallowing foods and/or liquids, a condition known asdysphagia.

Everyone knows what it feels like when a bite of food "gets stuck" or a sip of liquid "goes down the wrong pipe." It's an uncomfortable but rare problem that can be corrected by coughing or drinking a small amount of liquid.

However, when dysphagia begins to occur with greater frequency (generally, more than once per month), you should see your doctor to determine the cause. Prompt treatment will help you avoid serious complications, such as dehydration, malnutrition, choking and aspiration (when food or liquid leaks into the airways), pneumonia and even death.

Caution: If a swallowing problem leads to an obstruction that interferes with your breathing in any way, have someone perform the Heimlich maneuver on you.

What to do: While standing behind you, the person should place the thumb side of his/her fist just above your navel...grasp his fist with his other hand...and give four quick inward thrusts. This should be continued until the obstruction is removed. If this technique does not help, have someone call 911. If you are alone, you can perform the inward thrusts on yourself.

ARE YOU AT RISK?

Aging can affect our ability to swallow. That's because our muscles, including those in the mouth and throat, weaken as we grow older. Even healthy adults may begin to notice subtle swallowing and eating problems, such as difficulty swallowing pills or eating dry or crunchy foods, by age 60. However, serious problems are not a normal sign of aging and should be promptly evaluated by a doctor.

Several medical conditions can cause dysphagia. Chronic heartburn increases risk for dysphagia—stomach acid backs up into the esophagus, sometimes damaging esophageal tissue, which may lead to swallowing difficulties. A stroke or head injury may affect the coordination of the swallowing muscles or limit sensation in the mouth and throat. Neurological disorders, such as Parkinson's disease and multiple sclerosis, also can cause swallowing problems.

A tumor in the esophagus can narrow this passageway, making it difficult to swallow. Surgery, radiation and chemotherapy for head and neck malignancies also can irritate the esophagus and/or lead to a buildup of scar tissue that interferes with swallowing.

Related problem: About 2,000 medications, ranging from diuretics (water-excreting drugs) to drugs used to treat such conditions as insomnia, can cause xerostomia, a drying of the mouth that often makes swallowing food difficult.

GET A CORRECT DIAGNOSIS

A primary care physician often is the first health-care professional to suspect dysphagia. Depending on the cause of the disorder, you may be referred to an otolaryngologist (ear, nose and throat specialist), a gastroenterologist (specialist in diseases of the digestive system) or a neurologist (specialist in diseases of the nervous system).

A process known as video fluoroscopy is the most common and effective way to diagnose dysphagia. This test videotapes the entire swallowing process so the doctor can see how a patient's tongue and throat movements affect the flow of food, fluid and medication.

BEST TREATMENT OPTIONS

Treatment for dysphagia depends on what's causing the disorder. People with heartburn can make lifestyle changes, such as not eating for at least two hours before bedtime, and/or take medications, such as *ranitidine* (Zantac) or *omeprazole* (Prilosec), to reduce stomach acid. People who have suffered a stroke may be asked to perform muscle exercises to strengthen weak facial, tongue and throat muscles.

Dysphagia improves for some people when they follow certain practices while eating, such as turning the head to one side or looking straight ahead with the chin tucked toward the chest. These steps help direct food and fluids away from the airway and into the esophagus.

TIPS ON EATING AND DRINKING

What helps one individual with a swallowing difficulty may not help another. However, there are many basic strategies that allow people to swallow food and drink with greater ease. *For example...*

- **Sit upright in a chair while eating**—do not eat in bed.
- **Swallow a single bite or sip before taking another,** and put eating utensils down between bites.
- **Limit bite sizes (to one-half inch or less) and the amount of liquid taken with each swallow.**
- **Eat one type of food texture at a time.** Swallow a bite of mashed potatoes, for example, before chewing and swallowing a piece of chicken.
- **Choose soft foods,** such as cooked cereal, mashed potatoes, soft-cooked eggs, cottage cheese, applesauce, yogurt and soups.
- **Thicken thin fluids,** such as tea, apple juice and water, if necessary. This allows more time for throat muscles to get into position to ensure safe swallowing.

Natural thickeners include many flours (tapioca flour is often used), instant potato flakes and oats. To determine the amount of natural thickener to be added to a liquid, ask your doctor for a referral to a nutritionist or speech and language pathologist (a clinician with expertise in swallowing problems).

Sounding "Old" Is Not About Age

Study titled "Voice Changes in Elderly Adults: Prevalence and the Effect of Social, Behavioral, and Health Status on Voice Quality" by researchers at Research Institute and Hospital, National Cancer Center, Gyeonggi, and University of Ulsan, Seoul, both in South Korea, published in *Journal of the American Geriatric Society.*

If you read *Little Red Riding Hood* aloud to a child, you probably make Grandma's voice weak and quavering to sound "old." But the truth is you can have a strong voice at any age—unless you have a specific health problem...one that affects your whole health, not just your vocal chords.

In a recent study of 420 seniors (average age 72) with dysphonia, the medical term for decreased ability to produce a normal voice, South Korean researchers found that, compared to statistical averages, they were 300% more likely to have a particular medical condition—low thyroid function.

The condition, called hypothyroidism, is easy to overlook because many of the symptoms—constipation, fatigue and sensitivity to cold—are also symptoms associated with aging. While the new study doesn't prove causation, it does suggest that in an otherwise apparently healthy 60-plus person, a weakening voice could be a clue—perhaps the only clue—to this health-compromising condition.

So if you have a "grandmotherly" or "grandfatherly" voice or know someone who does, speak up—to a doctor. Ask him/her to test your thyroid function.

15

Staying Safe

Agility Exercises That Prevent Falling

Michelle Gray, PhD, assistant professor of kinesiology, department of health, human performance and recreation, University of Arkansas, Fayetteville, and codirector, Office for Studies on Aging, College of Education and Health Professions, also at University of Arkansas.

Agility, meaning the ability to quickly change speed and/or direction, decreases with age. That, in turn, increases the odds of falling—for instance, when someone darts out in front of you unexpectedly—setting the stage for the bone fractures that can rob you of your mobility, your independence and even your life.

Self-defense: Safeguard your agility with an easy and fun workout that you can do at home using an inexpensive type of exercise equipment called agility cones. And if you think you're too young or too fit to benefit from agility cones, think again. Pro football players do versions of this workout all the time—and they know what works!

Agility cones look like those orange traffic cones you see on the highway but smaller. They are typically six to 12 inches high and can be purchased at sporting-goods stores or online for as little as $2 apiece. You'll need four cones—but if you want to give this agility workout a try right now, you can start out by using overturned plastic drinking cups or empty plastic jugs. Then if you like the workout and want to stick with it, go ahead and invest a few dollars in the cones—with their bright color and stabilizing base, they'll be easier to see and less likely to topple than a cup or jug.

The workout below was suggested by Michelle Gray, PhD, assistant professor of kinesiology at the University of Arkansas. The movements promote agility because they require the vestibular (balance) system of the inner ear to work in concert with the muscular systems, especially the very fast-twitch "type IIx" muscle fibers that allow you to move suddenly, Dr. Gray explained.

Do the following workout at least twice a week. Use a long hallway or large room indoors...or go outdoors. Make sure that you're on a surface free of any objects you could trip over.

Throughout: Move as quickly as you can while still maintaining control—don't push any faster than you can safely go. Try not to knock over any cones, since object avoidance is part of being agile. For each exercise, complete two or three sets, taking a brief rest between sets.

If you have a history of falls: Stick with just the first easy exercise until your agility improves and you feel confident about moving on to the intermediate and advanced exercises...and check with your doctor each step of the way.

EASY: UP-AND-GO

Setup: Place one agility cone eight feet in front of a sturdy chair.

Sit in the chair.

Move: Rise from your seated position, walk quickly to the cone, maneuver around it in a clockwise direction, return to the chair and sit back down. Repeat 10 to 15 times—that's one set. For the next set, maneuver around the cone in a counterclockwise direction.

INTERMEDIATE: WEAVE IN/WEAVE OUT

Setup: Arrange four cones in a straight line, each about eight feet apart. Stand next to the first cone in the line.

Move: Walking quickly, weave in a zigzag pattern between the cones. When you reach the last cone in the line, walk around it and return, again weaving between the cones, to your starting position. Repeat two or three times—that's one set.

ADVANCED: SQUARE DRILL

Setup: Arrange four cones in a square, with each side of the square measuring 10 to 15 feet. Stand to the outside of any cone, with the cone next to your right foot (we'll call this cone number one).

Move: Facing forward and moving around the square clockwise, walk quickly toward the outside of cone number two. When you reach it, switch to a sideways walk or shuffle, moving to your right toward cone number three. When you reach it, turn your body and walk or shuffle sideways to your left toward cone number four. When you reach it, turn your body and carefully walk backwards toward cone number one. Repeat two or three times—that's one set. For the next set, start with your left foot at the outside of cone number one and move around the square counterclockwise.

After you've mastered these moves: Work on safely increasing your speed...try the drills with one eye closed, then the other...get creative and invent your own agility exercises...or watch a football team practice to learn some new agility drills you can try.

Catch Your Balance Problem Before It's Too Late: These Easy Exercises Could Save Your Life...

Jason Jackson, MSPT, a physical therapist in the outpatient rehabilitation department at Mount Sinai Hospital in New York City, where he specializes in balance training, along with prosthetic training, manual therapy and neuromuscular disease.

No one expects to get seriously injured—or even die—from a fall. But it happens all the time. And while older adults are at greatest risk for falls, there are no age requirements for taking a tumble.

Surprising statistic: Even among adults in their 30s, 40s and 50s, falls are the leading cause of nonfatal injuries (more than 3 million each year) that are treated in US hospital emergency departments. For adults age 65 and older, falls are the leading cause of fatal injuries.

Certain "fall hazards" are well known—electrical cords and area rugs...slippery floors...medications such as sleeping pills and blood pressure drugs...vision problems...and even poorly fitting shoes.

What often gets overlooked: Subtle changes in the neuromuscular system (the nervous system and muscles working together), which helps keep us upright. Regardless of your age, exercising and strengthening this system before you get unsteady (or fall) is one of the best steps you can take to protect your health. *Here's how...*

WHY OUR BALANCE SLIPS

Does your foot or ankle feel a little wobbly when you stand on one leg? Some of that is probably due to diminished strength and flexibility. After about age 40, we begin to lose roughly 1% of our muscle mass every year. As we age, we also become more sedentary and less flexible. These factors make the body less able to adapt to and correct a loss of balance.

The nervous system also gets less sensitive with age.

Example: Sensory receptors known as proprioceptors are found in the nerve endings of muscles, tendons, joints and the inner ear. These receptors make us aware of our bodies in space (proprioception) and can detect even the slightest variations in body positions and movements. But they don't work well in people who don't exercise them (see suggestions below)—and these people find it harder to keep their balance.

The other danger: Muscle weakness, even when it's slight, can lead to apprehension about losing your balance. You might then start to avoid physical activities that you feel are risky—walking on uneven pavement, for example. But avoiding such challenges to your balance actually accelerates both muscle and nervous system declines.

ARE YOU STEADY?

If you're afraid of falling or have a history of falls, a professional balance assessment, done by your doctor or a physical therapist, is the best way to find out how steady you are on your feet. *The assessment usually includes tests such as the following (don't try these tests on your own if you feel unsteady)...*

• **Sit-to-stand.** Sit in a straight-backed chair. If your balance and leg strength are good, you'll be able to stand up without pushing off with your hands.

• **Stand with your feet touching.** You should be able to hold this position for 15 seconds without any wobbling.

• **The nudge test.** Ask someone to gently push on your hip while you're in a normal stance. If you stagger or throw out your hands to catch yourself, your balance is questionable. If you start to fall, your balance needs improvement.

BOOST YOUR BALANCE

Balance, like strength and endurance, can be improved with simple workouts. Incorporate the exercises below into your daily routine—while at the grocery store, in the office, while watching TV, etc. Do them for about 15 minutes to 30 minutes a day, three to four days a week (daily if you have the time). *What to do...**

*Do these exercises next to a stable object, such as a countertop, if you feel unsteady. Also, they are more easily done while wearing shoes. When you feel comfortable doing these moves, you can perform them barefoot to add difficulty.

• **One-legged stands.** You don't have to set aside time to do this exercise. You simply stand on one leg as you go about your daily activities—while waiting in line, for example. Lift your foot about six inches to 12 inches off the floor to the front, side and back. Try to hold each position for about 15 seconds, then switch legs. This strengthens the muscles in the ankles, hips and knees—all of which play a key role in one's balance.

• **Heel raises.** This move is good for balance and strength. While standing, rise up on your toes as far as you can. Drop back to the starting position, then do it again. Try for 10 repetitions. You can make this exercise more difficult by holding weights. Start with three-pound weights, gradually increasing weight as you build tolerance.

FOR MORE BENEFITS

Once you have become comfortable with the exercises described earlier, you can up your game with the following to keep you even safer from falling...

• **Balance on a Bosu ball.** It's a rubberlike half-ball (about two feet in diameter) that you can use for dozens of at-home workouts, including balance and abdominal exercises.

Cost: About $100, on Amazon.com and in some sporting-goods stores.

Example: With the flat side on the floor, start by standing with both feet on the ball. Your muscles and joints will make hundreds of small adjustments to keep you balanced. When you get better at it, try to stand on one leg on the ball. When you're really comfortable, have someone toss you a basketball or tennis ball while you maintain your balance.

JUST FOR FUN

You don't always need formal balance exercises. *Try this...*

• **Walk barefoot.** Most of us spend our days in well-padded shoes that minimize the "feedback" between our feet and the ground. Walking without shoes for at least a few minutes each day strengthens the intrinsic muscles in the feet and improves stability. If you prefer to wear socks, be sure to use nonslip varieties that have treads to avoid slipping on wood or tiled floors.

Also helpful: Minimalist walking/running shoes. They're made by most major footwear companies, such as New Balance, Adidas and Nike, as well as by Vivobarefoot. Because they have a minimal amount of heel cushioning and arch support, they give the same benefits as barefoot walking but with a little extra protection.

10 Ways to Protect Yourself from Dangerous Falls

Marilyn Moffat, PT, DPT, PhD, professor of physical therapy at New York University, and author of *Age-Defying Fitness*.

With all the systems contributing to the ability to stay upright, problems in just one area can make people vulnerable to falls. For instance, loss of vision with age makes people fearful of falling—that anxiety itself actually increases the likelihood they'll fall. In addition, the brain and nervous system decline in function with age, which can lead to problems with depth perception and coordination and timing of movement. As a consequence of these and other changes, aging adults may move tentatively and slowly, taking smaller, shuffling steps and often keeping their eyes focused on the ground—all of which set them up for a fall.

However, the news is not all bad. With commitment, practice and time, fall-resistance training can absolutely turn the situation around. For people who are unfit or have serious problems maintaining their balance, a physical therapist should do an initial examination to determine where weaknesses lie and how extensive the problem is, in order to develop an individualized exercise program to do at home or at a fitness club.

AT-HOME TECHNIQUES

If you are reasonably fit, though, you can start your balance fitness training right now in your own home. *Here are some ideas on how to get going...*

- **Walk on tip-toes.** How long has it been since you walked on your tip-toes? Probably years, but this childhood diversion is excellent for strengthening your ankle and calf muscles and for improving balance. Marilyn Moffat, professor of physical therapy at New York University, suggests going up and down on your toes as often as possible, including as you brush your teeth each day and while you walk around the house.

- **Walk in all directions and different ways.** Since staying upright requires adapting to different types of movements, a good workout should include movement in different directions and ways. Try walking backward, both on your feet and your toes. Also try walking on your heels...tandem walking (one foot directly in front of the other)...sidestepping...and doing grapevines (walking sideways alternating front and back with the feet).

- **Look around.** Switch your gaze around, from side to side as well as up and down as you stroll. Be careful to avoid tripping—for instance, keep one hand on a hallway wall.

- **Balance yourself.** Soon you should be able to multitask while practicing balancing—several classic techniques are to cross your arms, then stand on one foot, then the other...another is to stand on one foot while holding onto a counter, then close your eyes. (For more on basic balance exercises, see previous article.)

- **Vary your gait.** Change it up, from long strides to short steps, suggests Dr. Moffat, who considers methodical gait training a very important motor skill.

- **Speed up, slow down.** Walk at a normal pace, accelerate, slow down, speed up...and do it again and again.

- **Exaggerate.** Deliberately exaggerate your typical heel-to-toe pattern... then try it with a high-step gait.

- **Vary your footwear.** Go barefoot, wear a variety of shoes.

- **Change the surface.** Switch from stable to unstable surfaces—walk on tile floors, carpeted floors, the beach, gravel...these are good ways to reinforce your ability to sense where your foot is on the ground.

•**Heads up.** It's crucial to break the habit of gazing at the ground while you walk. Looking down throws off your postural alignment, which makes correct body responses more difficult. After a short time, you will find that walking with your head held high feels good, and it is not at all scary.

Extra benefit: It may help you avoid neck/back problems.

Practice balance activities every day of the week, incorporating a variety of techniques into your usual routine. This should require no more than 10 to 15 minutes of your day and in about eight weeks' time, she says you should see a big difference in your balance, your gait and your confidence.

Surprising Medications That Increase Your Risk of Falling

Jack Fincham, PhD, RPh, professor of pharmaceutical and administrative sciences at Presbyterian College School of Pharmacy in Clinton, South Carolina.

Read the package insert for any medication and you'll likely see dizziness listed as a possible side effect. Still, few of us take dizziness seriously. But we should. Dizziness can lead to a fall...and that could lead to a serious injury.

MORE MEDS, MORE RISK

More than half of all Americans are taking two prescription medications—20% are taking five or more, according to Mayo Clinic research. So it's important to recognize that side effects, including dizziness, are more pronounced with every drug you take. The increased effects are not additive—they are exponential. After a while, the question is not if you will fall, but when. Falls are one of the leading causes of long-term disability in older adults.

Here are widely used medications that commonly cause dizziness and falls. Chances are you use at least one of the following medications.

PAIN MEDICATIONS

The risks of opioid pain medications (including disorientation and dizziness) are well known, but there is an increased fall risk even with over-the-counter (OTC) pain relievers. These seemingly benign medications influence many body systems, including the central nervous system (CNS), and can cause dizziness, even at normal doses.

Examples: Nonsteroidal anti-inflammatory drugs (NSAIDs), such as aspirin, *ibuprofen* (Advil) and *naproxen* (Aleve).

Surprisingly, aspirin may be the worst offender. In addition to its effects on the CNS, aspirin bombards the vestibular nerve that feeds balance information from the inner ear to the brain. Many people can't take aspirin (even the baby aspirin dose of 81 mg) without experiencing severe dizziness or even vertigo—the nauseating perception that the room is spinning or tilting.

Note: Muscle relaxers are also sometimes prescribed for pain. These drugs cause significant drowsiness.

Examples: *Carisoprodol* (Soma), *cyclobenzaprine* and *orphenadrine*. When paired with a pain reliever, the combination of dizziness and drowsiness is a perfect recipe for a fall.

SLEEP AIDS AND ALLERGY DRUGS

Diphenhydramine is an antihistamine recommended to clear a stuffy nose and induce drowsiness at bedtime.

Examples: Benadryl, Tylenol PM, Advil PM and Aleve PM.

Like aspirin, diphenhydramine affects the CNS and the vestibular system, causing dizziness. It also slows down mental abilities such as thinking and processing information, so you may be less able to recognize side effects.

Because this drug is included in medications as a sleep aid, many people assume that they can sleep away the side effects. But diphenhydramine has a long half-life—in older adults, it can stay in their systems for up to 18 hours. The medication-induced dizziness can cause a fall if you get up during the night, for example, to use the bathroom.

ANTIDEPRESSANTS

All antidepressants work at the level of neurotransmitters—the chemical messengers, such as *serotonin, norepinephrine* and *dopamine*, that allow us to think, act and experience emotion.

The most widely used antidepressants are selective serotonin reuptake inhibitors (SSRIs), which work by making serotonin more available to the brain, elevating mood and decreasing anxiety.

Examples: *Fluoxetine* (Prozac), *paroxetine* (Paxil) and *sertraline* (Zoloft).

Migraine drugs also work by affecting serotonin availability.

Examples: *Sumatriptan* (Imitrex) and *zolmitriptan* (Zomig).

Serotonin and norepinephrine reuptake inhibitors (SNRIs) are a newer type of antidepressant that makes both serotonin and norepinephrine more available to the brain.

Examples: *Duloxetine* (Cymbalta), *venlafaxine* (Effexor) and *desvenlafaxine* (Pristiq).

Bupropion (Wellbutrin) affects the availability of both norepinephrine and dopamine.

Note: The smoking-cessation medication Zyban also contains bupropion.

Besides affecting mood, these antidepressants carry messages to the brain from the balance centers of the inner ear, so they can affect your equilibrium. In addition, a faulty message can make the communication between brain and body less responsive. When you stand up or move, you may be less able to control your body position, increasing the risk of toppling over.

BLOOD PRESSURE DRUGS

There are many types of blood pressure medications, including…

- **Diuretics** ("water pills"), such as *furosemide* (Lasix).
- **Beta-blockers,** such as *propranolol* (Inderal) and *atenolol* (Tenormin).
- **Angiotensin-converting enzyme (ACE) inhibitors,** such as *enalapril* (Vasotec) and *lisinopril* (Zestril).
- **Angiotensin II receptor blockers (ARBs),** such as *losartan* (Cozaar) and *olmesartan* (Benicar).
- **Calcium channel blockers,** such as *amlodipine* (Norvasc).

All medications that lower your blood pressure can also diminish your ability to quickly adapt to changing blood pressure needs, such as when you change your body position. Therefore, a common side effect of these drugs is orthostatic hypotension—a sudden spell of light-headed dizziness that happens when you quickly stand up after sitting or lying down.

ANTICONVULSANTS AND NEUROPATHY DRUGS

Drugs for epilepsy, fibromyalgia and neuropathy can alleviate pain by putting the brakes on nerve impulse transmission. But this may limit the brain's ability to respond normally and quickly, significantly reducing alertness and increasing dizziness.

Examples: *Gabapentin* (Neurontin), *pregabalin* (Lyrica) and *carbamazepine* (Tegretol), all commonly used to treat diabetic nerve pain and fibromyalgia…and *clonazepam* (Klonopin) and *phenytoin* (Dilantin), both used as antiepileptic drugs.

WHAT TO DO

Literally every drug has the potential to cause dizziness and increase your risk of falling. *What to do…*

- **For occasional-use medications**—assess your level of discomfort. If you don't really need a drug, don't take it. If you must take a medication, develop an alternate plan that may include a medication change that is approved after consultation with your health-care provider.
- **For long-term medications**—never stop taking them without advice from your health-care provider. Many medications need to be tapered and will create rebound side effects if stopped abruptly.
- **For all new medications**—be alert for signs of dizziness or drowsiness. Are your body and mind as quick and responsive as usual? Do you feel alert? These side effects may be subtle or pronounced, but they should not be ignored. If they occur, avoid any activity that could result in a fall, including using stairs or ladders. If you must use stairs, steady yourself with handrails and move slowly up or down the stairs.

As your body adjusts to a medication, you may be prescribed a higher dosage to get the appropriate therapeutic effect.

Important: Watch for new side effects with each dosage change. They can appear even after the drug has been taken for an extended period.

• **If you experience orthostatic hypotension**—be sure to take your time standing up...and don't immediately start walking. Take a moment to steady yourself. If you become light-headed, sit down immediately. This practice is useful for anyone taking medication.

• **If you feel dizzy or have other troubling side effects while using any medication**—call your doctor...or talk to your pharmacist, who may be more accessible. Ask if there is another treatment that might have fewer side effects and less dizziness.

• **Before driving or exercising—observe how you are reacting to the medication.** Does an effect diminish in intensity after a while? If so, try to drive small distances and exercise carefully with companions to see how you are doing.

Natural Rx for Stronger Bones

Jamison Starbuck, ND, is a naturopathic physician in family practice and writer and producer of *Dr. Starbuck's Health Tips for Kids*, a weekly program on Montana Public Radio, MTPR.org, both in Missoula. DrJamisonStarbuck.com

---

Osteoporosis, a condition marked by weak and brittle bones, can't be felt and it isn't fatal by itself, but if you have it, you're much more likely to fracture a bone if you fall. And recent research points to greater risk for premature death following an osteoporosis-related fracture. Osteoporosis can't be seen either, but one possible tip-off is a loss of height. The condition affects both men and women, but most often postmenopausal women.

Conventional doctors often treat osteoporosis with calcium supplements and perhaps prescription drugs such as *alendronic acid* (Fosamax) or *raloxifene* (Evista). These medications can have side effects that range from joint pain to weakening of the jawbone with Fosamax...and hot flashes to chest pain with Evista.

Note: People with moderate-to-severe osteoporosis and/or a strong family history of osteoporosis may need medication.

I recommend calcium as well but prefer that patients get it from food. Although more research is needed, studies have indicated that getting too much calcium from supplements may increase risk for heart disease. Excess calcium can also cause constipation and lead to kidney stones. So if I do recommend a calcium supplement, I advise a calcium/magnesium combination (the magnesium reduces risk for constipation) along with 400 international units (IU) of vitamin D to aid absorption.

Many of my patients choose my protocol as their only treatment for osteoporosis, but it can be used in conjunction with prescription medication.

Important: It's also crucial for patients to not smoke (smoking increases risk for osteoporosis). *My osteoporosis prevention and treatment plan...*

• **Improve diet.** Studies show that people who eat foods that are low in minerals and vitamins are more likely to develop osteoporosis and experience a fracture than those who eat a diet emphasizing leafy greens, nuts, beans, whole grains, dairy and oily fish like salmon and sardines. That's because these foods contain lots of the nutrients necessary for healthy bone growth—calcium, magnesium and vitamins D and K. Get plenty of these foods in your daily diet.

Beware: Frequent alcohol consumption, diets high in meat protein and salt and drinking carbonated beverages daily all will increase your odds of osteoporosis.

• **Enhance digestion.** In addition to eating healthy foods, you have to be able to digest them effectively to get all of their benefits. Minerals and fat-soluble vitamins like D and K need plenty of stomach acid to be broken down and absorbed. Acids like fresh lemon juice and vinegar help speed up the breakdown of minerals and vitamins in your stomach so that they get absorbed into your bloodstream quickly. Just sprinkle some vinegar or fresh lemon juice (or any fresh citrus juice) on vegetables, fish and meat, and be sure to choose a vinaigrette salad dressing.

• **Optimize strength and balance.** Weight-bearing exercise helps build bone strength and stem bone loss.

Good options: Walking, dancing, lifting free weights and using resistance bands. Try to do weight-bearing exercise for 30 minutes, five times a week. Wearing a weighted vest when at home or when walking helps, too. Practicing yoga (even for just 15 minutes three times a week) gently develops muscles and balance.

Also: Practice walking on slightly uneven ground, like a footpath or dirt road—it will improve your balance and make you less likely to fall.

Your Bones Are in Danger

Neil Binkley, MD, professor in the divisions of geriatrics and endocrinology at University of Wisconsin (UW) School of Medicine and Public Health, Madison. He is director of the UW Osteoporosis Clinical Research Program and associate director of the UW Institute on Aging. Aging.wisc.edu

We've been told that the best way to prevent fractures is to prevent or treat osteoporosis—diet, exercise and, if needed, medications. But that approach has not been successful.

For people with osteoporosis, medications do prevent many spinal fractures—but fewer than half of hip and other fractures, according to a major study published in *The New England Journal of Medicine*. And many people who fall and break bones don't even have osteoporosis.

Example: An overweight or obese person may have good bone density (from carrying that extra weight) but still get fractures. Unless he/she has the muscle strength to carry that extra weight, mobility issues—such as difficulty getting up off the toilet or climbing stairs—can lead to falls that cause fractures. Rather than hip fractures due to weakened bones, they tend to get ankle or lower-leg fractures.

In the end, it's *preventing* fractures—from any cause—that really matters. Many of us think that if we break a bone, our friendly orthopedic surgeon will put it back together and life will go on as usual. But after age 50—and especially after age 65—a fractured bone can threaten independence and quality of life. And that's what we fear most about aging—losing independence...not being able to drive...and winding up in a nursing home. The classic example is a hip fracture, which often sends people to nursing homes and is linked to a shorter life span. But breaking an ankle, an arm or even a wrist can make daily life harder at home...and make it tougher to be mobile.

To find out what is really needed to prevent fractures, we spoke with geriatrician and endocrinologist Neil Binkley, MD. He started with a simple question—"What causes most fractures in older people?"

The answer: Falling.

Here's how to prevent falls—and the fractures that could end your independence...

• **Eat for muscle strength, not just bones.** Getting enough calcium and vitamin D—standard elements of osteoporosis prevention—still is important. But pay close attention to calories and protein, too. These are essential to maintaining muscle strength—and that's as important as strong bones in preventing fractures. After all, when our muscle strength declines, we fall. And when we fall on weak bones, guess what? They break.

Protein needs are based on your body weight. To calculate your individual needs, multiply your body weight by 0.45. For a 150-pound woman, that's 67 grams a day...for a 185-pound man, 83 grams. To get a sense of what that looks like, a three-ounce serving of tuna or salmon contains about 22 grams of protein and an egg contains six grams, on average. Aim to include good sources of protein—seafood, lean meat, poultry, eggs, nuts, seeds, soy and legumes such as beans and peas—at every meal.

For some older people, a waning appetite also can mean that they just don't eat enough calories. If you're not eating enough, a registered dietitian can help find practical ways to help you get enough protein and calories each day.

• **Get strong—and balanced.** Now that you're nourishing muscles, make them work. Exercise helps keep your bones and muscles strong, so it's vital for lowering your fracture risk. The best exercise is the one that you'll actually do, whether it's walking, biking, swimming or team sports. Beyond general fitness, exercises that improve core strength and balance are key to fall prevention. *Suggestions*...

• Join a tai chi class. This ancient Chinese set of gentle, slow-moving exercises strengthens lower limbs and improves balance. Several studies have found that practicing tai chi regularly significantly reduces fall risk in older adults.

• Yoga may help, too. It can strengthen bones, and while it is less well-studied for fall prevention, it has been shown to improve balance and mobility in older people.

• **Take fall-prevention classes.** One popular, evidence-based program is *Stepping On*, a seven-week, two-hours-per-week workshop, first developed in Australia, that now is offered in 20 US states. It is geared to healthy adults over age 65. One study, published in *Journal of the American Geriatrics Society*, reported that people who participated in Stepping On had 31% fewer falls over the next 14 months, compared with a similar group of people who didn't go through the program. To find programs like this in your area, check with the National Council on Aging's Fall Prevention website (NCOA.org/healthy-aging/falls-prevention).

• **Consider physical therapy.** If you've fallen and have been injured—even if you didn't break a bone—you're waving a red flag that a fracture could be in your future. A physical therapist can do a formal strength-and-balance assessment...show you exercises to strengthen muscles, bones, walking posture and balance...and help you find classes in your community.

• **Make your home safer.** A key part of fall prevention is taking a look at what you can do to make it less likely that you'll trip and fall...

• Do you have night-lights in your home? Consider putting a night-light in your bathroom for those middle-of-the-night trips.

• Are there throw rugs that you might slip on? Get rid of them!

• Is there clutter on the floor or stairs that you could stumble on? Declutter!

• Do you need to get on a chair or step stool to reach things on high shelves? Put everyday items on lower shelves that are easy to reach.

• Is it hard to get in and out of your bathtub without slipping? Consider installing grab bars or replacing your tub with a walk-in shower.

Some of your safety changes may need to be in your own behavior—such as drinking less alcohol. That's a fall risk that many older people don't consider.

And don't forget to get your vision checked regularly. If you can't see it, you can trip on it.

• **Review your medications.** Some medications (prescription or over-the-counter) or medication interactions can cause dizziness, light-headedness or low blood pressure, which can increase the risk of falling. Key medications to be aware of include antihistamines, sleep aids, pain pills, antidepressants and antianxiety medications. In addition, some medications, such as glucocorticoids (steroids taken for inflammatory and autoimmune conditions) contribute to bone loss. If you are taking medications that increase your fall risk, talk to your doctor to see if you can reduce the dose, find an alternative—or modify how you take it, such as only at bedtime.

It's not that strong bones aren't important—they're a key part of a fracture-prevention plan... but only one part. If your doctor has prescribed a diet, exercise program or medication for you to prevent or treat osteoporosis, continue following those instructions. Osteoporosis medications often are prescribed based on an individual's estimated risk for fracture. For individuals at high fracture risk, the benefits of reducing that risk far outweigh the risk of side effects. But just taking medications is not enough.

Now you know what else you need to do to protect yourself.

MORE FROM NEIL BINKLEY, MD

This Exercise Prevents Falls

One of the simplest and most effective exercises—and one that you can do almost anywhere—is the Chair Rise. Do this daily to strengthen the muscles in your thighs and buttocks, which can help keep you steady on your feet and prevent falls...

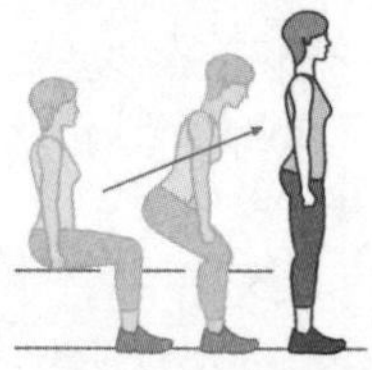

- **Sit toward the front of a sturdy chair,** with your knees bent and feet flat on the floor, shoulder-width apart.
- **Rest your hands lightly on the seat on either side of you,** keeping your back and neck straight and chest slightly forward.

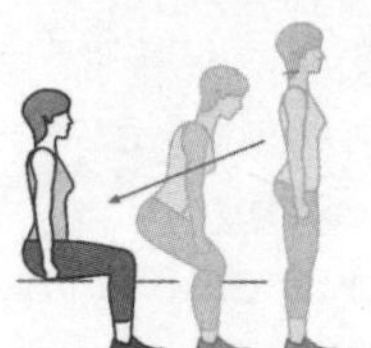

- **Breathe in slowly.** Lean forward and exhale as you stand up—feel your weight on the front of your feet.
- **Pause for a full breath in and out.**
- **Breathe in as you slowly sit down.** Try not to collapse down into the chair. Rather, control your lowering as much as possible.
- **Breathe out.**

Repeat for a total of 10 to 15 stand/sits. Rest and breathe for a minute, then do another set of 10 to 15. You may need to work up to this level over several days or a few weeks. The goal is to get to the point where you can complete two sets without using your hands at all.

Are Calcium Supplements Now Safe for Your Heart?

Connie Weaver, PhD, distinguished professor and head of the department of nutrition science at Purdue University in West Lafayette, Indiana. She is an expert on mineral bioavailability, calcium metabolism and bone health.

Until a few years ago, taking a daily calcium supplement was considered a safe, effective way to protect against the bone loss that comes with aging and to reduce the risk for fractures—especially for women, who are more prone to osteoporosis than men.

Then the standard advice came under fire...big time. Not only was serious doubt raised about calcium's usefulness in preventing fractures, but some studies suggested that calcium supplements actually cause harm—increasing the risk for heart disease.

Now a large new British study—with more than half a million subjects—appears to show that calcium supplements actually are safe for your heart. Should we believe this study? Are calcium pills suddenly safe again? And even if they are, do we really need them to keep our bones strong?

To get answers, we spoke with Connie Weaver, PhD, distinguished professor and head of the department of nutrition science at Purdue University in West Lafayette, Indiana. She is a world-renowned mineral and bone-health expert.

THE GREAT CALCIUM/HEART DEBATE

A little background: Until 2010, the only serious health concern from taking calcium was thought to be a very small increase in the risk for kidney stones. But that year, in a study published in *The BMJ*, New Zealand researchers analyzed several studies of people (mostly women over age 70) who took calcium supplements. They found that calcium supplements were associated with a 30% increase in the risk for heart attack and a smaller increase in the risk for stroke. Even calcium supplements that contain vitamin D, which other studies have suggested protects the heart, were associated with a small increased risk for heart attack and stroke, the same team reported in 2012.

Such statistical links can never be proof of causation, however, and from the start some researchers had their doubts about whether this danger would turn out to be real. The New Zealand researchers speculated that taking calcium supplements gives the body a surge in calcium all at once, which then ends up in our arteries and contributes to the formation of plaque, the substance that leads to atherosclerosis (hardening of the arteries).

Yet animal studies conducted at Purdue University (and elsewhere) showed no such mechanism, notes Dr. Weaver. When animals were given high levels of calcium as supplements (or as dairy products), "there was no increased calcification of arteries."

Even the statistical link was an outlier. In a comprehensive review of studies by the US Preventive Services Task Force (USPSTF), a government panel of 16 experts that evaluates health research and makes official health recommendations, none showed any increased cardiovascular risk.

The 2010 and 2012 calcium studies got plenty of press, though, and suddenly people were seriously worried that the calcium they were taking was hurting their hearts...and some stopped taking it.

The new British study, presented in April 2016 at the World Congress of Osteoporosis, Osteoarthritis, and Musculoskeletal Diseases, dealt a strong new blow against the heart-harm hypothesis. More than a half-million participants ages 40 to 69 were followed for seven years. Their use of calcium with or without vitamin D was tracked over the entire period of the study. Then the researchers analyzed their heart-disease–related hospitalizations and deaths, using hospital records.

Result: No link was found between calcium or calcium/vitamin D supplementation and hospital admissions or death related to heart disease.

Bottom line? To Dr. Weaver, this large new study—combined with the fact that nearly all other studies have found no heart risk and that careful animal studies find no plausible mechanism—make a compelling case. Her conclusion? "The new research adds to the now large body of evidence that there is no cardiovascular risk of calcium supplementation."

BUT DO YOU NEED A CALCIUM SUPPLEMENT?

Just because calcium pills are safe for the heart, though, doesn't mean you should take them. According to the USPSTF, there simply isn't enough evidence to recommended a calcium/vitamin D supplement for the prevention of fractures—even in postmenopausal women. It's true that in postmenopausal women, as well as in older men, calcium plus vitamin D supplements halt bone loss and modestly increase bone density, but there's no good evidence that any particular supplementation level will actually prevent fractures.

Still, there's no question that both calcium and vitamin D are important for bone health. For men age 71 and older and women age 51 and older, the Institute of Medicine's current recommended dietary allowance (RDA) for calcium is 1,200 mg.

To get enough, and to protect your bone health, Dr. Weaver recommends an approach that starts with dietary calcium and vitamin D and looks to supplements only if necessary...

- **Eat plenty of calcium-rich foods,** especially dairy foods such as milk and yogurt (by far the most calcium-dense foods)—but also nondairy calcium-rich foods such as kale, broccoli and turnip greens. Nuts, especially almonds and hazelnuts, also are good sources of calcium, as are canned sardines and canned salmon (be sure to eat the bones).

Tip: If you're a yogurt fan, eat some traditional American-style yogurt, not only Greek-style yogurt—traditional American has twice as much calcium, ounce for ounce.

- **Factor in fortified foods.** Many foods are fortified with calcium, including orange juice, breakfast cereal and soy foods such as tofu and soymilk. Remember to include these amounts when adding up your daily calcium intake.

- **If you're not getting enough dietary calcium, discuss taking a supplement with your health-care provider.** A typical serving of most dairy foods includes about 300 mg of calcium. Nondairy foods contribute, but you would need about three cups of cooked kale to get to that 300 mg. Add in the calcium in fortified foods that you eat daily (check labels), and if you're still below 1,200 mg, consider a supplement for just what you're missing.

For vitamin D, the RDA is 600 IU for people age 70 and younger. For those 71 and older, the RDA is 800 IU. It's very hard to get this amount without taking a supplement.

- **Eat a wide variety of whole foods.** Many nutrients contribute to bone strength and the prevention of osteoporosis, not just calcium and vitamin D but also boron, manganese, silicon, zinc, magnesium and potassium. Eating enough protein is important, as is moderating how much sodium and caffeine you consume and eating plenty of fruits and vegetables. To increase your body's ability to absorb calcium, especially if you are over age 50, Bottom Line's medical consultant, naturopathic doctor Andrew Rubman, ND, advises also taking digestive enzyme supplements that include betaine HCL.

Attention Men: This Bone Danger Can Kill You

Harris H. McIlwain, MD, founder of McIlwain Medical Group in Tampa and former chair of the Florida Osteoporosis Board. He is board-certified in rheumatology, internal medicine and geriatric medicine. He is the pain expert for Dr. Oz's ShareCare.com website and is a coauthor of *Reversing Osteopenia*.

If you're a man, here's something important you probably don't know—about 25% of men will have an osteoporosis-related bone fracture in their lifetimes, and a man's risk of dying in the year following a hip fracture is twice as high as a woman's.

Women try to protect themselves against osteoporosis because rapid bone loss is a hallmark of menopause. Men eventually will lose as much bone strength as women, but it happens more slowly and later in life—and the consequences of ignoring it can be terrible. *Here's what men need to know to protect their bones...*

MALE BONE LOSS

Bone is always breaking down and building up. This process, known as remodeling, depends on things such as exercise, vitamin D and calcium intake, hormone levels and other factors. Osteoporosis (or osteopenia, an earlier stage of bone loss) occurs when more bone is lost than gained.

Women can lose 20% or more of their total bone mass within just five years of menopause. Men are somewhat protected but only at first. They have more bone mass to begin with...are more likely to have been physically active, which builds bone...and don't have the same midlife estrogen changes that deplete bone. But men may lose bone when testosterone levels are low. Men tend to have their first bone fractures about 10 years later than women.

By the time men have reached their 70s, their osteoporosis risk is the same as women's. In severe cases, the bones can become almost paper thin. This can lead to fragility fractures—bone breaks that are caused by seemingly minor mishaps such as stepping off a curb in an unusual way or merely bumping into a doorframe.

RISK FACTORS

With a few exceptions (see below), men don't need to be tested for osteoporosis until about age 65. Before that age, they should assume that they'll eventually lose bone and start taking steps to prevent it.

The DEXA (dual-energy X-ray absorptiometry) test, which measures bone density at the hip and spine (and sometimes in the wrist), usually costs between $100 and $200 and often is covered by insurance. It assigns a T-score, a measure of your bone density. A negative reading (for example, a score of –1) indicates some bone loss. A score of –2.5 means that you have possible early osteoporosis. Anything lower indicates serious bone loss.

Most at risk: Older men who are underweight are up to 20 times more likely to get osteoporosis than heavier men. Smoking greatly increases bone loss. So does low testosterone, lung disease and a poor diet. Some drugs used to treat prostate cancer and other diseases (including some lung diseases) cause bone loss as a side effect.

Men with any of these risk factors should get tested earlier—say, at about age 50. So should men who have suffered fragility fractures. The fractures usually occur in the hips or spine, although wrist and shoulder fractures also are common. (Broken fingers and toes aren't considered fragility fractures.)

WHAT WILL SAVE YOUR BONES?

Men with early osteoporosis (or a high risk of getting it) can improve their diet, take calcium and vitamin D supplements, and get more exercise. Such men probably won't need medication right away—or ever. *Steps to take...*

• **Plenty of exercise.** Forty minutes a day is ideal. It's the best way for middle-aged men to build bone mass and for older men who already have osteoporosis to slow the rate of bone loss. Research has shown that people who exercise will have fewer hip or spine fractures than those who are sedentary.

• **Weight-bearing exercises—walking, lifting weights, playing tennis, etc.**—are the most effective at slowing bone loss.

My advice: Take frequent walks. Many people enjoy walking more than other forms of exercise, and it's foolproof. It doesn't matter whether you walk slow or fast—simply standing up and working against gravity stimulates bone growth in the hips and spine.

• **More calcium.** You can't build strong bones without calcium. Unfortunately, most Americans don't get enough. The problem is compounded in older adults, who absorb dietary calcium less efficiently. Men and women need a daily calcium intake of 1,000 milligrams (mg) up to age 50 and 1,200 mg thereafter.

Important: The guidelines include the calcium that you get from foods and supplements. There's no reason to take a high-dose calcium supplement if you also get plenty of calcium from dairy, fortified juices or high-calcium foods such as sardines with bones. For most people, a 500-mg calcium supplement is enough—take more if you tend to avoid calcium-rich foods. Your body absorbs calcium more efficiently when it is taken in smaller amounts (500 mg or less) several times a day. Taking 50 mg to 100 mg of magnesium a day also helps with absorption.

• **Add vitamin D.** You can't absorb calcium without enough vitamin D in your system, and older adults' bodies are not very efficient at using sun exposure to create the needed form of vitamin D.

My advice: I recommend taking 1,000 units of vitamin D-2 daily. Check with your doctor to see how often you should get your blood levels tested to make sure that you're getting enough.

• **Go easy on the colas.** Research has shown that people who consume a lot of cola (but not other carbonated beverages) tend to have lower hipbone densities. It could be that the phosphoric acid in colas reduces calcium absorption or that people who drink a lot of soft drinks tend not to consume calcium-rich foods in general and need to be aware of this. I agree with the National Osteoporosis Foundation recommendation to have no more than five cola soft drinks a week.

• **If you smoke, do everything you can to quit.** Smoking interferes with the hormones that you need for bone strength...decreases blood supply to bones...and slows the production of bone-forming cells. By the age of 80, smokers are about 71% more likely to have bone fractures than nonsmokers.

MEDICATIONS

Men with more advanced disease may need medication. Some of the same drugs used to treat osteoporosis in women also work in men. Bisphosphonates such as Fosamax and Actonel slow the rate of bone loss. The most common side effects include heartburn or an upset stomach. Using bisphosphonates for more than five years has been linked to two rare but serious side effects—thighbone fracture and osteonecrosis (bone death) of the jaw. Prolia, a different type of drug, helps prevent fracture and requires an injection every six months. Discuss this drug with your physician because it too has osteonecrosis of the jaw and thighbone fractures as possible side effects of long-term use. For men with low testosterone, hormone replacement will help increase bone mass and reduce the risk for fractures. Testosterone replacement should be done only under the guidance of a physician because too much testosterone has been linked to stroke and heart attack.

A Dangerous Birthday

Sita Slavov, PhD, professor of public policy at George Mason University in Fairfax, Virginia, reported by Bob Barnett, former editor, *Bottom Line Personal*, BottomLineInc.com.

If you're over 62, you've beaten the odds. In an analysis from Boston College's Center for Retirement Research, researchers discovered a 2% jump in male mortality at age 62. That early death risk was almost entirely concentrated in the 10% of men who quit working at age 62—early retirement. (Women are less likely to quit work at 62 and didn't face increased risk of dying at that age.)

Of course, one reason that some people stop working early is because they're in poor health, so their risk of dying young is higher. But other factors were at play, too. Leaving the workforce can be risky all by itself—men tend to drive more after retiring early, and there's a spike in fatal traffic accidents...some men become more sedentary...and smokers tend to smoke more, so deaths from lung cancer and COPD go up.

So is retirement unhealthy? I asked Sita Slavov, PhD, professor of public policy at George Mason University in Fairfax, Virginia, who has researched that topic.

Key finding: Ultimately, retirement increases both life satisfaction and health. Indeed, after retirement, people tend to get more physical activity, spend less time in sedentary pursuits—and finally get enough sleep. But not right away. Those healthy habits are actually stronger four years after retirement than in the first year.

What's tricky is the transition. Leaving the workforce—whether you're 62 or 72—is a time of enormous personal change, and many of us don't prepare for it enough.

Bottom line: The first year of retirement is a dicey time for your health and safety, so consciously use that year to take better care of yourself—so you can enjoy the fruits of your labor for many years to come.

How Not to Turn into an "Old Driver"

Richard A. Marottoli, MD, associate professor of medicine at Yale School of Medicine and medical director of the Dorothy Adler Geriatric Assessment Center at Yale-New Haven Hospital, both in New Haven, Connecticut.

As you buckle yourself into a two-ton metal machine and rocket down the road at 60 miles per hour or faster, you may ask yourself, "Am I as safe a driver as I used to be?" This can be a legitimate concern even if you're in robust health and still a long way from being a senior. For instance, you may no longer be able to turn your head far enough to look behind you.

Safety concerns become increasingly relevant as the years pass.

Consider: Compared with drivers age 55 to 64, those over the age of 65 are almost twice as likely to die in a car crash...drivers age 80 and older have higher crash-fatality rates than all other age groups except teens.

Aging affects driving ability in several vital ways...

- **Vision and hearing become less acute.**
- **Cognition slows,** impairing the ability to recognize and react appropriately to a hazard (such as a child dashing into the street).
- **The physical ability to operate a car** may be impaired by stiff joints, muscle pain, nerve damage and other maladies.

Advancing age also brings increased frailty. This means that, even if driving skills remain sharp, the ability to recover from accidents decreases.

The modern world also presents hazards that older drivers may not be accustomed to. More than ever, drivers around you are likely to be distracted by cell-phone calls, text messages and GPS devices. These distractions greatly increase the risk for accidents.

NEW RULES OF THE ROAD

Avoid dangerous situations...

- **Use routes that minimize left turns**—they are more dangerous than right turns. When waiting to turn left, keep your wheels straight so you won't be pushed into oncoming traffic if hit from behind.

- **On the highway, stay in the right lane whenever possible.** There's less risk of being tailgated, and you probably won't need to change lanes to exit.
- **Minimize travel on congested or poorly lit roads.**
- **Do not drive in rain or snow or when you feel tired or stressed.** Stay home or call a taxi.

See and be seen...

- **To determine if you're tailgating**, pick a spot that the car in front of you passes, then count the seconds until you reach that spot. If it's less than three seconds—or six seconds in rain or fog—back off.
- **Use your window defroster on high heat to clear window fog quickly...**then switch to cool air (not cold) to keep fog from coming back. This works in all weather.
- **Keep your windows clean inside and outside.**
- **Be on the watch for distracted drivers.** Stay focused yourself, too—don't talk on the phone or eat or fiddle with the CD player or have emotional conversations with your passengers.
- **Keep headlights on, even during the day**—it makes you more visible to others. Clean headlights often.
- **If you have poor night vision, drive only in daylight.**

Master new car technology...

- **Put your seat as far back as you comfortably can to avoid being injured by the air bag if it deploys.**
- **Tilt the steering wheel so that the air bag points toward your chest, not your head.** If your steering wheel telescopes, move it closer to the dashboard to lessen air bag impact.
- **If you skid, do not "pump" anti-lock brakes**—just brake steadily.

HEALTH CHECKS

Work with a health-care team...

- **Ask your doctor if any of the medications you take can cause drowsiness or light-headedness.** If you start a new drug, avoid driving for a few days until you see how it affects you.
- **Have your vision checked every year or two.**
- **Get a hearing test every three years.** If you have hearing loss, watch dashboard indicators because you may not notice strange engine noises.

Also: Be vigilant about watching for emergency vehicles.

SHOULD YOU TAKE A CLASS?

The more of the following factors that apply to you, the more advisable it is to take a refresher course in driving. *Take it as a clue if you...*

- **Often are honked at by other drivers.**
- **Sometimes have trouble staying in your lane.**
- **Occasionally think that vehicles or pedestrians have appeared out of nowhere.**
- **Caused a recent accident.**

Many insurance companies offer discounts to drivers who pass a refresher course. Contact your insurance agent for more information.

Some classes can be completed in one or two days...some you do at your own pace.

Bonus: Classes review your state's laws, which may have changed—for example, many older drivers are unaware of certain states' requirements to signal at least 100 feet before turning.

Refresher courses are given online and in classroom settings. A course that includes several hours of behind-the-wheel training is most beneficial, though this can add significantly to the cost. For schedules and pricing, contact AARP (888-227-7669, AARP.org/drive) or your local AAA club (AAA.com).

PUTTING DOWN THE KEYS

It's time to consider leaving the driving to others if you have taken a refresher course and yet still experience any of the following...

- **Often feel lost or confused on familiar roads.**
- **Occasionally hit the gas when you mean to hit the brake.**
- **Hear that other people worry about your driving or are scared to ride with you.**
- **Have been advised by your doctor to stop driving.**

If you stop driving...

• **Find out about public transportation options**, including discounted fares for seniors.

• **For referrals to civic groups that provide rides**, contact your local council on aging (800-677-1116, ElderCare.gov).

• **Ask nearby friends for rides (and offer to pay for gas).** Many people are happy to help out.

How to Survive 6 Deadly Driving Emergencies

Ben Collins, author of *How to Drive: Real-World Instructions from Hollywood's Top Driver.* He is a professional race-car driver and stunt driver based in Bristol, England. BenCollins.com

One moment you are driving down the road, the next moment your brakes fail...your throttle sticks...or a tire blows out. Respond wisely and quickly to automotive emergencies such as these, and there's an excellent chance that you and your car will escape unharmed.

Unfortunately, drivers' initial panicked responses often make these situations worse. Even drivers who remain calm sometimes do the wrong thing—the conventional wisdom on how to handle certain driving emergencies is dangerously flawed.

Here are simple and effective strategies for dealing with six worst-case driving scenarios...

TIRE BLOWOUT

A tire comes apart as you drive down the highway. Suddenly it feels as if you are driving on a rumble strip. Many drivers' first reaction is to slam on the brakes, but doing that is likely to put the car into a spin, making a bad situation much worse.

Response: Hold the steering wheel firmly so that you stay in your lane—the car might try to pull to the side of the blowout—and slowly lift your foot off the accelerator. Keep your steering slow and steady. Then ease your vehicle to the shoulder and coast to a stop. Don't brake until your speed is below 50 miles per hour.

Exception: If you experience a blowout with a heavily loaded vehicle while going quickly around a sweeping curve, there might be no way to avoid spinning out. If you already are in a spin, slamming on the brakes could be your best option.

Warning: Keep in mind that run-flat tires are not designed to run flat forever. If they are not repaired or replaced soon after going flat, they, too, can blow out. If your car is equipped with run-flats, your vehicle owner's manual should provide details about how far and fast your run-flats can be safely driven after a flat.

STUCK ACCELERATOR

You take your foot off the accelerator, but your car continues to go faster and faster. This could be the result of an electronics issue, though more often the problem is a rusted accelerator pedal hinge or a dislodged floor mat pressing down on the pedal. Whatever the cause, it is one of the most terrifying experiences a driver can have, causing many drivers to freeze up.

Response: Get the car out of gear. If it has a manual transmission, this is easy—simply depress the clutch pedal. If it has an automatic transmission, you will have to shift into neutral. It might take some force to get the shift lever out of gear while the vehicle is moving. The engine will make an ugly over-revving sound when it is taken out of gear, but this can be done and it typically won't hurt the motor.

If you're the passenger in a car with a stuck throttle and the driver freezes up, you can reach over and shift the car into neutral yourself.

Meanwhile, brake hard. Brakes alone often are not sufficient to stop a car when its accelerator is stuck, but they can bleed off much of the vehicle's speed and bring you to a stop once you get the car out of gear.

If the cause of the stuck throttle is not something you can easily diagnose and correct—you can fix an out-of-place floor mat, for example—have the car towed to a mechanic before driving it again.

Warning: Do not turn off the ignition in response to a stuck throttle unless all else fails. This ends the acceleration, but it also turns off the power steering and power-assist braking, rendering the speeding car virtually uncontrollable.

BRAKE FAILURE

You press down the brake pedal, but your car won't stop—and you're rapidly approaching an intersection...stopped traffic...or some other danger.

Response: Pump the brake pedal several times quickly. This should build up hydraulic pressure in the brake line and/or dislodge something that is jammed underneath the pedal.

If that doesn't work, downshift into increasingly lower-numbered gears if your car has a manual transmission...or shift into "low" if your car has an automatic transmission. The engine will make noises of protest when you downshift, but the damage caused should be minimal.

Meanwhile, gently engage the hand brake (or parking brake) until it is fully engaged, and alert other drivers by using your hazard lights or honking your horn.

Have the vehicle towed to a mechanic unless the problem is easy to identify and correct, such as a bottle lodged under the brake pedal.

If your brakes fail as you descend a steep mountain road, however, brake overheating is probably to blame. Once again, downshift through the gears as described above, and engage the hand brake until it is fully engaged. The hand brake is attached to the car's rear brakes, which likely are still working well—it is the front brakes that tend to overheat. Do not engage a hand brake abruptly, however, or you could put the car into a slide or spin.

After you come to a stop, let your brakes cool for at least 20 minutes before driving.

STEERING FAILURE

Your power steering fails, and suddenly your steering wheel feels extremely heavy. Modern cars are tremendously difficult to turn without power steering.

Response: Use all your strength to maneuver the car to the shoulder or any other safe spot, then park and call for a tow truck. You can brake to reduce speed, but often the steering will get even heavier as the car slows. If you don't have the strength to steer the car, put on your hazard lights and stop the vehicle.

Better yet, prevent this emergency before it occurs. Power steering usually does not fail all at once—if your car's steering seems to be becoming heavier, take it to a mechanic as soon as you possibly can.

BLOCKED WINDSHIELD

You're driving down the highway when suddenly your hood flies open and completely blocks your view...or a rock hits your windshield causing it to spiderweb so badly that you cannot see through it.

Response: If you're on an open stretch of road with no cars following closely, hold the wheel straight and brake hard. But if you're on a busy road, slamming on the brakes could cause an accident. Here the best option is to hold the wheel straight, lift your foot off the accelerator, lower your window and stick your head out far enough so that you can see the road ahead. That should provide sufficient visibility to steer the car to a spot where you can park and correct the problem or call for a tow.

SINKING CAR

You crash off of a road or bridge into deep water. The conventional wisdom is to wait until the car is nearly full of water before trying to open your car door and escape—we're told that water pressure will pin the doors shut until then—but following that advice could kill you.

Response: Disconnect your seat belt as soon as your car hits the water, unlock the electronic car-door locks and immediately try to force the door open. Urge any passengers to do the same. Cars sometimes float on top of the water for a moment or two before beginning to sink, so it might be possible to push the doors open before external water pressure builds.

If you can't quickly get your door open to escape, immediately lower your windows and escape that way (if there are passengers in the car, lower their windows, too, if you can do so from the controls on your driver's door). Electric window controls often fail when cars go into deep water, but they don't necessarily do so immediately.

If you can't open the doors or windows, try to break a window. If there is something heavy within reach, such as a steering wheel lock, use that. If not, remove one of the car's headrests (if the car has removable headrests), jam one of its metal posts into the seam where the window emerges from the door, and then pry upward until the glass shatters. (You may want to keep in your car an emergency escape tool that cuts seat belts and breaks windows, such as LifeHammer. This is available online and at stores that sell auto supplies.)

Only if all of these options fail should you follow the conventional wisdom of trying to open the car door once the car is nearly full of water, equalizing internal and external water pressure. This should be considered the last-ditch option because if it fails, there are no more backup plans—you'll be out of air.

Gadgets That Make Driving Easier and Safer

Donna S. Stressel, occupational therapist at Sunnyview Rehabilitation Hospital in Schenectady, New York, a certified driver rehabilitation specialist and a driving instructor in the state of New York.

No longer being able to drive and losing your feeling of independence can be traumatic, and you're not likely to hang up your keys without a fight. Well, maybe you don't have to! If you're not as capable and confident behind the wheel as you used to be, whether due to a physical issue such as arthritis or to diminished vision, there are many devices that can help you stay on the road longer—safely. We talked to Donna S. Stressel, an occupational therapist and certified driver rehabilitation specialist, who recommended products that can help remedy the most common issues facing older drivers, as well as drivers of any age with disabilities or mobility issues...

- **Larger mirrors.** If you have trouble turning your head or are regularly vexed by blind spots in your side-view or rearview mirrors, clip-on or replacement mirrors can help. Blind-spot side-view mirrors from AutoSportCatalog.com that attach on top of existing side-view mirrors are a good choice. With these add-on mirrors, you can continue to use the mirrors you are used to but expand their view. $20 to $50.

- **The HandyBar.** For anyone who has a mobility issue or is recovering from an injury, this assistive device provides support as you get in and out of your vehicle. It's especially helpful for people who have difficulty getting out of a low vehicle, such as a sedan, or getting into a high vehicle, such as an SUV or pickup truck. $35. Stander.com/Handy-bar

- **Steering-wheel cover.** A soft foam or leather cover can help when arthritis or carpal tunnel syndrome makes it difficult to hold the steering wheel properly. The most important consideration is that it fits the steering wheel of your vehicle's make and model—this is not as easy as it used to be because today's steering wheels tend to incorporate lots of unique contours and buttons, so read reviews about fit before purchasing. $10 to $20.

- **Seat cushion for height.** On average, people lose a half-inch of height every decade after age 40 and even more than that after age 70. If you don't have much height to spare when it comes to seeing over the steering wheel and dashboard, a seat cushion can help...and ensure that the center of the steering-wheel air bag is safely facing your chest and not your face. Visibility—your sight line—should be at least three inches above the steering wheel. A firm foam wedge-shape cushion (higher in the back and lower in the front) can increase your height without raising your legs too close to the steering wheel or too far from the pedals. An orthopedic gel cushion also can help with back or hip pain. These kinds of cushions can be found for about $13 to $80.

- **Swivel-seat cushion.** This type of cushion makes it easier for people with stiff joints or limited mobility to pivot to get in and out of the driver's seat. $15 to $60.

ADAPTIVE-DRIVING EQUIPMENT

The following items are adaptive-driving equipment that should be prescribed by a certified driver rehabilitation specialist to be sure that you're getting the best equipment for your needs and can be trained in how to use it. This ensures that you'll be able to safely drive with the modifications and are compliant with all license-restriction procedures in your state. Only a certified mechanic specializing in installing adaptive equipment should make the modifications so that the equipment and installation meet all regulations. Note that not all vehicles can be modified in all ways, but if what you need is possible, the vendor will ensure that the appropriate equipment is used.

You can find a certified driver rehabilitation specialist through the Association for Driver Rehabilitation Specialists (ADED.net) or the American Occupational Therapist Association (AOTA.org)...and a certified installer through the National Mobility Equipment Dealers Association (NMEDA.com).

• **Swing-out swivel-seat replacement.** If a swivel cushion isn't enough of an accommodation, consider a swing-out or swivel-seat replacement. This involves completely replacing the seat that came with your car with a seat that stays anchored to the vehicle but moves in and out so that you can enter and exit without twisting or rotating. Cost can run several thousand dollars with installation.

• **Steering-wheel spinner.** This simple attachment, often a knob, is secured to a steering wheel to enable drivers with limited or no use of one arm to steer with their working arm. Price is about $100, including installation.

• **Left-foot accelerator.** People who have very limited or no use of their right leg, whether because of amputation, stroke or another condition, may be able to operate all the car pedals with their left leg. Prices range from about $500 to $2,000 depending on style (mechanical or electronic), including installation.

• **Pedal extenders.** If you can't comfortably reach the gas and/or brake pedal, professionally installed pedal extenders can help. They eliminate the need to sit too far forward in the seat, which can be dangerous. Price with installation is between $300 and $800 depending on the type of control (whether it is permanently fixed or one that tucks out of the way for other drivers).

• **Hand controls.** If you've lost the use of your legs from a condition such as paralysis, spinal stenosis or peripheral neuropathy, this device allows you to control the accelerator and brake using your hands. Price is about $1,500, including installation.

IF YOU'RE IN THE MARKET FOR A CAR...

Consider paying extra, if necessary, for certain features that will keep you more comfortable and safer on the road...

• **Power everything**—steering, windows, lift gate, door locks and seats that move up and down as well as forward and backward

• **Tilting and telescoping steering wheel**

• **Rearview camera for backing up** (now required on any new vehicle as of May 2018)

• **Factory-installed adjustable foot pedals** for the brake and accelerator

• **Large dashboard controls with buttons,** which are easier to manipulate than knobs

• **Warning systems to alert you to objects in blind spots,** especially while changing lanes, merging and parking

• **Lane-departure warning system** to warn you if your car is veering outside your lane

• **"Smart" headlights with glare control that automatically pivot during turns** and adjust the range and intensity of light based on oncoming vehicles

• **Crash-mitigation systems** that sense when you might be in danger of a collision and automatically stop the car.

Editor's note: Unless noted, the products mentioned in this article are available on Amazon, at department stores and through specialty automotive and assistive-device sites such as IndependentLiving.com and LiveOakMed.com.

Also: The products typically are not covered by insurance but may be tax-deductible. See IRS Publication 502, *Medical and Dental Expenses*, for details.

Pedestrian Safety

Study led by researchers at Université de Bretagne-Sud, France, published in *Safety Science.*

Staring at drivers keeps pedestrians safer. When study subjects stared at drivers in approaching cars, the cars were more likely to stop for the pedestrians to cross the street—instead of driving past them—than when the subjects looked only in the general direction of the car.

Possible reason: Eye contact may trigger a driver's desire to make a good impression on a pedestrian by stopping.

Hands-Free Is Not Safe

Md. Mazharul (Shimul) Haque, PhD, senior lecturer, Queensland University of Technology, Brisbane, Australia.

In a surprising new finding, both handheld and hands-free cell phones caused a 40% increase in reaction time during a simulation of a pedestrian entering a crosswalk from the driver's peripheral vision compared with drivers not using a phone.

Explanation: The cognitive power needed to hold a conversation can decrease the ability to process some visual information.

Takeaway: Don't assume that hands-free calls are safe—stay off the phone altogether when driving.

Get Out Alive! Strategies to Survive 3 Deadly Emergencies

Clint Emerson, a retired Navy SEAL who spent 20 years conducting special-ops missions. He is also author of *100 Deadly Skills: Survival Edition* and founding partner of Escape the Wolf, a crisis-management and risk-mitigation company based in Frisco, Texas. EscapetheWolf.com

When emergencies occur, you don't always have the time or opportunity to call 911 and wait for someone to come to your rescue. It pays to plan before an emergency occurs so that you know just what to do when one does. Here, Clint Emerson, a retired Navy SEAL who spent 20 years conducting special-ops missions, shares his strategies for surviving three terrifying emergencies…

EMERGENCY: CARJACKING

Before there's a problem: If you are in a high-crime area, leave at least one car length's space between your vehicle and the vehicle in front of yours when you come to a stop at a red light or stop sign. This greatly improves the odds that you will have sufficient room to speed away in an emergency. While stopped in traffic, keep your car doors locked, windows up and transmission in drive (or in first gear if the car has a standard transmission). Monitor your side and rearview mirrors, and glance out the side windows. Drivers who focus only on the traffic light or who become distracted by their phones or radios at stops are more likely to be targeted by carjackers.

Also, pay close attention to your surroundings when in parking garages and when pulling up to drive-through ATMs—these are common carjacking locations. If you see anyone lurking, drive away and find a different parking place or ATM. After using an ATM, don't stop to count your cash or put it in your wallet—drive away quickly.

During an emergency: *The best response depends on how the carjacking occurs…*

- **If you are walking in a parking area when someone demands your keys,** locate an exit for an escape on foot and then toss the keys as far as you can in the direction opposite this exit to allow yourself time to run. What you hope will happen is that while you are making your escape, the criminal will go in the other direction to pick up your car keys and then simply will take your car. If there is no nearby exit, toss the keys and take cover behind a solid obstacle such as a concrete pillar. The carjacker will get your car, but removing yourself as a factor as best you can decreases the odds that you will be kidnapped or harmed.

- **If you are stopped at a stop sign or red light when you see someone approaching with a**

weapon, drive away even if this means going up on a sidewalk or running a red light (assuming that you can do so without causing an accident or running over a pedestrian).

- **If a carjacker gets into the passenger seat of your car while you are stopped,** immediately jump out and run. If he shows a gun and orders you to drive, offer to surrender the vehicle. If this offer is rejected, speed up, then slam on the brakes and quickly get out and run, ideally toward nearby people or into a building.

- **If a carjacker sticks a gun or knife through your driver's side window while you are stopped,** offer to surrender the car. If the carjacker refuses and orders you to slide over to the passenger seat, raise your arms slowly as if in surrender and then suddenly use your raised arms to push the carjacker's arm forward into your dashboard while simultaneously flooring the gas. The carjacker will not expect this, and his attention will immediately shift from stealing your car to not being hurt by your car.

EMERGENCY: HOME INVASION

Before there's a problem: Identify escape routes from your home. These should not just lead out of your house but also off your property. The ideal route exits your home only a short distance from a tree line or a neighbor's home that can shield you from view. Your escape route should conclude at a "rally point"—a predetermined place where family members can gather safely.

Keep your car keys, cell phone and flashlight near your bedside at night. These can come in handy (see below).

During an emergency: Resist the urge to turn on a light if you think someone has broken into your home at night. Light might make you feel safer, but turning on a light actually shows the home invader which room you are in. It also robs you of a tactical advantage—you know your home's layout better than the home invader does, so you can navigate it in the dark better than he can.

Grab your cell phone, car keys and flashlight... gather other members of the household...and head for your escape route. Sometimes it is not possible for everyone to move together as a family, so everyone, including children, should know that escape is the priority. What you don't want is your family waiting around while Mom or Dad confronts the intruder. If your car keys have a fob with a panic button, press this—the sound of your car alarm might scare off the home invader. Even if it doesn't, the alarm may provide a distraction that buys you time to escape while also alerting your neighbors. If you have a home-security system with a panic button, press this, too. (You should have a wall keypad or remote alarm button in your bedroom.)

Dial 911 as you proceed along your escape route or when you reach a safe spot—do not halt your escape to make this call. Do not hide inside your home unless you see no way to escape and/or there is a secure safe room in the home. Running is better than hiding because people who hide usually are found.

Warning about guns: If you are proficient with a gun, use it. But if it sits in your nightstand and you never use it, you should run rather than pull your gun—the last thing you want is to shoot a round through a few walls and injure or kill a family member or have the gun used against you.

EMERGENCY: OFFICE FIRE

Before there's a problem: Learn the location of the primary and secondary fire escape routes from your office.

In your desk in a backpack or some other easily carried "bolt bag," keep a flashlight, a bottle of water, a dust mask (douse the mask with the water to make a short-term smoke filter), a whistle (to alert others of your location) and chemical lights (sometimes called glow sticks).

During an emergency: Grab your bolt bag and your phone, and head for the closest emergency exit. If fire blocks your escape, try the secondary exit. Encourage other people to join you—bigger groups have more eyes, ears and brains to help them locate a way out. Use the glow sticks to mark your escape route to help other people follow you out...or help emergency services personnel find you if you cannot escape.

FLASHLIGHTS CAN BE TACTICAL TOOLS

A flashlight can do more than light your way during an emergency. *You also can…*

- **Shine a flashlight into a neighbor's window or at passing cars to signal for help if,** for example, you are pinned down inside your home.
- **Disorient a home invader by shining a flashlight in his/her eyes in a dark room.** Then quickly turn the flashlight back off and run—the light burst should temporarily rob him of his ability to see in low light.
- **Use a flashlight as a club.** This requires a big metal flashlight loaded with heavy D-cell batteries. It can be an effective weapon or can be used to break a window.

Index

G

H

K

W